Ethics in Clinical Practice
An Interprofessional Approach

Edited by
Dr Georgina Hawley

Contributors:

Helen Aveyard · Jill Barr · Stewart Blake · Dan Butcher
Georgina Hawley · Sue Hutchings · Gail Lansdown
Brenton Lewis · Phil Maude · Roger A. Newham · Moira Nigam
Angelica Orb · Kevin Reel · Elisabeth Settelmaier
Louise M. Terry · Catherine Ward

PEARSON
Education

Harlow, England • London • New York • Boston • San Francisco • Toronto
Sydney • Tokyo • Singapore • Hong Kong • Seoul • Taipei • New Delhi
Cape Town • Madrid • Mexico City • Amsterdam • Munich • Paris • Milan

Pearson Education Limited

Edinburgh Gate
Harlow
Essex CM20 2JE
England

and Associated Companies throughout the world

Visit us on the World Wide Web at:
www.pearsoned.co.uk

———————————————

First published 2007

© Pearson Education Limited 2007

ISBN: 978-0-13-201827-2

British Library Cataloguing-in-Publication Data
A catalogue record for this book is available from the British Library

10 9 8 7 6 5 4 3 2 1
11 10 09 08 07

Typeset in 9/12.5pt Interstate by 35
Printed in Great Britain by Henry Ling Ltd., at the Dorset Press, Dorchester, Dorset

The publisher's policy is to use paper manufactured from sustainable forests.

X
4.03.08

Ethics in Clinical Practice

PEARSON
Education

We work with leading authors to develop the strongest
educational materials in nursing, bringing cutting-edge
thinking and best learning practice to a global market.

Under a range of well-known imprints, including
Pearson Education, we craft high quality print and
electronic publications which help readers to understand
and apply their content, whether studying or at work.

To find out more about the complete range of our
publishing, please visit us on the World Wide Web at:
www.pearsoned.co.uk

Brief contents

Contents

Supporting resources

Visit **www.pearsoned.co.uk/hawley** to find valuable online resources

Companion Website for students
- Extra case studies with assessment questions
- Examples of reflective diaries, with hints on writing your own

For instructors
- Teaching tips and guidance on structuring your classes
- Suggestions for seminar activities

For more information please contact your local Pearson Education sales representative or visit **www.pearsoned.co.uk/hawley**

Foreword

This book invites health and social care students to explore the ethical issues of clinical practice. The writings reflect that it is a professional responsibility for health and social care practitioners to care for each person, whom they might call clients, in an ethical manner. For a health and social care professional to ethically care for someone they must provide quality care. This should reflect evidence-based practice, be culturally competent and be performed in collaboration with an interprofessional team.

Learning to care ethically is evident throughout this book in several ways, from the student or reader recognising their own uniqueness through to understanding the need for allocation of resources. The reader is guided through an engaging journey of professional development. The reader starts by identifying their own uniqueness with individual values and beliefs, before exploring the different uniqueness of clients or patients who also have different values and beliefs. It moves the reader onto an understanding that the health and social care professional can themselves cause moral problems or dilemmas. These reflect the student's professional moral development and personal values and beliefs.

Ethical rights are emphasised and the student is able to embrace and enact the values and beliefs of their professional body. Finally the components are combined together with critical reflection to enable the students to develop sound ethical standards that meet those of their professions' Code of Ethics or Standard of Practice Conduct.

The interactive layout of the book takes the reader on a stimulating and enjoyable journey to challenge their own thinking and to develop their practice in a more informed and critical manner.

Elizabeth Westcott, Director of Pre-Qualifying Learning and Development,
School of Health and Social Care, Oxford Brookes University, UK

Preface

The need for health care professionals to understand the subject of ethics has dramatically increased in the past ten years. The development of health care ethics or bioethics is closely associated with the advancement of the different professions, the advent of people's rights, and demand for improved health care. Ethics is what a person regards as right or wrong behaviour and so if we look at a few of the major situations in health care, when things were wrong, and how improvements were made so that these would be right (in the future), you will be able to understand as to how ethics has developed in relation to health care.

The first event that was instrumental in the development of health care ethics was the outcome of the medical research performed by the Nazi doctors during the Second World War (WWII) of 1939-1945. This research had been performed on men, women and children who had not volunteered nor given the choice to take part. This resulted in the formulation of the Nuremberg Code at the end of the war. The Code stipulates the standards by which any research in the health care must meet - most importantly, that people must be volunteers and that they consent to taking part in the research trial or study. The Nuremberg Code was first used as the standard by which the Nazi doctors were judged for war crimes.

The Declaration of Geneva closely followed the Nuremberg Code. That is, in 1948 doctors from the World Medical Association adopted the Declaration of Geneva, as the basis to provide medical care. This included their duty to protect life, and be non-biased in relation to religion, race, nationality, politics and social standing in providing patient care.

In the same year (1948), the International Council of Nurses (ICN) was officially recognised by the World Health Organization (WHO) and since that time nurses have been part of those meetings. In 1950, the first edition of Nurses Code of Ethics, was developed and this was adopted by nurses worldwide in 1953 (ICN Code of Ethics).

Although we take for granted the rights of children, it was not until 1959 that these were validated by the United Nations, in the Declaration of the Rights of the Child. Fourteen years later, in 1973, the American Hospital Associations developed and implemented the concept of patient rights in the 'Patients Bill of Rights'. Instrumental in the development of these rights was the 1965 court case, *Charleston Memorial Hospital* v. *K Darling*. In this case, the nurse and the doctor were deemed responsible for neglecting the patient. This was the first time that health professional other than a doctor had been charged with negligence. The court found that had the nurse reported her observations that she performed on 18-year-old Darling, his leg would not have needed to be amputated (due to gangrene). The Darling case demonstrated to all professions, including physiotherapists and occupational therapists, that they have the responsibility of making decisions for effective patient care.

With the increasing legal rights of women (such as the right to vote, etc.) women wanted to have more freedom in relation to their health care. In 1973, legal cases of *Roe* v. *Wade* and *Doe* v. *Bolton*, gave women the legal right to have a termination of pregnancy, even if her life was not in danger. Inherent in the decision was the ruling that the unborn have never been recognised in law as persons, and that if a woman felt she needed to have an abortion, she had the legal right to do so.

Then, in 1983, Beauchamp and Childress argued that health professionals needed to use critical reflection when examining ethical problems (and dilemmas), in order to work out what was the right thing to do. That is, they needed to systematically examine the ethical or moral problem, by asking questions not only of proposed treatments but also care that had already been given.

Since then a massive amount of literature has been produced, ranging from a broad array of ethical issues and problems that arise within health research, the professions, and the institutions that deliver care services. Its reach extends from the legal and philosophical aspects of biological science and genetics at the beginning of life, to those at the end of life including respecting and maintaining the dignity of the dying person and their significant others.

The aim of this book is to provide any student in health care, with a basic, easy to understand text. Which at the same time reflects contemporary health care practice, by emphasising interprofessional care and cultural sensitivity. For each of the ethical issues we have provided both sides of the ethical and moral arguments. However, we have not discussed counter arguments to the various philosophical theories, as it was felt that this would be too confusing for some students to follow. What were more important for us, included the use of clarity, logical flow and style so that students with dyslexia and spLD could also enjoy reading the book.

The cultural sensitive approach has been emphasised as many people on entering the health service are denied basic client or patient rights. This is primarily because many health professionals assume that their own values and beliefs are ethically correct and right, and ignore those of clients or patients from another culture. Consequently, while we have included a chapter on Western Philosophy, we have also included a chapter on Eastern Philosophy, so that those who read this book will gain understanding of the needs of all people.

You will notice the book is in two parts. The reason for doing this was to provide you with all the basic knowledge and understanding of health ethics in Chapters 1-10 whatever your profession might be. Then, Chapters 11-17 add on to the basic building blocks of knowledge and understanding you have gained in Part 1.

I would suggest the first time you read the book, you do so as you would a fiction book – that is, quickly skim through to find the interesting parts. In this way you will have gained the basics. The following times you read the chapters you will gain the necessary knowledge of the concepts underlying the various topics to fully understand health care ethics. This when enacted in the various clinical areas will enable you to meet your profession's standard of ethical practice.

So, please enjoy reading the book!

The Rev'd Dr Georgina Hawley
2007

About the authors

Dr Helen Aveyard, Senior Lecturer, School of Health and Social Care, Oxford Brookes University, UK. Helen's PhD investigated informed consent in nursing practice. She lectures in health care ethics, including research ethics and research methodology to undergraduate and postgraduate students. Her research and writing interests are in the area of informed consent, and the education of ethics to health care professionals.

Jill Barr, Principal Lecturer, School of Health Care, University of Wolverhampton, UK. Jill has been a university lecturer in health visiting for many years. She has contributed to the development of several primary care curriculum within the UK.

Stewart Blake, Senior Lecturer, School of Health Care, Northumbria University, UK. Stewart has lectured in nursing ethics for many years.

Dan Butcher, Senior Lecturer, School of Health and Social Care, Oxford Brookes University, UK. Dan teaches primarily in the adult nursing programme. His specialism is loss-related illness and palliative care.

Dr Georgina Hawley, Principal Lecturer and Programme Lead, Adult nursing, School of Health and Social Care, Oxford Brookes University. Georgina has been designing ethics syllabus for health care curriculum since 1988. She has taught extensively in ethics in Australia, the UK and Hong Kong. Her ethics research has included where nurses and other health care professionals experience ethical problems in clinical practice. Consequently, these trouble spots or areas of difficulty are covered in this book. Georgina strongly believes in client and patients rights, and has gained insight into their problems through researching the patients experience of being ill. She is also an Ordained Priest and has worked as a hospital chaplain in a large tertiary institution, where she had the honour of sitting and walking beside many ill people and their loved ones.

Sue Hutchings is Principal Lecturer, Interprofessional Education, School of Health and Social Care, Oxford Brookes University, UK. Sue's specialism is the development of interprofessional education among health and social care students.

Gail Lansdown, Principal Lecturer, School of Health and Social Care, Oxford Brookes University, UK. Gail leads the school's overseas programmes, in South East Asia. Her priority is to provide high quality culturally appropriate education for health professionals.

Brenton Lewis, Lecturer in Behavioural Science, School of Nursing, Curtin University of Technology, Western Australia. Brenton, a psychologist, teaches behavioural science subjects including sexuality across the curriculum. He has a special interest in men's health and global poverty.

Dr Phil Maude, Senior Lecturer, Postgraduate School of Medicine, University of Melbourne and holds a joint practice development appointment with the Alfred Hospital. Phil's PhD investigated psychiatric illness and treatment. He is a strong supporter of client and patients rights, and his specialism is the protection of vulnerable people. Phil lectures in mental health, pharmacology and ethical research with vulnerable populations. His research focus is on developing evidence based practice in behavioural emergencies in mental health (violence and suicide) and sexual health.

Roger Newham, Senior Lecturer, Health and Social Care, London South Bank University, UK. Roger's PhD is in health care ethics and he teaches ethics to both undergraduate and post-graduate students. Roger has a special interest in postmodernist virtue ethics and believes they are highly applicable in how health professionals undertake their clinical practice and make ethical decision.

Moira Nigam, as a lecturer in nursing, studied for higher degrees in anthropology and sociology. Her specialisms include cultural sensitivity and competency in the provision of health care.

Dr Angelica Orb, Senior Lecture, Division of Health Science, Curtin University of Technology, Western Australia. Angelica's PhD investigated ethics in nursing practice. She has taught nursing ethics for many years and is a member of the University's human research ethics committee. Angelica has nursing interests in other countries besides Australia (South America and Africa) and has a special interest in how health professionals cope with small budgets and the allocation of resources.

Kevin Reel, Education Officer Board of Occupational Therapy, UK. Previously, a senior lecturer in the School of Health and Social Care, Oxford Brookes University in occupational therapy. Kevin has taught health care ethics to occupational and physiotherapy students for many years. He has strong ideals about interprofessional practice and how multiprofessional teams work together.

Guided tour

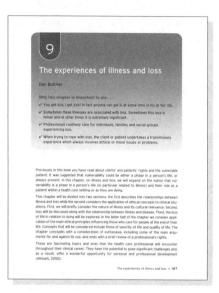

Chapter openers show the relevance of the topic to your own practice, and summarise what you will learn in the chapter

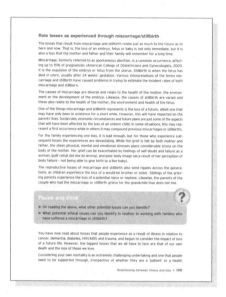

The **pause and think** symbol asks you to stop reading for a couple of minutes, and think about the item listed

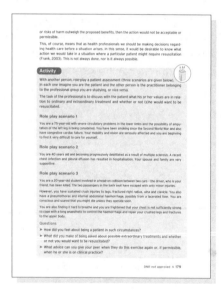

The **activity** symbol asks you to undertake the listed activity, either on your own, or with a partner

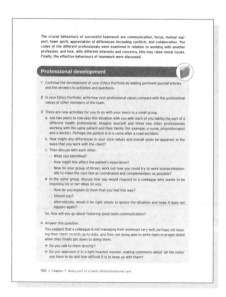

The **professional development** symbol shows you how you can enrich your knowledge and understanding of your own profession

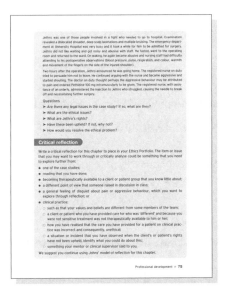

Critical reflection boxes explain how to reflect on your practice, and help you develop your own Ethics Portfolio

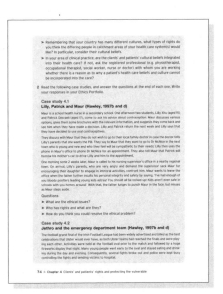

Case studies throughout the book show how the ethical theory applies to your own practice, and makes you question your own behaviour and beliefs

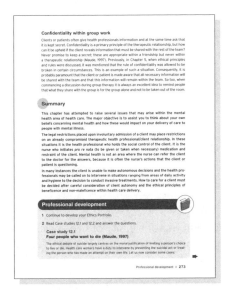

A chapter **summary** recaps and reinforces the key points to take away from the chapter. Useful for revision or quick reference

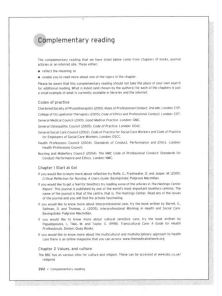

A **complementary reading** section at the end of the book enables you to explore and read around the topics discussed in the chapters

Author acknowledgements

As editor I wish to thank all those who assisted in the development of this book, namely:

- Kate Brewin, Commissioning Editor, Pearson Education for encouragement and support during the writing;
- Jan Taylor of Swindon for her help in preparation of the manuscript;
- Colleagues in the School of Health and Social Care, Oxford Brookes University, for their ideas and thoughts and support;
- The contributing authors for their hard work and diligence in crafting their chapters;
- The vitally important reviewers who, although busy university lecturers, took time to give such valuble constructive criticism;
- Rhian McKay, Publishing Editor, Pearson Education for her patience towards me in getting this book into the shops;
- Bill Hawley, best friend, par excellence husband, and lover, for his support during the whole writing and publication process.

Thank you all.

Georgina Hawley
(Editor)

Publisher acknowledgements

We are grateful to the following who acted as reviewers:

- Michael P. Connolly, the School of Nursing, Midwifery & Health Systems at University College, Dublin
- Shirley Goldstraw, School of Nursing and Midwifery at Keele University
- Mandy Mitchelmore, School of Health and Social Care at the University of Greenwich
- Lorraine Shaw, School of Nursing and Primary Care Practice at Liverpool John Moores University
- Pauline Stammers, the School of Health Sciences at the University of Birmingham

Part 1

The basic building blocks to understanding ethics in clinical practice

1

Start at 'Go'

Georgina Hawley

Board games such as Monopoly or Snakes and Ladders request that players begin the game at the designated place of 'Go'. There are possibly three reasons for this:

- First, the information provided for the players is in a set sequence, which tells the players what to do at each stage of the game.
- Second, that all the players commence at 'Go' means that they all have an equal opportunity to experience enjoyment of learning the game.
- Third, with all the players starting in the same place at the same time, there is more likelihood of them completing the game together.

Likewise, with this book we ask readers to start at 'Go' so that the sequential information can be readily understood. This indicates what to do at each stage of the game in a logical order. Second, commencing with other students or peers at 'Go' means that you all have an equal opportunity to experience enjoyment of learning! Third, with a group starting in the same place and time, there is more likelihood of you all successfully completing the ethics module or course that you are studying.

The logical order mentioned above is a series of building blocks of new knowledge. In this book these building blocks begin with the definition and concept of ethics, followed by the next building block of values and beliefs; ethical issues and problems come next, followed by clients' or patients' rights, protecting the vulnerable and so on.

When presented in this way the study of health care ethics is an enjoyable subject. Hence, the purpose of this book is to provide health care students with an easy-to-understand text which at the same time reflects contemporary health care practice by emphasising interprofessional practice, and is culturally sensitive to clients' or patients' needs. It is anticipated that students from different professions using this book will be provided with a common language in ethics which, in turn, will facilitate greater discussion of ethical issues and problems in interprofessional learning and collaborative practice.

Help along the way

The design of this book has been developed in such a way as to guide the novice learner in health care ethics through the various chapters. These include:

- Easy-to-understand language.
- Short paragraphs so that you are only reading about one item at a time.
- Frequent headings, for the reader who likes or needs these signposts to help their reading of the text.
- Gradual expansion of new knowledge: a word may be introduced in one chapter and then the concept expanded and discussed later where it is most applicable.
- The use of symbols, for the reader who likes or needs an alternative text to facilitate their learning.

The symbols used are:

Pause and think
This symbol asks for you to stop reading for a couple of minutes and think about the item listed.

Activity
This symbol asks you to undertake the listed activity. For example, 'Read the following case study and answer the questions at the end'.

Professional development
This symbol is displayed towards the end of each chapter. The concept of 'professional development' means to gain knowledge and understanding about your profession. Since your registration body or profession's council requires you to undertake clinical practice in a professional manner the aim of this section is to facilitate this development.

What does 'ethics' mean for health professionals?

In this chapter, first of all you will be introduced to the definition of ethics, followed by why we need to study ethics. Second, what is meant by multiprofessional and interprofessional. Likewise, what is meant by culturally sensitive care. You will notice that the words 'client' or 'patient' are used throughout the book, as some health professions use client and others use patient.

The word 'ethics' means the study of people's moral behaviour. By moral behaviour, we mean what is right or wrong, or what is good and bad. For example, being truthful is regarded as morally right, whereas being deceitful is wrong. As health care professionals we have an obligation to provide care that is ethically (or morally) right, good or correct to clients and patients. In this book we do not make a distinction between the words ethics and moral, as it would be out of keeping with the style of text. Consequently, sometimes the word ethics or ethical and at other times moral or morals will be used; please treat them as synonymous if you wish.

It is now time for you to think and list behaviours which you feel are ethically or morally correct and those that are wrong for health professionals to use (Table 1.1).

Table 1.1 What is right or wrong, good or bad?

Right or good	Wrong or bad
1 Telling the truth	Telling lies or being deceitful
2	
3	
4	
5	

How did you get on? Perhaps you needed more room to list all the behaviours?

The important thing with this task is to start identifying ethically right and wrong actions or behaviours. Later you will learn that ethics is not always this black and white, but you come to that after your confidence has grown through acquiring knowledge and understanding.

Why do we need to study ethics?

Quite simply, if we don't study ethics the people for whom we have been given a mandate to provide care will invariably suffer! There have been many tragedies over the years that could have been prevented if health professionals and the public who knew what was happening had spoken out about these situations. For example:

1 **Willowcreek School, USA** (1963–1966). This was a residential home for children with physical and mental impairments who were purposely infected (by injection) with hepatitis A to see how quickly the disease spread and whether or not the medication gamma globulin was effective.

2 **Tuskegee, USA** (1932–1972). This 40-year-long experiment was performed to study the difference between syphilis patients who were treated with penicillin and those who were not. A public health nurse (Eunice Rivers) helped to persuade some 400 African-American men with syphilis to forgo penicillin treatment, even though it had already been tested and was the available and standard treatment for the disease. As this experiment was exposed, its immorality towards people who were not aware of their rights and informed consent gained the reputation of being an 'horrendous evil' and gross violation of justice (Cranston, 1973). There is more about this type of ethical problem in Chapters 3 and 4.

3 **National Women's Hospital, New Zealand** (1958–1987), also known as the Cartwright Inquiry. The story of this dreadful tragedy is written by Sandra Coney (1988) in the book *The*

Unfortunate Experiment. Women with cervical cancer were not given the correct care. A total of 948 women who had the disease were divided into two groups: those who received treatment and those who received no treatment except to have their disease state monitored. As a result, many women died and others were traumatically disfigured so that they were unable to have sexual intercourse (Report of the Cervical Cancer Inquiry, 1988). As a result of the inquiry other substandard practices which had been allowed to continue for over 20 or more years came to light (Bromberger and Fife-Yeomans, 1991).

The ethical problems uncovered during this inquiry centred on clients' or patients' rights and research (see Chapters 4 and 16).

4 **Chelmsford Hospital, Sydney, Australia** (The Royal Commission Inquiry into Chelmsford Hospital, 1990). People with psychiatric illness were prescribed 'deep sleep' to cure their illnesses. This involved deep sedation for days on end. The full information about this can be found in the Royal Commission Inquiry into Chelmsford Hospital. Patients who survived gave evidence at the Royal Commission. The consequences of such immobility without appropriate adjunct care included bronchopneumonia, deep vein thrombosis, pulmonary embolism, decubitus ulcers, muscle wasting, contractures, etc. and death. This inquiry discovered that the rights of the mentally ill or psychiatric patient were abused (see Chapters 4 and 12).

5 **Bristol Royal Infirmary Inquiry** (1984–1995), also known as the Bristol Heart Inquiry. Babies and children requiring cardiac surgery were not provided with the correct standard of care, and many died as a result. This tragedy was not about bad or uncaring health professionals, but rather the ethical problems occurred because some lacked insight and their behaviour was flawed (Bristol Royal Infirmary Inquiry, 2001). This was compounded by some professionals in the cardiac surgical team failing to commmunicate with each other and work effectively together as a team (see Chapters 3 and 7).

6 **Alder Hey Hospital Inquiry** (Report of the Royal Liverpool Children's Inquiry, 2001). This inquiry centred on the different collections of babies' and children's organs. During the inquiry it was discovered that the first collection commenced in 1948, with others being added over the years. Central to the investigation was Professor van Velzen who, shortly after his appointment as Professor of Foetal and Infant Pathology, issued an order that no human material was to be disposed of (including returning organs to a body at the end of a post-mortem examination) without his permission. Instead, it was to be retained for his research. This activity is illegal under the Human Tissue Act of 1961. The inquiry also uncovered unethical practices within Alder Hey and Liverpool University, including the collection of children's body parts at the Institute of Child Health (responsibility of the University), the Eye collection (held by the University), the Heart collection (joint responsibility between Alder Hey and the University), and the Foetal and Cerebellum Collections at Myrtle Street (responsibility of the hospital). The types of ethical problems uncovered during the inquiry are explained in Chapter 3.

All of these tragedies demonstrate that there is no place for ignorance in health care, and that it is imperative for all professionals to have a high degree of knowledge and not simply be prepared to follow what other members of the team are doing or the orders of another professional.

These scandals are all well known and perhaps outstanding in the degree of unethical behaviour; it would be easy to think that ethical problems and dilemmas are only high profile. This is not the case; there are many small and less well-known incidents that occur everyday in health care. It is when these incidents are allowed to continue unabated and grow that they become publicly known. It is the little ethical problems or dilemmas that professionals need to remain vigilant, because once the little problems are identified, the big ones will be lit up as 'neon lights' and be very easy to recognise.

Why it is important for *you* to act when little problems occur

Because the big ones all commenced as little problems and became huge because the health professionals didn't recognise the inherent problem or, if they did so, were blocked from doing something about it. Sometimes, a junior person will think 'well I don't think that is right, but surely "the powers-that-be" know about it and are doing something'. My advice is, if you feel that something is wrong, do not assume anything, and tell whoever it happens to be who needs to know.

We need to study health ethics or bioethics not only for the clients and patients that we care for now, but also in the future (not forgetting all the clients and patients who suffered in the past because of unethical care). Surely, this is ample reason why it is imperative that health professionals today are educated in health ethics in clinical practice!

Interprofessional health care

In contemporary health care, a team consisting of different professionals invariably provides the treatment and care to clients and patients. This team approach is called 'multiprofessional' (that is, meaning involvement of two or more academic disciplines or professions). For example, the team at the primary health care centre may consist of the practice nurse, a physiotherapist, several general practitioners, a midwife and, depending on the population, perhaps a podiatrist or social worker. When this multiprofessional team change their working relationship with each other, then it becomes interprofessional. The term interprofessional implies that there is learning from each other about each other's roles in a collaborative relationship to provide an improved quality of care to clients or patients.

All health professionals are accountable for their own standard of practice and all different registration bodies or councils emphasise the importance of providing care that is ethically correct or good; some will de-register professionals whose conduct is unethical. In the UK recent reported examples have been a general practitioner who sexually assaulted patients, and in nursing, a practitioner who verbally and physically abused elderly patients.

Sue Hutchings and Kevin Reel write more about working in a team in Chapter 7.

Culturally sensitive care

In today's world there are very few countries that are not affected by faster communication, shorter travelling times, employment transfers and migration for socioeconomic reasons (including war). Therefore, the idea of one country having one specific philosophy and culture (including religion), compared to another country, has, or is, disappearing.

Inherent within a person's culture are not only their own personal values and beliefs but also their society's. It is that society's values and beliefs that become encoded into politics, law, government, education, health care and religions. That is, the values and beliefs of a country are communicated and transmitted through the legal process, the government's action or inaction, and cultural practices (which in many cases include spirituality or religious practices).

Earlier, ethics was described as the study of people's moral behaviour of what is right or wrong, good or bad. Therefore, we can understand that what one culture might regard as ethically or morally right may be regarded by another culture as wrong or bad. For example, as an Australian I am quite used to people using certain words when talking with each other. However, in the UK these same words are frowned upon and termed 'swearing'. That is, what might be acceptable (or right) in Australia may be unacceptable (or wrong) in the UK.

Similarly, in some cultural groups it is quite normal to lie or be deceitful, whereas in others it is not. Likewise, in some cultural groups young women are expected to abstain from sexual intercourse prior to marriage (as it is regarded as morally right and good), whereas in other cultural groups this is not an expectation (and therefore not classified as morally right or wrong). Take that behaviour pattern (of a young woman being expected to abstain from sexual intercourse) and place it in another country where that standard is encoded in the legal system; this could mean that the young woman might be punished by the courts (if she was found guilty of having sexual intercourse prior to marriage).

In health care, as professionals providing ethically competent care, we need to be mindful that we are not insensitive to clients' or patients' cultural beliefs. Therefore this book will provide the reader with the tools (to gain knowledge and understanding) to provide care which is culturally sensitive. Dr Elizabeth Settelmeir and Moira Nigam write more about values and beliefs and our connections with other people in Chapter 2.

Ethical care in clinical practice

It would be easy to treat the subject of ethics as a separate entity divorced from clinical practice. That is, learn about the ethics *per se* in a purely theoretical way. However, this would not assist you as a practitioner who will need to make ethical decisions both as an individual and as part of a team. Consequently, in this book there is an emphasis on tying the theory of ethics with case studies that illustrate ethical or moral problems and/or dilemmas from clinical practice.

For example, Case study 1.1 is about a man who has had a cerebrovascular accident (CVA). Therefore, to know what is ethical or not in providing care, the practitioner needs to know also about that type of CVA. That is, for the care provided to be ethically right or good, current practice standards for your profession must be reflected. For example, for a physiotherapist to be ethically correct the standard would reflect current evidence based on CVA rehabilitation. Likewise, for nurses care would reflect evidence-based nursing practice.

Part of the tragedy of the Bristol Heart Inquiry was caused by this lack of current practice standards; the same applies to the ethical problems uncovered during the National Women's Hospital Inquiry.

The following scenario, entitled 'Mr Chui and the physiotherapy students', is designed to see if you can begin to discern what could be regarded as ethically right or wrong.

Activity

Read the following case study and try to answer the questions at the end.

Case study 1.1
Mr Chui and the physiotherapy students

Mr Chui has experienced a stroke and has left-sided hemiplegia. He is receiving treatment in a stroke rehabilitation unit, which has won accolades for its interprofessional approach to care.

One day, a group of physiotherapy students come to observe the team. Among other activities that they observe, they watch Mr Chui as he is instructed how to move from a chair back onto the bed. He is being helped and taught by a physiotherapist and a nurse.

Mr Chui is feeling tired from the exercises he has done in the gym that morning, and tells the physiotherapist and nurse that he can't do it and wants them to lift him onto the bed.

The physiotherapist tells Mr Chui, 'I think you should at least try standing up and straightening your left leg'.

Mr Chui starts to stand with their assistance, but when they try to straighten his left leg, he tells them to stop as they are hurting him.

The nurse responds 'Mr Chui, your leg is nearly straight, and I think in the long term you would rather have a little bit of pain now than not being able to walk later on'.

No! No? He shouts 'Leave me alone! I will sit in the chair if you won't lift me onto the bed!'

One of the observing students, named Peter, states in a loud critical voice to the physiotherapist and nurse 'Why are you so cruel to Mr Chui by causing him pain? It is unethical!'

Questions

➤ Do you think the physiotherapist treating Mr Chui was acting in an ethical manner? If yes, why is that? If no, why?

➤ Do you think the nurse treating Mr Chui was acting in an ethical manner? If yes, why is that? If no, why?

➤ Do you think the student acted ethically? If yes, why is that? If no, why?

Exploring case study 1.1 – Mr Chui and the students

In answer to the previous questions, you may have decided that both the physiotherapist and the nurse were not acting in an ethically correct manner towards Mr Chui. This could have been because you felt that they should have been kinder to him. After all, he was tired and they could have lifted him up onto the bed. In this way Mr Chui would not have had to do anything, including straightening his left leg.

On the other hand, you might have decided that both the nurse and physiotherapist were acting ethically in that the patient should, as part of his rehabilitation, do some of the work himself to get back on his bed.

In relation to the student Peter, you may have said that what he did was not appropriate. In fact, it may even have been bad manners to voice his opinion in front of the patient and health care professionals when his role was to observe. However, you may feel that what Peter did was right, by being an advocate for Mr Chui.

Your perception based on your values and beliefs

How you answered the questions above will have depended on your own perception of the scenario, your knowledge of health care, and your professional education to date. However, the most important influence on the way in which you answered these questions comes from your own values and beliefs, drawn from both your life experiences and education. Your values and beliefs are very powerful components of the whole 'you' as a person as, up until now, you made all your decisions based upon your values and beliefs. These values and beliefs reflect:

- the culture in which you live;
- what your parents taught you;
- what you learnt at school; and
- what society said was right and wrong when you were growing up.

You will learn more about how your values and beliefs are part of you in the next chapter. For now, you only need to realise that the way you interpret situations and make decisions at present is based upon your own values and beliefs. Consequently, this book will help you to utilise other methods to make ethical or morally correct decisions in your professional practice.

Behaviour of health professionals

In health care, professionals interact with clients and patients to make decisions about the care and treatment required. Consequently, they have the potential power to do good or harm. For this reason it is imperative that they learn and understand ethics so that they use only those behaviours which their profession regards as good or correct, and refrain from those behaviours which are wrong, bad or incorrect.

Summary

Ethics is the study of moral behaviour, which can be regarded as good and correct or bad and wrong. As health professionals we have an inherent responsibility to provide care that is good and refrain from that which would be regarded as wrong or harmful.

Health professionals, as with ordinary people, have learnt what is right and wrong within their own society. Equally they are ordinary people, and are not exempt from the human frailties of making mistakes and bad behaviour. However, on becoming a registered health professional, it is necessary to undertake clinical practice which can only be regarded as 'professional'. This professional standard is made mandatory by each of the different professional councils (for example, the Nursing and Midwifery Council or Chartered Society of Physiotherapists). Therefore, it is important for you as a student to learn what standard of conduct and behaviour your profession regards as ethically correct or good. Similarly, you need to learn what behaviour and standard of practice would be regarded as unprofessional. In this way, learning about professional standards of practice and all the other topics that constitute health ethics or bioethics also assists in improving the standard of care clients or patients receive.

Since health care is invariably provided within a multiprofessional setting there is a need to approach the learning of ethics from that same perspective. That is, learning the different disciplines of health and social care together. Most countries are multiracial, multicultural or multiethnic and therefore there is a need for health professionals to be able to include these cultural perspectives in treatment and care plans.

If the team do not know what is culturally acceptable for a client or patient there is the possibility that they could recommend a treatment which is unacceptable, and therefore immoral or unethical, and with which the client or patient does not comply. In such circumstances the client or patient may wonder 'Why don't they know about my culture? And do they have no respect for me?' When such questioning occurs this can lead to mistrust and the breakdown of the therapeutic relationship. For example, a client or patient who has values and beliefs of the Hindu culture may not comply with taking medication that is in capsule form. This is because cows and pigs may be used in the manufacture of some capsules.

Professional development

The aim of this professional development session is to:

- introduce you to the concept of developing an ethics portfolio that will demonstrate your professional learning over the next few months as you work through this book;
- raise your awareness of some of the ethical issues and problems that can occur in health care.

1 Commence an Ethics Portfolio. Ideally this needs to be a large lever arch file in which you can keep the paper work that you use from the professional development section. File dividers could be used for each of the chapters so that when you collect papers such as the codes of practice from your professional body or journal articles these can be filed in the appropriate section that corresponds to that chapter. It is in the portfolio that you will write the answers to questions and discussions. You might also like to write about incidents that occur in clinical practice or at university.

Alternatively, instead of a file, you could have a folder on your computer with a file for each chapter. The articles could be collected via electronic copies and stored in the files.

An important part of your Ethics Portfolio will be your reflective journal writing. The purpose of writing the reflective journal is for you to examine in a systematic manner the journey or process of moral learning that you are now undertaking. One of the advantages of keeping the journal is that at the end of a course or in 2-3 months' time you can look back and see how you have grown professionally.

In summary, your Ethics Portfolio will be:

- A large file or folder, either hard copy or electronic.
- Divided into sections, one for each of the chapters.
- In each of these sections you will add:
  - readings, such as journal articles;
  - answers to questions that are raised in each of the chapters, discussions, incidents or situations;
  - reflective journal writing.

2 Your next task is to answer the following questions and write your answer in your Ethics Portfolio in the section for this chapter.

> ➤ Is it right or wrong for a health care professional to treat the Professor of Immunology from the USA who is on holiday in China and injures his back, with the same care and attention as a travelling backpacking student who sustains the same injury?

> ➤ Should the professor, because of his status and importance to the medical world, receive preferential treatment?

> ➤ Should a mental health nurse inform the police after reading about a horrific murder in the newspapers, when the description exactly fits the bizarre and secret wishes expressed by a patient?

The idea behind asking you to consider these questions is that you start to think about such issues and in due course discuss such questions with your peers and colleagues in order to develop appropriate ethical standards of care.

3 Next, access your university library catalogue and identify the code/s for books and journals on ethics (Hawley, 1997a and b). This may be ethics *per se* or bioethics; perhaps nursing ethics if you are a nurse or, if you are a medical student, look to see what you can find on medical ethics. You might like to list these codes in your portfolio for when you need them at a later date. For example, the Dewey classification number for ethics is 174, and the various disciplines and topics have numbers related to 174. However, not all books and journals related to ethics will be found at this number; others may be in the 600s or elsewhere.

When exploring the catalogue for information about ethics:

- Examine the range and extent of the ethics books and journals.
- Write down the names of books and journals by topic (e.g. research ethics or interprofessional ethics).
- Also include those journals that have a regular ethics column or feature.
- Now, examine the range of books and journals on transcultural, multicultural and intercultural care.
- See if any of these combine ethics and culture.

- Listing these books and their identifying numbers or codes will assist you in the future when you are preparing answers to the questions contained in the Professional Development sections at the end of each chapter (Hawley, 1997a and b).

4 If you don't already have a copy of your professional body's standards or codes of ethics of professional practice, contact the organisation so that you can understand your obligations and responsibilities.

Critical reflection

Write your reflective journal entry for this chapter. This writing will help you to gain insight into the world of ethics in relation to your own values and beliefs, knowledge and understanding of various situations and personal behaviour.

- Reflective writing is a process that can be used as a means to help us learn from our experiences. This involves a person engaging in and completing a reflective cycle of writing.

- This type of writing is different from essay writing in that the aim of the reflection is for the sole purpose of learning.

- This reflective way of learning will enable you to come to a different or deeper understanding of knowledge and understanding of ethics and professional behaviour in clinical practice. This writing process requires you to describe, analyse, evaluate and write an action plan. The success of your reflective writing will be demonstrated by your engagement in the process and your completion of each full cycle so that you have the opportunity to grow as a professional.

- If you are not familiar with the stages of reflective writing, you will find instructions on how to do this at the end of this chapter.

- If you are familiar with reflective writing, do not just list your feelings and values and beliefs about a specific situation, but continue through the reflective cycle so that learning occurs (Johns, 2000; Gibbs, 1988). For example, when using Gibbs (1988), not only would you describe the situation/reading/discussion and identify your feelings and thoughts, but you would also try and make sense of the situation through evaluation and analysis, and then finally identify your learning in an action plan or steps that you will undertake. This action plan needs to list strategies that you will undertake to increase your learning, or of adjustment to a situation or of coping.

- The types of things you will write about in reflection are those issues which are personal to you. For example, this might include something that you read in this book or an issue that arose when doing one of the case studies or as a result of a discussion with other students, or even something from clinical practice.

For example, say you are assigned to an intensive care unit (ICU), and your mentor or preceptor attends a quick team meeting to decide which patient should be transferred out of the unit to make way for a new patient to be admitted from the emergency department (ED) or Accident and Emergency. You observe the meeting and you become shocked at the necessity to transfer someone out of the ICU. When you mention this to your mentor, he says 'yes, I can understand that you are upset, but this is life, and the unit can only hold 16 patients. Therefore, for us to take the new patient from ED someone needs to be transferred out; this happens all the time in health care – in ethics it is called the allocation of resources'.

Such issues in clinical practice need to be explored systematically through reflection, so that you can learn from the experience.

- You will be asked to complete a reflection journal entry for each chapter of this book.
- For this reflective journal entry you might like to consider any of the following possibilities:
  ○ Commencing an ethics course. For example, how you feel about reading this book (if you are not using it as a text) or undertaking this module or course/unit on ethics. Think of possible outcomes that could occur, and then in the action plan section how you might cope or adjust to these outcomes or changes.
  ○ An issue from the case study, or from the questions raised in this chapter.
  ○ Something from clinical practice. Perhaps it was something that you saw or perhaps was mentioned as a comment to you.

(N.B. When writing about incidents, please do not name the hospital or organisation or people's names, as that would be breaching confidentiality.)

2

Where did you get your values and beliefs?

Elisabeth Settelmaier and Moira Nigam

Why this chapter is important to me . . .

✔ To grasp the difference between values and beliefs, culture and world views.

✔ Realise the impact of values and beliefs on behaviour and therefore ethics.

✔ Know how values and beliefs are formed, including those of an organisation.

✔ Realise that values and beliefs (can) change.

✔ Recognise the importance of providing culturally sensitive and/or culturally competent care.

Health professionals interact with people of all ages, cultures, languages, religions and spiritual beliefs, political persuasion, class, education and socioeconomic groups (Nigam, 1997). In this way, the health care is not restricted to one place, or indeed to one individual or group (Nigam, 1997). In reality, health care is a very cosmopolitan and essentially a public occupation. Knowing how values and beliefs influence not only your own behaviour, but also those to whom you will provide care, will assist you in developing what your profession regards as the professional standards of ethics and/or codes of conduct.

Primarily, to be a health care professional is to identify yourself as a healer and a person of the people. Your role is to acknowledge and care, not only for your own uniqueness, but also for the uniqueness of those with whom you work, as well as those who seek you out to assist in their healing (Martin, 1989).

In this chapter, you will be introduced to the notions of your uniqueness and independence as a person, your interconnectedness with others and interdependence. Also discussed are not only your own values, beliefs and cultural practices but those of others, and how these values develop and change. You will next be introduced to the concepts of culture, subcultures and the dangers of cultural stereotyping. Finally, you will have the opportunity to engage in Professional Development.

Who said they lived on an island by themselves?

When we think about ourselves as health care professionals we need to develop 'double vision'.

Pause and think

➤ What is meant by double vision?

There is no doubt that we are unique beings with unique qualities and talents. Yet we do not exist in isolation – as an island by ourselves – we are deeply interconnected with everybody else. Why and how is this?

Your uniqueness: that is, your individuality

Being unique has a strong relationship to our identity, and to our thoughts and feelings about who we are and what we understand is our place in the world (Schechtman, 1990). However, our identity is not static. This is because, as we grow from being a baby, through childhood, adolescence and adulthood, we experience the world and each other (Nigam, 1997). This is what is known as socialisation.

Growth of identity through socialisation with others

All through life, our thoughts and ways of living change and incorporate new images and realities of ourselves, and of the other people we meet and with whom we interact. This process of socialisation starts with you, and your understanding of your own identity as a person (Nigam, 1997).

Activity

Write down a description of your uniqueness.

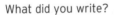

➤ If someone asked you, how would you describe yourself – what would your answer be?

What did you write?

- Perhaps you started with your name, which was given to you by your family, where you were born, and your position in your family
- You may have described what you do
- Where you work or where you live now

- Your physical appearance
- Your interests

What in fact you have been describing is your concept of your own identity! (Nigam, 1997.)

Looking at the order in which you have placed your descriptions, the way you have included some elements and left out others, and what meanings you have given, all adds up to how you perceive yourself!

In other words, the concept of your identity may integrate a number of understandings, which you have come to know about yourself. For example:

- you have a sense of the physical nature of yourself;
- a geographical sense of yourself;
- a sense of your relationships with others – what you value in, and about, life.

That is, your concept of your identity is a representation or a composite image of your past, present and future (Nigam, 1997).

In this way, we can say that your image of yourself is complex and merges many of your concepts, memories, projections and values.

Your interconnectedness with others

In the description of your own uniqueness, you might also have referred to your relationships with others. That is, to the way you relate to others and how they relate to you. To understand how people relate to each other it is worthwhile to consider for a moment what we can describe as 'interconnectedness'. The concept of interconnectedness consists of three phases: dependence, independence and interdependence (Figure 2.1).

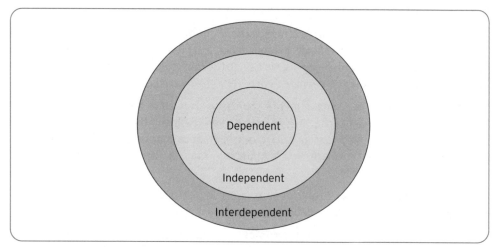

Figure 2.1
Nested circles of interdependence and interconnectedness

The first stage of interconnectedness: dependence

When you were a little child, you were very dependent on other people. You could do nothing for yourself: you could not walk, you could not talk, you could not feed yourself, and you could not get dressed without help. You were very dependent on other people's love and kindness. This stage represents the inner core of Figure 2.1.

The second stage of interconnectedness: independence

The next period of your life was dedicated to becoming independent – with the help of parents, teachers, friends and many others, you developed all the skills and knowledge you needed to become increasingly independent.

We can regard ourselves as an independent person only if we have developed 'true independence of character'. Stephen Covey explains that 'true independence of character empowers us to act rather than be acted upon. It frees us from our dependence on circumstances and other people . . .' (1989, p. 50). This stage is represented in Figure 2.1 as the middle circle of growth that comes after dependence.

The third stage of interconnectedness: interdependence

In our environment and in life in general it can be said that everything and everyone is interdependent. This means that, if we were to remain at the developmental level of independence only, we would be ineffective in our interactions with our interrelated environment. In Figure 2.1, the outer circle is strongly connected with others and the environment.

While you and I and others in our society are encouraged to develop independence and individuality, this does not mean that everyone will become a strong interdependent person. This is because people have a choice of becoming interdependent or not. As Covey states, ' . . . only independent people can become interdependent . . . Dependent people cannot choose to become interdependent . . . they don't own enough of themselves' (1989, p. 51).

In summary, our socialisation with others through interconnectedness with other people consists of the stages of dependence, independence and interdependence. It is important to remember that, as health professionals, we need to develop to the stage of interdependence so that we can provide care to people at each of the three stages.

In both health care and teaching, effective professionals need to be aware of the interconnectedness and interdependence that exists between them and the people for whom they care. As a student, it is important for you to reflect on both your uniqueness as well as your interconnectedness. Furthermore, you are not one singular identity but in fact 'multiple identities'.

To realise the penetration or extent of your interconnectedness with others, consider, for this day alone, how many roles you been played so far?

I asked the editor of this book to list her roles and she was amazed at how many she had. Her list for interconnections for the day is as follows (in brackets is the role and the running total of people with whom she interacted in that day):

'Waking up in bed at 6 am with husband/lover (family 1); went for a walk and spoke with people from the village walking their dogs (community 3); breakfast, received two phone calls (priest 6); mail person delivered mail (community 7); village shop to buy newspaper on the way to work (community 8); bought petrol on the way to work, and chatted to the person (community 9); parked the car at work and asked the general assistant emptying the rubbish bins if he had a nice weekend (lecturer 10); spoke to the two cleaning staff (lecturer 12); answered emails (lecturer 49); interviewed prospective students (lecturer 61); had lunch with some of the staff (work colleague 66); conducted an ethics seminar (lecturer 80); had a meeting (lecturer 90); made some phone calls (lecturer 95); went to the hospital for an NHS research ethics meeting (lecturer 105); went home and had dinner at the local pub and spoke with friends there (community 109); went to a meeting at 8 pm (priest 121); went home at 9.30, answered personal emails from children, grand-children and friends (family 130); went to bed 11.30 pm.

Total roles seven; interactions or interconnections with others for that day 130.'

You will find that the number of people with whom you interact and interconnect will be similar; it may not be the same sort of people or situations, but it will still be a large number.

Activity

Do the following exercise to explore your uniqueness and interconnectedness.

First, look at your uniqueness: if you were asked to list your identities or roles, what would you say? You could start with:

- I am the daughter of ..., the student of ..., the mother of ..., or the father of ..., etc.
- Currently, I work as ... In the past I have worked as ...
- That is, how many identities do you have?
- Write a list of your many identities.
- Now state how your roles have changed over time. For example, if you were a Girl Guide or Boy Scout as a child, but now you are a Scout leader. Likewise, if you have had children, the map would be different for when they were children to when they became more independent.
- You might like to draw a map to show how these roles intersect.

Values and beliefs – where do they come from?

The process of acknowledging uniqueness and interconnectedness is at the heart of the role of the health care professional. This process is based upon what we commonly refer to as our values. Values are what we hold dear to ourselves. They are those principles about which we feel strongly enough to defend, and which, over time, become incorporated and norm-alised into our daily lives (or way of living) (Nigam, 1997).

Values determine what we appreciate in life, what we reject and what we feel neutral towards. Examples could be valuing honesty in our dealings with others, or prizing the quality of being non-judgemental, or being accepting of cultural and spiritual diversity.

We tend to organise our values into some sort of hierarchy. This relates to the levels of importance that we attach to each of the values. The way in which we built this hierarchy is usually the result of our cultural socialisation as children, and by our changing ideas and life experiences (Nigam, 1997).

There may have been people whom we admired, or perhaps we read something we found inspiring or enlightening. Perhaps we have had certain life experiences that left us with 'conclusions' about what is valuable and what is not, what is good and what is bad. Usually families, towns, schools, nations, etc. share certain values. Values are like 'connective tissue', the glue that holds individuals together in an invisible web. Values help us to develop a feeling of belonging to a group.

We all have sets of values developed during our life. Some of these values have been adopted from people around us, while others have been formed through our experiences.

Activity

In this activity, I want you to identify your own values.

At this point in time, you have your own list of values. Take some time to visualise your list, write it down and put your values in order according to their importance in your life (Nigam, 1997; Nigam and Hawley, 1997).

1 Value: _____

2 Value: _____

3 Value: _____

4 Value: _____

5 .... _____

The uniqueness of other people

You have now reached a number of understandings about the complex nature of your own identity, which includes your roles and values. Likewise, the clients or patients to whom you will be providing care also have their own complex identities, comprising their many different roles and values. In addition, just like you, your clients' or patients' lives will involve change and therefore their values also have the potential to change (Purtillo, 1990).

The values of clients or patients, and those of work colleagues, have arisen from similar processes to those that you have experienced: the influences of childhood, family and the vacillations of daily life, through which they have learned to perceive themselves in terms of their relationships, geography and time (Milner, 1991). Like you, they too change and are constantly in the process of becoming. This is something important for health professionals to realise, this potential for change.

Too often, it is assumed that what was written in a client's or patient's notes 10 years previously still holds true. However, much could have happened in the mean time to that person. For example, the teenager with Attention Deficit Hyperactivity Disorder (ADHD) whom you last saw when he was in trouble with the law at 15 years old, when he was brought into

Accident and Emergency (Emergency Department) following a car accident, is no longer the same person. At the time, he was drunk and aggressive. However, over the years things have changed - he is now taking his Dexamphetamine 20 mg three times a day and is in stable employment. Today when you see him in the Emergency Department, it is because he has injured his hand at work and requires sutures, followed by physiotherapy to regain full movement, and an occupational therapy assessment.

Activity

How much are you aware of the uniqueness of others?

Ask someone who is culturally different from you to tell you how they would describe themselves (Nigam, 1997).

Hint: Take notes!

Other people's values

Earlier you considered your own values and constructed a list of values in order of their importance to you. You will remember that your values were the result of a process we call socialisation in childhood and your subsequent life experiences.

Activity

Ask the same person you interviewed before to list their five most important values in order of significance. As you did for yourself, you will need to list them according to their importance in that person's life (Nigam, 1997).

Other person's values:

1 Value: _____

2 Value: _____

3 Value: _____

4 Value: _____

5 .... _____

The role of personal socialisation – how do we 'learn' our values?

When we are children, we learn values through imitation, i.e. what is valued in our families and the societies to which we belong. In moral education, there are a number of theories as to how moral learning (the learning of values or what is right and wrong, good or bad) occurs.

The most commonly quoted theories are those developed by Lawrence Kohlberg (1980, 1984) and that developed by his student Carol Gilligan (1982). In his research, Kohlberg was able to demonstrate that moral development occurs in stages from wanting to please mum and dad, to being concerned about the relationships within a group, and to fairness at a level of moral maturity that is guided by self-chosen ethical principles. The people at this highest level would include Mahatma Gandhi and Dag Hammarskjöld.

Carol Gilligan applied a feminist viewpoint to Kohlberg's theory and, while she agreed that moral development occurred in stages, she stated that women were more focused in their moral development on relationships and care (which Kolhberg had not recognised). Hence, for women their moral development (and judgement) emphasises relationships and the interrelatedness of other people. Men, on the other hand, appeared to base their moral judgement on what is 'fair' and just.

More recent research in this area has shown that the gender boundaries in moral development are not as clearly defined as Gilligan had assumed; there are girls/women who base their moral decisions on fairness while some boys/men are very concerned with relationships among people (Gilligan, 1982; Blum, 1988; Hoff Sommers, 2000). However, Gilligan's research has led to the formulation of an Ethic of Care as distinguished from an Ethic of Fairness, as described by Kohlberg.

As health professionals, we need to make decisions about what is 'right' or 'wrong' and, unless we learn differently, these decisions depend on our values, beliefs and world views (that is, the ways we approach or think about the world). However, our values and beliefs can change through socialisation and we can learn to make ethical decisions based on moral philosophical theory and ethical principles (which are discussed in Chapters 5, 6 and 10).

How our values change

Values and beliefs are passed on through verbal and non-verbal communication – from one individual to another, from one generation to the next, and from culture to culture (Settelmaier, 2002, 2003). However, they can also change.

According to Kohlberg (1980, 1984) we change our values if confronted with a situation in which our existing values prove to be inadequate. We engage in a process referred to as *reflection*. As independent adults, we make decisions by applying a particular form of reflection called *critical reflection*. That is, we assess critically our current values and, depending on whether they appear useful to us, we either keep or discard our old values. The process of learning new values can be regarded as *transformative learning* because it transforms the way we think and how we approach the world (Mezirow, 1991).

Critical reflection and the resulting *moral disequilibrium* (i.e. our mind is out of balance) provides the opportunity for change. According to Kohlberg (1980, 1984), this state of moral disequilibrium opens the door to change. That is, we need this state of 'imbalance' to open up to new possibilities and to reflect on our existing values and revise them.

➤ How do we enter this state of imbalance?

Often it is through our communication with other people that we discover that there are other possibilities of thinking and valuing. It is through conversation, discussion and confrontation with others on topics and subjects that are based on values that we are forced to reconsider our own.

Over years of teaching ethics, I have noticed that students will quite often have a firm view on a topic. Then, in discussion, this student will say something like 'Gosh, I have never thought of that point of view before' and so the 'door to disequilibrium' opens and there is the opportunity for change and transformation to occur.

Activity

Remember the case study in Chapter 1 about Mr Chui and the physiotherapy students. Here this has been extended; read this, and then answer the questions at the end.

Case study 1.1
Mr Chui and the physiotherapy students *continued*

Later, when the students were having lunch in the hospital café and discussing the care and treatments they had observed that morning, Jonathon said to Peter (this student was the one who had been critical of the physiotherapist and nurse) 'What got into you this morning?'

Peter replied 'I have a ghastly hangover and was so irritated by having to observe all morning in this horrible place.'

Another of Peter's peers said 'I think you need to reflect on your behaviour.' With that, Peter scowled and got up, saying 'Go to hell the bloody lot of you,' and then walked away.

Questions

➤ What are Peter's peers trying to do?

➤ What is the name of the concept and/or process?

➤ Think about when someone has tried to do a similar thing to you, and identify what it felt like.

➤ Consequently, how should we care for peers and/or colleagues when we want them to consider their actions and behaviour?

Culture, values and beliefs

Previously it was mentioned that specific groups of people can hold and share certain values. What we didn't say at the time was that the term we use for this sameness is 'culture'. That is, culture consists of values and beliefs that a specific group hold in common. These are communicated and perpetuated (or driven by) those values which the specific group hold as desirable human experiences. Just as you have values and beliefs and act these out in everyday life through various behaviours, so too a group of people can have common values and beliefs, and manifest these through behaviour. In this way, we can define culture as a system of learned beliefs and customs that characterise the way of life for a particular society.

Culture can also be regarded as the acquired knowledge that people use to interpret their world and generate social behaviour. However, it is not the behaviour itself, but the knowledge used to construct and understand behaviour. When we talk about 'culture' we can mean those issues related to race and ethnicity, religion, social class, gender and language.

Culture might also be described as a system of knowledge by which people design their own actions and interpret the behaviour of others (Banks, 2004; Nieto, 2004).

Within any one nation, there might be many different ethnic, racial and religious groups. Within each of these groups we might find so-called *subcultures*, e.g. bikers, single parents, lawyers, medical doctors and drug addicts that form part of the so-called *mainstream* culture. What all cultures have in common is a certain set of shared values, practices and a common 'language', i.e. a set of terms used by a particular group as a means of communication (Banks, 2004).

Pause and think

➤ What are the different cultural groups that live in your town or city, or attend your university?

➤ Now think about 'subcultures' - what cultural subgroups can you think of?

Culturally sensitive health care practice – what is that?

As a health professional, you deal with people from diverse backgrounds, all with varied needs. Consequently, it is necessary to reflect on how you can cater to all these diverse backgrounds sensitively. Problems will occur in both professional and everyday life if we do not reflect on our own values and beliefs to recognise the difference between our own uniqueness and that of other people.

This will happen if we do not identify our own values and beliefs, and engage in critical thinking of the meanings we attach to these before we start to attend to the needs of others from different cultures. We are flirting with danger if we simply accept our own values and beliefs as right and correct! That is, if we assume our values and beliefs are correct and those of the other person are wrong or bad. Even though we may not verbalise this to the other person, it will show in our non-verbal communication (usually in our facial expressions or body stance).

Problems also occur if we do not reflect on our own uncritically accepted views of 'others', that is, our *cultural stereotypes*. It is crucial for health care professionals dealing with people from diverse backgrounds to reflect on these stereotypes, which they unthinkingly hold (Nieto, 2004).

As a health care professional you need to not only be aware that you hold a set of values, beliefs and world views, but recognise that the client or patient also does, as one person to another. Hence, there is the potential for problems to occur if your value system is different from that of your client or patient. The difficulty is that we can be unaware of this difference unless we undertake specific strategies to minimise the occurrence.

What is culturally sensitive practice? It is when a health professional recognises a client's or patient's culture is different from his or her own and engages in an equal partnership of negotiation when facilitating care.

According to Papadopoulos (2006), health professionals need to progress through three stages of learning to reach the fourth stage of cultural competence. The first stage is cultural awareness, when we recognise another person's cultural identity, heritage, ethnohistory and stereotype. The second stage is gaining the necessary cultural knowledge to understand the client's or patient's health beliefs, anthropological, sociological and biological differences, and health inequalities. The third stage is cultural sensitivity, when the professional uses empathy, interprofessional communication skills, trust, respect, acceptance, appropriateness, and awareness of the barriers that impede sensitive practice. The final stage is cultural competence, when a health professional uses appropriate assessment and diagnostic and clinical skills to challenge prejudice, discrimination and inequality to provide quality care.

Activity

All of us hold cultural stereotypes. Most of the time we are not even aware that we have them – these are the most insidious. Consider the following statements. (Please note that you are not being tested for your political correctness in these statements – most cultural stereotypes are *not* politically correct.)

Women cannot drive.

Men cannot multitask.

Women cannot read maps.

Men cannot cook.

Fat people are lazy.

People with psychiatric disorders need to be locked away.

Babies born with severe disabilities need to institutionalised.

Now let us consider particular groups. Without censoring yourself, describe the following.

- A typical Australian
- A typical Scotsman
- A typical biker
- A typical scientist
- A typical obese person
- A psychiatric patient
- A typical baby with severe disabilities
- A typical . . . . .

You will probably come up with a list of attributes that 'describe' particular groups of people. However, on careful consideration, how many members of this particular group do you know personally that actually fit these descriptions?

We know from our own experience that even within our own families not one person is like another. So, why do we hold on so strongly to the stereotypical views that we have of others? That is, why haven't we analysed these assumptions we hold?

It is because we have not challenged our own views and values. Such unchallenged cultural stereotypes often results in 'fear of strangers' or *xenophobia*. Alternatively, is it because we will not listen to other people's view points or that we dismiss them as wrong or bad?

Pause and think

How can we challenge our taken-for-granted assumptions?

First, by recognising that we all have 'stereotypes' in our thinking. Second, by learning as much as we can about those cultural groups that are different from our own.

Cultural stereotypes are based on the assumption that culture is something that does not change, something that has essential, immutable characteristics. According to Nieto (2004) this is a mistaken belief. It is a bald assertion to maintain or say that all those who share a culture behave or think in the same way.

Activity

Read the case study and answer the questions at the end.

Case study 2.1
Mai Lee and her drug overdose

Mai is a 19-year-old who is admitted to hospital after some university students found her lying naked and unconscious with her handbag outside in the grounds of their hall of residence at 7 am in the morning. They phoned for an ambulance as they could not rouse Mai.

At breakfast some of her friends talk of them coming back to the Hall at 6 am after being out all night clubbing to have a shower, breakfast and then go to class. They said that Mai was all right then, so they can't understand why she would have gone back outside again and why she was unconscious.

In hospital it is discovered that Mai has toxic levels of a recreational drug, plus Panadol and Nitrazepam within her system. There are also multiple lacerations to her thighs where she has been abusing herself. Following aggressive treatment in the emergency department, Mai regains consciousness and is transferred to the psychiatric unit.

Next day she asks one of the nurses to phone you and ask that you go and see her in hospital as she wants to tell you something.

You really don't want to go as you are embarrassed by what she has done. But, taking another friend with you, you go.

Questions

➤ Why might you and the other student be embarrassed to go and see Mai in hospital?

➤ Why do you think Mai might have taken the drugs?

At the hospital Mai says to you that she asked you to come so that she can give you the key to her room so that you can remove some drugs she has in there. She says that her parents are coming to take her back home, and they will be packing her bags at the Hall when the warden gives them access to her room. She also says that she fears that if her parents know she has been taking drugs, they won't let her come back to study at the university.

Mai then opens her handbag and takes out the key and gives it to you.

You ask Mai why she has drugs in her room? She replies 'But everyone in our group has drugs; you said that you take drugs'. You reply, 'but that was something I just said; I don't actually do it!'

Mai starts crying and yells at you for making her take drugs. The nurse hurries into the room and asks you to leave, saying 'You must leave now, drug overdose patients such as Mai who have severe liver damage need to have a lot of rest and not get upset'. You look at the nurse and say 'Mai has severe liver damage?' 'Yes' she says, 'didn't she tell you that she was silly and took 48 Panadol tablets, plus good-ness knows how many Nitrazepam?'

Questions

Discuss the case study with a peer or peers. Then:

➤ List what you think might be some of Mai's values and beliefs?

➤ What cultural aspects can you understand from the case study?

➤ Do you have an ethical obligation to go to Mai's room and remove the drugs before her parents arrive?

➤ You know that Mai's personal tutor in the School of Health and Social Care would not be aware that Mai is talking drugs and self-abusing. Do you go and tell the tutor?

➤ What do you think of the nurse telling you that Mai was silly in taking the Panadol and Nitrazepam?

Identity and equality

Your understanding of your own identities and those of others also contains an appreciation of the social processes which link people who have, through their cultural socialization, those interconnections of thought, images, feelings and attitudes (Blum, cited in Barrett and Keeping, 2005). Just as you have an emotional attachment and a cognitive understanding about how you fit in with particular cultural and language groups, and what your roles and obligations are there, so too do those people that you meet and help in clinical practice (Breton *et al.*, 1990).

Learning and caring as one person to another

Consequently, because you will encounter so many people in different contexts during your career, you will be presented with many opportunities to extend your knowledge and appreciation of the many dimensions of cultural life. This is because the connection with those who require your help will be an extension of yourself, of your own identities, and that caring relationship will be one that forms a partnership or therapeutic relationship. This includes an equal connection with the identities of the person whom you are helping. Essentially, the therapeutic relationship which follows will be mutual because, while you will assist that person, they will also assist you to a deeper understanding of what it means to be human.

Health professionals' values

It seems then that to be a health care professional is to be one who connects with other people at the point where identities intersect and connect (Nigam, 1997). This intersection transcends your own cultural conditioning because the focus of your attention in health care is the other person (not yourself), while you simultaneously remain cognisant of that which makes you 'you' (Nigam, 1997).

Professional values are the tool which enable you to become open to this type of connection (Nigam, 1997). It will be your level of commitment to these professional values that others will see manifested in how you approach, communicate and care for clients or patients in a culturally sensitive or competent manner that is vitally important. Such values are, and will be, core competencies or outcomes for your registration to your professional board, council or body. No doubt you have already discovered that these are built into your education (theory and competencies for clinical practice). These professional values represent the values of the collective body of that discipline or profession. They identify the principles that a particular group of health care professionals regard as important and which guide your clinical practice.

Each profession has their own standard of ethical practice, and the names of these standards will vary from one profession to another. In the UK:

- osteopaths have a Standards of Conduct;
- physiotherapists, occupational therapists, nurses and midwives each have a Code of Professional Conduct;
- social workers have a Code of Practice;
- operating department practitioners have the Practitioners' Code of Conduct; and
- those health professionals who belong to the Health Professionals Council have the Standards of Conduct, Performance and Ethics.

So, while the names of these documents may be different, they all aim to represent the professional values of each of the different disciplines.

The purpose of these documents is to act as part of the standards for professions and communicate to people in the community or society what they should be able to expect from their interactions with that particular group of health professionals (Nigam, 1997).

Responsible ethical behaviour

Ethical behaviour for health professionals is inclusive of culturally sensitive and competent care. This is a responsibility for all practitioners. However, it is also a privilege, as it enhances the experience and knowledge of the health professional, allowing them to become a better person. When culturally competent care is embodied in the therapeutic relationship, the client or patient feels secure and appreciated as a unique human being, and mutual trust is fostered.

The key to this sensitive cultural connection is to:

● understand the nature of your own complex cultural identity;
● be open to appreciating the same in others;
● gain knowledge and understanding of the client's or patient's health beliefs, anthropological, sociological and biological differences, and health inequalities.

The often publicised media notion that culture is like a suitcase that one is given at birth and which one carries about unchanged until the end of life is a simplistic notion, and shows a completely inaccurate understanding of human experience. It is also devoid of any understanding of human nature and of how we change through life experiences (Nigam, 1997). The press may also use classifications and stereotypical group labels as convenience tools as they create the idea that the person or group are 'the other', with which they have no connection (Nigam, 1997). But such concepts have no place in a health professional's practice.

Don't mislead

Sometimes you will find terms such as 'cultural background' being used. These need to be fully explored and in some instances discouraged as the words can invoke a misleading statement. This is due to the inference that a person's cultural background is of primary concern (which it is). However, so too are a person's life experiences, especially if the client or patient has since left that culture. Therefore a term like 'cultural background' is only useful if the person still holds those values and beliefs from that culture or if these impinge on their health problem.

Models of cultural care

There are now many models of care, which professionals can use to provide culturally competent care. The Giger and Davidhizer's transcultural assessment model (2004) is manifest in a series of concentric circles, with the central core component as 'Client: unique cultural being', with the six phenomena of culture surrounding the centre. The six areas for assessment are areas of communication, space, time, social organisation, environmental control and biological variations. Once these have been identified, the health professional is in a position to facilitate and negotiate care with the client or patient.

It should be remembered that a health professional's level of competence needs to be dynamic and constantly developing. Your ability to work as a health professional depends on your commitment and willingness to listen to other people, actually hear their words, and accept that their cultural realities are just as legitimate as your own (Nigam, 1997).

If you can do this, then you have internalised the critical values of caring, and you have started the journey of becoming an ethical practitioner of your profession.

Summary

You have gained knowledge and understanding of your own uniqueness and interconnectedness with others, which includes the necessity to become interdependent to function as a health professional. You have also identified your own values and the importance you place on these. Just as important is that you have recognised that these change with life experiences through communication with others. Likewise, you have explored your own culture and that of someone who is different from you. You then became aware of how the collective values of the various health professional councils or bodies reflect the necessary standard of ethical conduct which members are required to adopt and practise.

Professional development

Your aim in this professional development session is to:

● examine yourself;

● examine the culture in which you live and work.

In this way you will be able to separate your own values and beliefs from those for whom you will be providing care, and at the same time be empathetic and sensitive to their situation.

In your Ethics Portfolio write answers about the following questions so that you increase your self-awareness and that of possible clients and patients.

(Note: there is no need for you to write a reflection on these, simply list the answers to the questions. It is item 4 that you will need to critically reflect upon in your journal – that is, including all the stages of the cycle.)

1 Access one of the cultural assessment tools and, using the questions, document your own cultural perspective. Suggested models include:

● Campinha-Bacote, J. (1998) *The Process of Cultural Competence in the Delivery of Health Care Services. A Culturally Competent Model of Care*, 3rd edn. Cincinnati: Transcultural Care Association.

● Giger, J. N. and Davidhizer, R. E. (2004). *Transcultural Nursing. Assessment and Intervention*, 4th edn. St Louis: Mosby.

● Leininger, M. M. and McFarland, M. (2002). *Transcultural Nursing, Concepts, Theories and Research*, 3rd edn. New York: McGraw-Hill.

● Andrews, M. M. and Boyle, J. (2003). *Transcultural Concepts in Nursing Care*, 4th edn. Philadelphia: Lippincott.

Although these models might state their use in nursing, they also have a universality that allows most health professionals to use them. The Giger and Davidhizer assessment model has been found useful by the majority of different health professionals in their clinical practice (midwifery, psychiatry, radiology, dentistry, perioperative surgery, education and training).

2 Your next task is to locate the government statistics about the people who reside in the geographical region in which you undertake clinical practice. These statistics will provide you with the information you need to discover about the people, e.g. their country of origin, language, religion, annual income per household, type of housing, etc. Such information is necessary for you to become culturally competent to the needs of your clients or patients. That is, this information will enable you to achieve the first stage of cultural competence which is 'cultural awareness' (see p. 25 if you have forgotten about the different stages). Then answer these questions:

➤ What are the different cultures of people where you undertake clinical practice?

➤ What languages do the people use?

➤ What spiritual beliefs do these people have?

➤ To what political persuasion do they belong?

➤ What socioeconomic groups are there?

3 Now, use the internet to find all the necessary information needed to care for a client or patient from at least one of these cultural groups (which is different from yours). Include their values, beliefs and customs (including religion or spirituality).

Some of the following points will help you in writing down how to provide care and treatments.

➤ What is the religious identity and authority (does this need to be strictly adhered to)?

➤ What are the important values and beliefs: especially those related to dress, modesty, diet, fasting and sex?

➤ What is the cultural expectation of marriage and family life: meaning of marriage, family relationships, care of the children, education and marriage breakdown?

➤ What are the values and beliefs in relation to quality and value of life (including abortion, those that are vulnerable, the older person, dying and death)?

This will take time, but you need to do the same for all the different cultural groups that you might come across in clinical practice. Consequently, you could start with those cultures that have the highest population and/or those known to have a significant health problem.

Once you have this information you will be prepared with knowledge and understanding to provide care that is culturally sensitive.

Critical reflection

Reflective journal entry. For this chapter, you are asked to be critical of your own values and beliefs. Begin by asking yourself:

➡

➤ Why do I have these values?

➤ Are they important to me?

➤ Which ones need changing?

➤ Why do they need to change?

➤ How will I change these values and beliefs?

We suggest that you use Johns' (2000) model for structured reflection for this, as it will enable you to work through these questions. Johns' stages are (p. 47):

Looking in

● Find a space to focus.

● Pay attention to your thoughts and emotions.

● Write down those thoughts and emotions that seem significant.

Looking out

● A description of the situation.

● What issues are significant.

● Aesthetics, that is:

○ What was I trying to achieve? But in this case, it will be what I am trying to achieve?

○ What were the consequences to the patient/others/myself? Or in your case, what are the consequences for the patient/others/myself?

○ How were others feeling? In your case this will be, how will others feel about this; and

○ How do I know this?

● Personal:

○ Why did I feel the way I did with this situation? For your exercise, this will be why do I feel this way?

● Ethics:

○ Did I act for the best? Or will this be for the best?

● What factors (either embodied within me or embedded within the environment) are, or were, influencing me?

● Empirics:

○ What knowledge did or could have informed me?

● Reflexivity:

○ Does this situation connect with previous experiences?

○ How could I handle this situation better?

○ What would be the consequences of alternative actions for the patient/others/myself?

○ How do I now feel about this experience?

○ Can I support myself and others better as a consequence?

○ How therapeutically available am I to work with patients/families and staff to help them meet their needs?

If you know of another reflective model that will enable you to answer the questions about your values, then please feel free to use that one.

If you are going to use Johns' model, I suggest you ask the questions during the looking-in stage. That is:

Looking in

- Find a space to focus.

- Pay attention to your thoughts and emotions.

- Write down those thoughts and emotions that seem significant. For example, are you quite happy to ask yourself these questions, or have you asked a friend to do this with you.

- What am I trying to achieve; in this case you are critically reflecting on your personal values so that you can identify which ones need to change. So, list your values:

  1 _____

  2 _____

  3 _____

  4 _____

  5 _____

- Then ask yourself: why do I have these values?

- Which ones are important to me as an individual? Why?

- Now ask yourself, which of my personal values will conflict with those of my profession?

- Which values will conflict with providing culturally sensitive care?

The values that will conflict with you being able to provide culturally competent care are the ones that need to change. The values that conflict with your profession may also need to change (depending on what they are, some people are able to keep their personal values separate from their professional values).

So write down the values that need to change.

Looking out

- What am I trying to achieve (trying to change my values)?

- What are the consequences for the patient/others/myself?

- How will others feel about this?

- How do I know this?

- Personal:

  ○ How do I feel now that I have identified those values that need to change?

- Ethics:

  ○ Will this be for the best?

- What factors (either embodied within me or embedded within the environment) can help me change?

- Empirics:
  - What knowledge and resources can I use to change my values (that is, those that you have identified that need to change)?
- Reflexivity:
  - Does this situation of needing to change connect with a previous experience of needing to change?
  - If so, what helped you then?
  - Can you use those same methods in this situation?
  - What alternative actions are there that can be used?
  - What will be the outcome of this change in relation to being therapeutically available to patients/families and staff to help them meet their needs?

Don't be surprised if this exercise takes you a while to do. The length of time will depend on:

- how in touch you are with your values; and
- being able to express your feelings and thoughts on paper.

Just keep going until you reach the end.

If this exercise raised too many feelings of disquiet, make an appointment with your personal tutor at university to discuss the issue. Alternatively, seek a counsellor at the university to talk through the issues raised.

3

Ethical issues and problems in health care

Georgina Hawley

Why this chapter is important to me . . .

✔ To understand ethical or moral issues.

✔ Learning what ethics is not!

✔ How to discern if a situation is an ethical problem.

✔ Types of ethical or moral problems that can occur, including dilemmas.

The purpose of learning about ethics is so that you will be able to identify what is regarded as right and wrong in clinical practice. Health care has seen many dreadful tragedies where professionals unthinkingly provided care that they supposed was satisfactory, when in reality it was not. This was caused because decisions were based on their own values and beliefs. Take, for example, the Tuskagee experiment (which was mentioned in Chapter 1).

At the time, the doctors conducting the trial believed that syphilis developed differently in the black population than the white. That is, as the American-Africans in the study developed the disease it would not damage the brain during the tertiary stage as it did with the white population. These men did of course go on to develop tertiary syphilis and die the agonising death that it brings, when they could have been cured at any time from the 1940s onward when penicillin became available as the successful treatment. This whole study reflected the racist premise of the US public health doctors who were involved at the time.

In the previous chapter you learnt the importance your values have in defining your own uniqueness, and that decisions you make will reflect your values and beliefs. You also learnt that these values might not be the same as another person's and that problems can arise because of this. At the very heart of all of this are the very people for whom we have been charged to provide care: the patients or clients. That is, we need to protect the sick and vulnerable in our society, so that they can access the most appropriate care, and then provide care that respects their dignity and self-worth (and is therefore ethical). These ethical standards of care are embodied in the various health professional councils or registration boards as standards of conduct and/or codes of ethics.

In this chapter, you will learn more about ethics in relation to health care, that is, what is involved. First, you will learn more about what health care ethics is and is not. This includes a description of an ethical or moral issue, problem and dilemma. Second, moral problems will be discussed in greater detail, so that you can be aware of when and how they can occur. Third, you will be introduced to a model or framework that you can use when faced with a situation that you think may be an ethical problem or dilemma, to help you decide if it is. Fourth, the model is applied to the case study 'Mr Chui and the physiotherapy students' step-by-step, so that you can fully understand how to do it yourself. Fifth, different types of ethical or moral problems (including a dilemma) and how they occur will be described. Finally, at the end of the chapter is the Professional Development section to facilitate your understanding of ethics.

Ethical health care

In Chapter 2 you learnt about the need to reflect upon your values and beliefs, and to be critical about the positions or importance these have in relation to your professional practice. This was necessary as the subject of ethics in relation to health care is a critical reflective activity (Beauchamp and Childress, 1983).

Today, the very nature of ethics requires professionals to be concerned with the systematic examination of issues, problems and/or dilemmas. This critical reflection should show us what we ought to do by asking us to consider and reconsider actions, the rationales or reasons for those actions, and the judgements made (Beauchamp and Childress, 1983). You were introduced to writing a reflective journal so that you can start this systematic examination of situations involving problems and/or dilemmas.

Issues, problems and dilemmas

In this book, ethical issues in health care are defined as those phenomena or behaviours that have the potential to become a problem. For example, the ethical issue of abortion (the phenomenon) has the potential to become an ethical problem, as does resuscitating a terminally ill patient. Most people recognise obvious ethical issues such as abortion and euthanasia, but there are many more including patients' rights, working as a team, pain, resuscitation, dying, allocation of resources and research.

Ethical problems are those incidents or situations that have arisen from a moral or ethical issue which are vitally important in the life of the patient. On the other hand, ethical dilemmas are more than just a problem as these, when examined, have two possible ways or options of solving the problem; however, neither of these options appear to be correct (Hawley, 1997c).

To resolve ethical problems and/or dilemmas the whole team needs to be involved, using communication, understanding and reflection to identify and plan a resolution in the best interests of the patient. This discussion needs to examine the context of the situation and the available options, the available resources and then, with the client or patient as part of the team, a decision is made.

Historically, ethics in health care has been thought to be, written about and described as etiquette, good manners, law, codes of practice, organisational policy, etc. Today, it is none of these things. However, some of these are part of ethics.

What ethics in health care is not

Many people think they know what ethics is in relation to health care, and so it frequently becomes confused with hospital or professional etiquette, being good and following the orders of a superior, codes of practice, legal issues, hospital or organisation policy, public opinion and gut response.

Hospital or professional etiquette

Although historically hospital or professional etiquette was regarded as ethics, this no longer applies. Etiquette can only advise as to how to behave in certain circumstances. That is, it seeks to guide the demeanour and behaviour of health professionals in good manners and courtesy (Hawley, 1997a, b). For example, a student may be told to place their hands behind their back when talking to a senior person and to respond with only 'yes sister' or 'no sister'. I can remember being reprimanded as a student for saying 'Okay' instead of 'yes sister', and not waiting for the male consultant to walk through the door first! Good manners and politeness are necessary, but etiquette does not help a health professional resolve a specific moral or ethical problem.

Following the orders of a superior

All health professionals are legally responsible for their own standard of practice (Hawley, 1997a). The old legal precedent of the doctor being 'The Captain of the ship', with nurses, physiotherapists and all other allied health professionals obeying the doctor's orders, has gone.

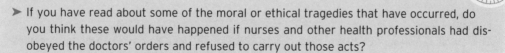

Pause and think

➤ If you have read about some of the moral or ethical tragedies that have occurred, do you think these would have happened if nurses and other health professionals had disobeyed the doctors' orders and refused to carry out those acts?

The Tuskegee situation was one of the turning points in US nursing in that it became glaringly apparent that nurses could no longer blindly follow the orders of doctors.

So, when health professionals deem that ethics is just being good and following the orders of a superior, they are incorrect.

The Liverpool Children's Hospital Inquiry heard that, in 1988, Professor van Velzen gave the order that children's organs set aside during autopsies for further examination were not to be returned to the body. This order was followed by the pathology staff, even though it was in direct opposition to the Human Tissue Act. So, staff broke the law on the orders of the doctor not only during that year but until 1998 – 10 years later!

Today, no health professional should carry out a treatment order from a superior that s/he does not think is correct or approve. In such circumstances, hospitals or organisations need to have a policy and guidelines for professionals to follow when they do not want to perform a superior's order. Basically, this needs to stipulate that the person explains to their superior why they can't undertake the order. If the superior insists that the order is performed, then the subordinate can go to the superior's line manager and ask for them to intervene (Wallace, 2001).

Codes of practice or ethics

Although codes of ethics or codes of conduct are part of ethics, they are not the whole of the subject. That is, while each health profession has their own code or standard, which lists the ideals each member should maintain, these can only guide moral conduct in particular situations (Hawley, 1997c). For example, the nurses' code of ethics does not provide nurses with a rigorous set of principles that they can use to seek resolution to an ethical problem (Singleton and McLaren, 1995).

Legal issues

Although ethics and law do overlap, there is a distinction between the two. Law and ethics are quite separate action-guiding systems, and care must be taken to distinguish between them (Johnstone, 1996). The law for the UK, Australia, Hong Kong and New Zealand consists of civil and criminal law, acts and statutes. Such laws can be enforced and the person that perpetrated the crime punished (criminal law) and/or the defendant compensated (civil law).

Civil law
The knowledge and understanding of civil law that health professionals need to acquire includes assault (and battery), consent, negligence, false imprisonment, defamation (and libel) and confidentiality (Hawley, 1997c). There may also be other areas, depending on the area of clinical practice.

Criminal law
The criminal law about which health care professionals need to have knowledge includes theft, criminal assault, criminal negligence (both of these are different from civil law), grievous bodily harm, sexual assault, rape, manslaughter, murder or homicide, assisted suicide and abortion.

Acts and statutes
The various Acts and Statutes about which knowledge is required include those that govern the profession and those that stipulate care. Statutes include the Medical Act, the Nursing and Midwifery Act, Physiotherapy, etc. Specific treatment Acts include mental health, human tissue and transplantation, infectious diseases and HIV/AIDS (Hawley, 1997c). Allied to these are child protection, discrimination and disabilities. The actual names of these Acts

are not recorded here as the names differ from one country to another. Again, the health professional's knowledge of these will depend on their area of clinical practice.

It was the Human Tissue Act 1961 upon which the Alder Hey scandal centred (The Report of The Royal Liverpool Children's Hospital Inquiry, 2001). This inquiry was undertaken to discover the extent of organs being retained from post-mortem examinations of neonates who had died (including stillborn), and also miscarried fetal remains. During an autopsy or post mortem it is normal practice for tissue and organs to be removed from the body and examined microscopically. However, these organs should be returned to the body for the funeral. The difficulty arises when tissues from the heart and brain need to be examined as they require fixing before the microscopic examination can take place (which, at the time of the inquiry, could have taken up to 6 weeks). What happened at Alder Hey was that the parents were not told that these organs had not been returned to the body, but in fact retained on the orders of Professor van Velzen. He stated that these now became the property of the hospital for him to use in research. He also valued his research more highly than the rights of the parents whose baby (or fetus) had died. These parents had not consented to these body parts being stored for research – in some case the whole intact fetus (Report of The Royal Liverpool Children's Inquiry, 2001).

Hospital, institutional or organisational policy

Policies cannot be written to cover every scenario that arises, even though there may be an extensive list (human resources, clinical protocols, infection control, etc.). Most are written in quite general terms and are certainly not meant to guide ethical behaviour. However, health professionals sometimes hide behind these hospital policies or use them to defend their own inadequacies when ethical problems arise (Veatch, 1989).

Public opinion or the view of the majority?

If ethics was just the matter of what most people think, then an opinion poll could be conducted each time an ethical decision needed to be made. What needs to be remembered is that, when seeking an ethical resolution to a problem, the rationales for proposed actions and judgement are steeped in ethical principles or moral theories (Thompson *et al.*, 1992).

Gut response

Just because a health professional feels good about doing a specific action does not make it ethically right (Bandman and Bandman, 1997). This means that a professional might think that they have been ethically correct. However, unless that action is critically and systematically reviewed (or reflected upon), it cannot be assumed to be ethically correct.

We have just done a whirlwind tour of what ethics is not: etiquette, following the orders of a superior, hospital policy, codes of practice, law, public opinion and gut response.

Case for studying ethics

There are times when the health professional needs to make decisions, especially in those areas which are important, but for which a legal Act or Statute has not yet been developed

(Hawley, 1997c). For example, when *in vitro* fertilisation (IVF) first became a treatment, there was no law regarding management of cycles, sperm or embryos or care of patients. At the time it was felt that the medical professional could self-regulate. It was not until 20 years later, after many unsatisfactory incidents had occurred, that the laws regulating the use and management of IVF were introduced. Likewise, the Misuse of Drug Act is there to assist with the detection and management of those people who are addicted to Class A drugs. Prior to the introduction of this Act, doctors, hospitals and the police tried to cope with the ever-increasing problem.

Consequently, knowledge and understanding of ethics is useful when a practitioner needs to make decisions which primarily rest upon their own integrity. According to Hawley (1997b and c), ethics can be used when the law cannot offer direction as to what is right and wrong. That is, a health professional first obeys the law for direction; however, if no law exists, they use their knowledge and understanding of ethics to decide the correct course of action.

Ethical problems and/or dilemmas

There are many problems that occur every day in health care, but not all of these will have an ethical or moral component. Sometimes health professionals think they have an ethical problem that needs to be resolved, or they think another health professional is acting unethically, when in reality this is not the case.

To help you understand whether there is an ethical problem or not the following framework has been developed. It will help you to think systematically about the various aspects of the problem, so that you can explore and discuss the situation with others in the interprofessional team in a calm, rational and non-judgemental manner.

Using a framework to understand potential ethical problems

This framework consists of three easy stages: communication, understanding and reflection.

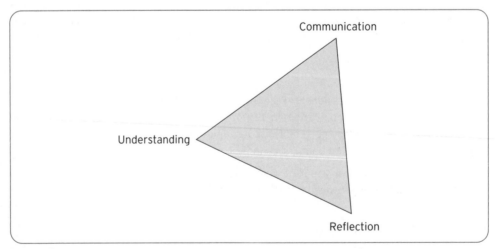

Figure 3.1
Ethical framework

In this framework, all three sides of the triangle are the same length, indicating that the three stages of communication, understanding and reflection are equally important. The triangle is tipped over more on one side; that is, it is skewed downwards. This indicates that the three stages take place one after another, starting with the stage at the top of the triangle and working down to the bottom. Notice that communication is at the top of triangle, indicating that communication is the first thing you need to do. Next is understanding, indicating that this is the second stage you need to undertake. Finally, the lowest of the concepts is reflection, indicating that this is the third stage of the framework.

Each of the three components interconnects with each other, and need to be considered both individually and together as a whole.

In the first stage, communication, the health professional finds out as much information as they can about the issue that is troubling them. The second stage is understanding the roles of the different people involved, such as the other health professionals and the patient (and their family or loved ones). The third stage is to reflect on all the information, to decide if there is an ethical problem or not. If there is, then follow hospital or organisation guidelines to deal with it; however, if these do not exist, the multidisciplinary team (including you) could follow one of the models of decision-making mentioned later in this book.

Since you are a professional who respects other roles in the team, and they in turn respect your role, it is important to be clear about the potential ethical problem. It would not do your professional credibility any good if you complained that someone in the team was unethical when in reality you did not have all the facts. Consequently, using this framework will help you to gather all the facts and consider them when examining a potential ethical problem.

The first stage: communication
The first stage in understanding a potential ethical problem is communication; that is, gathering as much data as possible about the situation. In doing this you need to remember what you have learnt about the communication process in other subjects. As you know, the communication process involves more than talking to someone or at them. It involves the other person being able to understand, and their perception of, what is being said.

This whole process has many twists and turns and, as health professionals, we learn about these intricacies. However, as co-workers we are sometimes not good at communicating with each other. Because of this lack of communication, we may think there is an ethical problem when in reality we may not have all the information and, as a consequence, jump to a conclusion without fully clarifying the situation with the other health professionals. For example, another member of the team may have some information about the patient which, when taken into consideration, justifies the decision that was made about that patient's treatment. Therefore it is not an ethical problem at all, but rather miscommunication.

The second stage: understanding
The second stage of the process of understanding a potential ethical problem is that of understanding. The term understanding means the ability to question and talk about the subject knowledgeably. Therefore, in this stage comprehension of the situation (including the communication) is required, along with the ability to ask questions of the other professionals and the patient or client involved. That is, an understanding of the roles of the other

members of the team and the patient is required. This stage is a continuation of the communication stage, in which you gain more knowledge, ask questions, and talk openly about the problem you perceive with the members of the team.

The third stage: reflection

The third stage is to reflect as a professional about the problem, examining each of the previous steps. Question yourself about:

- What is the perceived problem?
- Do you have all the information to support your perception of the problem?
- Do you need to go back to other members of the team to ask questions in relation to their knowledge and understanding of the situation?
- Clarify with others how they feel about the issue.
- Be honest with yourself and ask 'Is it just my feelings that have caused me to perceive this situation as an ethical problem?'
- Ask yourself 'Do I perceive this to be an ethical problem because my values and beliefs are different from the client's or patient's?'

Once you have been through this three-stage process of seeking information, understanding other people's roles (asking further questions as necessary, clarifying with others to understand the problem or situation fully), and then reflecting on your own values and beliefs, if you still believe there to be an ethical problem, then the right thing to do is to follow the hospital or institutional policy and guidelines on ethical problems. If there is no policy or guidelines, discuss the situation with your line manager. If you believe that the situation is being ignored by your line manager, then you have the moral responsibility to report the situation to a more senior person in the hospital who has authority to investigate and take action. In all this it is your role to act professionally and non-judgementally.

Applying the framework to the case study of Mr Chui

We will now go through the model, using the case study of Mr Chui and the physiotherapy students (p. 9), step-by-step so that you can understand how it works.

Case study
Mr Chui and the physiotherapy students *continued*

Another student, Jonathon, observing the same situation with Mr Chui, waited for the physiotherapist and nurse to settle Mr Chui back into his chair and then go and wash their hands. When they were out of hearing of Mr Chui, Jonathon asked them 'Why didn't you just straighten Mr Chui's leg and ignore his complaints of pain?' The physiotherapist replied that they wanted Mr Chui to have choices with some aspects of his care at this stage of his rehabilitation. This way he would feel in control of the situation, in order that he might try the alternative of having some pain and try to get into bed with their help. The nurse added, 'This way, we hope that Mr Chui can empower himself to move forward in his rehabilitation.'

The first stage: communication

1   Did Peter wait and gain further information from the physiotherapist and the nurse about the patient's treatment so that he could clarify or validate his information?

He did not, so can he legitimately say that what they were doing was ethically incorrect?

He cannot, as it was his lack of communication that was at fault; that is, he didn't find out about the treatment of this type of stroke rehabilitation.

2   Jonathon, on the other hand, did. He waited until he could communicate with the physiotherapist and nurse about the situation privately. By doing so he gained information to help him gain a more accurate perception of the situation. He not only learnt more about physiotherapy and rehabilitation, but also about being professional; that is, by not interfering in a situation in which his role was one of observer.

The second stage: understanding

1   Did Peter have a full understanding of the situation? No.

2   That is, in the scenario Peter did not have an understanding of physiotherapy treatments for this type of stroke, or knowledge of muscle wasting, and the need for active and passive exercises to maintain movement and assist rehabilitation. Consequently, we can see that interprofessional understanding is essential to work harmoniously together.

Case study
Mr Chui and the physiotherapy students *continued*

Later, the students were having lunch in the hospital café and discussing the care and treatments they had observed that morning.

Jonathon said to Peter (this student was the one who had been critical of the physiotherapist and nurse) 'What got into you this morning?'

Peter replied 'I have a ghastly hangover and was so irritated by having to observe all morning in this horrible place.'

Another of Peter's peers said, 'I think you need to reflect on your behaviour.'

With that Peter scowled and got up, saying, 'go to hell the bloody lot of you' and, without saying anything, walked away.

Stage two continued: understanding the roles of others involved

1   In the first part of the case study, it can be recognised that Peter did not understand the roles of others and the treatment involved.

2   In this part of the case study we now see that the other students are trying to communicate and understand Peter's role in the morning session. That is, in this part of the scenario, we see the students trying to understand his angry behaviour, and giving him the opportunity to communicate his feelings and his reasoning. If perhaps his behaviour towards the physiotherapist and nurse had been about the treatment or pathophysiology

of the stroke patient, his peers could have assisted him with the information he needed (so that he would know and understand the next time). Instead, his behaviour was due to his hangover and irritability.

Stage three: reflection

1 From the scenario, we don't know whether Peter reflected on the situation and his behaviour, even though his peers recommended this action to him.

2 However, no doubt his clinical supervisor or university lecturer would hear of the situation and request that he do so. Hopefully, he would then realise the consequences of his hangover.

3 This case study highlights a serious matter; that is, the effect of alcohol on behaviour and ability to undertake clinical practice. In most countries different professional registration boards (or bodies) have standards that stipulate that a member must not practise while under the influence of alcohol or dangerous drugs (this time frame also includes the morning after, when the blood alcohol level can still be raised). Such a serious misdemeanour by a professional is cause for investigation. For a student on clinical practice this situation may warrant his/her suspension from clinical practice and/or other disciplinary measures. For example, the university investigating committee may give a written warning to the student; for a repeat offence, a fail grade may be awarded for that module or clinical practice.

When using the framework to work through the case study we have discovered that, although Peter thought there was an ethical problem in relation to the care and treatment Mr Chui was receiving, this was not the case. Therefore there is no responsibility for anyone involved to report the treatment and actions of the physiotherapist or nurse as an ethical problem. The scenario does demonstrate the following:

1 Communication is vital to have all the facts about a situation.

2 Understanding the role of other health professionals and treatments is necessary to work together as an interprofessional team.

3 Reflection can assist in professional growth by increasing personal and professional awareness.

4 As a student there are correct ways in which to ask questions, especially when observing on clinical practice.

5 It is a serious misdemeanour for a student or health care professional to be so influenced by alcohol as to not be able to undertake their role. Such behaviour could warrant disciplinary measures by the hospital or professional body or, in the case of the university, the Dean of the faculty or school, and also the hospital.

6 Is there anything else? What about culture? Did you realise that what Mr Chui or another patient thinks is ethically correct may not be what the practitioner may regard as correct or right? Or what might be considered an ethical problem in one country or culture may not be in another?

It is possible that Mr Chui might think that the physiotherapist and nurse were incorrect or bad in not helping him get onto his bed. Likewise, Peter may have come from a culture that reflects values and beliefs differently from his peers. Not all cultures approve of a woman providing care for male patients. Neither do some cultures approve of a female telling a male what to do or causing him pain. If these cultural differences were in the case study then, when you are working through the framework, it is necessary to take them into consideration.

Providing culturally sensitive care includes valuing inclusion and diversity. As professionals in health and social care we need awareness of the different cultural influences on health behaviours, illness and recovery, and to be able to translate that awareness into culturally competent care. Cultural diversity encompasses issues perceived and real differences with respect to age, ethnicity, disability, religion, life styles, family and kinship, dietary preferences, traditional language or dialects spoken, sexual orientation, educational and occupational status, and other factors (Leininger, 1998).

In valuing diversity, the awareness of cultural differences and acceptance of values, beliefs, behaviours and orientations is essential. Most universities provide education in this respect to health care professionals. If you have not yet reached this stage in your education, some self-directed study in this area is suggested.

The obvious way to find out whether the care and treatment given to patients and clients is appropriate or not for them is to assess their culture, values and beliefs, etc. during the assessment phase of diagnosis and care. This needs to be done to clarify existing knowledge and understanding. To know nothing of the client's or patient's cultural system would appear rude and disrespectful. As previously stated there are several models that health professionals can use as a framework to collect the necessary information, e.g. the Sunrise Model by Madeline Leininger (Leininger, 1998).

Types of ethical problems and/or dilemmas

Now that you understand how to discern whether a problem has an ethical or moral component, it is time to think about the various types of problems and how these can occur. When reading various texts about ethics, it becomes apparent that there has not been extensive research into how and why ethical problems occur. However, by analysing the knowledge and understanding gained from the psychology of moral development and team behaviour, pertinent information can be gained as to how these problems can occur.

Pause and think

➤ Consider the types of problems such as Tuskagee, The National Women's Cancer Treatment Inquiry, The Bristol Royal Infirmary Inquiry and The Royal Liverpool Children's Hospital Inquiry. What do you think may have caused these?

Of course, none of these were caused by one factor alone, but rather by a cluster of contributing factors. However, when we examine the behaviour of the health professionals involved it can be seen that different types of moral behaviour can give rise to these problems.

These include those caused by:

1 Professionals who have a genuine knowledge deficit about ethics.
2 Autocratic behaviour of committee or an authoritarian professional.
3 Groupie moral standards.
4 Insensitivity of the professional/s involved.
5 Amorality when the group lacks moral standards or concern for others.
6 Health professionals having different values and beliefs from each other.

It is useful to outline these so that you have an understanding of why education in ethics is important.

Problems caused by knowledge deficits

This type of problem occurs when the professional lacks education in health ethics or bioethics and consequently is unaware that a problem could occur or is occurring, e.g. undergraduate students who have not received any education in ethics.

This is manifest when the health professional does not see a situation as being an ethical or moral problem. Instead they think it is solely a clinical problem. An example is 'Do not resuscitate' orders on hopelessly or chronically ill patients. Many health professionals think these orders are solely a clinical decision and do not see the ethical or moral basis to the situation.

If professionals receive training in recognising moral problems and also in how to be assertive and negotiate the correct standard of care, the ethical or moral problems arising from knowledge deficits would in all probability not have occurred.

Examples of ethical or moral tragedies that have occurred because of this knowledge deficit include 'The Unfortunate Experiment', otherwise known as the National Women's Hospital Cancer Inquiry, and the Chelmsford Hospital deep sleep therapy (see Chapter 1). However, this does not apply to all staff involved, as some did not have a knowledge deficit but had 'groupie' morality or were ruled by autocratic or authoritarian behaviour.

Problems caused by authority or an authoritarian professional

This type of problem occurs when a professional or a group of professionals have placed themselves in a position of power and authority so that they can use this position to enforce their moral standards on others. These professionals have moral beliefs that are black and white, and they do not take kindly to others questioning their opinions or beliefs. These people are unable to see different points of view even when decisions are discussed with them. This rigidity occurs not only with moral problems but also sometimes with other aspects of their professional or personal life (Wright, 1971). Because of their positions of authority these professionals have the power to avoid being found out when they have done something wrong. However, when they do get found out they will deny all knowledge or responsibility.

This type of problem can be controlled by hospitals and health care organisations having a Clinical Ethics Committee that reviews situations, incidents and standards, making appropriate decisions. Such committees are common in many overseas hospitals, where clinicians can refer an ethical problem and the committee makes the decision. These committees are often also available to patients and their relatives when needing impartial advice to make decisions, e.g. whether or not to refuse treatment. The committee structure is such that they are able to provide impartial advice but also have the power to make changes at the highest level in the organisation.

This type of Clinical Ethics Committee is different from a Research Ethics Committee where research proposals are discussed and approval is given for the study to proceed or not. You will learn more about Research Ethics Committees in Chapter 16.

Problems arising from 'groupie' moral standards

This type of problem occurs when the health professional is so much a group player that they do not question the behaviour, care and treatment provided by other members. That is, belonging to the group is far more important than anything else. For such individuals, their whole life revolves around the group, and they live and breathe whatever the group does. When this group is a ward or unit in health care, the professional does whatever the rest of the group (or team) does, including social activities. The professional's standard of ethics comes from what the rest of the group does or does not do; that is, they are 'group centric' (Wright, 1971).

These professionals do not express their opinion that something immoral or unethical is occurring or likely to occur. Examples of the groupie (Wright calls this the moral conformist) include those staff who, when a team member says a client or patient is DNR, do not question the decision. Part of the tragedy at The Bristol Royal Infirmary stemmed from this group behaviour. Although the cardiosurgical team and ward staff were caring and motivated, they did what the rest of the group did, and did not question the actions or behaviours of others in the team: in particular the standard of care provided by two cardiac surgeons (Bristol Royal Infirmary Inquiry, 2001).

This type of moral problem can be controlled by continuing interprofessional development in health ethics, better unit or ward leadership management, and coaching team members to voice their opinions.

Problems caused by moral insensitivity

Moral insensitivity problems arise when a professional who is thoroughly convinced that they are right, that they undertake the action without considering the feelings of the client or patient. Examples of moral insensitivity include the doctor who is convinced that all life should be saved irrespective of the cost or the patient's quality of life and their wishes. Another would be a nurse who believes all clients or patients must be told the truth, even those who are not yet able to cope with that information or those who have requested not to receive certain information at that time. The unfeeling nature of this type of care is insensitive and does not conform to any professional standards.

Moral insensitivity can also cause ethical problems when health professionals are not vigilant about patients' rights and the ethical principles that need to be upheld, e.g. not respecting the dignity of the client or patient or not protecting their confidentiality. The extent to which this moral insensitivity occurs could be classed as incompetence or incompetent professional behaviour or standard. That is, the health professional concerned did not meet the competency expected for professional behaviour.

The problem can be controlled by identifying these professionals, having them undertake sensitivity training. However, they will usually only listen when given verbal warnings about their conduct in relation to their employment (such as verbal or written warnings), and then they will undertake the training.

Problems caused by amoral behaviour

These problems occur when a professional does not display any moral concern for anyone else but themself. In this situation the professional lacks complete moral concern and rejects any moral position, except for their own gain.

When trying to decide in which category to place the Alder Hey scandal at first I was undecided. That is, on reading the report published by the Crown Law department, I did not think Professor van Velzen had a knowledge deficit (as he was a pathologist and would have received the education), neither was he a groupie, or insensitive. Instead he occupied a position of power and authority, and that was where I categorised him first of all. Then I changed this to amoral as, on re-reading the report, he appeared to be without any moral standards of right, good and correct. I based this upon his ability to tell parents and staff lies and falsify post-mortem results, records and statistics (Report of The Royal Liverpool Children's Inquiry, 2001).

It is these behaviours of deceit and lying to parents about his methods and findings that I find completely amoral. I think of the parents to whom he must have told lies about why their child died, or why the fetus aborted or was stillborn; they believed him and based their future plans about whether or not to have additional children on his so-called facts. I find such behaviour disgraceful, as did the UK General Medical Council.

Problems caused by differences of opinion

Moral problems caused by a difference of opinion have been extensively written about and described in the field of business, marketing and also management whereas very little has been devoted to this subject in health care. However, the knowledge gained from these areas can be transferred into health care.

The moral problems arising from differences of opinion occur when health professionals disagree about their values and beliefs towards client or patient care, incidents or situations. These occur when professionals can agree that something should occur but their reasoning is different to each other. For example, they might agree that bed numbers need to be decreased, but their values and beliefs as to why the bed numbers need to be reduced are different from each other.

This is the type of moral problem seen most frequently and is the cause of endless debates and arguments in hospitals and other health organisations. Another example of this is the allocation of resources and about which department or unit gets what and how much of the budget needs to be spent on Y and how much on X.

Problems caused by oppositional views

These are moral differences between health professionals when they cannot agree about what should be done in a given situation or only partially agree. Again, the professionals' values and beliefs are different. For example, a professional might believe that terminations of pregnancy should not occur. These people are allowed to conscientiously object to being involved in the treatment and care of women seeking a termination. However, if the situation should have implications in other areas (such as a resource issue), then the professional who would not primarily be involved in the care, now needs to be. Hence the oppositional views.

When moral problems are dilemmas

As previously stated, these are more than a moral problem as, when examined, there are two possible ways or options of resolving the situation; however, neither of these appear to be correct. They can also occur when there is incompatibility between ethical principles, competing moral duties or conflicting interests (Johnstone, 1996).

Resolving ethical and moral problems and/or dilemmas

Unfortunately, many health professionals try and resolve problems by gut response and make a quick decision or rely on organisational policy which is usually not effective. Prevention is always best, and so problems that could arise through knowledge deficit, authority, groupie behaviour and insensitivity can be prevented to a certain extent by rigorous ethical education. However, when a moral problem or dilemma does occur this needs to be resolved by undertaking a systematic approach involving:

- assessment of the situation;
- identification of the problem;
- planning - thinking of ways to resolve the situation (including options) and deciding which way would be the most ethical;
- implementation;
- evaluation.

In trying to discern which action is the most ethical, health professionals need to consider the resources available, alternative options that could be used and, using ethical principles or philosophies, discern which action is the correct one to undertake (Hawley, 1997d). These ethical principles and philosophies are discussed in Chapters 5 and 6. However, before you gain that knowledge and understanding it is important to examine the subject of human rights and clients' or patients' rights. This is because underpinning all ethical behaviour in health care are those we care for, the clients or patients.

Summary

Ethics is concerned with questions of right and wrong, of duty and obligation, and of moral responsibility. When ethicists and philosophers use words such as good or right to describe a person or patient, they usually mean that the person or action conforms to some moral standard and that the good person or the right action has desirable qualities.

However, ethics in health care is more than identifying what is right and wrong as, to do this, the professional needs to reflect critically on the situations and/or problem. Hence ethics is a critical reflective activity that requires us to be concerned with the systematic examination of issues, problems or dilemmas. That is, this reflection needs to guide what we ought to do in a specific situation by asking us to consider and reconsider ordinary actions, the rationales or reasons for those actions, and the judgements made (Beauchamp and Childress, 1983, p. xii).

In addition, we have defined ethical issues as those phenomena or behaviours that have the potential to become a problem, along with those situations which are vitally important in the life of the patient. Ethical or moral problems occur through knowledge deficit, authority, groupie behaviour, insensitivity, amorality and differences in opinion. There are also types of moral problems such as moral or ethical dilemmas, the latter being a type of moral problem that, when examined, has two possible courses of action, neither of which appears to be correct. Such problems require the use of ethical principles or theory to resolve them and to ascertain which is the most ethical option to use.

Professional development

1 Continue to develop your Ethics Portfolio. Remember to start a new section for this chapter.

2 Read Case study 3.1 and write your answers to the questions at the end, in your Ethics Portfolio, so that you can refer to these at a later date if needed. Do not use reflection in writing the answers, as this is not what is being asked for.

Case study 3.1
First year nursing student Mary Jones and her mentor

Mary Jones had just started her first clinical placement in a large acute hospital. She had been assigned to an acute medical ward which was very busy with admissions of seriously ill patients. She found her mentor/preceptor/supervisor to be abrupt and rude to her at times, but dismissed this as part of the culture and thought perhaps it was because the ward was so busy, and she herself was probably not much help to the mentor or supervisor.

One morning the mentor/preceptor/supervisor went to see her assigned patients. Mary was a little way behind her and, as she entered a room with four patients, she saw the mentor talking very angrily to a patient, and then she poked the woman in the chest, saying 'you bloody foreigners, you come into my country, and expect everything to be done for you. Well, don't expect anything from me, as I have had the bloody lot of you,' and hit the woman on the upper arm and left the room.

Mary followed the mentor out into the corridor and asked her 'I don't understand what happened; what was that all about?' to which the mentor replied 'It is not your bloody business, and I am not going to be looking after that lot in there, nor have you hanging around me all day. I have had enough! I am going home, I will go and tell the charge nurse I am sick, and they can get some other poor sod to come and look after this lot.'

With that the mentor went to the charge nurse and stated that she was sick and going home and without giving the charge nurse time to reply, walked out the door of the ward.

The charge nurse quickly arranged for additional help and reallocated the patients to whom the mentor had been assigned.

Mary Jones was shocked about the whole situation; the ward was busy and she didn't want to be seen as making a fuss, so at morning tea she left the ward and phoned her tutor at the university.

The tutor was gravely concerned about the situation and went to see Mary on clinical practice. After speaking to Mary he visited the patient who explained what the mentor had said and done to her. The tutor then sought out the charge nurse and stated what had occurred.

Questions

➤ Is this an ethical problem?

➤ Use the model to discern if it is or not.

3 Read the following case study and answer the questions at the end. To do this, you need first to understand the situation. Consequently, you will need to read about brainstem cerebrovascular accidents (CVA) in a textbook. Then read the case study and answer the questions.

Case study 3.2
Mrs Xhung Hu

Mrs Xhung Hu is a 90-year-old lady admitted to a general medical ward following a brainstem CVA. She was given a high standard of nursing care but received no active treatment. The hospital staff have explained to the relatives that the prognosis is poor and wish to know what Mrs Xhung Hu's wishes might be in relation to her care.

Questions

➤ From what culture do you think Mrs Xhung comes?

➤ What do you think her values and beliefs might be in relation to her care?

➤ Try and identify the ethical issues and the problem.

Critical reflection

Write a critical reflection for this chapter to place in your Ethics Portfolio. The item or issue that you may want to work through or critically analyse could be something from the following.

● One of the case studies.

● Reading that you have done.

- A different point of view that someone raised in discussion in class.
- Something arising from the types of moral problems that you want to reflect critically.
- A general feeling of disquiet about how you will cope with ethical or moral problems which you want to explore through reflection.
- Clinical practice:
  - such as your values and beliefs in relation to caring for clients or patients who are different from some members of the team;
  - how you have realised that the care you have provided for a patient on clinical practice was incorrect and consequently unethical.

Johns' (2000) model (p. 47) for structured reflection (MSR) is provided to guide you:

Looking in

- Find a space to focus.
- Pay attention to your thoughts and emotions.
- Write down those thoughts and emotions that seem significant.

Looking out

- A description of the situation.
- What issues are significant.
- Aesthetics, that is:
  - What was I trying to achieve? In this case, it will be what I am trying to achieve.
  - What were the consequences to patient/others/myself? In your case, what are the consequences for the patient/others/myself?
  - How were others feeling? In your case this will be, how will others feel about this?
  - How do I know this?
- Personal:
  - Why did I feel the way I did with this situation? For your exercise, this will be, why do I feel this way?
- Ethics:
  - Did I act for the best? Or will this be for the best?
- What factors (either embodied within me or embedded within the environment) are, or were, influencing me?
- Empirics:
  - What knowledge did, or could have, informed me?
- Reflexivity:
  - Does this situation connect with previous experiences?
  - How could I handle this situation better?

○ What would be the consequences of alternative actions for the patient/others/myself?

○ How do I now feel about this experience?

○ Can I support myself and others better as a consequence?

○ How therapeutically available am I to work with patients/families and staff to help them meet their needs?

4

Clients' and patients' rights and protecting the vulnerable

Phil Maude and Georgina Hawley

Why this chapter is important to me

✔ Health professionals care for others.

✔ All of us are vulnerable at some period of our life.

✔ Some people are, however, vulnerable all their life.

✔ What ethical responsibilities do we have as health professionals?

✔ How should health professionals respect client and patient rights, dignity and integrity?

All people are vulnerable at some time in their life! This time usually occurs when a person is dependent on others, such as at the beginning and end of their life. Other times at which this vulnerability and dependency can occur is when a person is seriously unwell or ill. In such circumstances, we can say that vulnerability can be a phase in a person's life. It is at these times that we, as professionals, need to plan and implement care so that the client's or patient's health needs are met. However, we need to be mindful that, for specific groups within our communities or societies, vulnerability is not a phase in life, but does in fact extend throughout their life. These people have a severe or gross physical, mental, cognitive or emotional impairment.

Irrespective of whether dependency is a phase or a permanent state, people who are vulnerable require care from health professionals. It is because of the very nature of their vulnerability that others can take advantage of them. People in the community, the health care system and individual professionals can do this! It is not surprising then that this group of clients or patients suffer the result of nearly all the ethical or moral problems that occur in health care.

In previous chapters, it became apparent that your values and beliefs are manifested in your actions and attitudes to others, including when providing client or patient care. You have also gained knowledge about how you can change your values and beliefs to adopt those of your profession so that you meet the required standards or outcomes as described in the codes of practice or ethics. As discussed in Chapter 3, even knowing what is regarded as the correct ethical behaviour does not stop ethical or moral problems from occurring.

With this background knowledge and understanding it is time to learn about clients' or patients' rights and how to protect those in need. First is an activity in which the myriad of situations when clients or patients need protection can be identified. Second, you will consider what your values and beliefs are in relation to clients' and patients' rights and what you think these need to be. Third, the types of right that clients or patients have and are entitled to are discussed, followed by the ethical or moral problems of vulnerable people.

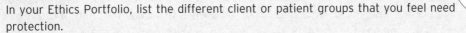

Activity

In your Ethics Portfolio, list the different client or patient groups that you feel need protection.

If you are having difficulty thinking about who these may be, cast your mind back to the ethical tragedies mentioned in previous chapters. What were the different patient groups?

- The Tuskegee syphilis experiment involved racially oppressed, poorly educated men of low economic status, who believed what the nurse Eunice Rivers and the public health doctors told them. They were vulnerable to believing that they would receive free medical treatment and, when they were dying, were offered a free funeral as long as they died in hospital (this was so that an autopsy could be performed for the research).
- Both the Bristol Royal Infirmary Inquiry and the Royal Liverpool Children's Inquiry involved sick or ill paediatric patients and their parents.
- The National Women's Cancer Inquiry involved women who did not know that they had been included in a research programme without their consent. It also included anaesthetised women who had not consented to having medical procedures performed on them without their knowledge.
- The Chelmsford Hospital Inquiry involved mentally ill patients who had not consented or who were coerced into consenting.

In each case, the clients or patients were either women or children, socioeconomically indigent or mentally ill. Other groups that are also vulnerable are the homeless, prisoners, refugees, illegal immigrants and older people.

Health professionals provide care and treatment to clients or patients in a myriad of settings, including primary, secondary and tertiary care, so it is not always possible to think of all who have the potential to be vulnerable. However, if you gain knowledge and understanding of clients' or patients' rights then your awareness of those who are vulnerable or have the potential to be vulnerable will be heightened.

Clients' or patients' rights

These rights come from a variety of sources, namely human, legal and ethical. First, there are the human rights that are contained within the United Nations Declarations (Protection of Human Rights) and those of the World Health Organization (for example, availability of primary care worldwide). For those living in Europe there is also the Council of Europe (which is based on the United Nations declaration). Then there are the legal rights provided by the government of the country in which you live. Finally, there are ethical or moral rights.

Human rights

The United Nations Declaration of Human Rights has had a profound influence in gaining obligatory rights for people worldwide. It has also strongly influenced health care for vulnerable groups in our societies. For example, these human rights underpin the American Constitution, and it was this document that enabled women to access a legal termination of pregnancy for health reasons other than when their life was in danger. That is, the legal case of Roe and Wade in the USA were based on women's rights within the constitution to appeal to the courts and have the grounds of abortion broadened to include the concept of serious ill health (Bandman and Bandman, 1990). Before this, women could only have a termination of pregnancy if they were definitely going to die because of the pregnancy. With the legal cases being successful, the Abortion Act was changed in various US states and other countries, including Canada, Australia, New Zealand, the UK and some European countries, followed suit shortly thereafter. It needs to be remembered that a termination of pregnancy is still not legal in some countries of the world, and the grounds vary from one country to another.

Legal rights

In Chapter 3 you learnt that ethics is not law and this is correct. However, a country's legal system provides the basis of clients' or patients' rights in relation to health care. This means that the legal rights of clients or patients are embedded within the legal system of each country. In the UK, Australia, New Zealand, Hong Kong, USA and Canada these include: access to health care and medical assistance; the receipt of reasonable care; power to consent to or refuse treatment; access to health care records; confidentiality; and the protection of identity and information through a Data Protection Act.

In the UK, Hong Kong, Australia and New Zealand, The Statutory Acts of Medicine and the Law of Tort of Negligence (in particular, duty of care) provide the legal rights for access to health care and medical assistance (Hawley, 1997d). As to the standard of reasonable care, this is also covered by the Law of Tort of Negligence, where the bench mark (or standard) is described as what any other reasonable person would do in the circumstances; that is, whatever another doctor, nurse or other health professional would do in the same situation, given the same circumstances. (However, there is more to this topic than that mentioned here, and so consultation of appropriate law texts is required to gain the additional knowledge and understanding.)

The right to consent to or to refuse treatment is also covered by the civil Law of Consent and Assault. If consent is not obtained, the nurse or health professional has trespassed on that patient (Hawley, 1997d). In some countries, various Medical Treatment Acts are in place which protect the health professional if the patient desires to refuse treatment. There are times when it is necessary to treat a patient without their permission to do so; such incidences are emergencies and situations covered by the legal Acts of Mental Health and Infectious Diseases. Other countries may have additional legal Acts. However, although different countries may have similar Acts, the words and conditions may vary. For example, the

Mental Health Act in England is different to that in Western Australia. To become familiar with such information (which is outside the scope of this book) refer to an up-to-date law text for health professionals. The right to confidentiality is covered in civil law, as are staff employment contracts (Hawley, 1997d).

The legal right of Data Protection means that some information cannot be disclosed to others. This is closely associated with the Law of Confidentiality, and extends the protection of the identity of the patient and information pertaining to them even further. Depending in which country you are practising could mean the difference between patients' names being displayed on a notice board in a hospital or not.

Development of bills or charters of patients' rights

Since the mid 1970s most governments in developed countries have instructed their Departments of Health to develop and implement a standard of health care, embedded within the ethos and name of 'Patients' rights'. Some of these are termed 'Patients' charter', and others 'Patients' bill of rights'. Irrespective of the name, the concept is to inform clients or patients of the standard of care that they can expect and/or request. These rights are derived from the Declaration of Human Rights and the laws of that country.

The idea of these clients' or patients' rights, bills or charters is to ensure that the standard of care is made explicit and so that clients or patients know what to expect. They are also a reminder to staff of what to provide so that the provision of health care is more effective, and so that the client or patient gains greater satisfaction from the care and treatment.

Although these charters of patients' rights differ slightly from one country to another, there are similarities in the basic concepts. These rights are listed as follows.

1   Right to access health care.
2   Right to make an informed choice and consent to treatment.
3   Right to refuse treatment.
4   Right to reasonable care.
5   Access to information regarding treatment and of patient's own health.
6   Privacy and confidentiality.
7   The right to know the hospital rules and regulations, guidelines, policies, etc. (Hawley, 1997d).

Even though we have said that these are common rights, the extent to which these rights are practised differs from country to country. For example, some countries and health care systems allow clients or patients full access to their own health care records, whereas other countries and systems may not. In the USA, the Patients' Charter states that a patient has a right to know the cost of the treatment and/or hospitalisation irrespective of whether it is being paid personally or sent to an insurer or government department for payment.

Allocation of resources

A major factor that impinges on whether or not clients or patients have access to the types of care they might want or need is the allocation of resources (Hawley, 1997e). In each country in the world, the government will have made an economic decision as to how much of the gross economic or national product (GNP) the country earns will be spent on health care.

You will find that no country spends more than 13% of their GNP on health care. The UK and Western European countries spend 8–9%, with the USA spending 13% (van Delven *et al.*, 2004; van Gelder, 2005). Consequently, access to health care is limited, taking into consideration the many areas that the capital needs to be divided into: primary, secondary and tertiary care, mental health, research, and the education of future health care professionals.

Activity

In your Ethics Portfolio, list all the ethical or moral rights you would like as a client or patient. That is, what would you like!

Pause and think

Here is an example of a Patients' Charter. Read it through and think about the contents.

1 The right to considerate and respectful care.

2 The patient has the right to obtain current information concerning diagnosis, treatment and prognosis in language and terms s/he can understand.

3 The right to receive all information in order to make an informed consent, except in emergencies when the patient is unconscious, or if critically ill, only the crucially important facts are told to the patient.

4 The patient has the right to refuse any treatment (as permitted by law), after s/he has been informed of the medical consequences of that action.

5 The right to culturally sensitive care.

6 The right to privacy during all care, including examination, treatment, case discussion, diagnostic tests and procedures. Furthermore, confidentiality of all information and record-keeping arising from the above.

7 The right to know of the relationship between the hospital and universities, and of the presence of students. The patient has a right to limit the students' observation of their care and treatment, and also the right to refuse treatment and care provided by the student/s. They have a right to request a trained or registered health professional to undertake that care and treatment.

8 The right of the patient to be informed of other types of care and treatments suitable for his/her diagnosis but not available at the present hospital.

9 The right to continuity of care between department, wards and units within the hospital, but also if the patient wishes to be transferred to another facility.

10 The right to information in relation to health promotion resources related to his/her diagnosis.

11 The right to printed information of care notes (including knowledge of possible complications), and when and where to return to the hospital if further treatment is indicated (this to also include outpatient appointments, etc.).

Rights for clients or patients

Ethical or moral rights are complementary to the human and legal rights afforded by the law. That is, health professionals need to go further than the human and legal rights to ensure that ethical rights are met. Such types of behaviour are sometimes implied in codes and professional standards as required by different professional bodies, and also in the vari-ous bills or charters of patients' rights. However, we believe that there is something more that needs to be added.

Consequently, we begin with the philosophical understanding of a right and then, moving forward, we can gain greater understanding of what may be needed.

A right implies that a person has a liberty to do something if they wish (Hawley, 1997d). The English philosopher Thomas Hobbes (1588-1679) proposed this notion. He proposed that if someone has 'a right' they have the right and liberty to do whatever it is, but also the person does not have to do it if they so desire. An example of the liberty right is that I can go to my family doctor for immunisations and vaccinations, or I can go to the Government Department of Health Immunisation Clinic (Hawley, 1997d).

Another philosopher, Carl Wellman, argued that a right had certain characteristics, which included the notion that it is something which is, or ought to be, respected by other indi-viduals and protected by society (Barry, 1982). This would include religion, attitudes to women, children and the elderly (Hawley, 1997d). These are behaviours which are primarily governed by our race and culture.

Activity

What would need to be added to a patients' charter or bill so that it becomes the ideal for clients' or patients' rights? List these in your Ethics Portfolio.

Perhaps you listed words such as caring, compassion and empathic care. However, are these rights that clients or patients should expect?

If you think *yes*, then how would we state these?

Perhaps, if we take them and turn the rights around so that they become the responsibil-ities of the health professional, then that standard of care could be provided. That is, caring, compassion, advocacy, accountability and collaboration as the ideal expectation of moral care. We also need to highlight that clients or patients are equal partners in the care that we provide; perhaps that could be included in collaborating. That is, we will collaborate with the client or patient to facilitate his/her care. This would be essential in order to be culturally sensitive and provide culturally competent care.

Ideal moral behaviours of health professionals

So what do we mean by advocacy, accountability, collaboration and caring (including compassion).

Caring
The moral concept of caring has had a long tradition in nursing (it is not restricted to nursing – it is just that it has been written about extensively in nursing). The concept of caring indicates a commitment to the protection of human dignity and the preservation of health. First, caring is a natural human sentiment and is the way all people relate to their world and to each other (Noddings, 1984). Second, caring is entwined or inextricably linked with to the social need for/of love, and so there is the need by the health professional to show compassion and kindness. According to Bishop and Scudder (2001), ethical caring includes valuing caring for a client or patient so that there is a shift from just wanting to be caring to actively fostering the wellbeing of others. This means that, for a health professional to be caring in the moral sense, their actions need to demonstrate or manifest the caring behaviours of respecting dignity, compassion and kindness.

Advocacy
Advocacy can be defined as the active support of a client or patient or a cause. When health professionals adopt this role as part of their ethical behaviour it can greatly influence the standard and quality of care. This is because the advocacy role involves assisting in the self-determination of clients or patients.

The two ethical moral concepts of fidelity (being honest and truthful) and respect for human dignity are rooted in the role of advocacy. Respecting the human dignity of clients or patients also extends to privacy and choice. This means that the health professional taking on the role of advocate assists in the truthful self-determination of a client or patient. They ensure that other professionals and the information provided is accurate and honest, and that the client's or patient's integrity and their dignity (and privacy) is respected so that they can make their own choices.

Accountability
The health professional who is morally accountable is not only responsible for their own behaviour but also answerable to the client or patient. This means that when the professional does something wrong, they need to apologise to the client or patient and explain their actions. They also need to do so to their employer. Although hospital insurers do not like health professionals apologising to clients or patients, there is growing evidence that, when the client or patient knows the reason and how a mistake occurred, they are less likely to take legal action against the organisation and professional.

Collaboration

Collaboration is twofold. The first is the collaboration with the client or patient as equal partners to facilitate and negotiate the delivery of their care. The second part of collaboration is the participation with other professionals to achieve the best possible outcome for the client or patient. It is going beyond multiprofessional care to achieve the gold standard of interprofessional practice (or provision of care). It certainly does not mean participating in moral problems caused by groupie behaviour or authority (as described in Chapter 3).

These moral behaviours of caring (including protection of human dignity and the preservation of health, and demonstrating to fellow human beings compassion and kindness); advocacy (ensuring that the client's or patient's integrity, and their dignity, privacy and choice is respected); accountability (to client or patient, their employer, the legal system and also their professional body or council); and collaboration in interprofessional provision of care will improve the standard and quality of client or patient care.

Vulnerable clients or patients

Having listed the basic health care rights for all clients or patients, and also the ideal moral behaviour of health professionals, it is possible to identify those whom we could class as 'vulnerable' and to whom we need to provide extra attention and care.

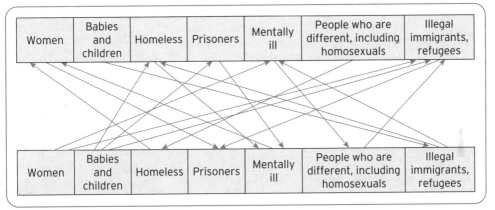

Figure 4.1
Vulnerable clients or patients

Health professionals can come across many different patient and client groups in their clinical practice, and it is difficult to identify who requires special care for vulnerability. The authors of this chapter have decided that, for the purpose of this book, the groups will be:

1 Women, babies and children.

2 The homeless.

3 The person with a learning disability or who is mentally ill or suffering from psychiatric disturbance.

4 Both men and woman held on remand or serving a prison sentence.

5 People who are different, such as new arrivals in the country, such as illegal immigrants and refugees. Other people may be different because of sexual orientation and this can make them vulnerable.

6 The older person.

Is that all? You might ask. In reality these groups are rarely discrete entities, rather they can be combinations of these same entities. Consider Figure 4.1 (p. 61) to realise how many different possibilities there may be. For example, the older or mentally ill person may also be homeless. Likewise, a woman prisoner may need to give birth, or it could be an illegal immigrant in the detention centre who gives birth and then becomes mentally ill. There are many combinations.

Each of these patient groups will be discussed separately.

Babies, children and women

The United Nations Declaration of Human Rights states that babies, children and women have the same rights as everyone else. However, because of their vulnerability and in different cultures these rights are often abused. In the legal sense a baby does not have legal rights until s/he is born. However, we quite often want to provide ethical rights to those who are unborn. The difficulty with attributing rights to the unborn raises the question of when should these begin?

People have different ideas as to when human life begins, and when these rights commence. That is, when does the embryo or fetus become a human being, and have claim to these rights?

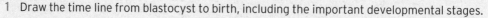

Activity

In your Ethics Portfolio:

1 Draw the time line from blastocyst to birth, including the important developmental stages.

2 Now, state on that time line when you think:

   a. Human life has begun.

   b. When the embryo or fetus is a human being.

   c. When you think the embryo or fetus is a person.

The activity that you have just attempted is the same problem that everyone seems to have. That is, what is a human being? In addition, when can this status be conferred on an embryo or fetus? When does a human being become a person?

It is the basis of the answers to these questions that underpin people's values and beliefs of termination of pregnancy and/or abortion. That is, if a person believes that human life begins at fertilisation and before the blastocyst becomes attached to the uterine wall, then they will oppose all terminations of pregnancy (including the morning-after pill).

However, if a person believes that a human being exists once implantation has occurred then they might say that abortion should not occur from then onwards. On the other hand, another person may believe that the embryo is not a human being until it is fully formed or a fetus, or until a mother feels the baby moving *in utero*.

We are not going to discuss the issue of termination of pregnancy fully, as it is so complex. Instead, we have given an overview of the complexity of the issue. To understand the basis of the moral argument, read additional literature to extend your knowledge and understanding.

Pause and think

It is difficult to imagine abuse of an unborn child but Hulsey (2005) suggests that every 1.5 minutes an infant is born to a mother who has been using substances during pregnancy.

This leads us to consider the question: if society agrees that unborn children need to be protected from harmful substances, should we be testing pregnant women? If we were to find positive testing in a pregnant woman, then ethically, legally and morally what would society be able to do about this? Many of you will be on the side of the fetus and several will take the side of the mother. We need to find common ground in this argument and consider harm minimisation strategies. In reality, a country's legal system is not always best placed to impose sanctions when it comes to the rights of the unborn child.

Rights of children

The ethical problems that occur in relation to health in children arise from the fact that it is frequently forgotten or ignored that children are afforded the same rights as adults. This is especially so in relation to consent for treatment, pain relief and participation in research. This means that children are sometimes overlooked, and all communication conducted through the parents.

In reality, children have their own views and these can be taken into consideration when planning care and treatment. It is too easy to say that a child would not understand. However, when communication is geared at the developmental level of the child they can understand. Consequently, it is important for the health professional to treat the family as a unit, not just respecting the parents' wishes in consenting issues.

This consent to treatment is different for adolescents. The law states quite clearly that, if a teenager has shown evidence of being able to understand what a specific care and treatment will involve and that if the parent/s were informed, the relationship between the health professional and teenager would be destroyed or damaged, then the parents do not need to be involved. Consequently, care and treatments arising from sexuality, alcoholism and drug dependency do not need the consent of the parent.

We are perhaps stating the obvious here; that is, babies and children feel pain just as much as adults but, because they are unable to articulate their needs to receive pain relief, this right is often ignored.

Rights of women

In previous chapters, there has been discussion of tragedies that have involved women and earlier in this chapter it was mentioned that the Declaration of Human Rights has been instrumental in changing women's rights. The whole issue of women's rights stems from the cultural perception that women are inferior to men and that men can make decisions on behalf of women. For many years, physiological and psychological testing has proved the former concept to be incorrect, and the latest developments in neuroscience have supported this and verified the different ways in which men and women think and act.

In some cultures, the notion of superiority of the male over the female (including children) still exists and, for the health professional, interacting with such a family needs sensitive handling and care. However, the law is quite clear that the abuse of women and children is not to be tolerated and that health professionals have a mandatory obligation to protect and report these activities.

The latest UN report on child abuse (WHO 2006) has uncovered that, while children have rights, these have failed to guarantee protection. While the worst-case scenarios exist in developing countries, no country is guiltless. The report states that violence can be perpetuated by governments, criminals and family. Some of the violence is perpetuated under the guise of health care treatment. 'In some cases children as young as nine are subjected to receiving electric shock treatment without an anaesthetic, sedation or muscle relaxants.'

The homeless

In every large city or urban area across the world, you will find the homeless. They are an extremely vulnerable population with diverse needs. Many people who are homeless lack the social skills to obtain accommodation. A high proportion of the homeless have associated mental health or psychiatric problems. Some have drug-related problems or are escaping abusive relationships, while others are illegal immigrants. Consequently, as a health care professional you cannot say that, because a person is homeless, they will have 'health problem X', as the variety of people is so diverse.

You may find people sleeping by day; this is so they are alert at night when it is not safe to sleep on the street. Irrespective of whether they are in a large city or small town there is a great deal of violence perpetrated towards the homeless.

In the UK and Australia models of case management and assertive outreach have been implemented to meet the health care needs of these people. There is debate as how best to meet the needs of the homeless, and these pertain to the ideas of over- and under-servicing. Some models of care have been very effective and others have not, and this does not appear to be dependent on the amount of financial resources invested for health care of this nature.

In Australia, psychiatric nurses visit the homeless 'in their patch' on the streets (that is, where they are likely to be found), instead of waiting for the client or patient to go to the clinic to see them. In this way, they keep in touch, provide medication and monitor the patient's condition. In Bristol, UK is another successful outreach programme, which finds accommodation for those who lack the social skills to do so themselves.

When health professionals provide such care, ethical problems can readily arise. These occur because of the relationship between the health care professional and the homeless person. This is because of what is known as 'dual responsibility'; that is, the health professional has a responsibility to the client or patient, but also to their employer. These ethical problems are similar to those mentioned in Chapter 3 under conflicting opinions, but more pronounced. This is because the human rights of the client or patient are sometimes ignored by the organisation. The areas where this is most likely to occur are prisons, the military and the mentally ill.

Learning disablity and mental illness

A person who has a learning disability has a permanently reduced or impaired cognitive ability. This is different to the person who is mentally ill and may have a chronic illness, as they do not usually suffer from a permanent state of reduced or impaired cognitive ability.

However, owing to the long-term nature of chronic mental illness this type of patient may have impaired cognitive ability. Consequently, people with learning disabilities and also those with long-term chronic mental illness are grouped together as both groups need extra protection and care. This is because the law may not recognise them as legally competent and therefore not able to give consent to treatment.

For the client or patient with a learning disability this is of special significance. Chapter 12 discusses mental and psychiatric illnesses.

Prisoners

We tend to forget that once a person goes to prison they still have health care needs. They may go to prison with existing health care problems or develop problems because of the new and restrictive environment. Providing care to clients who are restrained with shackles on their wrists or ankles can prove challenging in any health care setting.

Providing patients who are incarcerated with treatment and care is especially challenging. For health professionals providing this care to a prisoner the challenges can be ethically unique as we are faced with the contradiction between causing harm (the purpose of imprisonment) and acting for patients' good (the purpose of health care). The answer to this problem lies in a professional's duty of care and the responsibility to care for a patient no matter what the presentation is and remain therapeutic.

Many of us need to consider carefully whether we are able to attend to a person who presents with a confronting history and provide them with equity as well as promote their rights and responsibilities.

People who are different

Historically, societies worldwide are not tolerant of those who are different from the majority. That is, when someone is different, the difference (be it sexual orientation, physical appearance or race) becomes the means to belittle or abuse the other person. In health care, those who are different include clients and patients with physical deformities or impairments, those who are homosexual, and new arrivals in a country, especially refugees.

New arrivals

The health provision for immigrants and refugees differs from country to country, but an important ethical consideration is the access to appropriate health care. In relation to refugees the rules and regulations for the acceptance and removal of refugees varies from country to country and is outside the remit of this ethics book.

Refugees

Health professionals providing care for refugees may want to consider the concept of appropriate health care. For example, the socioeconomic refugee might only need temporary health care for a couple of years while their home country is experiencing economic devastation. This person may be in good health and may only need screening for disease, immunisation and vaccination.

Another refugee may have suffered extreme torture before escaping from their home country. For this person, mental and emotional care will need to be provided and perhaps medical and surgical care for injuries. It should also be remembered that people that have been raped before escaping to a new country will not be able to unburden themselves by telling the full details of their story immediately upon arrival in a new country. This can affect their refugee status and cause unresolved health care problems (sexual and reproductive).

Through the United Nations, each of the developed countries of the world states how many refugees they will accept each year. The amount of refugees each country accepts varies. Some countries, e.g. Australia, will give priority to refugees from certain countries close by (as the government believes that they have a moral obligation to provide refuge to countries close to Australia).

Illegal immigrants

These people arrive unannounced into a country, usually by illegal means. When found, they are assessed and some may be granted refugee status, while others are deported out of the country. However, it can take some months for their case to be assessed and actioned. Consequently, some people may spend months or years in an immigration assessment or detention centre.

During their stay, they will have the health problems that any normal person experiences. In addition, they may be suffering from illnesses that are caused by the conditions of their mode of transportation, and places they have stayed *en route*. Typical illnesses and conditions that arise are caused by unclean overcrowded environments (e.g. scabies, tinea, tuberculosis, hepatitis A, B or C, Hanson's disease, HIV/AIDS, sexually transmitted diseases, Dengue fever and malaria. Diseases may be more unusual in some, including elephantiasis, yaws (Frambesia), or having, or being carriers of, typhus fever, typhoid and cholera.

Whatever the condition or disease, treatment needs to be given not only to the person suffering but, if the disease or condition is communicable, the rest of the population needs protection. Therefore, the health provision here needs to be health screening and treatment of any illnesses.

Legal immigrants

These are people whom the government of the country knows are arriving on a specific plane, train or ship. That is, they have asked to be accepted by that country to live and/or work there, and have been given permission in the form of letter or visa to do so. Some countries have different categories of immigrants, such as skilled workers, assisted or sponsored migrants, family reunion, business and investment, etc.

These immigrants are not detained in their new country for assessment status, and usually do not have health problems on arrival. For example, a person (or their dependant) applying for immigration from the UK to Australia may be refused if their health problem is considered too costly for the Department of Health to treat and provide ongoing care. Others with a health problem may be allowed entry if they meet the cost of their own health care.

Health assessment for new arrivals

With a broad range of populations with differing health care needs and unknown health beliefs, Kemp (2006) has published a brief assessment tool which health professionals can use to discover the health beliefs and provide culturally sensitive care. The questions are:

➤ What do you think caused your problem?

➤ Do you know why it started when it did?

➤ What does your sickness do to you? How does this work?

➤ How strong is your sickness? How long do you think it will last?

➤ What problems has your sickness caused?

➤ What do you fear about your sickness?

➤ What kind/type of treatment/medicine do you think you should have?

➤ What good things will happen if you receive this treatment/medicine?

Perhaps these questions do not need to be limited to new arrivals, but could also be used whenever we need to assess someone's health beliefs?

Sexual orientation

Culture and family norms, in combination with other factors and priorities within a culture, determine the expression of sexuality. There are a myriad of influences on the development of a person's sexual orientation, including social class, ethnicity, religion, and when and how sexual behaviour begins. Although homosexuality exists in both men and women, it is mostly men that have been discriminated against by health professionals. This means that their health care needs are sometimes regarded as unimportant and not given priority in health care programmes. Until recent times, male homosexuality was considered to be a psychiatric disorder and treatment was prescribed to change sexual orientation to heterosexual.

If health professionals show or voice prejudice against homosexuals, it will cause these clients or patients to hide their sexual orientation and consequently not seek treatment for health problems. It should also be remembered that, in some cultures and countries, homosexuality is illegal. Therefore, if people arrive in countries such as the UK or Australia where homosexual behaviour is legally permitted, they may be fearful of seeking health care treatment for symptoms arising from sexual activities.

The older person

As people age they are more likely to have health care problems because of the aging process, which affects all bodily systems. For example, bones become weakened and therefore the older person is more likely to suffer from various fractures, some of which may lead to death.

Pause and think

➤ What other bodily changes occur in the older person?

Memory impairment can occur so that the person is no longer competent to give consent to treatment. With dementia and Alzheimer's disease behavioural problems can occur which can make caring for these patients difficult at times.

The ethical or moral problems that occur with providing health services for older people arise because of the debilitating health problems that the older person can experience, and physical and/or mental frailty. Work practices that prioritise tasks and doing for the person rather than engaging with and encouraging self-care no doubt raise ethical issues. Housing for the older person can vary immensely; some choose to stay in their own home, others want more security and so move into a retirement complex, and yet others become dependent and need constant care and attention. Many places call the person at this stage of their life a 'resident'. This title is used to infer that the person who resides in that environment for help and assistance is not a patient or client but a resident with rights.

In Australia, The Commonwealth Department of Health and Aging has provided a charter of residents' rights and responsibilities:

Each resident of a residential care service has the right:

- To quality care which is appropriate to his or her needs;
- To full information about his or her own state of health and about available treatments;
- To live in a safe, secure and homelike environment and to move freely both within and outside the residential care service without undue restriction;
- To freedom of speech;
- To maintain control over and to continue making decisions about the personal aspects of his or her daily life, financial affairs and possessions;
- To be consulted and to choose to have input into decisions about the living arrangements of the residential care service.

Activity

Find the charter or bill of rights for older people in residential care in your country, and compare it with the one from Australia.

➤ Is there a charter?

➤ If not, is there something else?

➤ If not, why do you think this is?

➤ If you do have a charter, which one (that of Australia or your country) is better in its overall ethical or moral breadth?

Imagine you are an older person in need of health care:

➤ How would you like to be cared for?

➤ Would you want the above charter, more or less?

Johnstone (2004) suggests that working with older adults requires us to consider ethical principles and value respect for others, promote dignity through autonomy and advocacy, and provide quality care that any other person would expect.

Pause and think

➤ Do you see those behaviours in residential care?

Common ethical or moral problems

It was stated earlier that, while vulnerable groups would be discussed separately, there was also commonality as some groups were combinations or mixes of two or more factors. For example, the refugee who is mentally ill, the illegal immigrant or older person who is homeless, and the woman who is pregnant and in prison. These are all complex scenarios which need the health professional to display sensitivity, tact, consideration of the client's or patient's humanity and empathic care.

Just as the scenarios are complex, so too can be the ethical or moral problems. However, there are common elements in all of these, which include:

● The individual client or patient and their feelings as a fellow human being who is suffering.

● The accountability of the health professional to provide a legal and ethical standard of care, irrespective of their own values and beliefs.

● The potential for abuse to which vulnerable clients or patients are susceptible, not only from people within the community in which they live, but also by those who have been employed or paid to care for them.

In providing care for vulnerable clients or patients, there are two ethical concepts that are readily used in these situations; these are autonomy and paternalism.

Autonomy

Autonomy means to self-rule, to be able to make decisions for oneself. That is, the client or patient is provided with all the information that they need to make their own decision (Hawley, 1997c). However, sometimes a vulnerable person may not be able to think clearly to make that decision. This can occur when the health professional uses specialised jargon that the client or patient cannot understand. At other times the professional and client or patient speak different languages, and the health professional needs to supply a recognised and licensed or authorised interpreter. Sometimes the client or patient may have pain and their judgement may be clouded and they may not be able to think properly.

Paternalism

The other concept is paternalism, and this is when the health professional makes a decision on behalf of the client or patient without asking their opinion (Hawley, 1997c). That is, they do what they feel is right for the client or patient in the particular circumstance. Consequently, if the vulnerable person is not able to make decisions or is not in a position to do so (e.g. too young or does not understand the language) and the professional makes those decisions without consulting the client or patient, there is huge potential not only for problems to arise but also mistreatment or substandard care. This can also happen when the client or patient is in pain or distress and does not understand fully what it is the health professional proposes.

Remember Willowcreek School and Chelmsford Hospital (see Chapter 1); these were clear examples of paternalistic actions by the health professionals. It is important to remember that these are not the only residential schools or mental health facilities (including hostels of people with learning disabilities) in which such situations have occurred; such cases will be found in every country in the world.

Rights and duties of professionals

Having outlined the rights of the people using health care systems, it is also worthwhile to consider briefly some of the rights and duties of the health professional. A right, as indicated earlier, is a claim that has weight or justification and results in the action of an individual or institution. This obligation to act is often referred to as a duty, and every individual in a society has a range of duties. Some are required by law, such as stopping when involved in a traffic accident, while others may result from religious affiliations or membership of a particular culture. Health professionals have rights and duties purely because of their role and which are a requirement of their professional membership (e.g. The Nursing and Midwifery Council or The Chartered Society of Physiotherapists).

Professional rights conflicting with patient rights

In the majority of situations, the rights of ill people and the duties of health professionals match to ensure an ethical service. However, there are situations in which rights and duties may conflict and result in the loss of choice. In Chapter 3, the nature of ethical problems and dilemmas was discussed, including when the possible solutions to a situation do not appear correct for all involved. Just as philosophers differ in their view points of what is right and wrong, so do health professionals and those for whom they care. As a result, it is essential that everyone involved with the care of people who are ill or experiencing loss is 'ethically sensitive'.

This does not require a detailed knowledge of every ethical theory, but a working knowledge of key principles and self-awareness of how your own values influence practice. The rights of health professionals in relation to caring and treating clients or patients includes the right to safety at work, the right to refuse to provide care or treatments on the grounds of conscientious objection or unsafe practice, and the right to support.

The right to safety at work

A particular issue for all health and social care staff is safety in their work environments. This includes not having violence directed at them, not being abused, being provided with the necessary skills and equipment so that they can do their job correctly, and not suffering personal injury. These are all provided under the Health and Safety and Employment Acts. However, sometimes the need of the patient and the professional may conflict.

Moving and handling patients is just one example of where the rights of professionals and the rights of the patient potentially conflict. In 1996, the UK Royal College of Nursing issued guidance that suggested that 'the manual lifting of patients is eliminated in all but exceptional or life-threatening situations' (Royal College of Nursing, 1996). This was used by a number of organisations to justify a 'no lifting' policy and resulted in a significant debate concerning the conflicting rights of health care staff not to be put at risk and the rights of patients to receive appropriate care. In 2003, a judgment was reached in the case of two women with profound physical and learning disabilities whose parents had been told that manual handling equipment must be used to reduce the risk to care staff (Mandelstam, 2003).

Reviewing a significant range of legislation, including the Health and Safety at Work Act (1974) and the Manual Handling Operations Regulations (1992), the judge made it clear that neither the rights of paid carers nor, in this case, of disabled people had precedence over the other. He concluded that these rights should be balanced and that simplistic policies that discriminate cannot be tolerated. Health care professionals must discuss the issues with those involved and use their expertise to arrive at fair decisions. In issues concerning patient moving and handling, the law is increasingly being used to adjudicate. The dilemma becomes somewhat more complex when it involves the moral standpoint of the parties involved.

The right to refuse to provide care

As previously stated 'autonomy' means that a person has the right to accept or refuse access to health care and treatment. Likewise, a health professional has the autonomy as a person to refuse to carry out specific duties if they can prove that they have a 'conscientious objection' to whatever that duty may be.

It is generally accepted that no-one should be asked to violate their ethical principles to carry out their professional role. As an example, midwives or nurses (in the UK, Australia, the USA, Canada, New Zealand and Hong Kong) with a moral objection to abortion have the right not to be involved in the practice. In many circumstances these events can be managed by relocating staff; however, with an increasing moral rights discourse throughout the world, the potential for direct conflict is growing.

Although the ethical principle of autonomy is the highest one and is paramount, the autonomy of one person cannot overrule that of another (Hawley, 1997b). That is, a patient cannot state and demand that they want a specific treatment when a health professional's autonomy would be overridden. Consider if physician-assisted suicide was legal and a client or patient requested this of a doctor. If that doctor felt that it contradicted their own morals, then the doctor could refuse to perform that treatment.

The right to support

As each employer has a duty of care, so the employee has a right to support. This is particularly the case in a situation where individuals are exposed to the daily stresses and strains of witnessing loss and suffering with commitment to improve the situation. The incidence of burnout among those working in health care settings is considerable (Maslach, 2000).

Burnout

A physical, cognitive and affective state can present with a range of symptoms, including depression, loss of energy and a sense of hopelessness. This stems from emotional exhaustion, a frequent consequence of sharing people's daily health traumas. Health care professionals have a right to work in a supportive environment. In some cases, this refers to the structures of the organisation but, in many situations, is more about the supportive attitudes of the colleagues and a commitment to be vigilant on behalf of others. Many health care organisations now provide their employees with access to counselling, cognitive therapy and massage.

Pause and think

Think about the rights you have just read.

➤ Are these rights sufficient for you?

➤ As a health professional, would you like more rights? If so, which ones?

Using an ethical grid to identify the rights of patient and professional

In Chapter 1, it was stated that quite often people thought something was an ethical problem when in reality they had not gathered sufficient facts about the situation. Once they had done so, the so-called ethical problem disappeared as it was discovered that it was really miscommunication, misleading or inaccurate information. In this chapter both clients' and

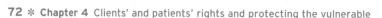

patients' rights and those of health professionals have been discussed; to identify the various aspects when examining an ethical situation, we suggest that you map out the facts.

To do this you can develop your own mind map or use one of the many available on the internet. However, you could also use the following ethical grid by Johns (2000, p. 187). You might also need to adapt the grid, adding additional rows or columns so that all the different perspectives can be mapped.

Client's or patient's perspective	Who has authority to act?	Other health professionals' perspective
Is there a conflict of values?	Situation	Ethical principles
Your perspective	Power relationship	Organisation's perspective

The advantage of mapping out the rights of those involved allows you to identify:

- what the client's or patient's perspective is;
- what the health care professional's perspective is;
- what the organisation's perspective is (usually found in policies and procedures, etc.); and
- identify who has the authority to decide what to do.

Once this is mapped out it is easy to see what the situation is and how it can be resolved.

Summary

In this chapter, we have explored clients' and patients' rights and those of vulnerable people. Patients' rights have been discussed in relation to several population groups that could be considered vulnerable. Ethical issues and problems that can occur have been considered. This is probably only the beginning of such discussion, as you will no doubt come across more complex presentations of vulnerable or potentially vulnerable people as you engage in clinical practice. Finally, the rights of health professionals were briefly discussed.

Professional development

1 In your Ethics Portfolio, write the answers to the following questions.

➤ In relation to your own profession, what rights are afforded to your clients or patients? Are these sufficient?

➤ How will you meet the moral or ethical ideals of caring, advocacy, accountability and collaboration?

➤ Remembering that your country has many different cultures, what types of rights do you think the differing people in catchment areas of your health care system(s) would like? In particular, consider their cultural beliefs.

➤ In your area of clinical practice, are the clients' and patients' cultural beliefs integrated into their health care? If not, ask the registered professional (e.g. physiotherapist, occupational therapist, social worker, nurse or doctor) with whom you are working whether there is a reason as to why a patient's health care beliefs and culture cannot be incorporated into the care?

2 Read the following case studies, and answer the questions at the end of each one. Write your responses in your Ethics Portfolio.

Case study 4.1
Lilly, Patrick and Maur (Hawley, 1997b and d)

Maur is a school health nurse in a secondary school. One afternoon two students, Lilly Xhu (aged 15) and Patrick Desraeli (aged 17), come to ask his advice about contraception. Maur discusses various options, gives them some brochures with the relevant information, and suggests they come back and see him when they have made a decision. Lilly and Patrick return the next week and Lilly says that they have decided to use oral contraceptives.

They discuss with Maur that they do not wish to go to their local family doctor in case the doctor tells Lilly's parents that she wants the Pill. They say to Maur that they want to go to Dr McNice in the next town who is young and new and who they feel will be sympathetic to their needs; Lilly then uses the phone in Maur's office to phone Dr McNice for an appointment. They also tell Maur that Patrick will borrow his mother's car to drive Lilly and him to the appointment.

One morning some 2 weeks later, Maur is called to his nursing supervisor's office in a nearby regional town. On arrival, Lilly's parents, who are very angry and demand the supervisor sack Maur for encouraging their daughter to engage in immoral activities, confront him. Maur wants to leave the office when the father further insults his personal integrity and safety by saying, 'I've had enough of you bloody poofters leading young kids astray! You should all be locked up! Kids aren't even safe in schools with you homos around.' With that, the father lunges to punch Maur in the face, but misses as Maur steps aside.

Questions
➤ What are the ethical issues?
➤ Who has rights and what are they?
➤ How do you think you could resolve the ethical problem?

Case study 4.2
Jethro and the emergency department team (Hawley, 1997b and d)

The football grand final of the Irish Football League had been widely advertised and billed as the best celebrations that Ulster would ever have, as both Ulster teams had reached the finals and were playing each other. Activities were held at the football oval prior to the match and followed by a huge fireworks display that night. Many young people went early to the oval and stayed eating and drinking during the day and evening. Consequently, several fights broke out and police were kept busy controlling the fights and sending victims to hospital.

Jethro was one of those people involved in a fight who needed to go to hospital. Examination revealed a dislocated shoulder, deep scalp lacerations and multiple bruising. The emergency department at University Hospital was very busy and it took a while for him to be admitted for surgery. Jethro did not like waiting and got noisy and abusive with staff. He fasted, went to the operating room and returned to the ward. On waking, he again became abusive and nursing staff had difficulty attending to his postoperative observations (blood pressure, pulse, respiration, and colour, warmth and movement of the fingers on the side of the injured shoulder).

Two hours after the operation, Jethro announced he was going home. The registered nurse on duty tried to persuade him not to leave. He continued arguing with the nurse and became aggressive and started shouting. The doctor on duty thought perhaps the aggressive behaviour may be attributed to pain and ordered Pethidine 100 mg intramuscularly to be given. The registered nurse, with assistance of an orderly, administered the injection to Jethro who struggled, causing the needle to break off and necessitating further surgery.

Questions

➤ Are there any legal issues in the case study? If so, what are they?

➤ What are the ethical issues?

➤ What are Jethro's rights?

➤ Have these been upheld? If not, why not?

➤ How would you resolve the ethical problem?

Critical reflection

Write a critical reflection for this chapter to place in your Ethics Portfolio. The item or issue that you may want to work through or critically analyse could be something that you need to explore further from:

● one of the case studies;

● reading that you have done;

● becoming therapeutically available to a client or patient group that you know little about;

● a different point of view that someone raised in discussion in class;

● a general feeling of disquiet about pain or aggressive behaviour, which you want to explore through reflection; or

● clinical practice:

○ such as that your values and beliefs are different from some members of the team;

○ a client or patient who you have provided care for who was 'different' and because you were not sensitive treatment was not therapeutically available to him or her;

○ how you have realised that the care you have provided for a patient on clinical practice was incorrect and consequently, unethical;

○ a situation or incident that you have observed when the client's or patient's rights have not been upheld, identify what you could do about this;

○ something your mentor or clinical supervisor said to you.

We suggest you continue using Johns' model of reflection for this chapter.

The relationship of ethics to philosophy

Roger A. Newham and Georgina Hawley

Why this chapter is important to me . . .

✔ To understand the relationship of ethics and philosophy.

✔ To gain knowledge of ethical principles and rules, and how to apply these.

✔ Become aware of some of the philosophical theories that people can use to identify actions that are correct or right.

In Chapter 1, you learnt that your actions or behaviours reflect your personal values and beliefs, and this is especially so when you need to make a decision. An example is when you need to buy a car. The person who believes a car should be nothing more than a vehicle to get them from A to B and who values thriftiness, will buy a different car from the person who believes a car should be an extension of their personality and values style. Likewise, values and beliefs impinge on our behaviour at all times.

In Chapter 2, you gained recognition of your uniqueness and the various stages of dependence, independence and interdependence; as a health professional, you need to be able to operate at the interdependent level when connecting with others. You also learnt how group values and beliefs are inherent within society's different cultures, and how other people's values and beliefs can be very different to your own, which can lead to differences of opinions and life styles. This chapter paved the way for Chapter 3, in which it was discussed that there can be many problems in health care, some of which are ethical or moral whereas others are not. The different types of ethical problems were discussed to enable you to understand how easily these can occur in any health organisation. The remedy to such problems is for health professionals to gain education in ethics, including the actions of critical reflection, negotiation, moral sensitivity and assertiveness.

In Chapter 4, clients' or patients' rights were discussed, along with the ethical or moral ideal standards that health professionals should aim to attain (caring, advocacy, accountability and collaboration). This chapter examines the relationship of ethics to philosophy. You will gain knowledge and understanding of how ethics is part of philosophy and how to use ethical principles, rules and theories to guide your ethical behaviour in clinical practice.

This overview of philosophy is brief compared to other books that have been published, but it will be sufficient to gain an understanding; if you wish to study further, you can use other texts to augment your knowledge and help you in communicating about ethics with other professionals in clinical practice. For it is to moral philosophy and ethical theories that we need to appeal for the words and language to use when discussing ethical issues and problems with our peers and colleagues in the interprofessional team.

The inherent value of this chapter is that it will enable you to use the language that other health professionals use when discussing ethical issues, problems or dilemmas. First, there is a brief discussion on the relationship of ethics to philosophy and the part in which we are interested. Second, ethical principles will be discussed; third, ethical theories; and, finally, the professional development section.

The relationship of ethics and philosophy

Ethics is just one part of philosophy and, if we examine the subject, we will notice that it has different branches, including meta-ethics and normative (or prescriptive) ethics (Hawley, 1997a). It is the latter in which we are interested, that is, normative ethics as it provides ethical theories which aim to guide our conduct or behaviour, to help us decide what we ought to do, and how we ought to live. It is these theories and inherent ethical principles that provide frameworks by which we can discern which action to take in clinical practice (Hawley, 1997a).

When a person uses the unqualified term 'philosophy' it usually refers to the philosophical tradition referred to as 'Western' which began with the ancient Greeks, and is used extensively in the Western world (Western Europe, the UK, Canada, the USA, Australia, etc.). However, there is another philosophical tradition; the Eastern philosophies, belonging to countries such as India, Pakistan, China, Japan and the general Eastern area.

Until recently, Western philosophy was the only philosophy taught in many universities in the Western world. Consequently, the Eastern tradition was frequently overlooked, even though a large proportion of the world exists in countries that use such philosophies. Since the cultural perspective is very important in this book, both Eastern and Western philosophical traditions will be discussed, the Western tradition in this chapter and the Eastern in Chapter 6.

The purpose of giving you this information about Western and Eastern philosophies is to assist you in becoming aware of people's roots, and the many differences. This will help you to understand the cultural background of your clients or patients, but also those of other professionals and staff with whom you work in clinical practice. That is, just because you have a specific philosophical view point that reflects your values and beliefs does not necessarily mean that another person will have the same. Nor can you say that yours is correct and theirs is wrong. We might like to think it is, but it ain't necessarily so!

Activity

➤ If you live in mainland Europe, the UK, Ireland, Australia or New Zealand, why do you think it is important that you become aware of Eastern philosophy as well as Western?

I hope that you said it was because so many people from the Eastern traditions now live in Europe, the UK, Ireland, Australia or New Zealand, and therefore their culture influences their health beliefs. Consequently, as health professionals the more we know about others' philosophical roots the easier it will be for us to provide effective ethical health care.

Consequently an understanding of philosophy is important for health professionals not only to understand people's cultural heritage, but also to be able to use those philosophical frameworks to facilitate ethical decisions which will be culturally congruent for them.

Western philosophies

The Western tradition of philosophies has formed the framework for culture, governments, health, education and industries in countries such as Greece, Italy, France, Germany, Spain, Portugal, etc., and Ireland and the UK. With migration of people to Australia from Europe and the UK, Western philosophy formed the frameworks there as those countries started to develop. Likewise, with New Zealand, Canada and the USA the migrants took with them their Western philosophical values and beliefs.

Although in this book Western and Eastern philosophies are presented as separate entities, these are not strict cut-off points. That is, many people will have a blend of values and beliefs that may have developed from their socialisation with people of these cultures.

We will be using Case study 5.1 - Mrs Smith and the students Annabelle and Adrian - to illustrate points of view in this chapter. Read it now, so that you start to familiarise yourself with the situation. You might like to answer the question at the end of the case study before moving on to the rest of the chapter.

Case study 5.1
Mrs Smith and the students Annabelle and Adrian

Mrs Smith is 69 years old and, until a recent fall, lived and managed by herself in her own home with a little social care. She is due to be discharged from hospital quite soon. She is classified as 'DNR' ('Do Not Resuscitate') should she have a cardiac arrest. This has not been discussed with her.

A student nurse, Annabelle, and a social work student Adrian are both familiar with Mrs Smith's case. Adrian thinks that Mrs Smith ought to be involved in the decision as to whether she wishes to be resuscitated. He feels that a sensitive discussion with Mrs Smith would allow the consultant to find out her views on the subject, and may then influence her care in a beneficial way. Annabelle thinks that Mrs Smith ought not to be involved in such discussion, and that she may become upset if she is asked the question, which could be harmful to her recovery.

Question

➤ Who do think is right, Annabelle or Adrian?

Ethical principles

In Western philosophy, four main principles are used to guide ethical practice. They are autonomy, beneficence, justice and non-maleficence.

Ethical principle of autonomy

The everyday meaning of autonomy is that a person has the right to and should make their own decisions in life, provided that the consequences do not violate another person (Hawley, 1997c). It should be remembered that just because an action is autonomous does not mean it is legally right and/or morally acceptable.

In health care, autonomy implies that people are self-governing of their own behaviour, and that they have the right to consent to or refuse treatment. This right implies that they are not to be constrained, coerced or impeded in any way (Hawley, 1997c). This recognition of individual autonomy is a relatively new idea in health care. Previously the doctor did what they thought best for the patient without giving the patient a choice (this is known as paternalism). Today, models of decision-making between doctors and patient emphasise open communication and discussion of consequences before a client or patient makes their own decision.

For clients or patients to make autonomous decisions in regard to their health, they need to be free of the control of others. That is, they must be able to deliberate rationally through various possible courses of action without being impaired by lack of time, incomplete information, mental illness and/or impairment (Hawley, 1997c).

Autonomy has the highest priority of all the ethical principles in Western health care, and should not be overridden except when it impinges on the autonomy of another person (Hawley, 1997c). When a client or patient cannot be autonomous, then a health care professional would need to use the principle of beneficence.

Ethical principle of beneficence

Beneficence implies that the intended care is aimed at what is good for the wellbeing of the client or patient. Beneficence is the deliberate bringing about of positive action/s or interventions (Hawley, 1997c).

There is a need to realise, however, that a health care professional's duty to do good towards a client or patient may be limited not only by those with whom they work, but also by the available resources. Consequently, it is not always straightforward to achieve.

Ethical principle of justice

Justice refers to what society's expectations are of what is fair and right. John Locke, a philosopher, considered the characteristics of justice to be such that it guaranteed equality with others (Hawley, 1997c).

Justice as fairness in health care does not imply that the client or patient should be offered all available treatment and service, and that everyone should be given identical service and treatment. Rather, the health care professional needs to proceed with planning and giving care that incorporates the notion of 'due care' so that all people, irrespective of socio-economic status, race, gender or religion, are offered and given the appropriate health care according to their medical, nursing and allied health care needs (Hawley, 1997c). See Chapter 14 for different theories of justice in relation to the allocation of resources.

Ethical principle of non-maleficence

The principle of non-maleficence means 'above all, do not harm' (Hawley, 1997c). Non-maleficence implies restraint from doing harm, or prevention or prohibition of some action, which would cause harm. According to Mitchell *et al.* (1996), the principle of non-maleficence involves not only the duty of care to avoid actual harm but also the risk of harm.

Sometimes health professionals consider it difficult to separate beneficence and non-maleficence, or that they are the same. However, it needs to be remembered that beneficence is actively doing good, whereas non-maleficence means active prevention of harm. That is why, in this book, the ethical principle of justice is inserted between the two so that readers do not think there is a similarity (Hawley, 1997a).

When health professionals discuss cases and ethical issues, they quite often say 'the principle of autonomy has been met'. This means that the client or patient has made their own decision and therefore the concept behind the principle has been achieved (Hawley, 1997b).

Another term that may be used is 'fulfilled'. That is, a health professional may say, 'if we do x, y, z, then the principles of beneficence, justice and non-maleficence will be fulfilled'. This means that those principles have been achieved (Hawley, 1997b).

Activity

Re-read Case study 5.1 again and then answer the following questions.

Questions

➤ In the case study was Mrs Smith allowed to be autonomous in her decision regarding resuscitation?

➤ Do you think her autonomy was upheld?

➤ Do you think Adrian's idea would fulfil the principle of beneficence?

➤ Do you think justice would be fulfilled?

➤ Do you think non-maleficence would be upheld?

Answers

Mrs Smith was not allowed to be autonomous, and therefore the principle of autonomy was not upheld. Mrs Smith is only 69 years old and no other health problems are mentioned; there was therefore really no need for a DNR order to be placed on her chart. Adrian is correct, this needs to be discussed with her, meaning that the principle of beneficence would then be met. In relation to justice, this principle has not been met as there is nothing fair and equal about not being resuscitated at such a young age with no other health problems. Likewise, with the principle of non-maleficence, to refrain from doing harm. It would be harmful to Mrs Smith if, for some unknown reason, she had a sudden cardiac arrest and was not resuscitated just because of the DNR order.

Can you see how using ethical principles allows you greater understanding of the situation?

Read the following case study and how you can apply ethical principles to gain an understanding of the ethical problem.

Case study 5.2
Mrs Mains-Johnston

Mrs Mains-Johnston was a 53-year-old Scot in agony with cancer of the kidney and bladder with bony metastases in her spine and pelvis. Her pain control, although originally satisfactory, is now unmanageable and, after becoming exhausted by the whole process, she decides she wants a peaceful end to her life. The consultant in charge of her case judged Mrs Mains-Johnston to be mentally competent and her husband and children agreed with her request. The doctor asked another oncology consultant to assess Mrs Mains-Johnston, who agreed with the decision.

The doctor inserted an additional intravenous (I.V.) line and administered further pain relief and sedation which resulted in Mrs Mains-Johnston going to sleep in the arms of her husband, surrounded by their children. When she lapsed into a comatose state, an anaesthetic drug was added to the I. V. This resulted in Mrs Mains-Johnston's respirations ceasing, and she was pronounced dead shortly afterwards.

One of the staff on the ward, although not looking after Mrs Mains-Johnston, did not agree with the doctor's actions and felt that she should report him to the police since euthanasia was not legal.

Although the names have been changed, the case occurred in Australia, and the doctor was charged with murder.

Application of ethical principles to the scenario

An individual who has cancer of the kidneys and bladder with bony metastases, all causing pain, asks the doctor to provide the means of peaceful death to end her suffering.

- The principle of autonomy is clearly relevant here as Mrs Mains-Johnston is mentally competent and therefore has a right to request and also refuse medical treatment. The right to one's own peaceful death would appear to be an area over which an individual has a right to be self-governing. However, the autonomy of one individual should not override that of another. Therefore, Mrs Mains-Johnston could not demand euthanasia from the doctor, as her autonomy cannot override that of her consultant.

- The principle of beneficence, to do good, could be interpreted as allowing a peaceful death.

- However, the principle of non-maleficence would imply that the doctor should not harm Mrs Mains-Johnston by causing her death. Equally, the principle could mean not to cause her any more suffering, and therefore, as much analgesia as required to ease the pain could be given.

- The principle of justice, of being fair and the equal distribution of benefits, is not really relevant in this case study. However, if other patients equal in their suffering to Mrs Mains-Johnston requested similar treatment, then the consultant should also consider their requests.

- It would appear that the staff member who reported the case to the police, in order to be fair and equitable to the doctor, patient and family, should only report the doctor to the police if they were going to report all cases where death had been caused or hastened by medication.

We now have a clearer understanding of the ethical problem by making the principles explicit.

Ethical rules

An ethical rule is a concept that, while it would be ideal for the health professional to uphold, it is not deemed absolutely necessary to do so. So, while ethical principles must be fulfilled or met for the health professional to be acting ethically, an ethical rule may be 'put aside' by the health professional if there are sufficient grounds to do so. The ethical rules usually referred to are confidentiality and veracity.

Ethical rule of confidentiality

This rule obliges all health professionals not only to refrain from disclosing information from clients or patients to others, but also to ensure that any records of that information remain confidential (Hawley, 1997d). This rule continues after the death of the client or patient.

Exceptions to this rule are when it is necessary to protect the client or patient from harm, or to protect another party or parties from harm. For example, a client may tell a social worker that they want to commit suicide and 'not to tell anyone'. Although the social worker has the obligation not to breach confidentiality, it would be in the client's bests interests for the social worker to inform the psychiatrist so that effective treatment could be given (Hawley, 1997d).

The ethical rule of veracity

In relation to the rule of veracity the health professional needs to strive to be honest, straightforward and truthful as possible (Hawley, 1997d). This means to disclose all information that a client or patient needs to make a decision, not to tell lies about care and treatment, and, when asked questions by the client or patient, to answer those truthfully. However, such issues of truth telling must be handled sensitively (Hawley, 1997d). For example, if Mrs Mains-Johnston was a client or patient of yours and she asked you to explain her diagnosis to her, you could do this. However, once you explained the diagnosis in a way that she could understand, you would not continue by stating 'and all the other patients I have looked after with this type of cancer died a horrible painful death'. Neither would you give her information unless she was ready. To do so would be ethically insensitive and this is a type of ethical problem (see Chapter 3).

Sometimes you might read in an ethics book of these two ethical rules referred to as ethical principles. This is not quite correct as principles must always be met, whereas rules, providing there is sufficient legal and ethical grounds, can be set aside or only partially met.

Activity

Re-read Case study 5.1 and answer the following question.

➤ Is the care received by Mrs Smith according to the ethical rule of veracity?

Activity

Read Case study 5.3 – Lorraine and Max – and see if you can identify where the different ethical principles of autonomy, beneficence, justice and non-maleficence are involved.

Case study 5.3
Lorraine and Max (Hawley, 1997a)

Lorraine (age 38) and Max (age 42) are a very busy professional couple who have left having a child until their careers are established. They have recently moved from Paris to live in London. They want to have a child, but because of Lorraine's PCOS and Max's low sperm count, need to embark on an *in vitro* fertilisation (IVF) treatment programme.

Lorraine is given treatment and her left ovary produces multiple ova which, when mixed with Max's sperm in the laboratory, results in five blastocysts that can be implanted in her uterus. The health care team decides that three blastocysts are to be implanted and the remaining two to be stored until needed.

The three embryos proceed to develop well; however, Lorraine and Max decide that they could not cope with the financial burden of bringing up three children and ask for a selective termination of pregnancy of one embryo at 14 weeks' gestation.

The remaining two embryos are threatened by the procedure, and this results in Lorraine having to spend the majority of the rest of her pregnancy in hospital.

Later, Lorraine develops pre-eclampsia and the babies (one boy and one girl) are delivered early by an emergency Caesarean section. The available intensive neonatal equipment in the hospital is already in demand by other multiple births. Likewise, other London hospitals cannot help. This means one baby (the girl) has to be flown to a neonatal unit in Glasgow for care.

After a month the baby girl is flown back to the home city where the other baby, that is, the boy, is fighting for his life. The girl baby continues to do well, but the boy's condition further deteriorates and, despite extraordinary efforts, he dies.

This means that Lorraine and Max can only take home one baby girl. However, they have also learnt that it was a boy that was removed through selective termination.

An explanation of how these ethical principles and rules related to the case study is given below and overleaf.

● The principle of **autonomy** (being self-governing): it is Lorraine's and Max's own choice to delay having a family; likewise, for the implantation of three blastocysts. Later, it is Lorraine's and Max's choice that they have a selected termination; likewise, agreement for the Caesarian to take place.

- The principle of **beneficence** (to actively do good): the team decide to implant three blastocysts and store two. Implanting five blastocysts would possibly have caused health problems for both mother and children. However, the implantation of three allows the team to do good for Lorraine and Max by allowing them to become parents. The storage of two blastocysts allows for implantation at a later date should the first pregnancy fail, or if Lorraine and Max want additional children at a later date.

  It is the team's decision to do the Caesarian operation to do good for Lorraine in possibly saving her life and those of the babies. The principle of beneficence is also met by the transfer of one baby to Glasgow for care when there were no facilities in London at the time.

- The principle of **justice** (what is right and equal for everyone): one baby is transferred as the other baby needs to be allocated care in London. However, you could argue that justice has not been upheld as the team decided three blastocysts are transferred when it may have been better to use only one.

- The principle of **non-maleficence** (do no harm): the selective termination harmed one embryo by bringing about its death. Therefore, if you believe that an embryo has ethical rights, then you could state that the principle of non-maleficence has not been met.

- The ethical rule of **confidentiality** (to keep secret client or patient information): there is no evidence in the case study that this rule has been broken.

- The ethical rule of **veracity** (always tell the truth): there is no evidence in the case study that the team did not tell Lorraine and Max the truth. However, one needs to wonder why three blastocysts were implanted when the parents later decide that they could only manage with two babies?

Normative ethical theories

Earlier in the chapter we stated that it is normative ethics that can provide theories that offer guidance for making ethical decisions. When studying these ethical theories, you will find that the various philosophers have different views. In fact we can broadly allocate these theories into three main types, which are listed below (Table 5.1). The first type is what is known as 'teleological' theories; the second, 'deontological' and the third are the 'caring' type. Under each of these types you will find some of the philosophers' names and theories.

In this section teleological theories will be examined first, then deontological and, finally, feminine moral theory, care ethics and virtue ethics. In Western philosophy, teleological and deontological theories are often referred to as classical or rationalistic. That is, they were

Table 5.1 Types of ethical theories

Teleological	Deontological	Feminist and postmodernist
Theories of Egoism and Utilitarianism Philosophers: Hobbes, Bentham and Mill	Theories of prima facie duties and Natural Law Philosophers: Ross, Rawls, Kant and Aquinas	Pythagorean women Philosophers: Gilligan, Noddings, Blum, Sheldrick, Hursthouse and Slote

developed by classical philosophers hundreds of years ago, and they are rationalist in approach. This means that the concepts are purely objective, and therefore can be used as rationales or reasons for pursuing a course of action. On the other hand, they are divorced from patient care and do not consider the concepts of caring, compassion or empathy. It is not until feminist and postmodernist philosophies are considered that the rationalistic approach is dropped and the theories correlate more with the concepts of caring (such as advocacy, relationships, and the virtues of compassion and kindness).

Teleological theories

This is a group of theories that are judged to be ethically correct by the end outcome. That is, it doesn't matter how the outcome was achieved as long as the end result is ethically correct. Because of this emphasis on the outcome, teleological theories are sometimes called 'end-based theories' or 'consequential theories'. It is acceptable to use any of the three names: teleological, end-based and consequences or consequential (Hawley, 1997c).

Deontological theories

This group emphasises the way something is performed or carried out. That is what deems an action to be ethically correct or right (and that is what is most important). A deontologist has a duty to do what is right and to refrain from doing what is wrong, irrespective of what the outcome might be (Hawley, 1997c).

Teleological v. deontological

Teleology says that the outcome is correct, whereas deontological theory says the way in which something is performed or undertaken is what makes it correct. Can you see how these two types are different from each other? That is, in teleology the outcome or consequences resulting directly or indirectly are the most important. The manner in which the outcome or consequences were achieved is deemed unimportant. This is in direct contrast with deontological theorists who maintain that the method of the action is important (Hawley, 1997c).

Different types of teleological theories

There are two theories which fall under the type of teleological theories: these are Egoism and Utilitarianism.

Egoism
According to Egoism, people are and ought to be orientated and motivated only by self-love (Hawley, 1997c). In Plato's *Republic*, Thrasymachus was an Egoist who defined justice (where justice is a broader concept than our idea of law that includes the right way to live) as self-interest and that it is rational to act only in one's self-interest. As a model of ethical practice, Egoist professionals would do only those actions that would promote the greatest good for the professional themselves (Hawley, 1997c). The basis of modern Egoism was identified with Thomas Hobbes (1599-1679). He believed that the main drive of human nature was

self-preservation. For Egoists an act is moral when it is in a person's best long-term interests. If an act is intended to produce, or will probably produce, or will produce, more good or right than bad or wrong, that action is the right one to perform (Barry, 1982, p. 56).

There are two kinds of Egoism (Hawley, 1997c):

- Personal Egoists who would be most interested in their own best long-term interests. For example, if you were an egoist nurse, you would be more concerned about improvement of your own conditions and career than about others.
- Impersonal Egoists who believe that anyone and everyone should follow their own best long-term interests.

Utilitarianism

David Hume (1711-1776), Jeremy Bentham (1748-1832) and John Stuart Mill (1806-1873) are major names in the instigation of this theory. G. E. Moore (1873-1958), R. M. Hare (1919-2002) and Peter Singer (1946-) are more recent Utilitarian theorists.

Utilitarian theory states that there is only one basic ethical principle and this is 'the Principle of Utility' which, in rough terms, means that we ought always to strive to promote 'the greatest good for the greatest number' or we ought to produce 'the greatest amount of utility as value over disvalue' (Hawley, 1997c).

Classical Utilitarianism was developed by Jeremy Bentham and John Stuart Mill. Bentham noted that no matter what moral philosophers argued, people were all governed by two masters, pain and pleasure (the Principle of Utility). The basis of this type of theory is that voluntary actions should produce the greatest amount of good for everyone concerned, and is termed 'goal-based' (Hawley, 1997c).

The aim of Utilitarian ethical behaviour is to minimise the pain and maximise the pleasure. Today, this could be called the cost-benefit analysis or, as some would say, the cost-risk-benefit rate. According to Bentham, the basis for judging the pain and pleasure depended upon: intensity, duration, certainty (or uncertainty), remoteness, purity (is the pleasure being followed by more pleasure), fecundity (the chance the behaviour has of being followed by similar sensations) and the extent (the number of persons the behaviour/action is extended to) (Barry, 1982).

The advantage of Bentham's classical Utilitarianism is that it encourages health professionals to consider the client's or patient's feelings of pain and pleasure. It also includes the principle of sufferability, which includes the notion of the capacity of all sentient beings to suffer (Hawley, 1997c).

The disadvantage of this Utilitarianism is that it only considers the values of pain and pleasure, and disregards other values (Bandman and Bandman, 1990).

John Stuart Mill added to Bentham's classical theory of Utilitarianism by examining other values such as duty, love and respect. According to Mill:

- An action is right if it conforms to the greatest happiness principle.
- Actions are right in proportion to the extent that they promote happiness.
- Pain and unhappiness produce the reverse effects (Hawley, 1997c).

When assessing the good, the time span is irrelevant. That is, if in one action good will were produced immediately, but if in another action greater good will were produced in the long term, then the latter action is the right one (Hawley, 1997c). For example, if you are faced with two actions, and you don't know which one to choose, you could look at it this way:

Action 1		Action 2
Some good produced immediately	or	A greater amount produced at a later date

The second action is the correct one as it would produce the greater amount of good (Hawley, 1997c).

If, however, the good in the long term is uncertain, while good can be produced in an immediate action, then the immediate action is the correct moral action.

Action 1		Action 2
Some good produced immediately	or	Uncertain amount of good will be produced in the long term

The first action is the correct one (Hawley, 1997c).

Furthermore, unhappiness or pain must be considered. If the action could cause pain and unhappiness, these must be subtracted from the amount of good or happiness (Hawley, 1997c). If the actions being considered produce unhappiness or pain, then the action that produces the least amount of unhappiness or pain is the correct action (Barry, 1982). For example:

Action 1		Action 2
Some pain or unhappiness produced immediately	or	Lesser amount of pain or unhappiness at a later time

The correct action is the second one (Hawley, 1997c).

Mill maintained that Utilitarianism required a person to be 'strictly impartial' but also a kindly or 'benevolent' spectator (Hawley, 1997c). Mill cited the example of Jesus as the complete spirit of the ethics of Utility, 'to do as you would be done by' (of course a possible problem with such an idea is that different people like different things) and 'to love your neighbour as yourself', as the ideal perfection of Utilitarianism morality (Mill, J. S., Utilitarianism Act 22; cited by Barry, 1982).

The notion of it not mattering who does the action is related to the idea of 'agent neutrality'. Agent neutral reasons are such that it makes no difference whether it is you who kills one person to save 50 or that being one's wife is no reason to favour her over a stranger when they are both drowning. There is much current literature by recent theorists trying to show how Utilitarian theory can account for goods such as friendship or the importance of the health care worker-patient/client relationship.

There are two main types of Utilitarianism:

- Act: appeals to the principle of utility to particular acts to determine the rightness of the act. For example, a Utilitarian act may justify having a particular relationship with a client or patient only if it maximises the good outcome or consequences.
- Rule: applies the principle to general rules. For example, a Utilitarian rule may claim that the action is only good if it can be applied to everyone.

An advantage of Utilitarianism is its practical usefulness.

Deontological theory

There are several theories which fall under the type of deontological which we will consider. These are those by Immanuel Kant (1724-1804), perhaps the classic name associated with this theory; H. A. Pritchard (1871-1947), W. D. Ross (1871-1971) and John Rawls (1921-) are more recent deontologists. Theories discussed in this section are Kantian, Ross's prima facie duties, Rawls' Principle of Justice and Aristotle's Natural Law.

Kantian deontology

One of the most prominent of the classical deontological theories is that developed by the German philosopher Immanuel Kant (1724-1804). Kant's theory is not without problems, as he formulated the basic principle of his theory in a number of different ways. For the purposes of this book, Kant's theory will be viewed from a health perspective (Hawley, 1997c).

The first formulation of the theory tells us to 'act only on that maxim through which you can at the same time, will, that it should become universal law'. That is, a health professional needs to act in such a manner that their behaviour is so good that it could be a law for everyone (Hawley, 1997c).

Another part informs us to 'act in such a way that you always treat humanity, whether in your own person or in the person of any other, never simply as a means but always at the same time as an end'. In this way Kantian deontology is an ethic of respect for clients and patients. That is, the health professional needs to respect everyone's rational nature and their inherent dignity (Hawley, 1997c).

According to Kant, from this fundamental principle, a system of particular duties can be derived. This system of duties includes duties to self as well as to others. In each of these cases, 'perfect duties' must be distinguished from 'imperfect duties', thus becoming a four-fold classification of duties (Hawley, 1997c).

- Perfect duties to self
- Imperfect duties to self
- Perfect duties to others
- Imperfect duties to others

Perfect duties: these are actions that we must always observe. There are no legitimate exceptions to a perfect duty. Kant also called these actions 'negative obligations'; that is, we must refrain from doing these actions because we must have respect for all persons, e.g. not to injure another person and not to lie (Hawley, 1997c).

Imperfect duties: by contrast, these are actions that have 'positive obligations'. Imperfect duties require the promotion of certain goals – personal perfection for self, and happiness or welfare of others (Hawley, 1997c).

Kant believed that nothing is good in itself except a 'good will'. By 'will' he meant the uniquely human capacity to act according to the concept of law; that is, principles. A 'good will' to Kant is an action that is good, not because of how it is performed, the way the end is achieved, or the effect it causes, but by virtue of a health professional's conscious decision to take, and/or the intention of, the action: that is what Kant regarded as good (Hawley, 1997c).

It might be argued that Kantian deontology, by sorting out various duties into the categories of perfect and imperfect, and assigning priorities to perfect duties, provides us with a structure in terms of which ethical issues can be resolved (Hawley, 1997c). However, many health professionals have found difficulty when a perfect duty is in conflict with another perfect duty; e.g. confidentiality and not to lie. Nevertheless, Kantian deontology does emphasise the respect for all persons irrespective of race or socioeconomic status, and this is very important for health professionals to remember (Hawley, 1997c).

Kant believed that actions can be right and good regardless of the consequences. Some acts are 'good in themselves' or 'intrinsically good or right'. So, for example, the end never justifies the means.

Ross's prima facie duties

This theory was developed and presented in 1930 by W. D. Ross in his book *The Right and the Good* (Mappes and Zembaty, 1991). In this book Ross presents an ethical theory which attempts to join the ideas of Utilitarianism with those of Kantianism. Ross maintained that people are often aware of a number of obligations in situations, some of which are conflicting (Hawley, 1997c). Therefore, Ross believed that we must always weigh options when deciding which action is morally correct. In this way a health professional would weigh each course of action, and then observe if that action would fulfil a 'prima facie' duty or not (Hawley, 1997c). Ross insisted that there was nothing arbitrary about these prima facie duties; in fact, he believed that they were intuitive in all people, and at the same time conditional. He maintained that, if a moral action fulfilled a prima facie duty, then that duty became an actual duty and the person needed to carry out the action to be morally correct. For example, the duty to keep a promise while it is a prima facie duty can be overridden if a health professional holds the opinion that the duty was not in the client's or patient's best interests (Hawley, 1997c).

In addition, if more than one prima facie duty is recognised in a moral problem, the health professional needs to sort and weigh them all before deciding which action is morally correct. To make the correct decision when sorting and weighing these duties, the health professional needs to assign a relative weight to each, and the action that has greatest balance of prima facie rightness to wrongness is the morally correct action (Hawley, 1997c).

The prima facie duties are:

1 **Fidelity** - these are actions that rest on prior acts of our own; for example, not to lie, to be faithful, to keep promises and to repair incorrect actions, pay debts, etc.

2 **Gratitude** - these are actions we do for people with whom we have a relationship, such as friends and relatives; e.g. repaying a kindness.

3 **Justice** - these are actions which give us pleasure and happiness. Ross says care must be taken to make sure these are only gained in fair, proper or correct ways; that is, not from devious or illegal ways, and that the goods or benefits must be distributed rightly. Moreover, Ross contended that rules or duties which determine what is right from wrong are to be followed regardless of how the actions contribute towards the good.

4 **Beneficence** - there are actions for which other people depend upon us. In nursing, our patients rely on us and therefore we should use our virtue, intelligence and happiness to improve their lives.

5 **Self-improvement** - these are actions which would help us, or others, to strive for self-improvement.

6 **Non-maleficence** - these are actions in which we refrain from injuring someone and/or others (Barry, 1982, pp. 73-77).

According to Ross, the action that would be morally correct is the one that would fulfil the greatest balance of the prima facie rightness to prima facie wrongness, as shown in Table 5.2.

Table 5.2 Using Ross's prima facie duties in practice

Action 1		Action 2		Action 3
Prima facie duties • Non-maleficence	or	Prima facie duties • Justice • Beneficence • Non-maleficence	or	Prima facie duties • Fidelity • Self-improvement

Action 2 would be the morally correct action, or actual duties to be performed, as this action would fulfil the greatest balance of rightness to wrongness. Furthermore, Ross argued that if it was your considered judgement that a particular prima facie duty takes precedence over all others, it becomes your absolute duty to do it. That duty would then become 'an actual duty' and, as such, needs to be carried out (to fulfil its absolute claim on us) (Hawley, 1997c).

Ross believed that these duties were only 'prima facie' and could be overridden depending on the circumstance. For instance, honesty, while always a right, could be overridden by other principles such as beneficence; the principle or duty that was actually acted upon being the duty proper. Thus he paved the way for the idea of 'balancing or weighing' principles.

Rawls' maximum principle of justice

In 1971 Harvard philosophy professor John Rawls published his book *Theory* of *Justice*. The underlying concept of Rawls' theory is that justice is of intrinsic value. To determine what factors constitute justice, Rawls used the 'original position' as a base. The 'original position' is a hypothetical state in which a person is not aware of his or her own socioeconomic situation or talents (he also called this position the 'natural state'). Therefore, when people are in this original position they all share certain characteristics – self-interest, rationality, needs and capacities (Hawley, 1997c).

Rawls argued that if people were in the original position they would choose two principles to ensure their own justice. These two principles would be:

- The liberty principle: people in the original position would expect to have an equal amount to the greatest amount possible of liberty.
- The difference principle: people in the original position would allow inequality only if it was to everybody's advantage (Hawley, 1997c).

For example, let us suppose you had the task of allocating staff on a surgical ward at the beginning of a shift to look after patients at different preoperative and postoperative stages. You could morally allow an inequality in the amount of time spent by a nurse with a patient, as all patients need a lot of time spent with them immediately before and after surgery; this gradually decreases as each patient's condition improves and they are discharged home. In this way the inequality of time spent is morally correct according to Rawls, as it is adjusted to the particular nursing need of each patient. Likewise, the local Member of Parliament, while in hospital, should be nursed in the same way as the young juvenile delinquent (i.e. according to nursing needs, not socioeconomic status) (Hawley, 1997c).

Natural law ethics

This theory equates moral life with the life of reason, as discerned from nature or God's eternal law. Natural law theorists argue that, whether a person believes in God or not, moral agents share the same rational human nature and therefore the same human concept of morality (or what is right or good). In Natural Law the word 'law' is used to mean laws that apply everything to nature (God) as opposed to human constructed or government law.

These Natural Laws, from the Roman Catholic doctrines, have influenced our legal system, institutions and social policies over the centuries (Hawley, 1997c).

The two important doctrines or principles of Natural Law are those of double effect and totality; these are used today not only as ethical principles for moral behaviour, but also in law (Wallace, 1995). The principle of double effect implies that an action should be performed only if the intention is to bring about a good effect; if a bad effect occurs as a consequence this will be unintended or indirect and not occur before the good effect. The principle of totality is that individuals have the right to dispose of their organs or destroy their capacity to function only to the extent that the whole of the body demands it. The basis of this principle is that God has created our organs with a goal in mind and that we, as custodians of our bodies, must hold our organs in trust. When a diseased organ threatens our life we are morally and ethically justified to have an operation to dispose of the diseased part. But if there is nothing wrong with an organ or part of the body, then we must not destroy its capacity (Hawley, 1997c). You will learn more about these two doctrines in Chapters 7 and 8 when they are applied to pain relief and dying.

So far we have focused on the two main branches of Western philosophy, those of teleology and deontology. These types of theory emphasise the action of behaviour to determine if it was ethically right or correct. That is, with teleology the outcome (end or consequences) was the most important part of an action, and determined if the action was ethically right or correct. With deontology theory it was how the action was performed or undertaken that was important.

Feminist and postmodernist theories

In this section we are concerned with the third type of ethical theory, namely feminist and postmodernist. This third type of moral theory allows for the special relationships such as those between family members, friends or health care professionals to be taken into consideration when examining ethical problems to determine whether an action is ethically correct or not. In this section, we will chronologically examine three perspectives: early feminist, care ethics and virtue. What is common to all three perspectives are the underpinning moral values for feminist and postmodernist philosophy. These are:

- neutral power;
- respect for relationships;
- cultural sensitivity;
- integration showing holism or holistic care;
- the fluidity of the situation, that is, it is dynamic and constantly moving, and not static;
- there is emphasis on the human emotion of compassion and kindness to alleviate suffering; and
- collaboration in negotiating care.

Feminist moral theory

After reading about teleological and deontological theories of Western philosophy there may seem to be a quite noticeable gender bias. For example, many texts make little reference to the philosophical contributions of women. However, since early history women have contributed to philosophy and ethics (Hawley, 1997c). For example, the Pythagorean woman Theano emphasised the importance of working in harmony. Hence her principle of harmonia. For Theano, women's responsibility for maintaining harmony and order in the home extends to maintenance of harmony and justice in wider society. This was not intuitive thinking but rather it involved a critically reflective approach.

This was later developed by Perictone who said that the principle of harmonia should be applied to the actual and concrete circumstances of life and not in decontextualised and hypothetical situations. Then there was Arête of Cyrene who was head of the Cyrenaic School of Philosophy. Later, Aesara of Lucania developed a comprehensive Natural Law theory of morality. This emphasised:

- the virtues of love (including compassion for others and kindliness);
- justice that is fair and considers special needs and concerns, such as extenuating circumstances for non-compliance.

The list continues; in fact, Waithe (1989) argues that over 100 women philosophers have been omitted from the standard philosophical works of reference.

Principles of feminist philosophy

The central theme of philosophies that have been developed by women is the emphasis on kindness, friendship, compassion, harmony, justice, wisdom and the recognition of obligations incurred in immediate relationships. In early Greek culture, the family played an important part in defining moral obligations, and moral law was proposed on three levels:

- The individual
- The family
- Wider social parameters (Hawley, 1997c)

Moreover, these levels were characterised by the moral virtues of love, compassion, kindness, self-esteem and a justice that is fair and considerate of special needs and concerns (Johnstone, 1996, p. 104). Such a view is in direct contrast to the Western philosophical thought of deontology, where detachment of the individual from the family in moral issues is deemed necessary to make an objective opinion and decision (Johnstone, 1996, p. 115).

Care ethics

The ethics of care or care ethics is attributed to writers such as Carol Gilligan, Nell Noddings and Annette Baier, among others (Statman, 1997). In the 1980s researcher Carol Gilligan (1982) looked into the way children acquired moral beliefs and practices and made an important discovery. She found that girls were more likely to resolve social and ethical problems by seeking solutions that maintained the relationship, whereas boys were likely to appeal to rules and precedents. Furthermore, boys tended to be somewhat legalistic in their thinking and sought solutions from an impartial standpoint. Girls, on the other hand, considered how the people involved in the dispute felt, and therefore sought solutions that created fewer disharmonies for those involved (Hawley, 1997c).

Gilligan's and Noddings' care-based approach to ethics arises from the research outlined above. This was in direct contrast to Kohlberg's (1980) *The Philosophy of Moral Development*, in which he proposed six hierarchial levels of moral development. The highest level (level 6) occurred when people used the 'reasoning of universal ethical principles'. According to Kohlberg, actions are morally right insofar as they accord with these principles and moral reasoning results from their employment. Kohlberg's research to substantiate his theory contained a serious design flaw in that he only used males!

Consequently, we could say that the care-based approach to ethics is a reaction to, and rejection of, a rational principle approach evident in teleological and deontological philosophy. The proponents of care-based approaches to ethics claim that teleological and deontological philosophical ethics is:

- too callous and uncaring (Alderson, 1992);
- too simplistic (Hunt, 1994);
- too complicated and jargon-laden (Hunt, 1994); and
- an 'unjust' conception of justice (Okin, 1987).

In care-based ethics, emphasis is focused on giving attention to others and the relationship between the health professional and clients or patients. There are many writings on care ethics and so it is a little difficult to summarise; however, there are four general characteristics (Edwards, 1996). These are:

- Uniqueness of the situation: the need for the health professional to realise that no two ethical problems are the same, that there is always a difference; for example, a different client or patient the next time the problem occurs.

- The mandate to care: since health professionals engage in caring this in itself can give rise to moral problems.

- The emotional involvement of caring: the recognition that in caring the health professional experiences emotions.

- The privileged view: that is, the awareness that those directly involved in the care of clients or patients will have a different view of the ethical problem than those not directly involved or outside the immediate view. Hence the term 'privileged view', meaning that two view points can be obtained.

These common characteristics remove the rationalistic component from ethical caring.

Some women philosophers, writing about care ethics, have maintained that it is little wonder then that female health professionals face moral problems in practice, if intuitive in the moral make-up are the values of love, compassion and kindness (that is, care in the true sense). However, in reality women sometimes have to argue pragmatically and deconceptualise situations because the care focus is not an ingredient in Western philosophical thought (Johnstone, 1996).

The biggest difficulty arises when women health professionals are faced with situations that need them to be empathetic with clients or patients in moral situations. For example, this might include termination of pregnancy, contraception, genetic screening, allocation of scarce resources, treatment of defective neonates and organ transplantation (Johnstone, 1996). However, it could equally be argued that doctors also need to demonstrate empathy to clients or patients in such situations. Consequently, an understanding by a health professional of their own moral development and recognition of feminine philosophical thought, and care-based ethics may do much to support the health professional when making a moral decision.

Postmodernist philosophy

The term 'postmodernist' is difficult to define because, in many ways, it is a misnomer (Edwards et al., 1998). However, the term is often employed to cover a period of history and also a major transformation in Western societies. That is, postmodernism is a consequence of the failure of modernism, which assumed a logical and ordered universe whose laws could be uncovered by science. Acceptance of the modernism ideology disappeared during the time of the First and Second World Wars, arising from global development and social and health changes. This loss of belief in the modernist enterprise has bought about the post-modern response. This response includes a radical rejection of the possibility of rational and constant knowledge and a celebration of the diverse and ephemeral; on the one hand, a critical recognition of the limits and excesses of modernism, yet a willingness to continue to see understanding without the certainties of modernist assumptions. In analysing situations or incidents the postmodernist deconstructs the situation and then reconstructs meaning. Nietzsche, in his book *Beyond Good and Evil* (1972), describes a philosopher as a male creature who is snarling, quarrelling and who often runs away from itself, is often afraid of itself – but which is too inquisitive not to keep coming back to itself again (p. 292).

Bernard Williams (1985) argued that Western philosophical questions take too much for granted and that some moral theories 'may well turn out to be mere prejudices' (p. 117). In his books Williams discusses the crisis of modern philosophy and the need for new direction in moral thinking. He argues that the cultural, social, political and religious reality of a particular ethical life is crucial to any ethical analysis of it, and to any ethical theory that might be generated. Alistair MacIntyre (1985) also warned of the danger of traditional Western modern philosophy – that is, the 'barren armchair' approach that ignores the cultural, social and historical environment in which they were written. In other words, MacIntyre said that, because postmodernist culture with its different social and historical aspects is different to the time of Kant, Bentham and Mill, etc., their theories can no longer apply or be applied.

Blum, in his book *Friendship, Altruism and Morality* (1980), writes that attention must be paid to the human emotions of sympathy, compassion, human concern and to friendship 'as a context in which these emotions play a fundamental role' (p. 1). He says that these are equally important as the rational constructs found in earlier philosophy. Other postmodernist moral philosophers are also beginning to change their attitudes and are referring to those behaviours that have emotions. For example, Hare (1981) says that our moral thinking will be incomplete if we do not 'put ourselves in the place of the person who is suffering'.

Like feminist moral philosophy, postmodernist philosophy has not been able to develop a substantive moral theory capable of directing human activity. This leaves us with many questions in moral reasoning, such as where do we go from here?

It is people who matter, not the objective approach that is evident in traditional or rationalistic philosophy, and it is the love of people that directs the moral life. That is, a health professional who is therapeutically available to clients or patients with compassion, and not the love of abstract and decontextualised principles found in earlier classical and naturalistic philosophy.

Virtue ethics

There is some debate about the origins of virtue ethics; some writers say that it comes from the ancient Greek philosophy of Aristotle, while others say it is a new way of looking at philosophy (Edwards, 1996). In this chapter Aristotle's virtues are not listed; instead we will discuss the concepts of the postmodernist philosophers Rosalind Hursthouse and Michael Slote. Virtue ethics for these writers focuses on the person who performs the action, the health professional. With this type of virtue ethics the health professional asks themself before undertaking an action, 'How should I be?'

Virtue ethics focuses on humans-as-we-are-now, and concepts such as flourishing and excellence. Virtue ethics as a distinct moral theory has as its prime focus the health professional's character. The focus being on 'how should I be?' or 'what sort of person would I be if I were to do X?' rather than solely on 'what action ought I to do?' (Watson, 1997). These questions appear to emphasise a professional's moral development, which facilitates ethical decision making.

This association with moral development is not restricted to professional learning but also includes the moral development of childhood onwards. In using virtue ethics in decision making it is said that principles and rules are not sufficient to make an ethical judgement, and that professional intuition when making an ethical decision needs also to be considered.

Activity

Stop and think about the last two sentences concerning moral upbringing, and that this is necessary when making ethical decisions. Also, consider the statement that principles and rules are not sufficient to make an ethical judgement about what is right and wrong.

➤ Do you agree with these statements? If so, why? If no, why?

Document your answers in your Ethics Portfolio for this chapter.

Moral learning as a child

The justification of using this philosophy is that the virtues, or having the virtues, are essential to live a good, flourishing life and therefore, for this to occur, the professional needs to have gained a moral education as a child. A person's upbringing is where one learns the virtues. The learning is often via recognition; after having been given some examples of, say, kindness or honesty early on, the person, as *they develop*, can branch out on their own and recognise particular situations as examples of such. The emphasis on principles as guides to right action is much less (some may say no emphasis) than in other moral theories.

In virtue ethics the health professional, to be fully virtuous, requires the right use of emotions as well as reason. Consequently, maturity and experience both in being a health professional and also in using ethics is needed before the professional can be deemed ethically wise.

Likewise, practical wisdom is an ability that the fully virtuous person has to *get things right*, to know when to be truthful and in what way. In a sense, to have practical wisdom is to have all the virtues. One can be too generous or too truthful but perhaps one cannot be too wise. However, if one is too generous then perhaps they do not quite have the virtue of generosity. So having the virtues enables one to act well (Hursthouse, 1999). Acting well is not (just) following principles or weighing consequences but requires an ability or capacity for 'moral perception'.

Activity

To illustrate how virtue ethics can be applied to a case study, we will return to Lorraine and Max (Case study 5.3).

An important point to bear in mind in application of virtues to practice is the conceptual link between the virtues and living well. So, rather than the focus being on principles such as respecting autonomy or rights such as the right to have an abortion, a virtue account would ask is having an abortion in these circumstances a virtuous or vicious act, or neither (Hursthouse, 1991).

First, you need to question their choice to have children late in life. Was the selective abortion and the financial emphasis a selfish act or a prudent one?

Next, you need to raise questions about the acceptance of the three blastocysts and the change of mind after 14 weeks. Was this lightminded, or anguished, were they irresponsible or responsible as mature adults facing a huge and important decision about raising a family and its importance in regard to a fully flourishing life or living well?

The answers to these questions would allow insight into the 'how should I be?' from Lorraine's and Max's perspective.

Pause and think

➤ So, how would a virtuous person perceive the situation of Max and Lorraine?

The use of principles and theories when making decisions

At the beginning of the chapter the use of ethical principles and rules was discussed. If you want to use these to help you make a decision, then the ethically correct option would be the one that fulfilled the most principles. For example, if you had a problem and there were two ways of going about it, the option that fulfilled or met most of the ethical principles would be the one to use.

So what do we do with ethical theories?

When each of the theories was discussed, it was explained which option would the most ethical. This is fine if we only want to use one theory. However, we have explained that:

- teleological theories emphasise the outcome or end;
- deontological theories emphasise the means or manner of the action being performed;
- feminist theories emphasise love, compassion, kindness, self-esteem and justice;
- care ethics emphasises the individual nature of the client or patient, and the situation, and that those directly involved in the care will have a different perspective from others who are divorced from the situation. Also, that by the very nature of caring the professional will experience emotions related to the client or patient and the care. Consequently, this can cause moral or ethical problems;
- virtue ethics emphasises the behaviour of the professional.

This means that there are four or five different possibilities of what is ethically correct. Therefore, if you are faced with a complex decision to make it is suggested that you use at least two different theories to gain a more balanced perspective of what would be ethically right (Hawley, 1997b).

For example, when you have a moral problem you work out three options that you could take. Apply the first theory to the options and see which one is the ethically correct option to use. Use another theory with the same options and see which option is the ethically correct one. If it highlights the same option, then that is fine. However, sometimes, because the theories can be so different, you will find that a different option is highlighted, and you end up not knowing which one to use. If this happens, you can always use a third theory, and see what you find (Hawley, 1997b).

So which theories would we suggest you use?
If you are going to use teleological theory, this needs to be balanced with either deontology or feminist principles. Likewise, if you are going to use deontology, balance this with teleological or care or virtue ethics (Hawley, 1997b).

Do not be too concerned if you are unable to work out how to do this at present, as it has only be given to you to use if you want to start using the theories in decision making. There is a whole chapter later on decision making. However, the sooner you begin practising using philosophy to help you decide which options are ethically correct the easier it becomes.

Summary

This chapter has introduced the ethical principles of autonomy, beneficence, justice and non-maleficence, and the rules of veracity and confidentiality. The ethical theories of teleology, deontology, feminist care and virtue ethics have also been briefly explained to provide you with an overview.

Ethical theories can be difficult to understand properly but it is worth the time and effort to read them, and try and gain understanding of the different perspectives. The descriptions given here can only be regarded as basic or 'rules of thumb'. They are given to provide you with the beginnings of knowledge and understanding. At times these will be very useful, and great to work with. However, you may want to explore them fully by reading more comprehensive texts. Likewise, if you want to become a health care ethicist (or bioethicist) your learning would be far more detailed and your knowledge of ethical principles, rules and theories would involve greater understanding, especially of the numerous nuances that exist.

Professional development

1 Continue to develop your Ethics Portfolio – do not forget to start a new section for this chapter.

2 Answer these questions in your portfolio:

   a. What would happen if a health professional adopted a strictly teleological approach to ethics?

   b. What would happen if they adopted a strictly deontological approach to ethics?

   c. What do you think might have happened when migration from the countries that use Western philosophical traditions occurred and people brought a new way of thinking and new frameworks to that country?

3 Read and identify the ethical issues that are part of Case study 5.3.

Can you work these out? Now check these with the following.

The ethical issues that you identified possibly included:

- Clients' or patients' rights – the couple has a right to health care as consumers and therefore have rights and responsibilities.
- Allocation of resources:
  ○ Should IVF be offered to all patients who ask for the treatment?
  ○ Are Max and Lorraine married? Do you think only married people should have access to IVF?
  ○ Should people who want special treatments such as IVF have this provided free by the government or should they pay?
- Abortion or termination of pregnancy:
  ○ Selective termination of one or more embryos in a multiple pregnancy.
  ○ Informed consent – emergency treatment: with a Caesarean operation does a woman have the right to informed consent?
- Allocation of resources: one baby needed to be sent to another hospital, as there were insufficient resources in the hospital where Lorraine gave birth.
  ○ Does a hospital need to provide unlimited numbers of neonatal intensive care cots and specialist health professionals to care for the babies?
- Illness and loss:
  ○ The baby boy's illness leads to loss and death, which was preceded by the selective termination of a boy. What rights and responsibilities do you think health professionals have in caring for a dying baby?
  ○ What rights and responsibilities do you think the parents should have when their baby is ill and dying?

4 Read the following case studies (5.4 and 5.5) and then answer the questions at the end.

Case study 5.4
Mrs Thomasina and her daughters (Hawley, 1997c)

Mrs Thomasina is a 94-year-old lady who has told her relatives over the last few years that she wants to die, as all her old friends, including her husband, have long since passed away. Mrs Thomasina developed vaginal bleeding and, on investigation, it was discovered that she had widespread carcinoma of the uterus with secondaries. However, her daughters do not want her to be told the truth about her diagnosis.

Mrs Thomasina asks the nurse looking after her what is causing the bleeding and what is wrong with her. The nurse knows from Mrs Thomasina's daughters that she will become depressed if she knows her true diagnosis. Mrs Thomasina has the prospect of a few months to live with medication, which will control the pain. The daughters say to the nurse that it would be better for their mother to have these months without having to know the truth of her diagnosis. The nurse, however, has difficulty with this opinion, as she believes the patient has the right to know the truth.

Questions

➤ Have the ethical principles (autonomy, beneficence, justice and non-maleficence) been met?

➤ Check to see if the ethical rules of confidentiality and veracity have been met by the health professionals or not? Have they been discarded?

➤ Is there justification for the ethical rules not to have been met?

Case study 5.5
Demitri or Flora MacDonald (Hawley, 1997b and c)

Demitri is a 19-year-old Greek man studying in London. Demitri was injured in a motorcycle accident. He has a serious head injury plus fractures of both legs and arms. Mrs Flora MacDonald is a 48-year-old mother, also from London, who fell and hit her head on the kerb when alighting from a bus, which resulted in a severe head injury needing emergency neurosurgery. Both patients need care in the ICU; however, there is only one bed left.

Questions

➤ Clarify your own values and beliefs in regard to age and access to health care.

➤ Who do you think should have the ICU bed?

➤ What would be your reasons?

➤ Which approach are you using (ethical principles and rules, deontological, teleological, virtue, care or feminine) in deciding who should have the bed?

Critical reflection

Write a critical reflection for this chapter to place in your Ethics Portfolio. The item or issue that you may want to work through or critically analyse could be something that you need to explore further from:

● One of the case studies.

● Reading that you have done.

● A different point of view that someone raised in discussion in class.

● A general feeling that people coming to your country should adopt the philosophy, values and beliefs, and not cling onto their previous ways.

● Clinical practice:

○ such as your values and beliefs in relation to caring, compassion and kindness to clients or patients;

○ how you have realised that the care you have provided for a patient on clinical practice was incorrect and consequently, unethical;

○ another member of the team on clinical practice is ignoring the client's or patient's rights;

○ an issue your mentor or clinical supervisor suggested that you reflect upon.

6

Eastern philosophical traditions

Georgina Hawley and Gail Lansdown

Why this chapter is important to me . . .

✔ Eastern philosophy is possibly older than Western philosophy.

✔ There is a strong relationship between Eastern philosophy and traditional Eastern medicine.

✔ Many health professionals know very little about the Eastern philosophy, culture and spirituality.

✔ The Departments of Health in the UK, Australia and New Zealand all state that health care needs to be inclusive of patients' cultural and religious ethos.

In previous chapters we have learnt where people get their values and beliefs, and their culture, but also that we are unique and individual people. There has also been discussion that ethical or moral problems can arise when health professionals just assume that the way they want to do something is ethically right and correct. Never has this been more so than with health professionals with a Western philosophical view point, who wrongly believe that theirs is the only perspective to consider. This lack of cultural sensitivity and disrespect of other traditions seriously impairs a therapeutic relationship between the client or patient and the health professional, but also destroys the client's or patient's trust and faith in the professional's ability.

Eastern philosophy follows the broad traditions which originated from, or were popular within, India, China and Japan and South East Asia. With the migration of people from these countries, it is not unusual to find such philosophies being the basis of cultures in other parts of the world such as Africa, Australia, Canada, Europe, the UK and the USA. In this chapter it is not possible to present all the Eastern philosophies, and therefore only the main ones will be explained; these are Indian, Chinese and Japanese.

It is very important to understand that, with Eastern philosophies, there is extensive blurring between philosophy, culture, and religion or spiritualities. This means that, while you might be interested in the philosophy of Buddhism, you will find that the religion or spirituality of Buddhism is slightly different from one country to another. For example, when I lived and worked as a health professional in Western Australia, the Buddhist client or patient from Laos had slightly different spiritual needs to a client or patient who was an Indian Buddhist. That is, the culture of the country causes subtle changes in relation to their spiritual needs.

One of the reasons some people erroneously believe that they only need to consider Western philosophy is that there is a clear and documented relationship between philosophy and ethics, whereas with Eastern philosophy the relationship is not as distinct. This has occurred as there was no word for ethics until the 19th century within Eastern languages. Irrespective of this, the fact that a country's philosophies are the foundation to their legal, health, education and government systems, which forms their culture, means that we need to recognise and gain an awareness of their philosophy.

Pause and think

➤ Why is understanding a person's culture important in this book, and also for you?

If you answered that you need this knowledge and understanding to be a culturally competent health professional you are correct.

This chapter is divided into four parts: first, the common principles of Eastern philosophy; second, the philosophies of India will be discussed (these include Hinduism, Islam, Buddhism and Sikhism); third, Chinese philosophies; and fourth, Japanese philosophies. This will be followed by an overview of the effect of these philosophies on the provision of medicine in both India and China. Finally, the chapter will finish with a reflection on the differences between Eastern and Western philosophies and the Professional Development section.

Activity

In your Ethics Portfolio describe or list:

➤ What are your values and beliefs about caring for people from a different culture?

➤ What are your values and beliefs towards caring for people from an Eastern culture?

➤ How far do you think health professionals should go in meeting the needs of clients or patients from other cultures?

Principles in Eastern philosophy

The Western philosophical tradition started with ethical principles born out of the normative ethical theories. Eastern philosophy does not have these same ethical theories; instead, each country has philosophies that have influenced culture and health beliefs of the people.

While there are some similarities between Indian and Chinese philosophies, there are also differences. However, there are sufficient similarities to be able to surmise common values and concepts between the two. For this reason I have named these as principles that can be used in the same way as the Western ethical principles of autonomy, beneficence, justice and non-maleficence. Consequently, I propose the Eastern philosophical principles to be harmony, respect, hospitality, modesty and balance.

Harmony

Harmony is extensive and pervasive within Eastern philosophy. It means to 'fit well together'. Another way to describe this concept is working together as congruent parts for the benefit of the whole family or department at work. In other words, there is cooperation, good will and unity between family members or work colleagues.

When harmony is displayed (or manifested) there is order and congruity between individual family members within the whole of the family, resulting in agreement and compatibility. In work it means that team members will strive for harmony in a working relationship and not create antagonism, hostility and conflict. Harmony also implies not harming other people! Consequently, harmony would not be met by being openly disagreeable, disobeying one's parents, being unfriendly at work, being in disagreement with senior colleagues or authority, or harming or hurting someone or something.

When I first started to explore the notion of harmony and then needed to teach about it, I contacted colleagues at Chibu University in Japan who told me that harmony is as important in Eastern philosophy as autonomy is in Western philosophy. Moreover, it is vital in decision-making. My difficulty arose as I had automatically compared the two concepts (autonomy and harmony) and there was dissonance. However, I found harmony to be compatible with Western postmodernist philosophies of care and virtue ethics.

In fact, it is extremely compatible with the ethics of caring and the need to work collaboratively with clients, patients and peers in interprofessional teamwork.

Respect

Respect is regarded as essential in relationships with each other. It is respect that provides the connections in relationships that bring about harmony. Respect includes politeness and kind regard, and giving and exchanging salutations with each other.

In both Indian and Chinese philosophies, there is an attitude of deference towards parents. In early Chinese philosophy there was automatic obedience to the ruler, which was not to be violated. This was followed by those in authority, and then by those members of the family that were older and wiser. This respect was also given as veneration to the Gods.

Respect also involves modesty. That is, of respecting the hidden beauty of one's own body and respecting the physical form of another person, particularly that of a person of the opposite sex. For this reason, those aspects or parts of the body related to sexual behaviour are covered and are not displayed to anyone else except between husband and wife.

Likewise, sex and related topics are not discussed with other people, except between husband and wife.

This respect implies recognition of the humanness of one person to another: that a person would not ignore, abuse, hurt or neglect another.

Hospitality

Hospitality is showing consideration and right behaviour, warmth and welcome to other people. This will include guests in a person's home and the welcoming of strangers. Hospitality is also offering food to one another. In India particularly it involves welcoming strangers into the home and sharing a meal. Hospitality is also a way of demonstrating respect and love for one another. For example, when someone is ill in hospital the family and friends bring food for the person.

Hospitality would be the health professional offering a patient a place to set up their shrine while in hospital (on the bedside cabinet or locker, heart table or window ledge). Hospitality would also ensure that the Chinese family are told bad news in a private and quiet atmosphere.

Hospitality would not be met by ignoring someone, being ignorant of their feelings, intolerant, narrow-minded, or being unappproachable.

Balance

Balance is striving for equilibrium within the body, with family, with God(s), and with the environment.

Balance is closely related to harmony, but slightly different. For example, balance within the body is in relation to the positive and negative energies, of striving to maintain these in balance. It is balance between the self and the whole of one's family that brings about harmony.

Being in balance with God(s) means that worldly material aspects take second place to achieve being right with God(s). This is done through good actions, by shunning worldly excesses, perhaps meditating, prayer or doing yoga to control one's mind on the higher things in life, including karma and reincarnation. Consequently, balance can be achieved through meditation, yoga, food, and behaviours of being good and kind, and shunning material and worldly excesses.

Balance with the environment entails not harming living creatures and protecting the environment.

Balance would not be achieved or met through abusing one's body, through engaging in bodily excesses, by being disinterested in God(s), by being out of harmony with parents, or by deliberately harming those creatures that need protection (including those that are spiritual (cow) and may contain the soul of a reincarnated person).

The Eastern philosophies have ethical principles of harmony, respect (including modesty), hospitality and balance. However, when reading this chapter you might decide there are other moral principles.

Part A Indian philosophies (includes Pakistan and Bangladesh)

Activity

Read the following case study.

Case study 6.1
Raj, Joseph and Ingrid

Raj is a young man of 40 years. He is an industrious scholar who has minimum contact with society. Much of his day is spent praying, reading and practising yoga to conquer his mind and senses so that he can concentrate on the higher things to reach heaven.

People in the village in which he lives in southern rural India quite often leave food at his door, as they know he sometimes forgets to eat. They in turn pray that Raj will stay a long time in their village before moving on, as they regard him as a man of God.

One day a 20-year-old distant cousin Joseph from the UK comes to visit. Joseph is taking a break from his undergraduate studies in mental health nursing. He is accompanied by 19-year-old girlfriend Ingrid who is an occupational therapy student from the same university. They are backpacking around Asia and Joseph decided to come and see his distant cousin whom his grandmother told him lived some-where near this village. At first Joseph couldn't believe his luck in finding Raj, as he had become short of money and he and his girlfriend needed somewhere to stay for a while.

However, the stopover was not as Joseph and Ingrid had planned. First, Raj invited them to join him in prayer, yoga and offered them his religious books to read. These activities did not interest Joseph and Ingrid who, back in England, liked going to the Student Union bar and nightclubs. Second, Raj has little food in his simple hut and is not concerned with eating. Also, he said that Ingrid would need to stay with a family in the village as she was an unmarried woman and could not sleep in the same house as Joseph and himself.

As the days went by Joseph became appalled by the simple quiet way in which Raj lived and became convinced that he was mentally ill, and perhaps suffering from some psychotic illness. Ingrid agreed with him, and they tried to remove Raj from the village and take him to a major town for psychiatric treatment. Raj refused to go, saying there is nothing wrong.

Joseph confers with Ingrid and says, 'I think we have an ethical problem; there are two ways we can handle this, but neither of them seem right.'

The name or term Indian philosophy refers to any of several traditions including Hinduism, Buddhism, Islam, Jainism, Carvaka and Sikhism philosophies (Hayes, 1998). In this chapter, Hinduism, Buddhism, Islam (Muslim) and Sikhism are outlined. Indian philosophy is perhaps the most comparable to Western philosophy.

Hindu philosophy

For Hindu people in India the principles of Hindu philosophy are a way of life as they are embedded within the social and cultural systems, and reflected within the values and beliefs of the people and their religious practices. The Hindu philosophy has its origin in ancient Vedic culture at least as far back as 2000 BC. The Hindu understanding of being a person centres on the relationship between the body and the soul (known as atman). Hindus believe that a person's material world is responsible for their sorrows (because of their lust, greed and anger, and therefore the person would be destined towards hell). The main principles within Hinduism are:

- Live a natural healthy life – be like the birds and animals.
- Be non-violent.
- Give selfless service to others.
- Act with love and good conduct.
- Reincarnation, a person's soul or 'true self' returns to the material world after physical death, to be reborn in a new body.
- Karma: the law of cause and effect; that is, each individual creates his or her own destiny by thoughts, words and deeds. Karma can accrue over many lifetimes.
- As a result of reincarnation and non-violence meat is not eaten because it involves harming a living creature.
- Strong belief in astrology.
- Older people are valued as being wise.
- The concept of purity is important and this is related to washing (showers are preferred to baths).
- Engage in meditation (including yoga) and/or prayer, usually following morning and evening showers.

The largest Hindu community outside India is in the UK. These people have tried to maintain their cultural and spiritual identity using their temples to ensure that the languages of Gujurati, Hindi and Punjabi continue to be spoken. Hindus believe that their philosophy, culture, language and spirituality are inseparably bound together and that, if they lose the language, the others will soon be lost.

Hindu society – the caste system

Hindu society is traditionally divided into four classes and many interdependent subcastes. This system goes back thousands of years. The cast and subcaste system into which a person is born defines their social and religious status, occupation, social contacts, and social and religious duties. Although it is now illegal in India to discriminate on the grounds of caste, even with the demands of modern life the caste system is slow to change. For the Hindu person living outside India, especially an older person, aspects of the caste system, e.g. food restrictions and religious practices, may still be important (Helman, 2000).

The highest caste (varna) is the Brahmin (white). These are the priests who perform religious services, rituals and chant the scriptures. The second (red) varna is the Kshatriya. This caste are the rulers, warriors and armed service people. The third (yellow) varna is the Vaisya. This caste are the farmers and business people responsible for the economic and social life. The fourth (black) varna is the Sudra. These are the people who provide basic services for others. The last group of people is the untouchables, who do not belong to any caste. These people carry out the most menial and basic of tasks, such as burying the dead, tanning leather, working on the roads, etc.

For many centuries the untouchables were banned from social life (which also meant being excluded from Hindu temples). In 1950, the law changed and allowed all Hindu people, irrespective of caste, access to a temple. Although the caste system is banned, it still operates in village life and is part of the culture. Marriage is nearly always restricted to one's own caste.

Modern Hindu philosophies

1 The modern movements of ISKCON, sometimes called the Hare Krishna movement – this can now be studied as a theological discourse at some universities in the USA (Clear, 1998).

2 Different schools of yoga (based on the ancient Vedic philosophy) – these yoga exercises or systems lay down elaborate prescriptions for gradually gaining physical and mental control and mastery over the 'personal self', both body and mind. The aim is to gain a level of consciousness that has intensified sufficiently to allow for the awareness of one's 'real self' (the soul or atman), as distinct from personal feelings and thoughts. Achieving the goal of yoga is known as moksha, nirvana and samadhi (Clear, 1998).

3 A proliferation of Hindu Vedanta schools – each of these interprets the Hindu philosophy texts in its own way and has produced its own series of subcommentaries.

From the Hindu philosophies which are part of cultural life come various forms of Hindu spirituality or religions. However, it is important to realise that not all Hindus are religious. Their belief is in the order of the universe – that summer follows spring, day follows night, and harvest follows seed time.

Spirituality and religion

Hinduism is generally considered to be the oldest major world religion still practised today. It has its origin in ancient Vedic culture at least as far back as 2000 BC. Hinduism is said to be a monotheistic religion whose followers believe in one God, Brahman (the absolute spirit), who is beyond human reach and understanding. However, Hinduism is also characterised by a diverse array of belief systems, practices and scriptures. There is no specific religious founder, nor one Holy Book, nor central authority over the Hindu beliefs and practices (Helman, 2000; Knott, 2000). For many Hindus, there is not just one God; instead, they believe in a vast array of gods.

Today, Hinduism is the world's third largest religion, with approximately 1.05 billion followers worldwide, the majority of whom live in the Indian subcontinent, with others in the USA, Australia, New Zealand, Fiji, South Africa and the UK.

Religious law – the dharma

A Hindu person knows that to live by the dharma law or way is the method or way to reach the higher truths. That is, if they follow the laws they will be able to live in harmony with dharma and proceed quicker towards moksha, or personal liberation (Helman, 2000; Knott,

2000). Other Indian religions such as Buddhism, Jainism and Sikhism also use the concept of dharma (Ames, 1998).

Belief in reincarnation is very strong within the religion. Hindu teaching or doctrine states that a person's personality, spirit, soul, true self or 'I' (or critical parts of these) returns to the material world after physical death to be reborn in a new body. This is a natural process and includes all experiences from each lifetime (Helman, 2000; Knott, 2000).

Religious beliefs

Irrespective of which Hindu system a person follows, there are common beliefs (Helman, 2000; Knott, 2000). When you read these you will easily see the strong relationship of philosophy to religion.

- The existence of a supreme spirit (Brahma or parabrahma).
- An immortal soul that exists in all living things (the cycle of birth, death and rebirth through which everyone must go). That is, reincarnation, a person's soul or 'true self' returns to the material world after physical death, to be reborn in a new body.
- Release from the cycle of rebirth is the ultimate aim of life.
- A clear code of dutiful and right behaviour, including selfless service to others, and act with love, and good conduct.
- Compassion and non-violence.
- The supreme duty to seek truth.
- Care and compassion to older people, obedience to parents, and hospitality to visitors.
- Also included in this list are the main components of Hinduism (see p. 106).

Hindu religious practices which influence health care

The family is central to Hindu life and stresses the sanctity of marriage. There is an expectation to marry and have children, with both parents being active in their children's well-being and education. A Hindu woman must honour and obey her husband, and he must treat his wife with respect and kindness (Helman, 2000).

Birth
Noting the exact time of a baby's birth is important for the child's horoscope. While traditionally in India a husband would not be present at the birth, this is not the case in the UK and Australia. A Hindu baby is breast-fed and a boy is not circumcised. The baby is usually named at a celebration on the 10th day after his or her birth.

Illness, accident and injury
Hinduism adheres to the theory of karma (the law of cause and effect). Each person creates his or her own destiny by thoughts, words and deeds. Illness, accidents and injuries result from the karma one creates and are seen as a means of purification. Karma is said to amalgamate over many lifetimes. Hence, a person may be suffering an illness caused by behaviour in a previous life or the present. A Hindu client or patient will not normally refuse

medication, including pain relief. However, if the medication contains alcohol or animal products it may be refused (Helman, 2000; Henley and Schott, 2002).

Illness is said to be caused by imbalances within the three body humours:

- Wind (vata)
- Bile (pitta)
- Phlegm (kapha)

This is based on the hot and cold theory, which also relates to food and medication.

When someone is ill a large number of relatives may wish to visit, and they may pray and sing hymns of comfort to the person.

Protective jewellery or sacred strings may be worn, and a health professional should not remove these without discussing the importance of the removal beforehand.

Birth control and abortion
Birth control is both approved and practised. Abortion is frowned upon, with no exception for rape and known fetal deformities.

Dietary restrictions
Most Hindus are strict vegetarians, as this is what is recommended in the scriptures. However, they are free to choose their own diet, with the exception of beef and pork.

They may refuse capsules because they may be derived from beef or pork (contain gelatine made from the animal). Fasting is common among Hindus.

Prayer
Most devout Hindus pray at least three times a day (sunrise, noon and sunset). Physical and spiritual cleanliness are closely linked, therefore a person will need to be clean in order to pray. Some people will shower and put on clean clothes before praying, or at least rinse out their mouth (to get rid of impure acts or thoughts).

For prayer, the person will usually sit on the floor or stand. Women who are menstruating will not pray and neither will they do so until 40 days after the birth of a baby. To help with praying the person may use a mala (a string of beads), which they keep in a small cloth bag. At home or in hospital a Hindu person may set up a small shrine with a statue or picture, a candle or incense to help focus the mind during prayer, and may want to give an offering to their God (flowers, fruit or a glass of water or milk). Sometimes they may ring a bell to catch the attention of the gods (Henley and Schott, 2002; Knott, 2000).

Assistance with prayer
An ill person who cannot get out of bed will wish to wash before prayer and have the opportunity to rinse their mouth. Some may want to wash their anal area with water after each bowel action so that they are always clean for prayer (Helman, 2000; Henley and Schott, 2002).

The patient who is incontinent will not want to pray while soiled and therefore needs to be washed and have clean linen. Reassurances of their cleanliness will also help. When caring for the patient it is also important to protect their modesty at all times.

Use of holy water

Since water has special significance, Hindus like to go on pilgrimages to sacred rivers such as the Ganges and may bring back holy water for an ill person to use. At times, a pandit or pujura (Hindu holy person) may bring this to an ill person to use (Helman, 2000).

Dying person

A dying person may wish to be at home so they can be sure that everything is done correctly. If the person is dying in hospital, it is important that their loved ones are with them at all times and that their religious rituals are performed (saying prayers, sprinkling of water, wetting the lips with water, and placing a coloured mark on the forehead).

Traditionally the dying person wishes to be close to earth, so placing a mattress on the floor is believed to ease the departure of the soul (Narayanasamy, 2001). If death occurs suddenly (e.g. from accident or murder) this may be regarded as unlucky and may cause distress to the relatives (Henley and Schott, 2002).

Organ donation

There is no religious basis to refuse organ donation; however, some relatives may refuse to donate if they belief that the person should be whole and complete at the time of cremation or burial (Henley and Schott, 2002).

Activity

Re-read Case study 6.1 to determine how knowledge and understanding of Hindu philosophy, culture and religion helps you to understand the ethical problem. Document your answers in your Ethics Portfolio.

Questions

➤ What do you think of the problem now that you have an understanding of Hindu philosophy?

➤ Work through the problem using the ethical framework (Figure 3.1 on p. 40).

In answer to the activity questions, first we can apply the ethical framework (see Figure 3.1), which consists of the three stages of communication, understanding and reflection.

Stage 1 – communication

The first stage of the ethical framework is communication, which involves gathering as much data as possible about the situation, and also remembering the intricacies of the communication process itself. So what is happening in the scenario? Basically, Raj has led a peaceful life until Joseph and Ingrid come along and they think that the life he is living is not right; in fact they believe that he is mentally ill. This is a radical thought!

Have Joseph and Ingrid gathered information to support this diagnosis? So what do they have?

● First, there is very little food in the house and Raj is not concerned about eating. Now, although some people with mental illness are not concerned with eating, it is not the sole sign and symptom.

- Second, he said that Ingrid could not live with him and Joseph as she was an unmarried woman and must stay with another family in the village. Such behaviour is not a sign and symptom of mental illness.
- Third, the quiet manner in which Raj lives. Some people who are mentally ill are quiet and withdrawn, but it is not the prime sign and symptom of being mentally ill.

So how could Joseph and Ingrid get more information to support their view? They could ask Raj himself if he has any of the other signs and symptoms of mental illness. However, they did not do this. Perhaps they were not very far along in their degree and lacked full knowledge of mental illness.

Stage 2 – understanding

The second stage of the ethical framework is understanding. This is a continuation of communication, where a person gains more knowledge, asks questions, and talks openly about the perceived problem.

- Joseph and Ingrid could ask Raj's fellow villagers what they think? Since they are in southern India where the majority of people speak English, this should not be too difficult for two people from the UK. In fact, the villagers like Raj and regard him as a holy man of God.
- Joseph and Ingrid could also ask the village people about their social customs to assess whether Raj's behaviour was normal or if he did have a mental illness. However, it does not appear that this has been done.
- In fact, by talking to Raj and/or the other people of the village Joseph and Ingrid would have discover that Raj's simple way of life and behaviours are the manifestations of his Hindu religion. That is:
  - Raj was seeking the 'one unitary truth', through reading the divine word of Aum, praying to the divine (atman/Brahman) and the power of mantras. That is, to live by the dharma law or way to reach the higher truths.
  - He had adopted the simple clear code of Hindu religious life of dutiful and right behaviour, which included compassion and non-violence to others and hospitality to visitors. Consequently, his way of life of praying, reading and practising yoga to conquer his mind and senses was simply the manifestation or the acting out of his religious beliefs to concentrate on the higher things required to reach heaven.
  - Raj would have had a small shrine with a statue, picture, a candle or incense to help focus his mind during prayer, and may have given offerings to his God (flowers, fruit or a glass of water or milk). He may have rung a bell to catch the attention of the Gods. These prayers would have been said at least three times a day (sunrise, noon and sunset), and involved cleanliness in order to pray (washing and changing clothes). Raj may have practised washing his anal area with water after a bowel action to be clean for prayer.
  - He may also have used a mala during prayers (a string of beads which he would have kept in a small cloth bag).
  - Modesty would be important to Raj, and so would the sanctity of marriage. Therefore his arrangement for Ingrid to stay with a family in the village would be part of his religious beliefs.
  - Likewise, he would not drink alcohol or eat animal products.

Stage 3 – reflection

The third stage of the ethical framework is reflection about the problem, including examining each of the previous steps.

- What is the perceived problem? If at this stage of the process Joseph and Ingrid had asked themselves this question, they would have realised that there is no problem with Raj and that he just has a different way of life to what Joseph and Ingrid had seen or experienced in the UK.

- Another question Joseph and Ingrid needed to ask themselves was whether they have all the information to support their perception of the problem. In fact, they have no information to support their idea that Raj has a mental illness and psychosis; rather they should know that his way of life was that of Hindu religious behaviour.

- In the reflection question 'Is it just my feelings that have caused me to perceive this situation as I have?' the answer would be yes, but also their lack of knowledge and understanding of the Hindu philosophy, culture and religious practices contributed to their misunderstanding.

Summing up of Case study 6.1 – Raj, Joseph and Ingrid

In conclusion, the problem that Joseph and Ingrid perceived was not an ethical problem for them, but rather their lack of understanding of Hindu philosophy, culture and religious practices.

In this case study, we have two people with a Western philosophical tradition finding out how different the Eastern way of life is. However, it could have been the reverse. That is, someone from the Eastern tradition experiencing the Western way. Would they also have thought that their host was mentally ill and want to take him for treatment?

There are many models of cultural care available, such as those mentioned in Chapter 2. However, we will now mention another, and that is the Sunrise Model by Madeline Leininger. According to Leininger, mistakes such as those made by Joseph and Ingrid can be minimised if health professionals follow a model that depicts the different aspects of a cultural world view such as technological, religious, philosophical, kinship and social, cultural and values, political and legal, economic, and educational factors. The idea is that a health professional collects all this data to use when planning the care and treatment of a person (Leininger, 1998).

Activity

Answer these questions and write your responses in your Ethics Portfolio for this chapter.

➤ If you are not a Hindu, how different are these values and beliefs from your own?

➤ In what way are they different?

Buddhist philosophy

Buddhist philosophy is based on the teachings of Gautama Buddha (c. 563–483 BC). It includes the concept of ethics (just like Western philosophy). The basics of Buddhist philosophy and/or religion are respecting human relationships, non-violence, meditation and karma. Buddhists believe that Buddha gave many teachings, including:

- to do no evil (including lying, stealing and killing);
- to cultivate good (to be against greed, hatred and folly); and
- to purify one's mind (through self-control, meditation and reflection of personal behaviour).

Buddhists use the five precepts to guide their behaviour.

- Avoid harming any living thing.
- Avoid taking what is not given.
- Avoid all sexual misconduct.
- Avoid all unworthy speech, such as lying, rumour spreading and gossip.
- Avoid all contact with illicit drugs and alcohol.

Buddhism did not sink deep roots in India. Instead, it spread in different forms south into Sri Lanka and south-east Asia, and north through Tibet to China, Korea and Japan. In the process, Buddhism suffered the same fate as the Hindu philosophy in that it became a religion. Consequently, when providing health care to a Buddhist from Tibet, you will find that their beliefs will be slightly different from a Buddhist from Laos or South Korea.

Spirituality and religion

Buddhism is based on the same teaching as the founder of the philosophy. That is, Siddhartha Gautama, the Indian prince later known as the Buddha, or one who is Awake (the word being derived from the Sanskrit 'bud' – 'to awaken'). The question of god(s) is largely irrelevant in Buddhism, though some sects (notably Tibetan Buddhism) do venerate a number of gods drawn from local indigenous belief systems (Helman, 2000).

Beliefs
The four noble truths and the eightfold path are Buddha's teachings. The four noble truths consist of the following.

- All living things are characterised by suffering and unhappiness.
- It is the wrong desire and selfishness that has caused suffering.
- When a person gets rid of the wrong desires and selfishness then suffering and unhappiness will lessen.
- The middle way between asceticism and hedonism is the only way to remove this craving.

The means to remove wrong desires and selfishness are through the eightfold path to enlightenment.

The Buddhist needs to have a complete understanding of life, involving:

- right outlook and motives;
- right speech, and not to lie or gossip;
- be good, by not doing evil things and have 'perfect conduct';
- earn a wage or salary according to Buddhist teaching;
- develop self-discipline to make the right efforts in life;

- undertake mental exercises in self-awareness and concentration to develop and attain right mindfulness; and
- regularly meditate and undertake self-analysis, and Buddhist philosophy and teaching.

Most Buddhist sects believe in karma, a cause-and-effect relationship between all that has been done and all that will be done. Events that occur are held to be the direct result of previous events. One effect of karma is rebirth. At death, the karma from a given life determines the nature of the next life's existence. The ultimate goal of a Buddhist practitioner is to eliminate karma (both good and bad), end the cycle of rebirth and suffering, and attain nirvana (Carrithers, 2001; Hayes, 1998; Hopkins and His Holiness the Dalai Lama, 2002). When translated this is nothingness or blissful oblivion.

Balance is the key element in a person's approach to life, in which extremes are avoided, and loving kindness (in which the person identifies with oneself) is supplemented by compassion for suffering (Carrithers, 2001).

Today, Buddhism is a small minority, having been driven out of India through religious wars with the Hindus and Muslims. However, Buddhism in other Eastern countries continues to flourish.

Buddhist religious practices which influence health care

Birth and death
Buddhists believe that, since birth has occurred death will also happen, and that a Buddhist prepares for death from birth. There is also the belief in reincarnation, and therefore they would not see the need for extraordinary treatments in keeping themselves alive.

Since a Buddhist prepares for their death since birth, they are psychologically prepared for the event, which occurs with dignity and calmness. They like to have, and maintain, a clear mind and so will only use pain relief for the analgesia effects and will refuse stronger doses that would cause sedation.

Death
Death is to be calm and peaceful, surrounded by family and friends who chant prayers of comfort to the dying person. There are no wailing pleas for the person to stay alive or crying, as it is necessary for a peaceful death to occur to allow the spirit to ascend from the physical body to another life.

Diet
The diet is vegetarian, and family and friends will bring the ill person food while they are in hospital, as they believe that food affects both body and mind.

Prayer and meditation
The client or patient in hospital will want to remove their shoes before entering a room with a shrine or statue of Buddha. They then place their hands together before prostrating themselves in either a kneeling or standing position.

There are no prayers as such, as there is not a God or gods to pray to; instead silent meditation takes place to create the right mind. Buddhists will use a shrine to aid their thoughts and meditation; light, incense and flowers may be placed on the shrine. Flowers are a reminder of the impermanence of life. Light dispels darkness, and incense is used as a reminder of the lasting fragrance of the Buddha's teaching.

For the client or patient who is unable to get out of bed, a small shrine can be assembled on their locker or nearby table. It is helpful, if possible, to offer a small statue of Buddha, one or two small flowers, a candle to light and incense. However, with health and safety laws the last two might be a bit difficult.

Meditation has proven psychophysiological rewards in that it lowers blood pressure and slows the pulse and calms respirations; it also increases concentration and therefore improves learning.

Islamic philosophy

Islamic philosophy is not indigenous to India; instead, Arab traders introduced it into the Indian subcontinent. This began in the early 7th century. Muslims coming south from the regions of Mecca and Baghdad brought with them their ideology, their philosophy and religion, their beliefs and practices, expounding their understanding of the Qur'an, the Hadith and the Sunnah (Leaman, 1998).

Islam is an Arabic word meaning to submit, and a Muslim submits to the will of Allah (God), who is creator and ruler of the universe.

Teachings of the Qur'an (or Koran)

The Qur'an is a book essentially religious, not philosophical, but it deals with all those problems which religion and philosophy have in common. Both have to say something about God, the world, the individual soul, and the interrelations of good and evil, free will, and life after death. Muslims believe that the Qur'an is the word of God – eternal, absolute and incomparable. The Qur'an forbids Muslims to be money-lenders or to behave unethically.

Women are considered equal to men, but different and therefore there are complementary roles for each. Segregation between men and women exists primarily to minimise physical contact so that illicit relationships do not develop. Physical contact between members of the opposite sex is strongly discouraged, although this is relaxed if medical treatment is required.

In Islamic culture, respect and esteem increase with age. Elderly parents are respected because of their life experiences and their hierarchical position within the family unit.

Religion

Islamic beliefs usually have a central role in the lives of many Muslims. There are two main branches of Islamic belief, Sunni and Shi'ah (or Shi'te). For Sunnis (meaning the path) the Qur'an is a fundamental and absolute Holy Book, and so the group rejects the views and customs of minority groups. The Shi'te believe that they are the descendants of Muhammed and are therefore the spiritual leaders (hence perfect and infallible) of Islam.

The Islamic belief system is divided into internal and external forms of worship. The internal worship (imaan) has seven facets, which include:

● oneness with God (Allah);

● Allah's angels;

● Allah's books;

● Allah's messengers;

● the day of judgement (the hour of reckoning);

● destiny or fate (Al-Qadar); and

● life after death.

External worship consists of five basic duties or pillars. These include:

● Shahadah (deep understanding and acceptance of Allah and prophet Mohammed as the final messenger);

● Salah (five compulsory daily prayers);

● Zakah (giving charity to the poor);

● fasting (abstaining from eating during daylight hours in the month of Ramadan);

● Hajj (if a person can afford to do so, a pilgrimage to Mecca). Inherent within the philosophy or religion are the four noble truths.

Types of prayer

There are two types of prayer, Salab or ritual prayer, and du'a or private prayer. Salab is done five times a day after the believer has performed the necessary wudu or washing. Salab involves moving through a sequence of actions and reciting of prayers. Du'a can be offered to Allah at any time, and can include prayers for thanksgiving, cries for help or prayers asking for success.

Health beliefs

It is generally held that a Muslim's faith protects them from ill-health as well as helping to manage and cope with health problems when they do occur. Among Muslims, there is a strong tendency to conceptualise illness as occurring to the will of God (Allah), who is understood to be a higher power than can be perceived by the senses. Central to this is the belief in Al-Qadar. It is believed that everyone's Qadar is written at conception, and whatever happens in life cannot be changed, except through supplication, and it is within the grace of Allah whether to accept or not. All life events are under the control of Allah and can only be changed by him.

In many cases human suffering is also looked upon as being a means to an end. When a person is afflicted, they should not complain and instead endure the illness patiently, as this is the way of being forgiven for sins and balancing rewards. Illness is also a trial placed on people by Allah to test their patience, piety, devotion and reliance.

Modesty

Women are bought up to be modest and, during a medical examination, modesty should be respected and, if possible, the examination performed by a female doctor. While menstruating or having vaginal loss, a woman is exempt from ritual prayer, although she may request privacy for personal devotions. Matters concerning family (birth control, abortion, pregnancy) require both spouses to agree. Cultural taboos dictate that sex should remain a very private matter between husband and wife.

Birth control and abortion

Birth control is permitted if the prescribed method does not have any adverse effect on the health of either spouse and if does not lead to permanent sterilisation. Abortion is permitted prior to 120 days, when the woman's health is in danger, or if it means she needs to cease breast-feeding another child, or for rape.

Birth

All babies are gifts from Allah and, within minutes of the birth, the words of Allah are whispered in the baby's ear. When 7 days old the head is shaved and the equivalent weight is given in silver or gold to the poor.

Dying and death

Muslims strongly believe in the resurrection, and the dying person recites the Shahadah while relatives read passages from the Qur'an. The head of the dying person needs to be raised and the bed turned so that they can see Mecca. After death the body is washed three times and is wrapped in three white sheets. At the funeral no coffin is used; instead the corpse is placed directly in the grave (on the soil), with the body lying on its right side and head raised to Mecca.

Sikhism

Sikhism is not a philosophy but a religion that has become a way of life (and therefore a culture). The beliefs and values are not part of original Indian history. Instead, they were developed as a means to bring Hindu and Islamic philosophies and religions together. This occurred in the 15th century after centuries of fighting between Muslims and Hindus. The founder of this religion is Nanak, a Hindu by birth who refused to undertake the Hindu religious rituals (Helman, 2000).

Sikhism is the newest of the Indian religions and members follow a code of discipline that includes:

- the reciting of five hymns each day;
- no drinking alcohol or taking drugs;
- no stealing or gambling;
- no adultery;
- serve all members of humanity, especially the poor;
- be willing to serve God, the true guru, in any way;

- must wear the 5 Ks:
  - kesh, the unshorn beard which is the sign of holiness and dedication to God;
  - kirpan, the sword, symbolising willingness to fight against physical and spiritual oppression;
  - kangha, the comb, which is essential to basic cleanliness, one of the foundations of Sikhism;
  - kara, the steel bracelet worn on the right wrist as a reminder that God is one, and the link between God and the worshipper is unbreakable;
  - kaccha, the traditional shorts, worn to show that the person is always ready to defend Sikhism (Keene, 2002).

The word 'Sikh' in the Punjabi language means 'disciple'. Sikhs are the disciples of God who follow the writings and teachings of the Ten Sikh Gurus. The wisdom of these teachings in Sri Guru Granth Sahib is practical and universal in their appeal (Helman, 2000). When becoming a Sikh a male adds 'Singh' to his name and a female 'Kaur'. The Sikh creed they say is:

> I observe neither Hindu fasting nor the ritual of the Muslim Ramadan month; Him I serve who at the last shall save. The Lord of universe of the Hindus, Gosain, and Allah to me are one; from Hindus and Muslims have I broken free. I perform neither Kaaba pilgrimage nor at bathing spots worship; one sole Lord I serve, and no other. I perform neither the Hindu worship nor the Muslim prayer; to the Sole Formless Lord in my heart I bow. We are neither Hindus nor Muslims; our body and life belong to the One Supreme Being who alone is both Ram and Allah for us.

Beliefs

The three aspects of belief are intertwined: these are God, the search for truth and reincarnation. God is present in the world in the souls of people, and Sikhism stresses a highly personal relationship with God. Each person needs to discover God for himself or herself. All people are equal and there is no difference between men and women. Sikhism retains a belief in reincarnation and karma. It is only by meditating on God's name and by serving others that release from the cycle of birth, life and death can be achieved. Good karma means rebirth as a human being and bad karma leads to rebirth as an animal. The place of liberation is nirvana, a restoration of the unity that the soul once enjoyed with God. This can be brought closer by congregating with others and singing hymns and praying (Keene, 2002).

The temple or gurdwara is important for Sikhs, and the inside is considered holy ground (therefore the head is covered and shoes are removed). Here the Guru Granth Sahib (Holy Book) is available for anyone to read, or have it read to them. After the service is Langar, when people come together and eat karah parshad (holy food) together. Also, Nam or Sat Guru, repeating God's name over and over in their hearts. When a Sikh meditates continually on Nam they are bringing the essence of God into their lives (Keene, 2002).

In 1947 the Sikhs' homeland of the Punjab was divided into India and Pakistan, and many left to settle in the USA and Great Britain.

Indian health care

Given the differences between Western and Eastern philosophy, culture and religion, it is not surprising that there is also traditional Eastern medicine, which is different from Western medicine. In India today there are strong indigenous systems of healing alongside Western medical health care concepts. Both the traditional complementary ways of medicine are legitimate avenues for providing health care and both receive government funding (Helman, 2000; Henley and Schott, 2002).

Indigenous or traditional health care

There are 91 recognised Ayurvedic (Hindu) and 10 Urani (Muslim) medical schools in India, Pakistan and Bangladesh. In some areas Ayurvedic medicine is used as stand-alone treatment, whereas in other areas (particularly the rural areas) it is complementary to Western medicine. Ayurvedica is based on ancient Hindu texts and has been influenced over the years by ideas from other cultures. The Urani or Hilmat system originated in ancient Greece and the Middle East, and came to India with the Islamic culture. Another form of traditional medicine is the Siddha, which is mainly used by the Tamil people in southern India and Sri Lanka.

Although these systems have different emphasis and methods, all work on the premise that different elements can cause imbalances in physical, mental and spiritual health, and can therefore cause illness. Diagnosis is by observation, discussion and the taking of the person's pulses. The aim of treatment is to restore the balance, which can be through diet, exercise and life style. Medication derived from herbs is a common treatment. The advantage for the people in India is that consultation and treatment by these practitioners is cheaper than for Western medicine (Helman, 2000; Henley and Schott, 2002).

Like all cultures, Indian people have beliefs about what they should and should not eat to be healthy (Helman, 2000; Henley and Schott, 2002). These foods are either:

- Hot foods which are salty, sour or high in animal protein. These are said to cause increases in body temperature and blood pressure, and lead to overexcitement.
- Cold foods which are sweet, bitter or astringent. These are said to cause a decrease in body temperature and blood pressure, and calm the emotions. These help to make people cheerful and strong.

The care of the Indian client or patient

Although we have provided specific health beliefs for the main philosophies, cultures and religions, you may need to know more if looking after an Indian with health beliefs which have not been mentioned. Consequently, the following overview is provided that includes the smaller or less-well-known philosophies and cultures. While individual philosophies and cultural norms are not given, we hope that the health beliefs will be useful. However, when providing care and treatments for another culture 'if in doubt, ask and clarify'.

Diet and foods

Families and friends will demonstrate their love and friendship to the client or patient in hospital by bringing the foods which they believe will make the patient better. These foods are soft (mashed) mixtures, such as rice with ghee, lentils or potatoes. Light soups with bread or dry chapattis are also recommended. This is because the sick Indian needs to avoid very spicy, oily or rich foods (those named as 'hot' above). Such foods are thought to delay healing. Soft puddings such as tapioca and sago are welcomed. Fresh fruit (being a 'cold' food) will aid in the healing of the person (Helman, 2000; Henley and Schott, 2002).

Family and personal care

Modesty is vitally important in the Indian family. A woman will want to keep herself covered, and likewise a man (from the waist to knees). Hospital gowns that do not sufficiently cover the body are the cause of extreme embarrassment, especially if the patient is seen like that by strangers (health professionals). Consequently, many people will want to wear a lighter version of their traditional dress in hospital.

Shoes are regarded as dirty, and therefore will need to be removed on entering an Indian's home. Shoes also need to be kept apart from other possessions; therefore, they should not be placed in a hospital cupboard or locker with other possessions, but on the floor by the doorway (Helman, 2000; Henley and Schott, 2002).

An Indian wife will provide physical care for the males in her family, even including intimate care for her husband. However, it may be difficult for a husband to provide intimate care for his wife because she could feel humiliated and ashamed. These forms of modesty need to be taken into consideration by health professionals when caring and providing treatment. For example, the Sikh woman in labour; even though she is going to deliver the baby very soon she will still want to keep her underpants on. However, her cultural and religious beliefs can be respected by helping her to slip the underpants down until only one leg is inside. The woman's thighs are then covered with a loosely draped sheet. In this way the woman is not breaking her cultural rules, and her health and that of the baby are not compromised (Helman, 2000; Henley and Schott, 2002).

Water is associated with cleanliness and spiritual purity, consequently there is a need to wash or shower at least twice a day. Baths can be regarded as unclean, as contact with body fluids is regarded as unpure to physical, mental and spiritual faculties. Because of modesty some people will shower with their clothes on and put on dry ones after their shower.

After going to the toilet the washing of the perianal area is important, and many clients and patients worry if they are not able to do this. Hence, the situation and condition of lavatories and bathroom facilities needs to be pointed out early in a patient's admission to hospital otherwise it can cause great anxiety. Likewise, distress can be caused by inadequate and poorly kept facilities (Helman, 2000; Henley and Schott, 2002).

Washing before prayer is considered essential. For some people this may mean only washing their hands. However, others may also include cleaning of the senses (including some of the following: washing out the mouth, cleaning teeth and tongue, nasal passages, eyelids and outer ears) (Helman, 2000; Henley and Schott, 2002).

The family will always want to be close by the person who is seriously ill or dying. This is because one of them must always be at the bedside of the person. Difficulties can arise when large families arrive together and all want to be with the ill person. Not only can this cause problems for the health professionals providing care for that person, but also other patients in the same room can feel hemmed in and claustrophobic.

I can remember recovering in hospital after an abdominal operation, feeling very nauseated and uncomfortable. The Indian lady in the next bed was seriously ill, and so all her family came to see her. I can remember becoming ill with the cigarette smoke, the pungent smells of the food that the relatives brought with them, and people leaning on the screens around my bed so that they all could fit into the room. I knew it was important for them to see her and for her to see them. However, vomiting and having little children point to my urinary catheter bag (after they had crawled under the bed screens) and asking their mother what that was for made me feel distressed.

Therefore, while there is a need to allow philosophical, cultural and religious beliefs to be implemented in hospital they should not be allowed to overshadow the respect for another person (or in Western philosophy beneficence). The remedy in the situation I have just described would have been to provide the Indian lady with her own room.

Part B   Chinese philosophies

Chinese philosophy has a history of several thousand years. Its origins are often traced back to the Yi Jing (the Book of Changes), an ancient compendium of divination, which introduced some of the most fundamental terms of Chinese philosophy. Its age can only be estimated, but it certainly draws from an oracular tradition that goes back to neolithic times (Ames, 1998). In this part of the chapter, the concepts which are common to all philosophies are first discussed, followed by the individual philosophies of Confucianism, Buddhism and Taoism. This will be followed by Chinese health care and health beliefs.

Common Chinese philosophical concepts

Although the individual philosophical schools differ considerably, they nevertheless share a common vocabulary and set of concerns (Hall and Ames, 2006). Among the terms commonly found in Chinese philosophy are:

- Tao (the way, or one's doctrine);
- De (virtue, power);
- Li (principle);
- Qi (vital energy or material force).

The Tai Ji (Great Heavenly Axis) forms a unity from which two antagonistic concepts, Yin and Yang, originate. The word Yin originally referred to a hillside facing away from the sun. Philosophically, it stands for the gloomy, passive, female concept, whereas Yang (the hillside facing the sun) stands for the bright, active, male concept. Both concepts, though antagonistic, are also complementary and the present domination of one implies the future rise of the other, as with the moon's phases (this is one of the meanings of the well-known Yin-Yang figures) (Hall and Ames, 2006).

Confucianist philosophy

Historically, Confucianism is the earliest philosophical and moral framework in China (prior to the 3rd century BC). Its origins go back to the analects, the writings and sayings of Confucius. It is a system for the management of society. It was the mainstream ideology in China since the Han dynasty and a major element in Far-East culture.

Confucianism is a social ethic and humanist system focusing on human beings and their relationships. It emphasises formal rituals in every aspect of life, from quasi-religious ceremonies to strict politeness and deference to one's elders, specifically to one's parents and to the state in the form of the Emperor. Basically, it is the recognition that people are social creatures who live with others and therefore one has the obligation of 'Jen' (or human kindness) to others (Hall and Ames, 2006). Jen is expressed through the five relationships in order of priority as follows:

● sovereign and subject;
● parent and child;
● elder and younger brother;
● husband and wife; and
● friend and friend (Hall and Ames, 2006).

These relationships function smoothly because of 'li', which is the etiquette and ritual of respect. In relationships a person may be superior to some and inferior to others but, by applying the Golden Rule and treating his or her own inferiors with propriety, relationships will be harmonious.

Elements of Confucianism have survived in China and are part of behaviour in Taiwan, Hong Kong, Macao and among Chinese emigrants to other countries (prior to 1949) (Hall and Ames, 2006). In China, over the centuries Confucianism has often had to contend with other systems such as Buddhism and Taoism (Hall and Ames, 2006).

Buddhism within China

Buddhism spread to China from India and, because of its origin, is similar. According to Lusthaus (1998), by the 13th century Buddhism had spread from India to Tibet, Central Asia, China, Korea, Japan and Sri Lanka, and was making its way into south-east Asia.

Taoism

Taoism is centred around letting things take their natural course. Taoism's central books are the Tao Te Ching, traditionally attributed to Lao Zi (Lao Tse) and the Zhuang Zi (Chuang

Tse). The core concepts of Taoism are ancient, incorporating elements of mysticism dating back to prehistoric times.

Taoism emphasises nature, individual freedom, refusal of social boundaries, and was a doctrine professed by those who 'retreated in mountains' (Hall and Ames, 2006). At the end of their lives or during the night, many Confucian officers often behaved as Taoists, writing poetry or trying to 'reach immortality'.

Zen Buddhism

Zen is a fusion of Mahayana Buddhism with the Chinese Taoist principles, and this is why Zen Buddhism is not classified under Indian philosophies. However, its founder was an Indian named Bodhidharma, a legendary Indian monk who travelled to China in the 5th century. There, at the Shaolin temple, he began the Ch'an school of Buddhism, known in Japan and in the west as Zen Buddhism.

Zen philosophy places emphasis on existing in the moment, right now. Zen teaches that the entire universe is one's mind and, if one cannot realise enlightenment in one's own mind now, one cannot ever achieve enlightenment (Hall and Ames, 2006).

Zen practitioners engage in zazen (just sitting) meditation. Several schools of Zen have developed various other techniques for provoking satori, or enlightenment. These range from whacking acolytes with a stick to shock them into the present moment, to koans (Zen riddles) to force the student to abandon futile attempts to understand the nature of the universe through logic.

Chinese legalist philosophy

Legalism advocated a strict interpretation of the law in every respect. Morality was not important; adherence to the letter of the law was paramount. Officials who exceeded expectations were as liable for punishment as those who underperformed their duties, since both were not adhering exactly to their duties. Legalism was the principal philosophical basis of the Qin Dynasty in China. Confucian scholars were persecuted under legalist rule (Hall and Ames, 2006).

There is no modern equivalent to legalism, except that some of the older people are extremely law-abiding and in awe of authority.

Maoist philosophy

Maoism is a Communist philosophy based on the teachings of the 20th-century Communist Party of China's revolutionary leader Mao Zedong. It is based partially on earlier theories by Marx and Lenin but rejects the urban proletariat and Leninist emphasis on heavy industrialisation. Instead, it was a revolution supported by the peasants, with a decentralised economy based on many collective farms (Hall and Ames, 2006).

Many people believe that the implementation of Maoism in mainland China led to the victory of the communist revolution. However, it also contributed to the widespread famine, with millions of people starving to death. Chinese Communist leader Deng Xiaoping reinterpreted Maoism to allow for the introduction of market economics, which eventually enabled the country to recover.

As a philosophy, Maoism has remained a popular ideology for various Communist revolutionary groups around the world, notably the Khmer Rouge in Cambodia, Sendero Luminoso in Peru, and an ongoing (as of early 2005) Maoist insurrection in Nepal (Hall and Ames, 2006).

Given the varying philosophies that have influenced governments, culture and health beliefs, people's health care needs will be different. However, there is sufficient commonality to state overall basic concepts; these include belief in traditional Chinese medicine, and balance between the body and mind.

Caring for the Chinese client or patient

Within the Chinese government's provision of health care and culture there are strong indigenous systems of healing which are evident alongside Western medical health care concepts.

In China traditional complementary ways of medicine are legitimate avenues for providing health care and receive government funding (Helman, 2000). These include acupuncture, moxibustion and herbal remedies, which still provide a complementary system for much of the population, especially in rural areas (Henley and Schott, 2002).

Irrespective of whether the person chooses Western or traditional medicine there are several philosophical, cultural and religious ethical beliefs that need to be considered. These include: balance, good and bad luck, yin and yang foods, the importance of harmony, and family and personal care and space.

Traditional Chinese medicine

Diagnosis in Chinese medicine is through observation, discussion, palpation, percussion and pulse-taking. Treatments include changes in diet, exercise, herbal treatments, acupuncture and moxibustion (a collection of herbs attached to an acupuncture needle to burn slowly while the needle improves the flow of Ch'i along the meridian) (Hall and Ames, 2006).

Balance

According to Chinese medicine, illness is an impairment of balance or harmony in the body owing to internal, external, physical or mental causes. The mind and body are closely connected and affect each other. Consequently the aim of traditional Chinese medicine is to recreate balance and harmony (Hall and Ames, 2006).

Chinese medicine includes ch'i (vital energy needed for life), yin (energy force of earth, night, interior, contemplation, female, cold and death), yang (energy force for heaven, day, exterior, activity, male, heat and life), and five elements of matter that are believed to influence health and the proper functioning of organs (Ames and Hall, 1998).

Ch'i, the vital energy, circulates through the body along 14 meridians or channels. The strength, flow and distribution of Ch'i depend on the balance of yin and yang. Acupuncture can be used to stimulate the flow of Ch'i along the meridians. Excess of yin can cause infections, gastric problems and anxiety, whereas excess of yang can cause dehydration, fever, irritability and edginess. The yin and yang foods are also important to restore harmony in the body (Hall and Ames, 2006).

The importance of harmony and family

The issue of consent to treatment and operations is a family matter as the concept of harmony is important, and also because the Chinese family has the 'best interests' of that person at the centre of any decision-making. For example, if the patient is an elderly widow the final decision will most likely be taken by the oldest son after talking with his mother and all the family members. This communication and consultation between family members means that they will ask other family members for advice about health problems (Helman, 2000; Henley and Schott, 2002).

Depending on the demeanour of the health professional, some Chinese clients and patients may feel that they are unable to question proposed treatments and care. That is, if a consultant was regarded as a figure of authority, the client, patients and relatives may be reluctant to question his/her choice of proposed treatment. Likewise, they possibly will not complain about poor treatment. Consequently, the whole of the interprofessional team needs to be aware of the care and treatments that others in the team are giving, so that these clients or patients are not compromised (Henley and Schott, 2002).

This concept of harmony can also affect the group dynamics within the interprofessional team. That is, some members may feel that they can't question another professional. This can occur between consultants and nurses/midwives. Imagine then if the client or patient feels unable to question a consultant's choice of treatment, as do the nurse or midwife (Henley and Schott, 2002).

Good and bad luck

Good and bad luck has always been important in Chinese culture, with various numbers, dates, times and positions being more favourable than others. Some patients may not want to have operations on specific dates or times as they are regarded as unlucky; likewise, room or bed numbers. In relation to positions, some Chinese clients or patients will not wish to have their bed in direct line with a door or open window. Given the ethical desire for harmony it is wise for the health professional to ask the client or patient what dates, times and positions are satisfactory to him/her and family (Henley and Schott, 2002).

Food and diet

Yin and yang foods can either bring about healing or cause illness. For these reasons it is important for the health professional to find out how various proposed treatments and care are regarded within the client's or patient's culture. For example, if the patient regards their illness as being caused by too much yang, and you prescribe antibiotics (which are regarded as yang), the patient might feel that you are trying to make them more ill.

Cold Western food will usually be left by the Chinese client or patient because of the yin/yang effect. To show their love to a family member who is ill in hospital, food such as soups and various herbal teas are brought in to sustain the loved one. While these can be complementary to Western medicine, they can at times have the opposite effect. Consequently, the hospital pharmacist has an ethical obligation to be aware of possible incompatibilities (Helman, 2000; Henley and Schott, 2002).

Personal care

The Chinese client or patient is modest and will therefore not want to be seen undressed by other people, especially those of the opposite sex. Cleanliness is also important and the provision of very hot water in a bowl that they can wash over themselves is greatly appreciated (Helman, 2000; Henley and Schott, 2002).

Prayer

Prayer at the beginning of the day in a quiet room or in bed with the screens drawn can be very important to some clients and patients (Helman, 2000).

They may wish to have a small shrine (picture or statue) on their table or locker upon which they will focus their prayer. They may also like to burn incense or have flowers or water as part of the shrine.

Giving bad news and family

When a health professional needs to give a Chinese person bad news about a diagnosis, plan for privacy and a quiet atmosphere. A busy noisy hospital room with the patient sharing with others is not the place. The patient's task when receiving such news is to do so quietly and have the time for reflection. Also, their task is to let others take over, that is, the family and health professionals.

In some families, explicit discussions should not be with the person receiving the bad news but with the family. Even though the patient may not be directly told, the patient themselves has an implicit understanding of what is happening through non-verbal communication (without the family stating it in words to them) (Henley and Schott, 2002).

Need for secrets

When a Chinese person is very ill and perhaps dying, conversations with health professionals can be regarded as dangerous (yin/yang effect). Some families may want the matter of dying and death kept secret from outsiders. At times the person who is very ill will not be visited by their grandchildren or women (especially pregnant women) because of the likelihood that the bad luck associated with death will be caught by the children or women.

Some Chinese people may refuse to accept that death is imminent for their loved one, and may request health professionals to continue with treatment. Again, this goes back to the concept of bad luck (Henley and Schott, 2002).

Closure v. openness

Open discussion with the person who is dying by well-meaning health professionals who advocate 'facing the reality of death', can lead to discomfort, distress and distrust. However, Chinese clients and patients educated in and living a more Western life style will prefer more open and explicit communication. This can lead to disharmony and conflict within the family if not all the family share the same values and beliefs (Henley and Schott, 2002).

Dying and death

Chinese Buddhists will regard death as part of the process of living, and look forward to the next life after the death of this one. Buddhists who know they are dying will possibly want to pay any debts they may have, buy their coffin and pay for the funeral in advance (Helman, 2000; Henley and Schott, 2002). While prayers and chanting may be undertaken by the family and monks and nuns, emotional outpourings (loud crying and wailing) are frowned upon, and a family member engaging in such might be removed from the room by other family members. This is because quiet and peace are paramount as the person leaves one world to go to the next.

The use of prescribed opioids will be appreciated by the patient and family so that the person does not suffer. However, the dose needs to be such that they do not cause disorientation, confusion, loss of control or clouding of the mind. Occasionally, a Buddhist may feel that their suffering is due to past misdeeds, and would rather suffer now than having to do so in a later life (Helman, 2000; Henley and Schott, 2002).

In some families the person who is dying will want to say a message or words of wisdom to those they are leaving behind. Therefore, consideration for family members is something for which health professionals need to strive (especially those arriving from overseas in the middle of the night) (Henley and Schott, 2002).

Activity

Answer these questions.

➤ What do you think the effects might be if a patient had an operation on a date which, to them, can only bring bad luck?

➤ Similarly, what about the patient that you place in the last remaining bed in the ward but which is directly opposite the swing doors to the corridor. You hear the family members saying something along the lines of 'he will die, as the evil spirits will come sweeping down the corridor and over him in bed every time the door is open'. What can you, as a member of the interprofessional health team, do?

➤ How does the Western ethical principle of autonomy differ from the Chinese ethical principle of harmony?

➤ What might occur when the client or patient does not feel able to question a consultant? Likewise, when other members of the team also feel that they cannot question the consultant?

Read Case study 6.2 and follow the discussion, so that you gain an awareness of how Chinese philosophy can be applied to the case study. (You will remember the case study from a previous chapter, but with different names.)

Case study 6.2
Lilly Li and Maurice Yip

Lilly (age 38) and Maurice (age 42) are a very busy professional couple who have left having a child until their careers are established. They have recently moved from Hong Kong to live in Beijing. They want to have a child but, because of Lilly's polycystic ovarian syndrome (PCOS) and Maurice's low sperm count, need to embark on an IVF treatment programme. Lilly is given treatment and her left ovary produces multiple ova which, when mixed with Maurice's sperm in the laboratory, result in five fertilised oocytes that can be implanted in her uterus. The health care team decides to implant three, with the remaining two to be stored until needed.

The three embryos proceed to develop well; however, Lilly and Maurice decide that they could not cope with the financial burden of bringing up three children and ask for a selective termination of pregnancy of one embryo at 14 weeks' gestation.

The remaining two embryos are threatened by the procedure, and this results in Lilly having to spend the majority of the rest of her pregnancy in hospital.

Later in the pregnancy, Lilly develops pre-eclampsia and the babies (one boy and one girl) are delivered early by an emergency Caesarean section. The available intensive neonatal equipment in the hospital is already in demand by other multiple births. Likewise, other Beijing hospitals cannot help. This means one baby (the girl) has to be flown to a neonatal unit in Shanghai for care.

After a month the baby girl is flown back to the home city, where the other baby, that is, the boy, is fighting for his life. The girl baby continues to do well, but the boy's condition further deteriorates and, despite extraordinary efforts, he dies.

Lilly and Maurice take home one baby girl. However, they have also learnt that it was a boy that was removed through selective termination.

Question

➤ Identify the Chinese philosophical principles that you could use when discussing your perspective during an interdisciplinary team meeting.

In answer to the activity question above, first Chinese philosophical general principles, then Confucius, and then Buddhist principles will be applied.

Application of Chinese philosophical principles to the case study

Chinese principles cannot be applied to this case to say what was right or wrong, but they may provide insight into the situation.

Application of general philosophical principles

1 The tendency not to view a person as separate from nature. From this perspective, Lilly and Maurice might realise that, like all aspects of nature, the human body is frail and has imperfections.

2 The tendency not to invoke a unified and personified supernatural power. Questions about the nature and existence of God which have profoundly influenced Western philosophy have not been important in Chinese philosophies. If Lilly and Maurice were not Christian and followed the Chinese philosophical tradition, then in this respect they would not worry what they might have done wrong to upset a god as to have PCOS, low sperm count and to need IVF to gain a family. Neither would they be angry at a god for allowing their baby son to die.

3 Acceptance and optimism that what has happened to them is just something that occurs over which they have no control. In this respect, Lilly and Maurice may be philosophical that, although they wanted a family, they realised that they couldn't afford or manage having three babies or children at one time. Therefore, although it was not planned that they would only have one child at this stage, this is what they have, and now they are a family. There is also a possibility of having the other fertilised oocytes implanted at another stage.

Application of Confucius principles

Since Confucius philosophy emphasises a cultural social ethic of people's relationships with others, involving quasi-religious ceremonies, strict politeness and 'Jen' (human kindness to the ranking order of government and subject, parent and child, elder and younger brother, husband and wife, and friend to friend), it is possible that Lilly and Maurice may not have minded the baby girl being transferred to another city for treatment and care, and they could respect and be kind to each other during this time.

Application of Buddhist principles

By interpreting the four noble truths it could be said that if Lilly and Maurice believed in:

1 Dukkha: then they would accept that all worldly life is unsatisfactory, disjointed and contains suffering;

2 Samudaya: then they may realise that there is a cause to the suffering they are experiencing, which is their attachment or desire (tanha) to something;

3 Nirodha: that there is an end of suffering, which is nirvana;

4 Marga: that is, if they follow the noble eightfold path they will be led out of suffering.

Most Buddhist sects believe in karma, a cause-and-effect relationship between all that has been done and all that will be done. Lilly and Maurice may therefore believe that their experience of birth and death may be the direct result of previous events. One effect of karma is rebirth. At death, the karma from a given life determines the nature of the next life's existence. The ultimate goal of a Buddhist practitioner is to eliminate karma (both good and bad), end the cycle of rebirth and suffering, and attain nirvana, translated as nothingness or blissful oblivion, and characterised as the state of being one with the entire universe.

Case study conclusion

By reflecting on some Chinese philosophies, we have been able to gain some insight into how Lilly and Maurice might be experiencing the situation. The only way we would know would be to ask them. However, if I was to work in a hospital in China or Hong Kong I would now be aware of the philosophical view points of patients compared with those in the west.

Also, I am very much aware of how my own values and beliefs are different to those of Lilly and Maurice. Consequently, if I need to care for a pregnant woman of Chinese origin outside the Eastern geography, I will have some knowledge and understanding of the philosophy which is inherent within her values, beliefs, culture and humanist philosophy.

Part C Japanese philosophies

The single most distinctive characteristic of Japanese philosophy is how it has assimilated and adapted foreign philosophies into its world view. Historically there was the archaic indigenous religion, Shinto (a form of animism). Then Confucian and Buddhist philosophies were imported from China. This was followed by neo-Confucianism. Next came Daoism (also from China); this had an impact but more within folk medicine than in philosophy (Kasulis, 1998). After this, Zen Buddhism and, finally, Western philosophy was assimilated (Ames, 1998).

The philosophical impact of Buddhism, introduced around the same time as Confucianism, has been primarily in three areas: psychology, metaphysics and aesthetics. Buddhism helped to define the various Japanese senses of the inner, rather than the social, self. Buddhist metaphysics helped to develop rational ideals for the indigenous religion (Shintoism), while the Buddhist metaphysical studies developed Japanese psychology (Kasulis, 1998).

Neo-Confucianism became popular in Japan in the 16th century, contributing to the understanding of virtue and social self. In the 19th century, Western philosophy forced Japanese philosophers to reconsider fundamental issues, such as social philosophy and philosophical anthropology. Just as Japan has assimilated Asian traditions in the past, so it has been consciously assimilating Western thought since the early 20th century.

This development gave rise to the Kyoto School, which incorporated Zen Buddhism with the Western philosophy of phenomenology. Likewise, the development of Japanese ethics at Tokyo University (Kasulis, 1998).

Although it would appear that Japan has an eclectic mix of imported philosophies, this is not quite accurate. What has happened is that each of the imported knowledge bases has first been adapted before being assimilated. For example, Japan has criticised the Western philosophical ideals of rationalism and positivism, while accepting other concepts (Kasulis, 1998).

Shinto beliefs

Shintoism is indigenous to Japan and means 'the way of the Gods'. It was named in the 6th century to distinguish it from Buddhism and Confucianism which at that time were imported from China. Consequently, Shintoism has been a major part of Japanese life and culture throughout the country's history; for a greater part of that history, however, Shintoism has shared its spiritual, cultural and political roles with Buddhism and Confucianism.

The essence of Shintoism is the Japanese devotion to invisible spiritual beings and powers called 'kami', to shrines and to various rituals. Some people refer to Shinto as the religion of Japan, whereas others would say that it is a cultural tradition and beliefs (BBC, 2006; Keene, 2002).

In Shintoism, the Japanese people worship the gods and goddesses, who are known as kami. Worship can take place at home or at any of the 100 000 shrines around the country. The main kami are:

- Amerterasu the sun godess, who is regarded as the principal kami because she rules over heaven. Amaterasu is said to have shown the Japanese how to cultivate rice and to have invented weaving on the loom. She is worshipped as an ancestor as she is believed to have sent her son to found or commence the imperial family.

- Tenman is worshipped as the god of learning and his many shrines are popular with students, who pray there for success in their exams.

- Hachiman was originally the god of farmers, but in the 12th century became the kami of war and warriors.

- Inari is the god of fertility and prosperity. At shrines, Inari is represented as a fox made of stone. In Shinto legend, foxes that roam the countryside are Inari's messengers.

Festivals

There are many Shinto festivals. The primary ones are held at New Year, at the time of rice planting, Spring and during the Autumn harvest. Other festivals are held for ancestral, purification, exorcism or agricultural purposes. During the festival the kami is often carried through the streets in a portable shrine to assure everyone that it is protecting the community.

Although there are shrines and kami, Shintoism has no founder, no major scriptures, no creed and no religious or ethical laws. Neither is there a concept of heaven or afterlife. Because of this some would say that it is not a religion *per se* but a cultural belief.

Japanese ethics

Today Japanese ethics is a mixture of Confucian, Buddhist and Western philosophies (Ames, 1998). In caring for the Japanese client or patient, the wisest way to respect their culture when an ethical decision needs to be made would be to ask the person concerned. It would not be correct to assume that a Japanese person has a specific view point. To assume the health beliefs of a Japanese patient incorrectly could very easily cause distress and mistrust.

Part D Differences between Western and Eastern philosophies

Whether Eastern or Western philosophy started first is immaterial to this book. What is important is that both philosophical traditions are old and both need to be equally respected. (There is some evidence to suggest that the Eastern tradition does pre-date the Western tradition.)

The two main differences between Western and Eastern philosophy are:

- The lack of distinction between philosophy and religion in the Eastern tradition compared with the separateness of philosophy and religion in the Western tradition.
- The perception of God and gods.

Lack of distinction between philosophy and religion

The distinction between religion and philosophy is not so important in the east (Ames, 1998). One fundamental reason for the separation of the philosophies in academia is that Eastern philosophy tends to be marginalised or ignored in Western studies of the 'history of philosophy'. Eastern philosophy tends to be relegated to the world religion departments of Western universities, or to New Age non-academic works, though there are several notable exceptions.

This arrangement stands in marked contrast to most philosophies of the west, which have traditionally enforced either a completely unified philosophical/religious belief system (e.g. the various sects and associated philosophies of Christianity, Judaism and Islam) or a sharp and total repudiation of religion by philosophy (e.g. Nietzsche, Marx, Voltaire, etc.).

Perceptions of God(s)

In relation to the differences of perception of God(s) between Eastern and Western philosophy this includes God's relationship with the universe, and the role and nature of an individual (Kasulis, 1998).

Eastern philosophies have not been as concerned by questions relating to the nature of a single God as the universe's sole creator and ruler. The distinction between the religious and the secular tends to be much less sharp in Eastern philosophy, and the same philosophical school often contains both religious and philosophical elements.

Integration of Eastern and Western philosophies

There have been many modern attempts to integrate Western and Eastern philosophical traditions. German philosopher Georg Wilhelm Friedrich Hegel was very interested in Taoism. His system of dialectics is sometimes interpreted as a formalisation of Taoist principles.

Hegel's rival Arthur Schopenhauer developed a philosophy that was essentially a synthesis of Hinduism and Buddhism with Western thought. He argued that the Upanishads (primary Hindu scriptures) could have a much greater influence in the west than they have had. However, Schopenhauer was working with heavily flawed early translations (and sometimes secondary translations), and many feel that he may not necessarily have accurately grasped the Eastern philosophies which interested him (Craig, 1998).

Recent attempts to incorporate Western philosophy into Eastern thought include the Japanese Kyoto School of philosophers, which combined the phenomenology of Husserl with the insights of Zen Buddhism. Much of the work of Ken Wilber also focuses on bringing together truths of Eastern and Western philosophies into a coherent and integrated framework or integral theory.

Summary

Eastern philosophy and ethics is different from the Western tradition. This has occurred with the two civilisations (Eastern and Western) developing independently of each other. The Eastern philosophies of India, China, south-east Asia and Japan include Hinduism, Buddhism, Islam, Sikhism, Confucianism and Shintoism.

The Eastern philosophers view relationships between people differently and so the ethical principles proposed here are harmony, respect, hospitality, modesty and balance.

It is important to remember that, although a person may have been born and lived in a country with an Eastern philosophical outlook, they may have incorporated some Western philosophical ideas into their ethical perspective. Likewise, the person who was born and lives within a Western country may have incorporated Eastern philosophical views into their ethical perspective. It is thus important for health professionals always to clarify with clients or patients what their personal values and beliefs are in respect to health care and treatments.

Professional development

1 Continue developing your Ethics Portfolio. You have possibly already noticed a difference between writing about case studies compared with when you did this for Chapter 2.

  ● You may have found that you have needed to keep including additional cultures into the Ethics Portfolio as you begin to realise that the people who are your peers and those on clinical practice come from a greater variety of places or have a wider range of philosophical beliefs than you originally thought.

  ● No doubt the same thing is happening in relation to the different cultures and religions of the patients or clients who receive care at the health care organisation in which you work or undertake clinical practice.

2 Read Case studies 6.3 and 6.4 and write the answers in your Ethics Portfolio.

Case study 6.3
Caught in a quandary

Kristy Li is an experienced nurse working in an oncology unit in a large Hong Kong hospital. She has just started her Masters degree and her first study module is ethics. Kristy goes along to her first class, and listens as the lecturer explains about the module and what the assessment will be. For the assessment Kristy needs to identify an ethical problem or issue in her clinical practice and, working through this, reach an ethical resolution.

As the lessons go by and each of the students finds a problem to work through and resolve, Kristy seeks the advice of her lecturer. The lecturer asks Kristy in which clinical area she works and she replies that it is oncology. Her lecturer enquires, are there not ethical issues there?

Kristy replies that the patients receive treatment and go home and/or they come back into hospital and die.

'And how does that happen?' the lecturer queries.

Kristy replies, 'the patients are given pain relief to keep them comfortable, and if they stop breathing they are resuscitated until such time as they no longer respond to resuscitation measures – the staff then know that they have done as much as possible for the patient'.

This interested the ethics lecturer, as she had worked in Australian oncology units, where the patient's autonomy was paramount in any resuscitation effort. Therefore, the lecturer kindly asked Kristy why she wanted to resuscitate a patient who is terminally ill and going to die.

Kristy replied that she didn't know, and so the ethics lecturer suggested that she might like to look at that ethical issue for her assignment.

Questions

➤ Why do you think Kristy wanted to resuscitate a terminally ill patient?

➤ What values and beliefs do you think she is thinking about when providing care for the patients on the oncology unit?

➤ How would you go about changing the situation on the oncology unit so that the terminally ill patients were not resuscitated?

Case study 6.4
Dr Lionel Li and the midwife-led delivery unit

Dr Lionel Li had just arrived in Hong Kong to undertake an obstetric consultancy at Stairway to the Stars Hospital, from a New Zealand hospital that had a medical interventionist approach to childbirth. Stairway to the Stars Hospital was a magnificent structure overlooking Victoria Harbour and, if the midwives were not so busy, they might have liked gazing out at the sea view.

The midwives were all very competent and had been working together for a number of years. During that time they had worked out each other's strengths and weaknesses to form a cohesive team. Some midwives had gained extra expertise in alternative birthing methods, such as reflexology, acupuncture, homeopathy and massage. However, it was hospital policy that the midwives needed to notify the consultant for any breech delivery, any woman in second stage labour who was not progressing, or any indication of fetal distress.

One day the midwife Flora was assisting Dr Li at his prenatal clinic, examining Mrs Ng whose baby was in a breech position. Dr Li tried to turn the baby but was unsuccessful. He then said to Mrs Ng

'Well, there is only one way to fix it, and that is you need to come into hospital and have an anaesthetic to turn the baby'. He went on, 'but if you are going to have an anaesthetic you might as well have a Caesarean section to deliver the baby.'

Mrs Ng looked quite horrified.

Mrs Ng looked at Flora and pleadingly said to her 'You are a woman, can you not do something. I came to this hospital because I was told the midwives can do extra things to help the woman and baby'.

Flora took one look at the expression on Dr Li's face (which was flushed) and said she would think about it and discuss the issue with Dr Li, but that Mrs Ng needed to make the arrangement as the doctor had requested.

When Mrs Ng left, Flora followed her out and, when they were out of listening range of Dr Li, Flora told Mrs Ng how to facilitate the baby turning in the uterus by crawling up and down stairs.

When Mrs Ng came into hospital Flora made sure that she was on duty to give her a prenatal check. Flora discovered that the baby had turned and that she was in early labour. She informed Mrs Ng of this and she and her husband were delighted. As the labour continued Mrs Ng needed some pain relief and so Flora asked her if she wanted to try acupuncture, have conventional pain relief or an epidural. Mrs Ng said she would like to try the acupuncture. As Mrs Ng relaxed into the effect of the acupuncture, Flora realised that she had forgotten to page Dr Li and tell him that there was no longer any need for the anaesthetic to turn the baby.

Flora left the room and paged the doctor and told him that the baby had turned and that Mrs Ng was in labour. The doctor told Flora that he did not believe her, as there was no way that the baby could have turned without his intervention.

A little later when Flora was back in the room with Mr and Mrs Ng, Dr Li arrived and greeted the patient. He then palpated the fetal position, and found that the head was engaged and that Mrs Ng was progressing nicely in labour. He told this to Mr and Mrs Ng, and also commented that he couldn't understand how the baby had been able to turn itself, when he hadn't been able to.

Mr Ng said 'Oh, we just helped the baby along by my wife crawling up and down the stairs as Flora suggested'.

Flora noticed that the doctor did not look happy with her, and was not surprised when he asked to see her outside. Once outside he told Flora in no uncertain terms that he was going to report her to the Director of Nursing, and personally make sure that the Hong Kong Nursing and Midwifery Council were going to hear of his complaint that she had interfered with the treatment and care of one of his patients, when she had no right to do so. With that, he turned and left.

Flora returned to Mr and Mrs Ng where a little later she delivered young healthy Austin Ng.

Questions

➤ What are the ethical issues in the scenario?

➤ What is your perspective of Flora's care of Mrs Ng?

➤ Does the doctor have grounds for reporting Flora to the Hong Kong Nursing and Midwifery Council?

➤ Assuming that Mr and Mrs Ng have traditional Chinese philosophical beliefs, what can you interpret?

➤ If you were the unit manager how would you resolve the situation?

Critical reflection

Write a critical reflection for this chapter to place in your Ethics Portfolio. The item or issue that you may want to work through or critically analyse could be something that you need to explore further from:

- One of the case studies.
- Reading that you have done.
- A different point of view that someone raised in discussion in class.
- A general feeling of disquiet about your own values and beliefs in relation to Eastern philosophy, which you want to explore through reflection.
- Clinical practice:
  - such as your values and beliefs in relation to Eastern philosophy, culture or religion being different from some members of the team;
  - how you have realised that the care you have provided for a patient on clinical practice was incorrect and consequently, unethical;
  - another member of the team on clinical practice is ignoring a client's or patient's rights and needs in relation to the Eastern tradition and is therefore not being culturally sensitive and/or competent.

Acknowledgements
We are indebted to the students from the Eastern philosophy tradition who, over the years, have taught us so much about their beliefs, culture and professional values, in order that we could write this chapter. We would also like to express our gratitude to colleagues from The School of Nursing, Chiba University, Japan.

7

Being part of a team: interprofessional care

Kevin Reel and Sue Hutchings

Why this chapter is important to me . . .

✔ To understand the need for awareness about other team members, and that the ethics of teamwork is about how members work together.

✔ That being part of a team can cause ethical or moral problems.

✔ There is a need for the different professions to work together for the client's or patient's benefit.

✔ You need to be able to state what you believe is correct and right to other members of the team.

✔ Knowing that interprofessional thinking and working will help with difficult or unexpected ethical problems and/or dilemmas.

In previous chapters, you have learnt about the importance of providing good client or patient care so that ethical problems and/or dilemmas are minimised. In addition, by using critical systematic reflection in relation to situations, incidents and behaviours you can gain insight into your own behaviour. When doing this, the questions that you or others ask will highlight discrepancies in your thinking, which will then lead you to improve your professional practice. In this chapter, you will learn how working in a team impacts on ethical issues, problems and/or dilemmas, so that you can be aware of the potential conflicts that could lie ahead. This is important as, in today's health practice, it is usual for a team to provide the care and treatment of clients or patients.

Interprofessional working involves complex interactions between two or more members of different professional disciplines. It is a collaborative venture (McCray, 2002) in which those involved share the common purpose of developing mutually negotiated goals which are achieved through agreed care plans and procedures (Barrett and Keeping, 2005). For this to occur, teams need to pool their knowledge and expertise (Cook *et al.*, 2001), and make joint decisions based upon shared professional view points (Payne, 2000; Handy, 2001).

To gain knowledge and understanding of how this may occur we will start at the beginning: that is, first, what a health and social care team is; second, where these teams are likely to occur and the different types of health care (primary, secondary and tertiary care); third, the different codes of ethics that these differing team members follow; fourth, how team problems can occur; and fifth, what is needed for a team to be successful in working together. Finally, the Professional Development section will conclude the chapter.

Health and social care teams

Any list of people involved in delivering health and social care to the public grows as the complexity of the field increases. For example, in the UK, the National Health Service employs 1.3 million staff, making it the largest employer in Europe. The NHS careers website lists nearly 100 careers, most of which are qualified professionals. With such a diversity of professions, it is evident that coordinated patient care will require communication and joint decision-making between a group or team of health and social care personnel.

Advantage of working as an interprofessional team

In health and social care, team working has advantages in that some tasks and procedures do not need to be repeated by each individual practitioner, when one professional can do it for the whole team. An example is the development of single assessment processes (SAP) to innovative care pathways, with the explicit goal of improving the quality of a service.

Interprofessional teamwork can often provide a platform for discussing complex, longer-term client or patient problems to be considered from a number of different professional perspectives. At best, these can complement each other to provide a well-rounded seamless service that is successfully implemented and maintained over time. It should always be possible to anticipate overlaps in professional roles and responsibilities, and to discuss how to manage these in a way that suits any particular care situation.

The interprofessional team: many members and many roles

There is probably no 'standard' or 'usual' interprofessional team in health and social care anymore - although there are those members (such as nurses, doctors and therapists) that readily come to mind. In addition to the members mentioned above, it is probable that teams will include psychologists, nutritionists, dieticians, interpreters, spiritual/religious/pastoral support staff, administrators, paramedics, pharmacists and many others. There is also a distinction to be made between a 'core' team who will work together on a regular basis over time to a more informal and *ad hoc* network of professionals and services.

No list can be considered comprehensive, and no description of roles can be considered definitive or universal. There is a constant evolution of roles as services are changed to make them more efficient. The 'traditional' boundaries between many professions and their 'territory' are shifting in many cases. In the UK, prescribing medication was once the exclusive domain of doctors (and dentists). New initiatives mean that nurses and others may now prescribe many drugs in some contexts. This may require further training for some or it may be part of their original education.

The composition of any interprofessional team is dependent on the practice context. To discuss teams and their members a little further, we will look at services as they are grouped, in primary, secondary and tertiary care.

Primary care

A primary care team (the first port of call for most people when seeking health care) might have a group of GPs, a practice nurse, a practice manager, a health visitor, a district or community nurse and perhaps a phlebotomist. There may also be a counsellor and others, depending on the local arrangement. Here the staff are skilled in dealing with a huge variety of health and social care problems, often combining physical, psychological and social elements.

The GP will see patients in the surgery and may make home visits to diagnose medical conditions and discuss appropriate treatment. They will also arrange for the patient to see another specialist practitioner to provide further care or interventions. A general practice will usually have a practice nurse (a registered nurse) providing the nursing services, including immunisations, testing for various illnesses, conducting clinics to help patients manage their diseases, offer telephone advice and make initial triage decisions. The overall running of the surgery is the responsibility of the practice manager. In the UK, given that the vast majority of consultations in the NHS happen in GP surgeries, primary care teams are a significant part of the workforce.

In the community there are health visitors; these are registered nurses who undertake additional training to be able to focus on promoting health and preventing illness for children, usually under 5 years of age. You will learn more about the primary care in Chapter 11.

Secondary care

In secondary care - acute hospitals mainly - the teams will include specialist doctors, nurses, therapists, social workers, assistants, pharmacists and almost every other health care worker imaginable. Emergency services, including trauma and rescue teams, can also be part of secondary care. The specialisms range from the emergency department (or accident and emergency) to neurology, orthopaedics to psychiatry, perioperative care (operating suite or theatre department), obstetrics to gerontology, and many others.

Nurses and midwives

Nurses work throughout secondary care to provide care and treatments and to coordinate client or patient care between the different professions. This includes care in wards and outpatient clinics. Nurses here practise within their particular specialist field of children's, adult or mental health. They also develop further expertise within clinical areas such as orthopaedics, neurology, vascular, intensive care, gerontology, general surgery and many others. Midwives provide care in hospitals and in the community to women and their families during pregnancy and the first months after birth.

Therapists

In secondary care, you will also find physical, speech and language, and occupational therapists, among many others collectively known in the UK as the allied health professions.

Physical therapists treat the physical problems that arise after illness, injury or aging. They concentrate on the respiratory, muscle and skeletal systems. They specialise in neurology, respiratory and musculoskeletal areas among others. Speech and language therapists help people with communication problems, as well as related difficulties with chewing or swallowing. Occupational therapists help people manage the physical, psychological and social challenges that arise from disability, illness or aging by focusing on their everyday activities (the tasks and routines that occupy them daily). Therapists often work very closely within their specialist teams, e.g. neurology, paediatrics, gerontology or mental health.

Operating unit or department

Operating department practitioners use their experience and training in surgical teams to provide perioperative care to ensure that different operations (especially the long or complex ones) proceed safely and smoothly for the patient and the team.

Pharmacists

Pharmacists are experts in drugs and medicines, their use, preparation, effects (and side effects) and interactions with other drugs. They keep stores of, and dispense, controlled and uncontrolled medications. In hospital, they provide medications for inpatients, and for immediate need upon discharge. In the community they may work independently or for a larger retailer.

Social workers

Social workers assist in planning for discharge, either back home and into the community or on to another care facility. They work closely with family and friends and community services to enable people to return home where appropriate. They may work with other care providers to set up care packages or arrange for a client to move to sheltered or other supported accommodation. They often take on a pastoral or supportive counselling type role.

Chaplaincy

A hospital chaplain usually takes on the pastoral or spiritual care of patients. Given the frequent life and death nature of health care, there are many ethical considerations that the chaplain or similar other helps the patient to understand and navigate. Chaplains may be of the same or another religious denomination as the patient, but they can normally approach a situation from an ecumenical standpoint, working with any client within their own faith perspective. Many hospitals have a variety of such spiritual support staff available, especially in those areas that serve a wide variety of faiths in the local population.

Genetic counsellors

Increasingly, the ethical issues that arise in health and social care are born of the ongoing revolution in our collective understanding of genetics. Many hospitals now have very specialist roles such as genetic counsellors. The growing awareness of, and ability to detect, specific genes responsible for certain diseases such as breast cancer and Huntington's chorea means that people are now faced with decisions they did not have in the past. Genetic counsellors are specially trained to help explain the complicated details of inheritance and probability where clients are considering having children who could inherit such conditions. They also explain what genetic screening is available and what it might mean if one pursues such genetic testing.

Tertiary care

In tertiary care, the teams have a highly specialised focus. For example, uncommon diseases and illnesses, transplant operations and highly complex care. The team composition is tailored to the particular speciality, with many different professional groups working together. For example, a high-risk neonatal intensive care unit will have nursing staff, midwives, physiotherapist and neonatal consultants. These are augmented with neonatal neurologists, neurosurgeons, orthopaedic consultants, renal physicians and nephrologists, cardiologists and cardiac surgeons, plastic surgeon, immunologist and a lactation specialist. So, while the speciality team is to care for the very ill neonate baby, others are also needed on the team for assessment and management of the care. This means that, when this very ill baby arrives, a team assesses what is wrong, then a case discussion takes place to analyse the findings and plan possible treatments or palliative care. The options are then discussed with the parents, who make the choices about care and treatment.

Complementary care

In many situations, patients are also involved with practitioners of what is sometimes called complementary and alternative medicine. These are considered in the west to be beyond conventional care, and can include herbalists, reflexologists, acupuncturists and others. It is important to note two things about the involvement of these other practitioners. First, their interventions may have significant effects, side effects or interactions with mainstream treatments, so this should always be considered. Second, their involvement with the client is an indicator of the client's own system of 'health beliefs', their understanding of what makes them well or unwell and how to go about improving their health and wellbeing. It would be an oversight to think that any of us can work ethically and effectively with clients if we ignore these health beliefs and behaviours.

Clients and patients are also part of the team

This brings us to the clients (or patients, or service users) themselves, the key team members who we have yet to mention. The term you might use would depend on the person and their situation. In varying situations, a different term might be used; within any one context, some of the 'service users' might like to be considered clients, others patients or residents. You will normally take your cues from various sources to know which term is best for each person and situation. As mentioned, the client brings a system of beliefs and behaviours related to their own understanding of health and wellbeing. They also bring a set of preferences and ethical view points.

In addition to the client, their network of family and friends often become part of the team to varying degrees. They may help make key decisions, to relate important information, take a great part in preparing for discharge, or simply offer the emotional or other support that is so crucial to a good outcome. They may also present some additional complications – not always welcome, but all part of the whole that is the person requiring the care.

Interprofessional teams and problems

The common ethical problems that occur with interprofessional teams in health and social care are ineffective leadership, poor (or lack of) communication, mistrust, egos, and the various members having different values and beliefs.

Leadership

In relation to leadership, different team members will want different types of leadership; some may require very little from their leader and just want to get on with their job, and others may want more direction. Leadership becomes ineffective when the leader provides the same style for all the members. Consequently, the good leader supplies the different needs to the different team members. In doing so, the leader needs to be able to trust the members and they in turn need to be able to trust him or her.

Damage can occur in teams when egos get in the way of leadership, which then affects team working. If egos can be suspended then the effect on the team is more comfortable and professionals are more at ease with each other.

Different values and beliefs

With different team members, there are going to be different personal and professional values and beliefs. Also, quite often some team members do not bother to find out how another health care professional undertakes their practice and makes decisions about treatments. Let us look at the issue of various team members all trying to work together, but all having different codes of conduct.

Different codes of conduct?

Professional codes are usually presented as a set of principles or standards, written to reflect relevant expectations of practitioners as they carry out their work. The professional and/or regulatory bodies responsible for each discipline write them. In health and social care, we are often familiar with our own profession's practice codes but remain vague or partially informed about the codes of other professional bodies. As mentioned in Chapter 1, these codes have legal significance – a practitioner found to be violating their own code may be brought before a disciplinary committee and penalised in some way, or even denied the right to practise for a period, or permanently.

A detailed knowledge of all professional codes is impractical and unrealistic for an individual practitioner. However, an awareness of recurring themes or areas of contrast can help us understand the moral behaviour of professional colleagues and appreciate their approach to making ethical decisions in practice. Common to all professional bodies is the end purpose of providing service to the client or patient, and a responsibility to the wider community and society as a whole.

In health and social care, the four ethical principles of autonomy, beneficence, justice and non-maleficence, as mentioned in Chapter 3, are considered by some to be cornerstones to all codes of conduct. Codes of conduct often give a more specific benchmark – they attempt to translate ethical ideas into a set of expectations reflecting each profession's practice context. However, it is important to remember that, although the codes are usually presented in one simplified form (the list of standards), they also have accompanying documents that elaborate them more fully and apply them to practice. Whether thinking about codes or ethical frameworks, always remember there is much thought and detail behind the shorthand versions.

The prominence of each of these (and other) principles will vary across the professional bodies, and is reflected in the language of the written codes, in terms of style and tone, as well as the volume of supporting explanation. Such variance illustrates the richness of diversity within the health and social care professions, although this can also be confusing and unduly complicated. An obvious example here is that professional groups title their codes differently – nursing and midwifery refer to 'code of professional conduct' (Nursing and Midwifery Council (NMC), 2004), social workers refer to 'codes of ethics' (British Association of Social Work (BASW), 2003) and also to 'codes of practice' (General Social Care Council (GSCC), 2002), and doctors abide by 'duties of a doctor' (General Medical Council (GMC), 2001). Some codes of conduct are presented as a series of points; for example, the Chartered Society of Physiotherapy (CSP) (2001) lists eight rules, and includes an explanatory sentence for each rule.

Other codes provide more detailed explanation and description. For example, the code of ethics and professional conduct for occupational therapists (College of Occupational Therapists (COT), 2005) includes 23 points described under the four categories of client autonomy and welfare, services to clients, personal/professional integrity, and professional competence and standards. Even more detailed are the 'duties of a doctor', which describes a total of 60 ethical behaviours under seven main categories, including probity (providing information about services, writing reports and giving evidence, and research) (GMC, 2001). The code of practice of the General Osteopathic Council (GOC, 2005) consists of four main sections, 15 subsections and a total of 61 statements. The previous code (of 2002) was revised to reflect the changes in the law and regulation of health care – a clear reminder of the evolving nature of professional duties.

Endeavours to find common ground between the practice codes of different professional bodies are more feasible today because of the changing remit and structure of the professional bodies. In the UK, for example, we have seen the formation of the NMC for nursing and midwifery (replacing the UKCC), the establishment of the General Social Care Council for social workers and the Health Professions Council (HPC) for the allied health professions, which represents 13 distinct professional groups in total. Indeed, the HPC (2004) has devised its own standards, making 16 explicit statements about a health professional's conduct, performance and ethics. Such uniformity could be seen as a constructive move towards greater consistency across professional groups.

For the purposes of this chapter, a brief exploration of what the different professional codes say about teams and interprofessional collaboration is instructive. As presented by the professional codes, different professional groups define and describe the expected behaviours of a multiprofessional team member. Again, how the different codes of conduct refer to teams and team working varies. Some professional codes describe it as 'cooperating with others' (NMC); the CSP talks about 'relationships with professional staff and carers'; the COT uses the term 'collaborative practice' to include working with institutions and agencies, as well as other professions.

Particular features of the language of code of conducts aim to state clearly what is expected of practitioners. Examples of this can be seen in terms of respecting the skills of other health care professionals (GOC) or maintaining proper communication with patients, carers and professionals (HPC). Some codes are also explicit about what not to do and what behaviours are to be avoided. For example, the CSP states that physiotherapists should avoid any criticism of professional staff and the GMC echoes this by stating that doctors should avoid unfounded criticism of colleagues.

However, scrutiny of different codes of conducts for ethical principles that promote interprofessional collaboration is fraught with difficulties. It is not always apparent whether the practice context is an unprofessional team or an organisational network of autonomous practitioners as opposed to a deliberate strategy of shared working to achieve common goals. The onus in all codes of conducts is the behaviour and 'fitness to practise' of the individual practitioner. Understanding differing values and achieving effective problem-solving can benefit from dialogue and negotiation within the team. Such complexities of interprofessional team working are not necessarily reflected in the separate codes of conduct of individual professions (Irvine et al., 2002). This suggests that shared understandings are generated in the workplace and might be context-specific and relevant to each team.

Beyond codes of conduct – the issues that arise in practice

While codes of conduct represent more of a regulatory or legal approach to ensuring professional behaviour, they are drawn from ethical ideas at their root - the concepts of good or bad and right or wrong. The differing ways in which these codes are written suggest that the ethical concerns arising in practice are somewhat different between professions.

In health and social care, the overall goal of providing good care is a common one between all professions. However, the differing roles and responsibilities and the differing 'core values' between the professions, will mean that the issues arising in everyday practice will vary.

Some practitioners have the responsibility to diagnose a client's health problem and then select the appropriate intervention. These interventions can have various levels of risk associated with them. Some, such as surgery, internal investigations or potent medications, are very invasive. Other interventions are less invasive, but carry much responsibility and can have a huge impact upon the client's life; e.g. assessing a person's capacity for independent living. Still other procedures, such as ultrasound or venepuncture, carry certain risks and anxieties for the client as well. In addition, seemingly simple responsibilities - like administering medication or assisting with washing or toileting - can have a huge impact on a person's physical wellbeing or sense of dignity.

As a team, it is always important to understand and respect each other's roles, as well as each other's opinions, work stresses and responsibilities. While it is not always easy to be attuned to what others are feeling and what their perspectives might be in any situation, this awareness is the basis of good understanding and effective teamwork. It is made possible by good communication and regular reflection.

Such issues relate to treatment choices, but there are other daily issues that arise from the way in which we interact with each other, for both patients and professionals. Think back to the therapy students in the case of Mr Chui in Chapter 1. While the students may have had valid questions to ask the staff, there were very different ways to pursue these questions.

Specific ethical issues for different team members

The literature on ethical issues in practice identifies some of the variations in specific professions' day-to-day experience. There is also discussion of the context of care and the types of issues that might arise. An in-depth review of the literature is beyond our goals here, but a few examples of what one might find are useful.

Research shows that, while we may be aware of and value the fundamental principles of ethics in practice, we are not always able to live up to those principles in a day-to-day context:

- General practitioners were found to have difficulty in applying their own sense of ethical practice in situations where they had to ration services (Berney et al., 2005).

- Occupational therapists reported difficulty keeping their practice in line with the four principles when it came to discharge planning (Atwal and Caldwell, 2003).

- In the high profile case of Victoria Climbie, a young girl who died after extended abuse at home, there was poor communication between the many professionals and agencies involved. During the subsequent inquiry, one of the professionals admitted that senior staff had ordered cases be closed which should have remained open. Although this was in contravention of their professional standards, they neglected to report this unethical practice to an appropriate authority. The reason given was that 'the climate' in the team at the time left them feeling unable to do so (Victoria Climbie Inquiry, 2001).

- Social workers in one study found it ethically very stressful to assess the competence of older persons with dementia when deciding if they could continue living on their own at home (Kadushin and Egan, 2001).

- One study of doctors and nurses making end-of-life decisions found that, while both groups of professionals aimed to make decisions according to the client's wishes, this often became bound up with their own values.

End-of-life issues and the team

When considering the enormous emotional involvement surrounding and involved in end-of-life issues, it is not surprising that they are often cited as difficult. The doctors often make decisions that the nurses do not consider to be in the patient's best interests. One study concluded that communication of ethical issues was important to foster understanding and support of each other in a context of great ethical burden (Oberle and Hughes, 2001).

Read the following case study and answer the question at the end.

Case study 7.1
Mary Anne

Mary Anne is a 61-year-old woman who has suffered a cerebral haemorrhage. She knew that she suffered from vertebro basilar iinsufficiency and wrote an advanced directive that if she had a bleed and suffered a cardiac arrest she did not want to be resuscitated. Her husband showed the directive to the staff. Some of the team wanted to respect the document and others did not. Mary Anne's husband applied to the Court for the directive to be upheld.

Questions

➤ Why would some team members want to resuscitate Mary Anne and others not?

➤ Does the Court have any power to dictate what the hospital staff should do in caring for Mary Anne?

Interprofessional conflicts

Any teamwork gives rise to the possibility of complex interpersonal interactions. In health care, the main conflicts appear to arise because:

● there are different experts working together with different opinions;

● roles change;

● opposing views from different team members; and

● personal conflict.

Different experts

In addition to the team of professionals (who might be seen as the 'trained experts'), it is important to remember that the client and their network are 'experts' of a different sort. They often know about aspects of what they are experiencing and how it is affecting them better than any other member of the team. Sometimes, however, this may not be the case and problems owing to a lack of insight and denial do arise. None the less, the client and their 'significant others' should always be considered collaborators, part of the team, and working with the team for a good result.

Even when we do not arrive at a consensus opinion, there is value in the process and the way in which ethical problems are considered. The journey and the way in which we behave and relate to others are as important as the end destination (care and virtue ethics).

The involvement of clients/patients or service users can extend beyond the usual situation where they are part of their own immediate care team. Increasingly, it is becoming common to consult with and actively involve clients in the development of services, and their delivery to other clients. This kind of collaboration brings a raft of new challenges and a range of new benefits to the service and its recipients (Bramley and Cockshutt, 2005).

One of the difficult aspects of team working is respecting each other's roles, and maintaining an appreciation of the scope and contribution of each member's involvement. Some might be able to take a somewhat broader interest in the client's overall situation. Where there is a team with varying levels of interaction and 'connection' with the client, some professionals might be better placed for certain roles in the team where that connection is beneficial. This might include having to relate disappointing test results, sharing bad news, or communicating with family or friends.

This focus on interprofessional working may seem to contradict another notion linked to contemporary practice in health and social care – that of being an autonomous and independent practitioner. Are we suggesting becoming reliant on the views and contributions of others in the health and social care team? If we value a holistic approach, a team can be an ideal forum for making complex but interdependent decisions. Indeed, your unique professional contribution can be made more explicit by comparing and contrasting skills and knowledge with other members of the team. This does require a practitioner to make connections and see emerging patterns between experiences within a broad professional framework. This sense of 'connectivity' is a valuable asset not only for contemporary professional practice but also for your future employability (Robinson, 2005).

Changing roles

As roles evolve over time, it can be a challenge to some team members when it appears that others are taking on some of their profession's tasks. It could also be a relief, helping to clarify professional roles and boundaries. If the changes in responsibility are sensible, then it should feel right and proper to make such a shift in practice. It is useful, however, to remember that change in itself can be difficult to understand, can appear to be a threat, and can bring about conflict between people who are working to the same end.

Opposing views

While we may all share a central value, belief or philosophy that led us to be involved in providing care, we might approach that task from a somewhat different angle. Some professions may be more focused on 'caring', while others are more focused on 'curing'. Some professionals' work role allows them only a restricted amount of time with each patient, and so they must focus on specific problems. Other professionals, by virtue of the work they do, see clients more often, work with them for many years, or spend more time with fewer clients. When we cannot agree with another team member, it is important to remember the need to focus on communicating effectively among ourselves. Good communication skills depend on keeping our minds open to the view point of the other, whether we agree or not.

Grappling with such opposing views is all part of ethics – thinking methodically through a situation where a multitude of factors weighs in on the 'actors'. There is often a range of responses, each with better and worse outcomes. Being able to consider what course of action is best, and why, is the ethical task.

Personal conflict or self-conflict

At times, we may experience an inner conflict between our personal values and the demands of our professional role. A commonly discussed example is that of a doctor or nurse working in obstetrics and gynaecology services, which includes termination of pregnancies. In such circumstances, it is normally possible for an individual practitioner to opt out of such procedures if they wish, and other members of the team who do not experience this ethical problem will provide the service.

Activity

Read the following case study and answer the questions at the end.

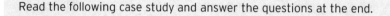

Case study 7.2
Alphonse Martinez

Alphonse Martinez has arrived by ambulance at the emergency department. He is quickly diagnosed to have suffered a severe anterior myocardial infarction and is at risk of having another within the next 8 hours, which could be fatal. Some of the team on the shift know Mr Martinez as he works at the local garage, where staff stop and buy petrol. From chatting to Mr Martinez in the past, you know that he is scared of death. You wonder if you should tell him that he could die if he has another heart attack.

Questions

➤ Does the professional have a right or obligation to tell the patient that there is a possibility of death?

➤ Which member of the team would have this authority?

➤ Should a professional make that decision on his or her own, or should (s)he talk it over with the rest of the team? Give your reasons as to why.

Belonging to a team

Team working has been variously defined and is seen as distinct from an informal *ad hoc* group of people who are not necessarily equally committed to the same goals or values or share a collective identity. A team is normally understood to be a relatively small group of people who share responsibility for planning and implementing agreed goals (Payne, 2000). It is accepted that a team approach is best actualised by the input of differing perspectives and skills of the members.

Given the myriad of places and situations in which health professionals can work together in teams, we cannot give explicit guidance as to how specific teams need to operate. However, we do know that ethical or moral problems can and do occur when the team does not function well together. The Bristol Royal Infirmary Inquiry Report (2001) detailed the poor teamwork which resulted in cardiac surgery children dying postoperatively. Consequently, we are going to present to you tips on working in a team so that, when you know how a team should work you can readily identify when this does not happen. The crucial behaviours of successful teamwork are willing participation, communication, focus, mutual support, team spirit, appreciation of differences including conflict, and collaboration.

Willing participation

Willing participation and a high level of motivation are necessary prerequisites for a team to function well together. Think about the teams who are successful in sport; they want to be there playing the game they love and they are motivated to win. Compare this with a team of people working together who do not want to do things together and are not motivated, and you gain an impression of a team who are losers.

Open and honest communication

There are several important factors to communication, including listening, seeking clarification, constructive criticism, and keeping other members informed.

- The team needs to listen to each other actively, and not tune out. If tuning out occurs then the member can miss something.
- Members need to ask questions of each other and, if something appears confusing, then that member needs to ask for clarification. When seeking an explanation always state the reasons why you need to know.
- Each team member needs to be able to give constructive feedback. Opinion should not be presented as fact! Instead, re-state the team member's original idea so that you can make sure you are responding to the correct concept; compliment another's idea; respond, don't react; don't interrupt; critique the idea not the person; be courteous; and avoid jargon!
- Effective teams keep each other informed. They discuss individual work and inform each other of changes. Lack of communication results in individuals working alone, unaware of how their work fits with that of others.

Focus

Good teams keep their ultimate goals and objectives in mind. Teams run into trouble when they do not allocate time well. In such teams, everyone notices the error but no-one is prepared to offer helpful solutions.

Mutual support

Team members need to give each other encouragement. Remember the successful sporting team – they rally round each other and celebrate the scoring of goals with much backslapping and great joy!

Good teams vocalise their support to each other, and compliment a team member on their success. They offer to help each other and are there to listen when one of them needs to let off steam or to talk things over.

Team spirit and mutual respect

An effective team takes pride in their work, and members are loyal to each other by speaking positively about the team and the success they have achieved together. At the same time there is a balance of participation, which also fosters encouraging individual achievements. An atmosphere of mutual support is needed so that team members feel sufficiently confident and safe to express their opinions without criticism or reprisal. In the successful team, members are able to raise concerns or errors without fear of hostility or retribution.

Trust and collaboration

Trust is an essential component of collaboration for, when team members do not trust each other or have respect, there is no collaboration. When a team collaborates, team members can be seen seeking information and opinions, offering information and opinions, and suggesting directions. Good leadership coordinates and manages the attainment of goals and objectives. This energises the team and stimulates the group to work to a high standard.

Appreciation of differences (including conflict)

Good teams know that there will be differences of opinion; that is, having differences of opinion is one of the essential benefits of teamwork. However, these differences must not be allowed to dominate discussions and impede the achievement of goals and objectives. Differences of opinion are not the same as conflict.

When conflict occurs within the team, this needs to be identified and a meeting scheduled to discuss the conflict. Huszczo (2004) groups conflicts into three types, those that arise from competition, those from misunderstandings, and those from historical events. Many people are surprised to learn that others do not share their thoughts and beliefs.

When conflict occurs

When conflict occurs this needs to be address by those concerned. This can be done individually with the team leader or at a team meeting. One of the most unproductive areas of conflict is the blame game! This is when team members focus on pointing fingers or finding someone in another group to blame for their problem. Bounstein (2002) identifies additional destructive actions that team members can use, and also highlights the constructive behaviours that can be used to work through conflict and maintain respectful relationships with others.

When conflict does occur during a team meeting (or when a meeting is held to discuss problems) the team leader or chair of the meeting needs to redirect the discussion away from blaming, to problem identification and how it can be resolved (Yoder-Wise and Kowalski, 2006). However, at the same time, the problem that is causing the conflict needs to be addressed as a shared need with both sides explaining their view point without interruption from the other party. If, once the issue has been aired, both parties cannot agree on a way forward, they need to accept that the rest of the team will decide on what needs to be done to resolve the issue and for the team to move forward. This can be addressed in an action plan.

Quite often, however, teams do not want to meet to discuss conflict. In these situations, there are several interventions that can be tried or used (Yoder-Wise and Kowalski, 2006):

- **Giving information**: provide information so that the person can understand that there is another perspective.
- **Give advice**: share your opinion to help the other person have awareness of your perspective.
- **Confront**: challenge the person's beliefs, attitudes and behaviour.
- **Being cathartic**: encourage the other person to express their emotion about the issue.
- **Being catalytic**: encourage the other person to talk through the issue with you.
- **Being supportive**: communicate your concern that the views are so opposed to each other and that you are available if the other person wants to talk about it.

Obviously, the intervention or interventions that we choose will depend on the nature of the team, the position of the other person and the role they have. Other approaches to resolving conflict include the four principles of win-win negotiations (Fisher and Ury, 1991), and Thomas and Kilmann's model (2002) of avoiding, accommodating, competing, compromising and collaborating.

Many health professionals are not open about conflict with each other. However, we hope that now you know the components of any successful team, you can now begin to understand about health and social care teams. Sometimes members of a team can have a tendency to use avoidance or accommodation (as described by Thomas and Kilmann, 2002); that is, avoiding the issue or working around the conflict. However, that is not always possible, and collaboration must be strived to maintain a standard of care to clients or patients.

Collaboration is a vital part of a team working together to provide quality care. Remember the Bristol Royal Infirmary Inquiry into the deaths of babies and children having cardiac surgery. There was no collaboration within the team; in fact, they hardly communicated with each other. If we are to prevent other such tragedies, we must learn to be open with each other and work through issues of conflict.

Effective interprofessional working in health care

Working together to be a successful interprofessional team involves knowledge of each other's professional roles, being a willing participant, having confidence and competence, open and honest communication, trust and mutual respect, recognition that conflict will occur and, should it occur, shared power and support and commitment at a senior level to resolve it (Barrett and Keeping, 2005). Strategies to support interprofessional working and dissipate the problems that may arise include group reflection and supervision, joint education and training, and managerial support (Barrett and Keeping, 2005).

Summary

This chapter has introduced the concept of working in a team and the ethical problems this can give rise to, while at the same time recognising, the benefits.

The crucial behaviours of successful teamwork are communication, focus, mutual support, team spirit, appreciation of differences (including conflict), and collaboration. The codes of the different professionals were examined in relation to working with another profession, and how, with different interests and concerns, this may raise moral issues. Finally, the effective behaviours of teamwork were discussed.

Professional development

1 Continue the development of your Ethics Portfolio by adding pertinent journal articles and the answers to activities and questions.

2 In your Ethics Portfolio, write how your professional values compare with the professional values of other members of the team.

3 There are now activities for you to do with your peers in a small group.

   a. Ask two peers to role-play this situation with you with each of you taking the part of a different health professional. Imagine yourself and these two other professionals working with the same patient and their family (for example, a nurse, physiotherapist and a doctor). Perhaps the patient is in a coma after a road accident.

   b. How might any differences in your core values and overall goals be apparent in the ways that you work with the client?

   c. Then discuss with each other:

   ○ What you identified?

   ○ How might this affect the patient's experience?

   ○ Now (in your group of three), work out how you could try to work interprofessionally to make the care feel as coordinated and complementary as possible?

   ● In the same group, discuss how you would respond to a colleague who seems to be imposing his or her ideas on you.

   ○ How do you explain to them that you feel this way?

   ○ Should you?

   ○ Alternatively, would it be right simply to ignore the situation and hope it does not happen again?

   So, how will you go about fostering good team communication?

4 Answer this question.

   You suspect that a colleague is not managing their workload very well, perhaps not keeping their client records up-to-date, and then not being able to write them in proper detail when they finally get down to doing them.

   ➤ Do you talk to them directly?

   ➤ Do you approach it in a light-hearted manner, making comments about 'all the notes' you have to do and how difficult it is to keep up with them?

> When might you consider bringing it up with your manager? (Alternatively, with your colleague's manager if you are from different professions?)

> What might be the consequences if you say something? Or, on the other hand, if you say nothing? What are the legal implications?

> Do these matter to you – or is it simply wrong on ethical grounds?

Critical reflection

Write your critical reflective journal entry for this chapter. Issues that you may want to consider (but are not restricted to) include your experience of:

- Working in an interprofessional team in clinical practice.

- Your experience of working with other students in an interprofessional seminar at university.

- A scene from a medical television programme that evoked issues about a team issue for you that you feel the need to work through.

- One of the case studies.

- Reading that you have done.

- A different point of view that someone raised in discussion in class, or something that your mentor or clinical supervisor said.

- A general feeling of disquiet about team working which you want to explore through reflection.

8

'Why do they make me suffer?' Pain and resuscitation

Georgina Hawley and Stewart Blake

Why this chapter is important to me . . .

✔ The concepts of pain and resuscitation raise similar ethical issues: respect and dignity.

✔ Pain is 'what a client or patient says that it is', not what the health professional assumes their experience to be!

✔ The pain experience is frequently misunderstood.

✔ Do not Resuscitate orders are not always clarified or communicated.

✔ Clients and patients have the right to refuse resuscitation, yet this can be ignored, causing them pain.

✔ Ignoring or not understanding clients' or patients' needs results in loss of trust.

The ethical issues of pain and resuscitation have been brought together in this chapter as they can give rise to similar ethical problems and/or dilemmas. These occur in relation to clients' or patients' rights and the potential power of the health professional to ignore these rights through lack of knowledge and understanding of pain and resuscitation.

In previous chapters, you have learnt how a person's culture and personal beliefs affect the way (s)he views health, care and treatments, and attitudes towards these. Consequently, when these are different from those of the health professional, the practitioners have the power not to recognise these beliefs as legitimate, or not transfer these into the treatment or care plan. That is, ignoring and/or not transferring these would not be ethical - it would be immoral or unethical.

The client or patient has certain rights in relation to health care: access to care, to be treated with respect and dignity, to be able to make autonomous informed decisions, to accept or refuse certain treatments and still receive care. These rights are important and need to be respected. They are underpinned by the ethical principles of autonomy, beneficence, justice and non-maleficence. That is, the ethical principles of beneficence and non-maleficence uphold the need for health professionals to actively do good to clients and patients, and refrain from doing harm or causing unnecessary pain.

In addition, you have learnt about the differences between Eastern and Western philosophy. Eastern theories emphasise the need for harmony in relationships, for calmness, respect and dignity of the person. Also, there is respect for that part of the person which, during life, is their connection with a God, gods or higher power, and at death will be reincarnated or go to another place, such as heaven. In Western philosophy there is emphasis on the need to do good on the basis of the end result or the means by which it is done.

This information will help you now to understand about pain and the ethical way to care for a client or patient who is suffering with pain. This is because pain is not just a physical process, but also a debilitating condition that can wreck a person's mental, emotional and spiritual life. In such situations the person has no dignity left, for they are just a hollow body that is racked by pain (or a shell of the person they used to be). In these situations their whole mind is clouded by the experience of pain to the extent that they may not be mentally competent.

Consequently, the person suffering pain needs the health professional or team to understand his or her experience and supply them with an analgesia and/or treatment to control the pain and the underlying cause. We could say this is a client's or patient's right, that is, to have their pain controlled (Johnstone, 1996; Rees, 1997; Tollison et al., 2002). Yet health professionals have the potential power to restrict that analgesia or pain-relieving treatment.

Likewise, with resuscitation, a client or patient may not want to be resuscitated, but, again, health professionals and the team have the power not to honour the patient's or client's wishes. This is despite clients and patients having the right to refuse treatment (Hawley, 1997b; Johnstone, 1996). This chapter discusses the phenomena of both pain and resuscitation in relation to the ethical concepts of respect for the integrity and dignity of the client and patient, so that you are not one of the health professionals who does not understand 'pain'.

The first section of the chapter highlights some ideas about ethical caring from various authors. Second is a definition and the classifications of pain followed by pathophysiology and responses to pain. Next, an overview of reliable and validated pain assessment tools and appropriate pain management is given and the ethical principles will be applied to pain to reflect upon the notion of respect for the integrity and dignity of the patient. The section on resuscitation begins with a definition of resuscitation and the relationship to ordinary/extraordinary treatments. This is followed by a discussion on issues relating to resuscitation, including witnessing resuscitation, withholding treatment, advance directives and possible conflicts. Finally, the Professional Development section will assist your knowledge and understanding of pain and resuscitation.

The placement of this chapter just prior to illness and loss is important because, although dealing with the loss that a person can experience during illness, it also discusses the greatest loss of all, death. Consequently, pain management important to a person dying who may need strong or large amounts of analgesia before death.

The first thing that you will need to do is to clarify your own values and beliefs about pain and resuscitation. This is so that you will be able to differentiate between your personal values and those required by your profession. That is, you may need to change your personal values on the subject to meet those of your profession. By identifying your own values and beliefs, when you care for clients or patients with pain or resuscitation issues you will be able to differentiate between your values and beliefs and theirs. This is important so that you do not become morally confused between those of your clients or patients and your own.

Activity

1 List your personal values and beliefs about pain in your Ethics Portfolio.

2 Likewise, do the same for resuscitation (or what you understand resuscitation to be).

3 Now explore whose rights are more important, those of the patients or those of the health professionals?

4 Finally, how are you going to demonstrate the ethical ideals of caring, compassion, advocacy and collaboration?

Caring and compassion

Edmund Pellegrino (1991) contended that the word 'profession' originally referred to a special promise to help humanity and to place this above one's own interests. William James (1948), like Pellegrino, believed that we are called to be moral by our interactions with others. The concrete call to care, for James, came not only from specific persons, but from the situations to which people respond. He was wary of idealistic versions of calls to morality that were divorced from specific situations.

Werner Marx (1992) developed an ethics of compassion that is not compassion from the Judaeo-Christian tradition, as he believed that this was no longer available to many people. Werner Marx's ethics of compassion is based on what he calls the shared mortality of all humans. He believes that, when we honestly face our mortality, we are confronted by 'horror . . . in the true sense of the word', shattering the comfortable everyday world in which we live. He argued that when people take life for granted (with no thought to possible suffering or pain), they are indifferent to others and to their own mortality. However, when a person is open to the horror of mortality they are open to the presence of others as fellow human beings.

We urge you to think about the above when considering pain and resuscitation, of the need to be open to the suffering of others.

The pain experience

You might be asking why pain is such an important ethical issue. The reason is, quite simply, that health professionals have the potential power to either disbelieve or misunderstand the client's or patient's pain. This can occur either through choosing to ignore the client or patient, or from having a knowledge deficit in relation to the concepts of pain classifications, pathophysiology, cultural competence and analgesia (or other treatments).

If asked what rights you would like to have met when suffering pain, you would probably ask for:

- Respect from the health professional, who demonstrates this by believing that you have pain.
- Respect from the health professional, who gives you information and choices in relation to analgesia.
- Protection of your dignity by the health professional insomuch that you do not lose your self-regard, self-esteem or self-respect by being destroyed by the anguish of unrelenting pain. Although the term anguish is used here, pain can also cause confusion, disorientation and irrational behaviour.
- Preservation of your dignity by the health professional providing timely and effective analgesia and/or other methods of pain relief that you have chosen. The health professional helps you to evaluate its effect so that you remain free from pain.

Definition of pain

The International Association for the Study of Pain (IASP) defines pain as 'an unpleasant sensory and emotional experience associated with actual and potential tissue damage, or described in terms of such damage' (Portenoy and Kanner, 1996a). From this description we come to realise that pain:

- is a perception, and not really a sensation;
- involves sensitivity to the chemical changes in the tissues and then interpretation that such changes are harmful (Ranney, 2001).

This perception is real (there is nothing imaginary about this) whether or not it has occurred or is occurring. Cognition is also involved, in that the brain and mind needs to formulate the perception. Therefore, there are emotional and behavioural responses to the cognitive and emotional aspects of pain (Ranney, 2001).

Conceptually, pain can be thought of as being composed of three hierarchical levels:

- Sensory-discriminative component (location, intensity, quality)
- Affective-motivation component (anxiety, depression)
- Cognitive-evaluative component (thoughts concerning the cause and significance of the pain) (Tollison et al., 2002).

Understanding these three interrelated components of pain will give you the knowledge to appreciate the 'holistic' nature of pain and how it can affect people's lives. For example, the person with chronic back pain due to osteoarthritis of the spine can readily become depressed with the persistent experience of pain and their inability on occasions to do the most simple daily living tasks of washing and dressing themselves, and who may ponder 'what have I done to deserve such suffering?'

Physiological and pathophysiological classifications of pain

There are several ways to classify pain:

- Peripheral pain: this originates in the soft tissues and involves the sensory nervous supply of the peripheral nervous system, e.g., a sprained ankle or Colles' fracture, etc. (Mense et al., 1997).
- Central pain: arises in the central nervous system (CNS) owing to structural changes in the CNS, e.g., spinal cord injury, multiple sclerosis, stroke and epilepsy (Boivie, 1996).

Another way of classifying pain can be related to the pathophysiology, such as:

- Nociceptive pain, in which the normal nerves (found in skin, muscle, joints and some visceral tissues) transmit information to the CNS about trauma to tissues. Only when the impulses reach the brain are they intellectually (cognitively) recognised as pain (Mense et al., 1997).
- Neuropathic pain, in which there are structural and/or functional nervous system adaptations secondary to an injury; this takes place either centrally or peripherally (Jensen, 1996). Much of what has been previously classified as psychogenic pain is now better understood as neuropathic pain of central origin (Portenoy and Kanner, 1996a). In fact, Covington (2000) states that psychogenic pain does not exist. The IASP defines central pain as 'pain initiated or caused by a primary lesion or dysfunction in the CNS' (Merskey and Bogduk, 1994).
- Note: neuropathic should not be confused with 'neurogenic', a term used to describe pain resulting from injury to a peripheral nerve but without necessarily implying any 'neuropathy' (Ranney, 2001).

If you are unfamiliar with the four processes of nociception (transduction, transmission, perception and modulation), we would suggest you research them for, until you do so, you will have no comprehension of the client's or patient's pain experience and suffering, including what was once known as 'phantom limb pain'.

When reading about pain, you will also find names or terms used such as acute or persistent pain, and characteristics such as intensity, quality, temporal, topography, and exacerbating and relieving factors (Portenoy and Kanner, 1996a). Again, finding out about these names and terms will help you to provide the care the client or patient requires.

Increasing a client's or patient's pain!

It is also well to remember that pain can be intensified by anxiety, depression, anger and fatigue. These may be caused not only through the client's or patient's disease or condition, but also when they perceive that the health professional treating them lacks knowledge and understanding or does not believe their statement of the pain (Spross, 1985). Consequently, responding to the client or patient with pain demands high standards of care.

Assessing pain

Pain is inherently subjective (that is, it is the way in which the client or patient describes it to you), and the patient's self-report is the gold standard in assessment (Tollison et al.,

2002). As such you need to acknowledge the information that (s)he is giving you. For, if the client or patient detects that you do not believe them, his or her trust and faith in you as a health professional is destroyed. Consequently, the therapeutic relationship is ruined, and the client or patient can experience increased or worse pain owing to anxiety.

How the client or patient may present for treatment or care

People respond to pain in many different ways. This response, to a great extent, may depend on the patient's cultural background, their age, gender, religion, past experience, or even as a learned response through family influence (Helman, 2000; Henley and Schott, 2000; Melzack, 1975). The health professional might also note that the client's or patient's blood pressure, pulse and respirations may be different from previous observations and the skin may appear pale and clammy, or cold.

Some patients may respond to pain by being either quietly or overly demonstrative; some will appear very quiet and withdrawn; other patients may be somewhat aggressive and demanding in requesting their pain needs to be met. Sometimes patients become very emotional when experiencing pain (Helman, 2000; Henley and Schott, 2000). Some patients may underreport their pain or remain in pain. This may result from cultural or religious beliefs (such as wrong done in the past) and therefore the client or patient believes that the pain needs to be experienced (MacLachlan, 1997).

While culture can affect the way in which a client or patient responds to pain it would be foolish to think that all people from that culture would respond in the same way (Helman, 2000). Such stereotyping through rigid ideas and mistaken beliefs can lead to unethical care (owing to discrimination and disrespect) when the health professional or team fail to recognise or acknowledge the patient's pain simply because (s)he did not respond in a predetermined or expected way (Henley and Schott, 2000).

Consequently, no matter which type of patient we are dealing with, or how the patient may identify their pain, it is not only our responsibility but also our duty to believe the client's or patient's description and expression of their pain, and accept that the patient may not simply be expressing the physical nature, but also the more holistic nature of the experienced pain.

Pain assessment tools

A variety of validated pain scales are available to assist in the measurement of pain. These include simple one-dimensional scales and multidimensional questionnaires. Commonly used one-dimensional scales include:

- Verbal Rating Scale (VRS);
- Numeric Rating Scale (NRS); and
- Pictorial Scale (such as a series of faces from smiling (no hurt) to grimace with tears (worse hurt) (Bieri et al., 1990).

The choice of pain scale may depend on the patient's age, ability to communicate or other specific circumstances. While the VRS (that is, 'none', 'mild', 'moderate' and 'severe') is the simplest measure, other scales can provide additional information (Bartel et al., 2003).

Multidimensional pain assessment tools have been developed to quantify the location and quality of the pain, and also the effects to mood and function. Multidimensional pain assessment tools take longer for the client or patient to complete than the one-dimensional scales (Bartel et al., 2003). Moreover, the socially indigent person or someone poorly educated or who is cognitively impaired may not be able to use the scale, or may need help in filling in the boxes. The advantage of using the scale is that the patient can select which descriptor best suits their pain. For example, burning, throbbing, aching, heavy, which can suggest underlying nociceptive or neuropathic mechanisms (Portenoy, 1991).

Multidimensional pain assessment tools include:

- The McGill pain scale assesses pain in three dimensions: sensory, affective and evaluative (Melzack, 1975). This scale may need to be modified for people who could be shocked and displeased at having to identify on the outline of an unclothed person as to where their pain is. It would be more appropriate if the body (both front and back views) were sketched with the cultural or religious clothes for that client or patient.

- The Memorial Pain Assessment Card, used with cancer patients for rapid assessment of pain, pain relief and mood includes a set of adjectives for pain intensity (Fishman et al., 1987).

- The Brief Pain Inventory is a quick multidimensional pain measurement tool with reliability and validity of the functional status of patients with cancer, HIV/AIDS and arthritis. This tool takes 5-15 minutes to administer and includes 11 numeric scales for pain intensity, as well as the impact of pain on general activity, mood, ability to walk, work, relationships, sleep and enjoyment of life (Daut et al., 1983).

- The Neuropathic Pain Scale assesses neuropathic pain once it has been identified (Galer and Jensen, 1997).

- The Comprehensive Health-Related Quality of Life Assessment (HRQoL) (Bartel et al., 2003).

- The Treatment Outcomes of Pain Survey (TOPS) is the gold standard of health-related quality of life. This tool is useful in patient monitoring and as a research tool to measure quality of life in relation to pain (Rogers et al., 2000).

Pain assessment is not simply a matter of asking how bad the pain is, but also of determining where it is, its description, its association (to the heart, muscles, stomach and abdomen), the type of pain (stabbing, gripping, aching or burning), the effect on daily activities, mood, the quality of life, and the cultural and religious values and beliefs (Portenoy and Kanner, 1996a).

Management of the pain experience

Although culture, religion and ethnicity may all influence a client's or patient's perception and response to pain, it is never possible to predict on the basis of his or her 'group' what pain relief (s)he may want or what concerns (s)he may have (Henley and Schott, 2000). Pain is by definition subjective, and understanding the client's or patient's own perception of their pain and what it means to them is the only logical starting point for planning pain relief and/or management.

As previously stated, the experience of pain involves the following three components: sensory-discriminative; affective-motivation; and cognitive-evaluative. It is important to provide treatment and care that encompasses all components to be effective.

When prescribing and administering analgesia you need to remember that the effectiveness and the effects of different medications are influenced by many factors. These include age, sex, diet, other medications, diurnal rhythms, menstrual cycle, and multiple disease states. Genetic differences in metabolism between ethnic groups can also alter the effectiveness and effects of medications (through slower or quicker metabolic rates). These genetic differences have been reported with the following medications: certain opiates, chemotherapy, immunosuppressants, antidepressants, anxiolytics, cardiovascular agents, antitubercular drugs, beta-blockers and alcohol. In these situations the client or patient may need a decreased or increased dose, or less or greater time between the doses (Henley and Schott, 2000).

None of the major religions forbids or advises clients or patients not to use pain-relieving analgesics, including opiates. However, sometimes clients or patients may refuse these because they fear it will affect their ability to make decisions, especially if they want to retain control of the situation or life. In such circumstances, ask the patient if there is something else you could do for them to help relieve the pain. This could be meditation and/or the use of a small shrine or lit candle, listening to music, and the reading of religious materials.

The following mnemonic illustrates the key elements for pain management – ABCDE pain management and assessment (Bartel *et al.*, 2003, cited by AMA, 2003).

A – Ask about pain regularly. Assess pain systematically.

B – Believe the client or patient and family reports of pain and what provides relief.

C – Choose pain control options appropriate for the patient, family and setting.

D – Deliver intervention in a timely, logical and coordinated manner.

E – Empower patients and their family. Enable them to control their course to the greatest extent possible.

Activity

It is now time to put into action the knowledge and understanding you have gained from the first part of this chapter by reading the following case study and answering the questions.

Case study 8.1
Alphonse and the pain that goes off the scale

Alphonse Martinez has been in the hospital for the past 24 hours following an episode of acute chest pain. Just as visiting time is coming to an end, he begins to experience another episode of pain. Staff are alerted and, as is routine, an ECG is required before treatment can be commenced.

Alphonse is asked to estimate his pain on a scale of 0–10 (0 being no pain, 10 being unbearable pain). He states the level of pain experienced is 5. Staff begin to attach the electrodes to his chest, but this proves rather difficult due to his clammy skin and it is not possible to get a good reading of electrical activity of the heart.

Again Alphonse is asked to estimate his pain level; by this time it has risen to 8. Staff are still having problems in attaching the electrodes and it takes a further minute to get a set that adhere to the chest. It is now some 3 or 4 minutes since he first complained of the onset of pain. A further assessment of pain level experienced by Alphonse reveals a level of 14. At this response staff reacted in a rather disapproving manner.

Questions

➤ What reasons might you think caused Alphonse to respond with a score of 14?

➤ Remembering the ABCDE mnemonic of pain assessment and management, what would have been the best way to respond?

➤ Would a different pain scale have been more appropriate? If so, which one?

Application of ethical principles

It is imperative that health professionals respect the integrity and maintain the dignity of the client or patient experiencing pain. The health professional remembering to uphold the ethical principles of autonomy, beneficence, justice and non-maleficence can do this.

Autonomy

When patients enter a hospital or health care facility they often lose their ability to be autonomous. As a result of this loss, the manner in which patients perceive their care and their involvement in the decision-making process about their care, will be different than if they had retained their autonomy. This, in turn, causes patients to have no knowledge of what information to ask for and creates a situation where patients are extremely vulnerable and in danger of losing the capacity to maintain their own dignity.

It is therefore important that we believe patients when they say they have pain and at what level so that appropriate treatment can be implemented. This may include explaining to patients the reason for the pain that they are feeling. Such information will allow them to understand and derive some control over the situation (and fulfils the principle of autonomy). For example, in the process of preparing patients for an operation, the health professional can inform the patient of what is to happen and what they may experience in respect to pain. This only provides patients with an estimate of the degree of pain they may experience and depends on how well they understood the information you gave!

Beneficence

The notion of beneficence is actively to do good for clients or patients. Consequently, to uphold or fulfil this principle accurate ongoing assessment is necessary. Acknowledging the client's or patient's experience and acting accordingly also demonstrates respect for the person.

Often linked with the term beneficence is the phrase 'best interests of the patient'. One problem that arises is how do we identify what in fact is meant by the best interests of the patient. It may be argued that to have an interest, or be interested, in something is a good thing. To have no interest whatsoever may be considered harmful or detrimental to the well-being of the person.

Interests are regarded as important aspects of life, the things that:

- we value (specific people, and the concepts of honesty, integrity, truth telling and kindness);
- things that appeal or are attractive to us, such as activities, hobbies and leisure.

Primarily, we are attracted to interests as they create and provide us with benefit and wellbeing.

When experiencing pain, anxiety, worry or distress, a client's or patient's interests may also be involved. Therefore, caution needs to be taken when trying to surmise what might be in the best interests of the patient in relation to beneficence. There is a danger in simply relating to what we might consider to be best interests from our own point of view if we were in that situation.

This is why, at the beginning of the chapter, you were asked to identify you own values and beliefs about pain. Therefore, there is the need to ask the patient what would be in his or her best interest. If this is not possible then, taking into consideration everything that you know about the patient (family, life style, culture, etc.), you could pose the question 'given all these, what would be in the best interest of Lynie or Johnnie?'

Justice

This is the principle that requires clients and patients be treated equally and with fairness in relation to resources provided for their care but also the quality of care. It does not mean that we treat one patient in exactly the same way as another, as there is the need to allow for individuality based on gender, cultural and religious beliefs. This might mean that some patients will get 'more' in the sense of treatment and care than someone else, but this should only occur based on their 'health needs', not because of who they are, or the position that they hold in society.

There is sometimes conflict between the health professional and the patient. For example, the health professional identifies and deals with what they consider the patient to need, while the patient identifies and requires a want to be satisfied, though both are calculated from a health perspective.

Pause and think

> Do you know the difference between a want and a need?

A need and a want are not necessarily the same thing. I may want a new computer, but do not need one. What I have is efficient and effective and does the job well. But what about the patient who wants a strong analgesic to relieve their pain; can the health professional justify giving a milder analgesic on the basis that is what, in their opinion, the patient needs?

- Is this unjust and unfair on the patient?

Consider the patient who has concerns regarding the use of pharmacological pain relief. The patient may be anxious that they do not become overreliant or addicted to the medication. How are you going to uphold the ethical principles?

Of course, it is also possible that the health professional has reservations regarding the patient becoming reliant on certain medication, which leads to undermedication and poor pain management.

Non-maleficence

This is the principle that informs us we must not cause harm, and must actively follow a course that prevents harm from occurring. When discussing pain relief with clients or patients it is important to explore possible side effects and also their beliefs and any possible fears about the different routes of administration, so that they are fully informed in the decision-making process and selection of the most appropriate pain management method(s). In this way, because of joint decision-making with regard to pain management there is less likelihood of intentional harm to the client or patient.

Activity

➤ If a health professional does not believe a client's or patient's response when assessing his or her level of pain, is this causing harm?

➤ Is it not upholding non-maleficence?

You might argue that this harm is not caused intentionally. However, if you consciously ignore a client's or patient's response (which is largely intentional in itself), then the harm caused could be categorised as being more intentional.

Consequently, if harm occurs to the patient as a result of something that you or I do or, in this case, fail to do, we still have to take responsibility. This is because we are accountable not only for our actions but also for our inactions. Therefore, every effort needs to be made to assist the client or patient to be without pain.

Activity

From an ethical perspective what would you do if a colleague* prescribes an analgesic that you know could cause harm to the client or patient for whom you are caring?

*The name colleague is used here for either a doctor or one of the health professionals that are now able to perform non-medical prescribing (nurses, physiotherapists and some other allied health professionals).

Pain management outcomes

The positive outcomes of pain management include the empowerment of clients or patients and also compliance and/or concordance.

Facilitating the empowerment of patients

By being beneficent and respectful of patients as people, health professionals can enhance patients' ability to maintain their dignity. As a result of this it is possible to facilitate their empowerment so that they can become more autonomous in relation to identifying the care required to meet their specific and more general health care needs. This is because the provision of good pain control increases patients' capacity to participate in their care (Bartel et al., 2003; Gamsa, 1994).

Patient compliance (or concordance)

When pain management is effective the client or patient feels more in control of the situation. This is turn may create potential for him or her to become more compliant with other medications required, but also other aspects of treatment.

In addition, if the client or patient is provided with information about his or her pain management (including medication usage and side effects, with issues discussed as they arise), then (s)he is less likely to worry about drug dependence, constipation, drowsiness, nausea or any other associated side effect (Helman, 2000; Henley and Schott, 2000; Portenoy and Kanner, 1996b).

Activity

Now that the positive outcomes of pain management have been discussed, list and describe in your Ethics Portfolio what the negative outcomes are (and what they might be).

Activity

Read the case study below and answer the questions at the end.

Case study 8.2
Sven and a case of drink?

Sven Zoderman, a 22-year-old factory worker, had injured his foot at work and, following surgery, is about to be discharged from hospital. He has been prescribed codeine phosphate tablets, an opioid analgesic, to control his pain. Owing to the extent of his injury, it is thought that he will be required to take these tablets for at least 3–4 weeks.

Sven has been told about the side effects of codeine phosphate and that he should not drink alcohol as, when taken together, these cause sedation and possible hypotension. Although he appears to have understood this information, you are concerned that he may not comply and that he will drink alcohol, as you understand his normal intake to be above 2 units per day.

Questions

➤ What obligation(s) does the health professional have in a situation like this?

➤ Taking account of the principles of autonomy, beneficence, justice and non-maleficence, decide how may the health professional approach this situation.

Paternalism and analgesia

In situations like the case study of Sven, it is quite possible for the health professional to become somewhat paternalistic in their approach to care (to make a decision on what (s)he believes is right for the patient) and to make assumptions as to what they believe to be in the patient's best interests. That is, the health professional limits the client's or patient's capacity for autonomy on the basis that (s)he knows best for the Svens of the world. This is sometimes termed 'beneficent paternalism' or 'paternalistic beneficence'.

However, it might not always be a case of paternalistic beneficence. Could it be the health professional trying to do what is right for the client or patient? If, for example, a patient in the terminal stages of illness has a fear of drug dependence, is this a legitimate concern for the patient? Would it not be correct to discuss with the patient that there is no danger of them becoming drug-dependent, and it is important for him or her to receive the correct amount of analgesia to control the pain.

Pause and think

➤ When terminally ill patients need to have a large dose of opiate analgesia to control their pain, is the giving of only a small dose in their best interest?

➤ When a patient with heart failure needs their opiate analgesia titrated, but the health professional keeps giving the same dose, is this in the patient's best interests?

We can recognise that, when health professionals do not provide effective pain management and the client or patient receives inappropriate pain control, not only are the ethical principles of beneficence, justice and non-maleficence not upheld, but also that beneficence and best interests have also been infringed. Consequently, the client or patient has been denied respect and dignity!

Clearly, such care is rude, crude and ignorant, and not worthy to be termed 'professional care'. Neither is the so-called health professional that provides the substandard care worthy of the trust that the client or patient and other health professionals have in his or her level of care.

Pain relief and dying

You will probably have noticed that, although we are discussing pain and analgesia *per se*, the condition and illness of the patient is intertwined and therefore the two cannot be separated. Consequently, there is some overlap between this chapter and the next in relation to the person who is dying and needing strong or large amounts of analgesia to control their pain so that they can die with dignity and be in control of their behaviours. There is nothing quite so distressing to relatives than to see their loved one in pain.

Read the following case study and answer the questions at the end.

Case study 8.3
Lady Sarah and morphine

Lady Sarah Bartholomew, aged 84 years of age, was admitted to hospital five days ago with pneumonia, and her condition is now deteriorating. She is semiconscious and clearly in distress.

Lady Sarah's breathing is laboured even though she is receiving oxygen via a face mask. She moans audibly on expiration, suggesting that she is experiencing a great deal of pain.

The interprofessional team meet to discuss the situation. An agreement is reached (though it is not supported by all staff) that Lady Sarah will be prescribed morphine to control the pain.

Some staff are concerned that the morphine will compromise the already weak respiratory system.

Others say that, although the morphine may cause respiratory depression, the effect of the drug will relax the patient's respiratory muscles and therefore Lady Sarah will not have to work as hard to breathe, and will therefore have less pain. Also, any anxiety she has owing to the difficulty in breathing will be dissipated.

Questions

➤ Are the first group of staff correct in their assumption that morphine will compromise the already weakened respiratory system?

➤ Are the second group of staff correct in their assumption about morphine?

➤ Do you think morphine is an appropriate treatment?

➤ Articulate your decision by using the ethical principles of autonomy, etc.

Doctrine of double effect or principle of double effect (as it is known within the Roman Catholic Church)

At times, as health professionals we can foresee that a particular act or treatment can be beneficial but may also have potentially harmful consequences. According to Ashley and O'Rourke (1989), at such times we can use the doctrine of double effect to see or ascertain if it would be ethical to provide that treatment. That is, the particular treatment can be used if the following criteria can be met:

1 The intended object of the act must not be intrinsically contradictory to a person's fundamental commitment to God and neighbour (including self).

2 The intention of the health professional must be to achieve beneficial effects and to avoid harmful effects as far as possible. That is, harmful effects should not be wanted, but only allowed.

3 The foreseeable beneficial effects must be equal to or greater than the foreseeable harmful effects.

4 Beneficial effects must follow from the action at least as immediately as do harmful effects.

In the previous case study of Lady Sarah, the intention is to relieve her of pain and discomfort and, in so doing, promote her dignity in dying. By following the doctrine or principle of double effect it can be seen that it is ethical to give morphine.

Pause and think

➤ How much analgesia can be given in these circumstances?

The answer is given in the criteria; that is, the third and fourth criteria. The third criterion states that the beneficial effects must be equal to or greater than the foreseeable harmful effects. That is, if the effect of the opioid analgesia (beneficial effect) is greater or equal to the drowsiness or lowered state of consciousness and/or respiratory depression (harmful effect), then the analgesia can be given.

If in such a situation a dose and strength of opioid can be given that does not cause loss of consciousness or respiratory depression then that is the dose that needs to be given. However, if this is not possible, then the dose and strength that possibly might cause loss of consciousness or respiratory depression can be given provided this meets the fourth criterion.

The fourth criterion states that the beneficial effects must follow from the action at least as immediately as do the harmful effects. This means that the pain relief (beneficial effect) needs to occur before or at the same time as any loss of consciousness or respiratory depression (harmful effect).

Activity

Read the following case study and answer the questions at the end.

Case study 8.4
Major Charles Wing (Rtd) and would you believe it?

Major Charles Wing (Rtd) has been on your ward for three days following a fall at home. He has complained consistently of severe pain in his back during this time, although on X-ray no cause can be found for the pain.

At a team conference Major Charles' care and treatment plan is discussed. Some of the nursing staff feel that Major Charles is simply seeking attention and they display an attitude of indifference towards him. However, an occupational therapist believes that he is suffering from pain.

Questions

➤ Compare the attitudes of the nurses and occupational therapist in the case study using the ethical perspectives of autonomy, beneficence, justice and non-maleficence.

➤ Find out the difference between the professional roles of occupational therapy and nursing? You could do this by asking students of these professions or accessing resources in the library or internet.

➤ Why might the occupational therapist have a different insight into Major Charles' pain experience?

Prescribing analgesia for other uses

Suppose a patient with a chronic long-term illness such as arthritis asks his or her doctor or a specialist nurse for a prescription for stronger and more frequent analgesia for pain relief.

Is the doctor or nurse obliged to supply this?

That is, if the gold standard of treatment is based on what the patient says the pain is, does the doctor supply the stronger, more frequent analgesia?

Obviously, the doctor or nurse needs to believe in and relieve the symptoms, but sometimes, although very rarely, the patient doesn't need the analgesia.

➤ What if the patient wants to use this medication for euthanasia?

➤ What if the patient is being threatened by someone to supply them with drugs?

➤ What if the patient is selling the tablets to a known drug addict down the street?

Let us hope that no doctor or nurse would be so busy that (s)he did not sit down and discuss appropriate pain relief with a patient, and if (s)he thought that the amount or type of analgesia requested was excessive to explore this with the patient.

Are doctors obliged to write a prescription for analgesia in the above circumstances?

In fact, it would be illegal to write a prescription that, in their professional judgement, was going to be abused. Many countries have laws specially dealing with misuse of drugs. In the UK, this is the Misuse of Drugs Regulations (2001). None the less, if we examine the criteria of double effect again, we can see that the doctor is also not morally obliged to supply the amount of requested analgesia.

If the doctor thought that the prescription was going to be used for euthanasia, the first criterion, 'the intended object of the act must not be intrinsically contradictory to a person's fundamental commitment to God and neighbour (including self)' would not be upheld. Neither would the second criterion, 'intention of the health professional must be to achieve the beneficial effects and to avoid the harmful effects as far as possible'. Likewise the third and fourth criteria would not be upheld.

So what can the health professional do?

- The doctor needs to explore the reasons behind the patient's wishes for the stronger analgesia. Is the request for stronger pain relief because (s)he is anxious about something else and feels lonely, isolated and scared and wants to end his or her life. Perhaps (s)he is clinically depressed. It is these background issues that need care and treatment.
- At the same time, the stronger analgesia is prescribed to ascertain the effect.

In all of this, the therapeutic relationship between health professional and patient can develop and the professional can discover the real reason for the request for the analgesia.

Supplying the medication to someone to sell

Again the criteria of double effect will be used. The first criterion would not be upheld, as this would be in contradiction to the professional's code of ethics and standard of practice as outlined by the Medical Act and Medical Board. Neither would the second criterion be met.

Only harm could be achieved by the supply of drugs for another person to sell. Similarly, the third criterion would not be met. The beneficial effects of supplying drugs is less than the harmful effects and, therefore, the harmful effects are disproportionate to the benefits. The fourth criterion would not be fulfilled because the beneficial effects might not be as immediate as the harmful effects.

Pause and think

➤ How could the situation be handled?

Supplying the medication to someone who is being threatened

If the patient was being threatened by someone to supply the drug or medication, much would depend on the context. For example, if in hospital an armed addict holds up a staff member, it is usually hospital policy to give the addict the drugs, rather than the staff member being seriously injured or killed.

In this scenario, if there was not sufficient confidence and trust between patient and doctor for the patient to divulge the information when the issue is raised, the doctor could say to the patient that (s)he could only have that medication under supervision at the doctor's surgery once or twice a day. Alternatively, the normal analgesia could be continued while the matter is investigated. If a patient is being threatened by someone to supply their medication, then their pain will not be controlled and so the doctor could hospitalise the patient for pain management (but also protection).

In each of these situations the health professional would need to work out for themselves what was appropriate.

Personal misuse

Sometimes a patient will obtain medications from multiple avenues, even to the extent of using false names to obtain prescriptions from more than one doctor. In the UK, doctors and non-medical prescribers are required to report cases of drug misuse to The National Drugs Treatment Monitoring System.

Although it does not happen very often, sometimes a health professional wants the medication for themselves. Doctors have been known to write prescriptions for patients who do not need the drug and then administer it to themselves. Likewise, other professionals who can prescribe medications can also do this. Nurses who have access to medication cupboards have been known to steal the drug of their choice. In these situations, whatever excuse the professional provides for their behaviour it cannot be condoned.

If you are faced with the situation of a colleague misusing prescribed drugs, the best way to help him or her is to report the situation to your superior so that the person can have sick leave and undertake treatment and rehabilitation for their addiction.

When the pain and suffering is too great

On 12 May 2006, the House of Lords rejected Lord Joffe's Assisted Dying for the Terminally Ill Bill (ADTI). The purpose of the bill was to allow a doctor who, at the persistent and informed request of a terminally ill patient who has the capacity to self-administer and is suffering unbearably, to prescribe medication for self-administration by the patient in order to end his or her suffering by ending his or her life (Hansard, 12 May 2006, col. 1184).

The idea or premise of this bill was so that patients, if they so desired, would not be dependent on someone else or at the mercy of someone else to effectively control their pain. That is, if a patient decided to go down this route the health professional would not need to calculate the fourth criterion of the doctrine of double effect each time they tried to control that person's pain. In this way, it would free the health professional of some of the guilt that many have regardless of whether or not they have brought forward the patient's death by prescribing or giving too much analgesia. This is a real and legitimate fear held by many nurses and doctors.

Although many assume a person's pain will be controlled during the dying process this is not always the case. If there was effective pain control, why would we need to devote a whole chapter in an ethics book to the subject, and why would we need to state so explicitly how to provide basic care for clients and patients in pain.

The reason is simple; that is, there remains a considerable level of ignorance about the effective use of treatments to relieve the distressing symptoms many people experience in dying. There is also a lack of skill in communicating with patients, causing them to feel isolated, lonely and in pain (Brazil and Vohra, 2005; Wells *et al.*, 2001).

A recent survey undertaken of patients and their carers in the UK found that less than 50% felt that the patient's pain had been adequately controlled. In fact, for the past 18 months there has been a shortage of diamorphine in the UK.

In your Ethics Portfolio, list the conditions, diseases or illnesses which a client or person could die from which could or will cause severe pain and/or distress. You may need to access textbooks to answer this question correctly. Why? Because some students and health professionals incorrectly think that it is only the cancer type illnesses that will cause severe pain in the terminally ill client or patient.

Assisted Dying for the Terminally Ill Bill

The argument in the House of Lords for Assisted Dying for the Terminally Ill Bill (ADTI) that day was epitomised in the following:

> all religious believers hold that there is no stage of human life, and no level of human experience that is intrinsically incapable of being lived through in some kind of trust and hope. They would say that to suggest otherwise is to limit the possibility of faithful and hopeful lives to those who are in charge of their circumstances or who enjoy a measure of control and success. Believers hold that even experiences of pain and helplessness can be passed through in a way that is meaningful and that communicates dignity and assurance'
> (http://www.publications.parliament.uk/pa/ld200506/ldhansrd/vo060512/text/60512-04htm/).

Pause and think

➤ What is this statement implying?

➤ Can a person in pain who is suffering unbearably (as that is what the bill was about) act and communicate with dignity?

➤ Can a person who is suffering unbearably in pain and is helpless find assurance in their faith?

➤ Can we say that a person who is in pain and a state of helplessness needs to seek assurance in their faith?

➤ Has a group of people (the House of Lords) the right to state how others (patients) should perceive their pain?

Professional obligation to be caring

At the beginning of this chapter Edmund Pellegrino's (1991) definition of being a professional in relation to caring was used, along with James' standard of morality. Likewise, Werner Marx's (1992) ethics of compassion argued that when people are indifferent to the suffering of others they are not being moral or ethical.

Many countries have laws that provide protection for doctors who feel morally obliged to provide the means of assisting death at the persistent and informed request of a terminally ill patient who has capacity and is suffering unbearably, to prescribe medication for self-administration. Such legal Acts provide for the very small percentage of people who are caught in the agony of uncontrollable pain and suffering to self-administer medication that will bring about their own death.

Not all patients suffering uncontrollable pain and suffering will want to avail themselves of ADTI as they are too fearful or it may be against their religious or cultural beliefs.

Activity

What is more ethical in your view?

➤ A doctor who legally prescribes a self-administered medication for a terminally ill patient who is suffering unbearably? or

➤ Watching someone who is terminally ill suffer unbearable pain and debility?

How does this compare with what is stated in your professional standards or code of ethics?

Pause and think

➤ If you live in the UK, how many people do you think might avail themselves of ADTI each year if it should become legal?

If thought about 35-50 people you are probably about right as this was the number that died using this method in countries with similar populations where ADTI has been made legal.

Mental and emotional pain

People quite often experience pain caused by life situations; for example, being bullied, bereavement, divorce, being caught in a war, being accused of something that they did not do, and being a refugee. Some health professionals believe that there is no actual physical cause for this type of pain and dismiss the client's or patient's pain experience. Identifying the pain with either psychological or psychiatric help and treatment would be more appropriate. Hence, we return to the gold standard of treatment, which is to acknowledge and understand that the pain is very real and even frightening for clients or patients. As health professionals, we should respect the integrity and maintain the dignity of the patient.

People who are clinically depressed also suffer from pain. They will say that they have a pain deep inside themselves. This pain is so bad that it causes insomnia and stops the person from thinking properly. Quite often, in trying to get away from the pain, which is so bad for them, they will commit suicide so that they do not have to feel the pain any more. (Dr Maude writes about this in Chapter 11.)

Summary of pain

Pain is a multifaceted physiological phenomenon. Conceptually, the experience of pain includes three hierarchical levels:

- sensory-discriminative component;
- affective-motivation component; and
- cognitive-evaluative component.

Together, these require empathetic assessment and management to achieve the 'gold standard', which is devoid of stereotyping and assumptions. The ethical duty of the health professional involves accepting the client's or patient's account of the pain experience and providing appropriate treatment care. In this way, respect for the integrity of the client or patient is achieved, and dignity is maintained. The bonus for the health professional is that trust will develop, and empowerment will be facilitated, as will concordance or compliance.

The prescription of analgesia for other uses, including personal drug addiction, has also been briefly discussed, as has assisted dying for the terminally ill patient who has unbearable pain and suffering.

Moral aspects of resuscitation

As discussed earlier, clients and patients have the right to refuse treatment. Consequently, they have a right to refuse resuscitation, and you might expect requests to be accepted. However, either individually or collectively as a team, health professionals have the power not to honour such requests. This can be done through either choosing to ignore or misunderstand:

- the client's or patient's health beliefs, including culture and/or religious beliefs;
- the client's or patient's health problem pathology and the pathophysiology that occurs with a respiratory or cardiac arrest; and
- the legal situation (or law of the country).

Ignoring the wishes of the client or patient could in some instances be unethical, and yet it frequently occurs. This part of the chapter discusses what is meant by resuscitation, why in some cases there is good reason to ignore the wishes of clients or patients and, finally, ordinary and extraordinary treatments, the pathophysiology of cardiac arrest and the potential outcome.

What is resuscitation?

The word 'resuscitation' comes from the Latin word *resuscitare* that means to revive or restore the person to consciousness. In relation to health care, it is important to establish what is meant by resuscitation. What do we actually mean when we refer to resuscitation of the patient or when considering a do not resuscitate (DNR) order?

Resuscitation is usually defined as the process of sustaining the vital functions of the person in respiratory or cardiac failure, using techniques of artificial respiration and cardiac massage, correcting acid-base balance, and treating the cause of the failure.

This means that, when the health professional or team are deciding whether or not the client or patient should be resuscitated, they need to consider why and how his might occur. That is, why would the respirations cease, or what would cause no cardiac output? Once this is known then the decision can be made whether or not it is in the client's or patient's best interests to be resuscitated. This decision also includes influential factors such as age, personal statements including religious and cultural beliefs, and allocation of resources.

Activity

Think of possible scenarios in which a client or patient may request not to be resuscitated and you believe that (s)he should be resuscitated.

In your answer did you include:

- The older person who, just because they are old, decides they need to make the decision.
- The depressed person who is likely to take an overdose or commit suicide.
- The person who is not mentally competent to make such a decision.
- The client or patient with a chronic illness (that has the potential to be terminal at some time in the future).

A patient's request for DNR needs to be specific

A DNR request must include details because, as health professionals, we cannot accept blanket written documents or statements unless they are specific and are regularly updated by the person concerned.

How a patient's views about DNR can change

In Chapter 2, you learnt how not only your values and beliefs change, but so can those with whom you work and those for whom you care. Naturally, then, clients' or patients' views about resuscitation also change not only because of their life experiences but also in relation to their illness or disease at the time. Research has shown that ill patients change their minds about whether or not they want to be resuscitated in relation to when they first become ill or diagnosed, when first admitted to hospital and when they are ready for discharge, and on returning home. Consequently, it would be erroneous to depend on a client's or patient's wishes without the team using specialist knowledge and understanding of the different perspectives of the health problem to make a collective judgement.

However, once this has been done and the collective decision concurs with the wishes of the client or patient, this needs to be clearly documented and upheld. In the case of the professional who feels this is not appropriate this should be grounds for them to refuse to care for that patient and they would therefore be allocated a different caseload.

DNR not approved

Many religious and cultural groups would not approve of a person being resuscitated and therefore to do so would cause that person emotional and/or spiritual pain if they survived. Therefore, these facts need to be obtained and documented on assessment.

Similarly, some people will only accept certain treatments and not others. Therefore, it is part of your professional obligation to the society in which you undertake clinical practice to discover who these people might be. Once you have done this you are then in a position to be able to enquire from a client or patient from this group if they want this same care and/or treatments. This is important as some groups collectively state that they have specific values and beliefs, but individuals within that group may differ. It would also be prudent not to assume that these values and beliefs are enduring, but to enquire each time that treatment would be suitable for the patient.

For example, a Jehovah Witness may say that they do not approve of blood transfusions. Yet, a client or patient may opt for an autologous blood transfusion and/or synthetic blood products for themselves or family. If it is their child that is involved, parents may consent to allowing a blood transfusion to be given (as long as this is not seen by the parent, friends of the family or by members of their religious community).

Sometimes people will say that they do not want any 'extraordinary treatment'; however, the difference between ordinary and extraordinary treatments is ambiguous and subjective.

Ordinary and extraordinary treatments

Ethicists sometimes divide possible treatments into ordinary and extraordinary. The difference between these is whether or not they are deemed to be:

- scarce or easily available;
- expensive or affordable;
- burdensome or tolerable; and
- invasive or non-invasive.

However, consideration of these factors will depend on the context or environment (including culture), the allocation of resources, the values and beliefs of the patient, and those of the health professionals looking after the patient.

The classification for ordinary treatments are those that would be considered for a specific condition to be:

- the usual or normal treatment for such a patient;
- what is readily available;
- what is affordable; or
- what is the everyday way to treat this condition (Hawley, 1997b).

For example, a nurse practitioner in a remote town in Western Australia admits a patient with a bleeding gastric or duodenal ulcer at 1 am in the morning. If this patient were in a city or large town (s)he would probably be sent to the operating theatre to tie off the bleeder as soon as possible (depending of course on how bad the bleeding is). However, in this remote town this is not possible, and so the nurse inserts an intravenous line for fluid replacement, gives the patient intramuscular analgesia for pain relief, inserts a nasogastric tube to aspirate the blood and connects the tube to low suction. The nurse then radioes through to the Flying Doctor Service requesting a plane to transfer the patient out of the settlement at first light in the morning to a hospital for surgery. Can you see how what is regarded as ordinary treatment for a large town or city may need to change because of the circumstances and the environment?

Extraordinary treatments are described as those which are complex, invasive, expensive, artificial or burdensome. Again we need to consider the context, the allocation of resources, the condition of the patient, and whether or not they would benefit from the extraordinary treatment. What one country might regard as extraordinary treatment might be regarded as normal in another owing to the expense of the treatment and the availability of resources. Likewise, what might be regarded as extraordinary in one country because of its invasive nature may be regarded as ordinary in another. Similarly, what may be regarded as extra-ordinary in a nursing home in the UK would be ordinary in a coronary care unit in a large hospital (Hawley, 1997b). For example, it is not normal to give cardiopulmonary resuscitation (CPR) to a patient with multiple chronic illnesses who dies in a nursing home, as it would be regarded as artificial and burdensome for the patient owing to their debilitated state. However, if the patient was 20 years younger and fit, and had just suffered a myocardial infarction, then CPR is ordinary treatment.

However, sometimes an attempt may be made to resuscitate an elderly patient in hospital irrespective of the futility of the procedure, especially if there has been no decision made to the contrary. Consequently, decisions regarding resuscitation need to involve the client or patient as part of the health team. They should be involved in discussing the facts about their disease, or illness and prognosis and if there is a likelihood of their respirations ceasing and/or no cardiac output.

These personal statements of clients or patients (including religious and cultural beliefs, and feelings about extraordinary treatments or means to keep them alive if the resuscitation is successful) are important as they provide the health professional or team with the right guidance as to whether or not to attempt resuscitation. Such statements save second guessing during a resuscitation attempt as to whether or not the treatment is in the best interest of the client or patient. Many hospitals have policies and protocols and patient information sheets about resuscitation, and these are distributed to specific patient groups when attending the hospital. Some of these hospitals place the responsibility for obtaining the patient's wishes about resuscitation within the first 24 hours of admission with the consultant.

It is sometimes difficult to differentiate between your own beliefs and those of the client or patient when discussing whether or not (s)he should be resuscitated. This is why you were asked to identify your own values and beliefs at the beginning of this chapter. Once these are documented it makes it easier for you to articulate these with other health professionals and also note the difference between yours and those of the clients or patients.

Activity

Pause for five minutes or so and identify your own values and beliefs in relation to ordinary and extraordinary treatments. Do the same for resuscitation if you did not do so at the beginning of the chapter, or you think your feelings might have changed since then. Write these in your Ethics Portfolio.

You may be aware of examples from your practice where you experienced moral distress resulting from a decision made regarding either the resuscitation or non-resuscitation of a patient in your care. This may have been an example involving CPR or the provision or withdrawal of treatment. This distress is natural as the process of resuscitation is an extremely emotional phase of providing health care.

It is also important to realise that there is a great deal of difference between discussing a case study objectively at university or practising CPR on a model, compared with being involved in the situation in clinical practice. These are two different contexts and therefore your physical, mental, emotional and spiritual feelings and responses will be different. In reality, CPR is a very exhausting process, not simply because of the physical factors and time constraints, but also the emotional and psychological circumstances.

Activity

1 By yourself or with a group of other people, reflect about similar situations in which you have been involved.

2 Discuss the issues that arise and explore any course of action that may be used in the future to resolve your distress.

You may have experienced varying concerns and conflicts that could have been dependent on criteria such as:

- The patient or family were not informed of the decision not to resuscitate.
- Was the act justified in the circumstances in which it was performed?
- Did those performing the resuscitation afford the patient any dignity?
- Was it respectful to the patient?
- Was the likely outcome beneficial to the patient or not?
- What would the patient want in this situation if given the chance to decide?

It is difficult to analyse these criteria in a hypothetical situation as they may appear so divorced from clinical practice.

If resuscitation is successful, irrespective of the age of the patient, we might consider it to be justified on the grounds of beneficence and respect for the value and worth of the patient's life. This could be further supported by virtue of the continuing best interests of the patient being enhanced. However, this justification may be contradicted if the success is limited and the patient remains in a subconscious state for, say, another five days before death intervenes.

Is there benefit from resuscitation?

It is prudent to examine 'a benefit v. harm' perspective, since all treatments and care that involve ethical issues need to consider this view point. This is due to the fact that all moral actions will contain possible benefits and risks or harm. An action is deemed moral or ethically permissible when the benefits outweigh the possible harm. Consequently, if the harm or risks of harm outweigh the proposed benefits, then the action would not be acceptable or permissible.

This, of course, means that as health professionals we should be making decisions regarding health care before a situation arises. In this sense, it would be desirable to know what action we would take in a situation where a particular patient might require resuscitation (Frank, 2003). This is not always done, nor is it always possible.

Activity

With another person, role-play a patient assessment (three scenarios are given below). In each one imagine you are the patient and the other person is the practitioner belonging to the professional group you are studying, or vice versa.

The task of the professional is to discuss with the patient what his or her values are in relation to ordinary and extraordinary treatment and whether or not (s)he would want to be resuscitated.

Role play scenario 1

You are a 75-year-old with severe circulatory problems in the lower limbs and the possibility of amputation of the left leg is being considered. You have been smoking since the Second World War and also have congestive cardiac failure. Your mobility and vision are seriously affected and you are beginning to find it very difficult to care for yourself.

Role play scenario 2

You are 40 years old and becoming progressively debilitated as a result of multiple sclerosis. A recent chest infection and pleural effusion has resulted in hospitalisation. Your spouse and family are very supportive.

Role play scenario 3

You are a 20-year-old student involved in a head-on collision between two cars – the driver, who is your friend, has been killed. The two passengers in the back seat have escaped with only minor injuries.

However, you have sustained crush injuries to legs, fractured right radius, ulna and clavicle. You also have a pneumothorax and internal abdominal haemorrhage, possibly from a lacerated liver. You are conscious and scared that you might die unless they operate soon.

You are also finding it hard to breathe and you are frightened that your chest is not sufficiently strong to cope with a long anaesthetic to control the haemorrhage and repair your crushed legs and fractures to the upper body.

Questions

➤ How did you feel about being a patient in such circumstances?

➤ What did you make of being asked about possible extraordinary treatments and whether or not you would want to be resuscitated?

➤ What advice can you give your peer when they do this exercise again or, if permissible, when he or she is on clinical practice?

Witnessing resuscitation

Many of the moral aspects of resuscitation may be magnified when the health professional is being watched by a loved one during a resuscitation attempt (or what is known as witnessed resuscitation). It is becoming increasingly common for relatives to be present as resuscitation is performed, especially in the emergency department or intensive and coronary care units. This may cause added pressure in an attempt to maintain dignity in what may well be seen as an undignified situation. This can be compounded if there is not sufficient staff to care for the relative(s) (who, understandably, are likely to be very anxious, frightened and emotional), and also provide them with ongoing information as the resuscitation continues.

Reaching a consensus to cease resuscitation efforts

How, then, does the team undertaking the resuscitation make the decision to cease when the outcome is not successful? Fortunately, hospitals have clinical protocols for what needs to be performed during resuscitation (including procedures, medications, recordings and observations), the process for these and how long the resuscitation needs to continue and under what circumstances. Consequently, when the person in charge of the resuscitation communicates these or lists these to the staff involved to obtain their consensus to cease, it also notifies the relative(s) present of the effort made to keep their loved one alive.

Communicating the ceasing to the witness

It could also be augmented with something like 'Mrs Jones, we have tried (and list the things done) to maintain your husband's life. I am sorry but there is nothing further we can do and therefore the staff and I now need to make the decision to cease our resuscitation attempts.' With that, the person in charge can turn to the staff and ask for their consensus.

Some staff may feel that having a relative(s) present during resuscitation causes problems. However, the relative may receive a great deal of comfort from knowing everything possible was done for their loved one.

Other issues related to resuscitation

These relate in many ways to aspects surrounding decisions not to resuscitate that may well infer stopping treatment, or refusal of treatment. These issues may include concerns such as:

- The use and acceptance of living wills/advanced directives.
- The notions of killing and letting die – is there a difference?
- Withdrawing and withholding treatment.
- Interpersonal conflicts related to resuscitation between the patient and relatives and health professional(s).
- Religious and cultural influences.

Although Dr Louise Terry discusses aspects of resuscitation in complex care (see Chapter 13), it is worthwhile looking at some aspects now.

Advanced directives

Some patients may attend a health care facility with an advanced directive, or living will, which states quite clearly how they want to be treated should certain situations arise, including resuscitation. This could be considered an expression of the patient's autonomous choice resulting from an understanding of information they have received in respect of their illness.

Accepting this directive from the patient may well be a demonstration of respect on behalf of the health professional as we show consideration for what the client or patient values.

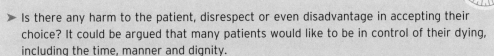

Pause and think

➤ Is there any harm to the patient, disrespect or even disadvantage in accepting their choice? It could be argued that many patients would like to be in control of their dying, including the time, manner and dignity.

➤ Do we need to consider whether or not the patient is making a statement expressing a wish to die, or to commit suicide?

➤ Do we need to question these directives, especially in light of what was previously stated in this chapter?

In answer to the point made immediately above; yes, as an advanced directive cannot be a blanket non-specific statement. Moreover, they need to be fully discussed and clarified with the client or patient. There is also the issue that it may be that patients have a right to die, but this is not an absolute right.

Questions of suicide and DNR

A person can commit suicide if they wish and are able to do so, as long as they do not cause harm or danger to any other person in the process.

➤ If a patient has lost the capacity to take his or her own life and considers that his or her particular circumstances are unacceptable should (s)he then not be allowed to request 'do not resuscitate'?

➤ Would this provide and uphold autonomy and beneficence through respecting the wishes of the patient?

This would allow the patient to die as natural and dignified a death as possible and not to prolong unnecessarily a life that the patient may see as not having any great value or quality.

Level of knowledge and understanding required

Concern is often expressed in situations where treatment is withheld, in the case of agreeing a DNR order. For example, a person might say that a DNR order is the same as killing someone - this is not the case.

Similarly, a person might say that not resuscitating is euthanasia - it is not.

Such suppositions demonstrate the depth of knowledge and understanding required by professionals to work through and analyse the issues and concepts involved to make informed and articulate decisions on the subject.

Once this process has occurred the professional is able to feel more comfortable in agreeing to a patient's request for active or extraordinary treatment to be withdrawn when both consider it to be futile and ineffective. This then allows for palliative care to be given and allows the patient to maintain dignity.

Interpersonal conflict within the team

Conflict may arise between patients, relatives and health professionals regarding resuscitation. At this point it may be important to note that it would be wrong for the health professional to believe that decisions regarding resuscitation are the sole responsibility of the doctor. Instead, the whole team need to be involved in these decisions, to encourage discussion of the concerns, to account for and acknowledge the patient's views and wishes as well as to express personal views. In doing this competing arguments can be explored and situations that may lead to distress or ethical problems and/or dilemmas can be avoided. It is important to realise the distinct possibility that personal distress and moral problems often result from a decision made by a senior member of staff that is unchallenged by the rest of the team. In such situations the professional can obtain benefit by being assertive and requesting justification of the decision. Discussing and questioning particular view points, possible outcomes and decisions is what Beauchamp and Childress (1983) regard as ethical! More importantly, such discussion encourages an interprofessional and even multi-agency approach to decision-making.

Interpersonal conflict with relatives

Relatives may request resuscitation on their loved one even after medical and health professionals have explained the futility of the treatment. Of course, relatives have their reasons for acting in such a way. One can imagine the feelings and emotions of the gentleman who, after 50 years of marriage, is faced with a situation where his wife is terminally ill. Consider also the views of children of a mother who, at 45 years of age, has made a living will refusing all forms of resuscitation.

There is also the fear of litigation among health professionals in situations where conflict arises regarding what might be considered to be the most beneficial treatment for a patient. These are conflicts that, as health professionals, we may face during clinical practice. Ignoring them is a great danger, yet exploring the reasons behind the conflicts can be very challenging, for this can take discussions into areas that are not easily communicated, or may be regarded by some to be socially unacceptable.

Not everyone is able to feel comfortable in discussing issues relating to health beliefs, spirituality and death. However, this needs to be done as health professionals have a responsibility or obligation to the family as well as the patient (especially when the patient is seriously ill).

Likewise, health professionals need to discuss the same issues among themselves so that they are aware of each other's values and beliefs to be able to work together in an inter-professional manner.

Activity

Consider the following case study and answer the questions.

Case study 8.5
Mazur Hussein and his journey into the unknown

Mazur Hussein, a 45-year-old stockbroker who has recently been diagnosed with cancer, informs the staff with whom he works that, if he should suffer a heart attack at work, he does not want to be resuscitated. Mazur explains that his prognosis is not good, although with chemotherapy, he may live a reasonably good life for another three years or so.

Some of the health professionals involved in his care believe Mazur could have a good quality of life for most of this time and question his decision in telling his work colleagues not to resuscitate him should the need arise.

Questions

➤ Is this questioning by the health professionals in the best interests of Mazur?

➤ Should a health professional interfere in an activity related to outside (that is, not pertaining to the hospital and the patient's treatment)?

➤ Could this be regarded as paternalistic?

➤ Are there any circumstances in which it might be considered that a patient should be allowed to die before a health professional thinks it is necessary?

Summary of resuscitation

In this section we have discussed a number of factors related to the moral aspects of resuscitation. This has included promoting or maintaining respect for the integrity and dignity of the patient as well as, in general terms, doing good and refraining from harm.

Case studies relating to clinical practice have been used to provide discussion and personal exploration of specific moral issues associated with resuscitation. These provide an opportunity to discover personal and professional values and beliefs that underpin your own moral view point, along with determining the moral stance of others.

Professional development

1 Document or insert your profession's standards in relation to pain and resuscitation in your Ethics Portfolio.

2 Find out about the different groups that access the health services in your area to discover:

  ○ their beliefs about pain and pain management;

  ○ their beliefs about resuscitation;

  ○ their beliefs about ordinary and extraordinary treatments; and about

  ○ living wills and advanced directives.

3 Answer these questions.

  ➤ What is drug addiction?

  ➤ What components must be present for addiction to occur?

  ➤ What is drug dependence?

  ➤ How can this occur?

4 Consider the following two case studies, and write the answers in your Ethics Portfolio.

Case study 8.6
Aminah Rashid – a risk worth taking? What benefit? What effect?

Aminah* was born in Singapore 40 years ago and moved to Hong Kong 10 years ago to take up her present employment. Until recently she held the position of personal assistant to the chief executive of American Express in Kowloon. Now Aminah is in the terminal stages of cerebral lymphoma. It is clear that the prescribed drug regime is not effective analgesia and she is becoming anxious and frightened about the pain. There are also increasing signs of cerebral irritation, when she just sits with her head in her hands and cries and whimpers, so much so that she is not able to express what is wrong, and is at the same time irritable with the staff.

Following discussion within the multidisciplinary team the medical staff have serious reservations regarding the use of different and more powerful analgesia. One doctor comments, 'It won't be too much longer now, she will die in the next three weeks.'

One of the nurses became upset at the comment, and said 'It is all right for you. You come in and see Aminah, and then leave the room. We are the ones that sit and hold her hand, and massage her head to try and ease the pain!'

The doctor replied, 'Now you are being emotionally involved with your patients; that will never do!'

The nurse by now was cross with the doctor and replied, 'And you are a patronising, condescending git who has no feeling for patients, and needs to learn about effective pain relief!' With that she got up and left the meeting.

The meeting then disbanded, with the doctors making the decision that treatment would continue as prescribed.

*Aminah is a female Muslim name meaning trustworthy and faithful.

Questions

  ➤ What has happened to Aminah's ethical rights to pain control?

  ➤ What is the Islamic approach to life?

> What is the Islamic way of dying?

> Now that you know more about Muslim practices, read about terminal cerebral lymphoma and, combining these (religious, physical, mental and emotional needs) identify the care that she should receive?

> Discuss your moral concerns raised in this case study.

Case study 8.7
Donny and the oncology team

Donny is a 45-year-old Malaysian nurse living in Hong Kong. He starts to suffer severe chest pain along the lower border of the lower lobes of his lungs. He sees the staff doctor in the hospital in which he is working. Chest X-ray reveals shadows along the border of the lower lobes with the pleural cavity. Later that day a computed tomography (CT) scan demonstrates cancer of the pleural cavity and lower lobes. Chemotherapy is instituted immediately. After a series of treatments Donny recovers and is in remission. He values the time he has with his wife and family, and his friend, a Buddhist monk.

Five months later a repeat chest X-ray and CT scan reveals widespread cancer of the pleural cavity. Danny is breathless and suffers a respiratory arrest. He is successfully resuscitated – namely, he is intubated and placed on a ventilator to assist his breathing. Later that day he is taken to the operating department for a tracheotomy, which is then attached to the ventilator to take over his breathing for him. Chemotherapy is once again commenced.

Several days later Donny signals for pen and paper and asks why the tracheotomy and the chemotherapy.

The doctor replies that the team want to do everything they possibly can for him.

When his wife and children come to see him, he writes on the pad to his wife that he is ready to die and wants to see his friend the Buddhist monk. His wife tells this to the team. However, they become extremely concerned as Donny is such a well loved nurse that they cannot think of him dying. When they convey this to him, he writes that he knows he will not recover and wants to go to a better life, and they are not to resuscitate him if he should have another respiratory or cardiac arrest.

The Buddhist monk arrives, greets Donny and then commences chanting prayers for him to be released from this world into the next.

The staff interrupt and say that the monk must leave.

The monk goes outside the door with the staff and explains about the Buddhist religion and their way of dying.

He then slips back into Donny's room, locking the door after him so that no-one can enter and interfere. Once more he sits with Donny and, quietly meditating, watches as his friend dies in the company of his family.

When Donny dies, the monk takes a note of the time and, when he has finished the ritual, goes to the door, unlocks it and tells the doctor and nurses waiting outside, the time of death.

The monk then asks permission from the staff to prepare the body for burial. Some members of the team ask the monk if they can help him prepare Donny's body for burial.

This case study occurred while the book's editor was teaching ethics in Hong Kong; the patient's name has been changed for confidentiality and anonymity.

Questions

➤ Why do you think that the Oncology team felt that they needed to do everything possible to keep Donny alive?

➤ What is the Buddhist approach to life?

➤ What is the Buddhist way of dying?

➤ Apply the ethical principles of autonomy, beneficence, justice and non-maleficence to the case study, and work out what would be the ethical way for Donny to die.

Critical reflection

Write a critical reflection for this chapter to place in your Ethics Portfolio. The item or issue that you may want to work through or critically analyse could be something that you need to explore further from:

● One of the case studies.

● Reading that you have done.

● A different point of view that someone raised in discussion in class.

● A general feeling of disquiet about pain which you want to explore through reflection.

● Clinical practice:

  ○ such as your values and beliefs in relation to pain and/or resuscitation are different from some members of the team;

  ○ how you have realised that the care you have provided for a patient on clinical practice was incorrect and, consequently, unethical; or

  ○ another member of the team on clinical practice is ignoring the client's or patient's rights and needs in respect to pain or resuscitation.

9

The experiences of illness and loss

Dan Butcher

Why this chapter is important to me . . .

✔ You get sick, I get sick! In fact anyone can get ill at some time in his or her life.

✔ Sometimes these illnesses are associated with loss. Sometimes this loss is minor and at other times it is extremely significant.

✔ Professionals routinely care for individuals, families and social groups experiencing loss.

✔ When trying to cope with loss, the client or patient undertakes a transitionary experience which always involves ethical or moral issues or problems.

Previously in this book you have read about clients' and patients' rights and the vulnerable patient. It was suggested that vulnerability could be either a phase in a person's life, or always present. In this chapter, on illness and loss, we will expand on the notion that vulnerability is a phase in a person's life (in particular related to illness) and their role as a patient within a health care setting or as they are dying.

This chapter will be divided into two sections: the first describes the relationships between illness and loss while the second considers the application of ethical concepts to clinical situations. First, we will briefly consider the nature of illness and its cultural relevance. Second, loss will be discussed along with the relationship between illness and disease. Third, the loss of life in relation to dying will be explored. In the latter half of the chapter we consider application of the main ethical principles influencing those who care for people at the end of their life. Concepts that will be considered include those of sanctity of life and quality of life. The chapter concludes with a consideration of euthanasia, including some of the main arguments for and against its use, and ends with a brief review of a professional's rights.

These are fascinating topics and ones that the health care professional will encounter throughout their clinical career. They have the potential to pose significant challenges and, as a result, offer a wonderful opportunity for personal and professional development (Allmark, 2000).

In your Ethics Portfolio answer these two questions.

➤ If ethics in health care is a critical reflection of incidents and situations that occur in clinical practice, what activity will facilitate this?

➤ What are your values and beliefs about illness, loss and dying?

What is illness?

We have all been ill at some point and are aware of the effects it has on how we feel both physically and emotionally, how we carry out our daily activities and the impact it can have on families and those who care for us. At its broadest level, the concept of illness refers to a lack of health (or wellness) as a result of disease and can affect the body or mind or both. Illness may be acute or long-term, mild or severe. We shall consider the loss impact of some forms of illness in more detail below; however, first let us consider the concept of illness (Figure 9.1).

The way in which we perceive illness, and so come to understand it as health care professionals, is fundamentally linked to the prevailing culture (Lawton, 2003). In Eastern philosophy the conceptions of illness are based on the principle of a disrupted balance. This contrasts with the Western perspective which is based on the medical model characterised by the presence of disease (which causes interruptions in people's lives).

This means that, in the Eastern tradition, people are more likely to understand their illness in relation to 'harmony' within their lives. When there is harmony, the body is understood to have the capacity to heal itself. Therefore illness in this perspective is seen as a result of ongoing disturbance in their life (either internally or between the person and their environment), which prevents the restoration of balance. At the heart of this perspective is a holistic approach to the individual's health.

The Western medical model, by contrast, may be considered a more reductionist and mechanistic approach to health. Illness is characterised by the presence of disease and the task of the physician is to diagnose the underlying cause, minimise symptoms and, where

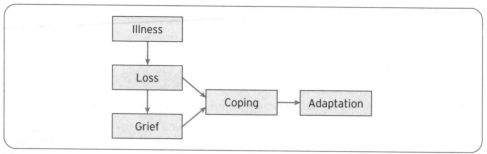

Figure 9.1
Illness, loss and coping

possible, offer a cure. In circumstances where a cure is not realistic it is necessary for people to adapt to and accommodate their illness.

Whether illness is perceived from an Eastern or a Western perspective, the challenges that result are frequently significant and can impact on the way we make sense of both our health and our lives in general. The reason for this is that illness or poor health often results in multiple losses, presenting us with an element of 'crisis' that we then have to manage. Health and social care professionals across a range of disciplines are routinely engaged in helping people to cope with the effects of illness, many of which can be understood in terms of loss.

Pause and think

Consider the last time that you were unwell, the effect this had on you and the impact it had on your life style.

What is loss?

Loss is something that happens to us all throughout our lives; however, it is not easy to define. The reason for this is that the significance and impact of a loss is a very personal experience and people react in many different ways. In some instances a loss may be developmental and necessary for personal growth, in others it may be traumatic and unexpected. The loss may be physical, emotional or social. In an attempt to draw together some of the diverse thoughts about this experience, Robinson and McKenna (1998) identified three critical attributes which they suggest are common to all forms of loss.

1 Loss signifies that someone or something one has had, or ought to have had in the future, has been taken away.
2 That which is taken away must have been valued by the person experiencing the loss.
3 The meaning of the loss is determined individually, subjectively and contextually by the person experiencing it.

(p. 782)

These critical attributes acknowledge the fact that loss can relate to a person (or part of a person), an object or a capacity with an orientation not only for the past but also for the future. There is recognition that the loss of potential, such as future roles, experiences and opportunities is significant and can prompt a sense of grief.

The extent of this grief reaction is dependent upon the value a person places on what has been lost, ascribed by the individual to the person or thing that they no longer have. This poses a challenge for anyone involved in the demanding role of supporting a person during and following a loss. While our own experiences provide us with a certain frame of reference, detailed reactions to loss are individual. Think back to Chapter 2 and about a person's individuality and their connectedness with others. Consequently, client or patient interrelationships with others can supply support and also meaning to their experience of loss.

Pause and think

➤ What was the last thing that you lost?

➤ How did it make you feel?

➤ What actions did it prompt you to take?

➤ How did you manage it or are you still managing it? If so, how?

Relationship between illness and loss

Illness, by its very nature, poses the risk of multiple and concurrent losses for the person and their family. To give an idea of how illnesses such as cancer, dementia, diabetes, HIV/AIDS, trauma and miscarriage/stillbirth can affect people's lives the following descriptions are given. It is when people are living with and being treated for these conditions that ethical issues and problems readily occur.

Physical losses experienced through cancer treatment

Cancer is the generic term for a range of diseases rather than a single condition. What links the various forms of cancer is that abnormal cells divide rapidly and without the usual control mechanisms. In most cancers this results in a 'growth' or tumour that causes a range of symptoms, many of which are dependent upon its location. The impact of a cancer diagnosis can also have far-reaching psychological consequences, often because of the way the disease is perceived. Our understanding of a condition is often a reflection of our own experiences and exposure within society. Media images of patients bloated by steroids, bald as a result of chemotherapy or generally frail and fatigued results in fear, not only of the disease and the risk to life, but also of treatment and the 'cancer journey'.

Over the past decade there has been a steady increase in the number of patient stories available to health care professionals. People have recorded their experiences of cancer treatment and in doing so frequently articulate the 'total' impact it has on their lives and those of their families.

● People's 'normal' routines become a distant memory as hospital appointments impose a totally new calendar on the future.

● Cycles of chemotherapy and/or radiotherapy require that regular periods of time be spent in hospital settings and even result in disruption to landmark events such as birthdays and holidays.

● The effects of treatment also bring about physical losses.

Chemotherapy can result in:

● Altered taste, persistent nausea and vomiting, altered bowel patterns that can ultimately remove the pleasure derived from eating.

● Hair loss and dry or discoloured skin, both very visible signs that can affect self-concept and body image.

- General fatigue that can make any physical activity seem like an impossible task.

Radiotherapy can:

- Affect the food that a person is able to tolerate.
- Cause skin irritation over the treatment site.
- Affect sex and fertility in both men and women depending on the area that is irradiated.

Surgery can result in:

- Scarring, a permanent reminder of the original disease.
- The need for prosthetics following the removal of a breast or testicle.
- Facial swelling caused by steroid treatment, along with the need for prosthetics, are both very visible signs of ongoing treatment.
- Pain which inhibits normal daily functions.

Clearly, the precise meaning of the losses that result from cancer treatment are individual, dependent upon the nature of the loss, its consequences and the person's mechanisms for coping. People are required to make choices that will have a permanent impact on their lives at a time when they are vulnerable and afraid. There is also a significant burden of responsibility on health care professionals to act in a sensitive and ethical fashion.

Activity

Read this case study and answer the questions at the end.

Case study 9.1
Liliana and her reaction to cancer treatment

Liliana is a 35-year-old model who travels the world for work and who regularly returns to her home in Singapore. The majority of her family are in the Ukraine but she shares an apartment with her partner and enjoys the 'jet-set' life style.

She begins to suffer breast tenderness during preparations for a photographic shoot but dismisses it as hormonal. A few months later she notices a small lump and attends the primary health care centre when she is next at home. Reassured that it is probably a cyst, she tries to forget about the lump but, after a few more months, notices that it is getting larger. Fearing the possibilities, Liliana talks to a colleague who advises her to arrange for a mammogram and chest X-ray as soon as possible. The results of this investigation indicate that Liliana has a breast tumour but it is not clear if it has spread. She is angry and upset that she was not advised earlier and aware that the surgery will mean she is not able to work for a few months. When talking about treatment options the oncologists suggest the need for surgery and chemotherapy to rule out the risk of metastases. Liliana is very distressed by this. She is aware of the need for the surgery but cannot contemplate chemotherapy because of the side effects.

Liliana undergoes a surgical procedure to remove the tumour and is very concerned that she will not be left disfigured. A prosthesis is inserted to minimise the impact of the surgery on her physical appearance. During the postoperative period, the oncology nurse attempts to talk with her about the need to start chemotherapy. Liliana becomes very upset, saying she cannot tolerate the thought of losing her hair and her livelihood, and refuses to discuss the issue any further. The following day, the nurse tries again and is told, 'Stop asking me about this. I have told you I don't want to have the chemotherapy and you keep on pushing me.'

Questions

➤ List the losses Liliana has experienced or may experience in the future.

➤ Think about the ethical issues that might result from this situation.

Relationship losses as experienced through dementia

Dementia leads to very different but no less destructive losses. Again, referring to a number of linked conditions, the various forms of dementia are progressive disorders of the central nervous system, the most common type being Alzheimer's disease. With an incidence that increases steadily with age, the disease causes individuals to experience confusion and disorientation in previously familiar environments. Short- and long-term memory are affected and, as a result, people may behave in erratic and unpredictable ways. These symptoms occur gradually in very many cases and result in what has been described as 'estrangement' from the everyday world. Periods of clarity become more fleeting as people experience what has been described as 'sailing into darkness' (Bayley, 1999).

Living independently can become increasingly difficult for people with dementia, as their daily activities no longer seem to make sense. A significant social impact affects long-term relationships that can change as partners are often forced to take on the role of carer. In addition, people lose contact with their friends and other acquaintances as the person's sense of reality alters.

The result is that many carers report a sense of bereavement, but bereavement without a death. The person they knew and loved is still alive but is lost to them, triggering feelings of grief, anger, guilt and frustration. Dementia represents a gradual isolation that impacts on entire families and potentially places considerable strain on the social support mechanisms upon which most people rely for their support.

Pause and think

➤ On reading the above, what losses can you recognise?

➤ What potential ethical issues can you identify related to dementia?

Life style losses as experienced through diabetes

Diabetes mellitus is a chronic condition of the pancreas, which leaves the body unable to utilise glucose in the blood effectively. The hormone insulin, which facilitates the uptake of glucose by the cells, is either not produced (Type 1) or does not have the required effect on the cells (Type 2). Both conditions impose significant restrictions on the life style of individuals and, as a result, often challenge their abilities to cope.

Type 1 diabetes frequently occurs during childhood or young adulthood. At a period in a young person's life when they are developing a sense of who they are (self-concept), this disease imposes diet and life style choices that can make people with diabetes feel very different from their peers. The challenge for health care professionals is to help minimise the long-term effects of poor blood glucose control (which impact on eyesight, renal function and the nervous system) while supporting people in making choices, where they can, about their own lives.

Type 2 diabetes generally affects people after the age of 40 years and, while there is a genetic predisposition, most cases are linked with being overweight. Like Type 1 diabetes, the disease results in a loss or restriction of choice so that effective blood glucose control can be maintained. The specific challenge for individuals coping with this form of the disease is that they will already have established a pattern of behaviour through their earlier life that they are now expected to modify to reduce health risks as they get older.

Pause and think

➤ On reading the above, what losses can you recognise?
➤ What potential ethical issues can you identify related to diabetes?

Social losses as experienced through HIV/AIDS

The diagnosis of HIV (human immunodeficiency virus) frequently has a catastrophic effect on individuals, their family and friends. The virus damages the body's immune system and potentially develops, over time, into AIDS (acquired immunodeficiency syndrome), an illness characterised by a range of symptoms including the presence of opportunistic infections, rare tumours, weight loss and fatigue.

As well as its physical consequences, HIV/AIDS often results in social losses with which people have to cope. The history of HIV/AIDS throughout the world indicates that there is significant stigma attached to the disease and consequently those who suffer from it. This is driven by fear and can result in prejudice and discrimination. For the sufferer, HIV impacts on both intimate relationships and social support networks. There is a potential that people are rejected and abandoned or that they choose to isolate themselves in their effort to cope with the disease (Kalichman, 1998). In both circumstances the loss of social support, frequently shown to be the most effective way of coping with stressful situations, is significant.

Pause and think

➤ On reading the above, what do you think might be the impact of the losses identified?
➤ What potential ethical issues can you identify related to caring for someone with HIV/AIDS?

Unexpected losses as experienced through accidents or trauma

Clearly not all losses related to health are a result of disease and illness. Many people experience loss following accidents or trauma and this can present its own particular challenges. The diversity of potential accidents and traumatic events leads to a huge range of losses physically, emotionally and socially. Fractures can result in loss of mobility and independence; burns can affect body image; physical assaults can lead to loss of confidence. In some circumstances an accident or traumatic event may lead to amputation of part or the whole of a limb, or some other form of surgery may be required.

Activity

Answer these questions in your Ethics Portfolio.

● What sort of injuries do you think a person would sustain if they accidentally trod on a landmine?

● What sports can cause injuries?

● How would you feel if your playing field had landmines?

The central characteristic of a traumatic loss is the sudden and unexpected nature with which it impacts. People find that their lives have been 'turned upside-down' without warning and there is no opportunity to engage in preparation activities to help them cope with or minimise the impact. In cases of severe trauma, there is also a potential risk to life.

Recovery, if possible, may take considerable time and energy but is guaranteed to disrupt most aspects of a person's life. Even in situations where the traumatic event is relatively minor, the consequences and potential losses remain significant, as the case study below illustrates.

Activity

Read the following case study and answer the question at the end.

Case study 9.2
Dalton Edwards and his loss because of a fractured wrist

Dalton Edwards is a semi-professional soccer player who fell awkwardly following a tackle during a training session. He was taken to the local emergency department where they confirmed that he had fractured his right wrist. The fracture was reduced, his arm was put in a 'back slab' designed to protect and immobilise the joint while also allowing for local swelling, and he was told to return for removal in four weeks. A self-employed plasterer, Dalton was unable to complete the project he had already begun at work and was unable to take advantage of the subcontract he had just taken on. He found it difficult to manage around the house and needed to ask for help from his girlfriend, much more than he had in the past. In addition, he was in intermittent pain and was upset by the fact that he had to watch his team mates rather than play out the last few weeks of the season.

Question

➤ What do you think might be the potential future short-, medium- and long-term losses of this situation?

Role losses as experienced through miscarriage/stillbirth

The losses that result from miscarriage and stillbirth relate just as much to the future as to here and now. That is, the loss of an embryo, fetus or baby is not only immediate, but it is also a loss that the mother and father and their family will remember for a long time.

Miscarriage, formerly referred to as spontaneous abortion, is a common occurrence, affecting up to 15% of pregnancies (American College of Obstetricians and Gynecologists, 2001). It is the expulsion of the embryo or fetus from the uterus. Stillbirth is when the fetus has died *in utero*, usually after 24 weeks' gestation. Various interpretations of the terms miscarriage and stillbirth have caused problems in trying to estimate the incident rates of both miscarriage and stillborn.

The causes of miscarriage are diverse and relate to the health of the mother, the environment or the development of the embryo. Likewise, the causes of stillbirth are varied and these also relate to the health of the mother, the environment and health of the fetus.

One of the things miscarriage and stillbirth represents is the loss of a future, albeit one that may have only been in existence for a short while. However, this will have impacted on the parents' lives. Social roles, economic circumstances and future plans are just some of the aspects that will have been affected by the loss of an unborn child. In some situations, this may represent a first occurrence while in others it may compound previous miscarriages or stillbirths.

For the family experiencing one loss, it is bad enough, but for those who experience subsequent losses the experiences are devastating. While the grief is felt by both mother and father, the sheer physical, mental and emotional stresses place considerable stress on the body of the mother. Her grief can be exacerbated by feelings of self-doubt and failure as a woman, guilt (what did she do wrong), and poor body image (as a result of her perception of body failure – not being able to give birth to a live baby).

The reproductive losses of miscarriage and stillbirth also send ripples across the generations, as children experience the loss of a would-be brother or sister. Siblings of the grieving parents experience the loss of a potential niece or nephew. Likewise, the parents of the couple who had the miscarriage or stillbirth grieve for the grandchild that does not live.

Pause and think

➤ On reading the above, what other potential losses can you identify?

➤ What potential ethical issues can you identify in relation to working with families who have suffered a miscarriage or stillbirth?

You have now read about losses that people experience as a result of illness in relation to cancer, dementia, diabetes, HIV/AIDS and trauma, and begun to consider the impact of loss of a future life. However, the biggest losses that we all have to face are that of our own death and the loss of those we love.

Considering your own mortality is an extremely challenging undertaking and one that people need to be supported through, irrespective of whether they are a 'patient' or a health professional. It is not within the scope of this chapter to explore this in detail, but it is essential to recognise that the values you hold will impact on the way in which you care for others. For this reason, if you have not already identified your own values and beliefs (as requested earlier in this chapter), it is important that you now do so.

In Chapter 2 you came to realise that your values and beliefs may not be the same as others. Hence, it is not surprising that in this chapter there is a reminder once again to be aware that your values and priorities may not be the same as those held by clients or patients for whom you provide care. Similarly, other people in the interprofessional team may have different values and beliefs from you. Recognising this and the resulting potential for ethical problems is essential self-awareness in clinical practice.

Loss of life

For the vast majority of people, bereavement is a life-altering loss that impacts in an array of ways depending on the nature of the relationship, the circumstances of the death, and the person's ability to cope. In much the same way as miscarriage, bereavement has the potential to impact on every aspect of an individual's life, resulting in a major reaction as people work to cope with and adapt to their new circumstances.

Numerous authors have attempted to identify the nature of grief, developing models to help identify the normal patterns of coping with an all-consuming loss (Bowlby, 1980; Parkes, 1986; Worden, 1991). Contemporary theories acknowledge that, rather than achieving a point where the loss is accepted, instead the loss is coped with and 'dealt with'. In this way the loss becomes part of a person's life and who they are (Stroebe and Schut, 1999).

Consequently, they are able to continue with their daily lives in a way that has been shaped by their losses rather than in spite of them. This notion of accommodating loss is currently driving therapeutic efforts to support people who are bereaved as well as those experiencing illness-related losses such as those mentioned in this chapter (cancer, diabetes, accidents and trauma, dementia, etc).

Loss of control

In all of the examples identified so far, a central feature of loss related to health, illness and disease concerns the concept of control. Self-determination, or the ability and authority to influence our own lives, are much valued throughout the world and serve to cement together our personal and social lives.

Activity

Reconsider your own responses to the loss and illness that you identified during the earlier part of this chapter.

➤ How many of your responses relate to the issue of control?

➤ How do you feel when you do not have control over a situation?

➤ How similar is this to your reaction to loss?

Losses frequently remove options and opportunities but prompt people to make decisions concerning their current and future lives. It is this feature that makes working with people who are experiencing loss an ethical arena. In relation to health, people may choose to give up control voluntarily, deferring to those with knowledge who are able to advise and guide. We are all likely to have been in situations where clients do not want to exercise control and ask for assistance, be it physical or emotional.

In these circumstances, giving up control is an autonomous act and does not have the same impact as when control is removed as a result of an illness or treatment process. This places a significant burden of responsibility on health care professionals and an expectation that they will act in the person's best interest. Fundamentally, loss of control as a result of illness requires the person to place trust or faith and hope in others. It is this vulnerability that demands a sound understanding of the ethics in relation to clinical practice.

Loss of hope

Placing trust or faith in others and having hope for the future is an essential feature of coping in a range of situations. A former colleague used to encourage people to 'plan for the worst and hope for the best'. Implicit in this is the notion that, regardless of the circumstances (and this related to caring for people at the end of their lives), maintaining hope is essential in order to have a quality of life. For, without hope, life becomes miserable and the person experiences the devastating consequences that can cause (Moore, 2005).

However, hope is an elusive concept – we cannot reach out and touch it, and quite often even explain what it means. However, we can all feel what hope is like, and recognise its presence and share a sense of its impact on our living. When hope is lost as a result of illness it impacts on a person's behaviour, including their adjustment to the illness, their subsequent reactions, and even ideation of suicide, and committing suicide.

People who experience this level of hopelessness may feel there is nothing that can be done for them and that there is nothing they can do for themselves. Reports of the value of hope illustrate how, when numerous other losses have occurred, it can serve as the vital basis for living even under the most difficult of circumstances.

For health professionals, fostering or the 'unfolding' of hope is a critical component of caring in whatever environment or setting they may be working. Kylma (2005) suggests that 'factors contributing to folding possibilities should be minimised' while 'factors contributing to unfolding possibilities should be nourished' (p. 628).

Professionals must also be aware that they can often be the agent responsible for diminishing hope, particularly when they do not critically evaluate their own practice. Focusing on procedures and excluding patient priorities can be particularly destructive. Rushing a clinical task to get on to the next activity when a client or patient is keen to explore their concerns and anxieties is a common example of this. People look for hope-enhancing messages in their interactions with health practitioners all the time. Failure to recognise this can result in clipped, blunt and thoughtless communication, even if the intention was not to cause distress.

Truthtelling, or veracity, is a generally accepted principle of everyday life; however, this can frequently conflict with the principle of maintaining hope, particularly when the prognosis or outlook for an individual is poor. Being honest may have negative consequences for both professionals and patients and be the cause of moral problems. Depending on the level of understanding and insight on the part of the practitioner, this may be an example of knowledge deficit, authoritarian or moral insensitivity as discussed in Chapter 3.

It is therefore essential that we are able to recognise and analyse such situations to make considered and justifiable decisions rather than destroying hope through lack of knowledge and understanding, assuming that we are correct (authoritarian), or insensitivity.

Activity

Read the case study and answer the questions at the end.

Case study 9.3
Sandra Shah: truth and hope

Sandra Shah is a married mother of three who has recently undergone a radical mastectomy following a diagnosis of breast cancer. She has struggled to come to terms with the events of the past year and has been referred to a counsellor but prefers to manage the situation by avoiding talking about the cancer. Sandra has undergone more tests just recently and, along with her husband, is visiting her oncologist for the results.

In the waiting room, her husband catches the attention of the clinic nurse and suggests he is aware that Sandra may have developed 'other tumours'. He says that he does not think Sandra will be able to cope with any more bad news and that their marriage is already 'on the rocks'. He asks that she not be told the full extent of the test results so that they will be able to carry on 'hoping for the best'.

Questions

➤ What are the likely effects of telling Sandra that the tumour has metastasised?

➤ What are the likely effects of withholding information as the husband has requested?

➤ What are the professional responsibilities for the staff involved?

The notions of control and hope have a huge bearing on the ethics of situations involving loss through health and illness. This is particularly so when a person is approaching the end of his or her life and is endeavouring to find a meaning for the experience. In the following section, we shall consider the general rights of people when they are a 'patient', before focusing on the rights of individuals as they are dying. However, we should first briefly consider what a 'right' actually is.

Rights

In Chapter 4, you were introduced to the ethical issue of clients' or patients' rights. There was discussion that these are best thought of as a claim that has some weight or justification and they come in various forms. Some are fundamental to all humans while others only really operate in certain circumstances or when we occupy particular roles.

Rights result in specific and particular actions on the part of others. Using the example of patient rights discussed below, each one requires the action of health care professionals, health care services and those responsible for deciding health and social care policy. The obligation on the part of each of these institutions or individuals forms their duty, which we will touch upon at the end of the chapter.

The rights of the person who is dying

The specific rights of patients vary from country to country and depend on the existing cultural and social norms. The fundamental rights of patients, irrespective of the location, setting or the nature of their physical or mental illness, include the rights to privacy, confidentiality, to consent or refuse treatment, and to have information such that they can make informed decisions (see Chapter 4). Without these rights, people are disempowered, vulnerable and risk abuse on a number of different levels. These rights are considered as part of other discussions within this book; however, they also inform the ethical considerations of working with and caring for people at the end of their lives.

Activity

➤ What are the rights of people when they are being cared for by health and social care professionals?

➤ What are the specific rights of people who are at the end of their lives?

Statements of the rights of people who are dying, and there are many forms available throughout the world, serve to raise awareness of issues that may be overlooked by health professionals who do not routinely work with people at the end of their lives. Clearly the fundamental rights of patients apply, including the right to autonomy and information, confidentiality and privacy, truth and protection from neglect; however, these do not always protect people at a very significant stage of their lives. What follows should not be viewed as an exhaustive list but an illustration of the principles upon which practitioners can base care when working with people who are dying.

The right to 'appropriate' treatment

The medical model has as its basis the aim of curing people of illness and disease. This is often challenged in situations where removing the illness is not possible or where death is inevitable. One significant risk and fear for people in these situations is that they will be subjected to increasingly heroic measures at the expense of a peaceful death. To reduce this risk, greater numbers of people are making use of living wills, statements indicating that they do not want to be resuscitated if their heart stops. In recognition of the increasing input of people in their own care, advanced care plans are now more widely used to ensure greater consistency between the treatment priorities of patients and practitioners.

A contrasting scenario sees the dying person neglected because of the limited knowledge and skills of those caring for them. These may be technical or interpersonal skills deficiencies but they result in distancing between client and carer. Some fear that their pain and other symptoms will not be controlled adequately or in a way that allows them to maintain a sense of control over what is happening to them.

There remains a considerable level of ignorance about the effective use of treatments to palliate distressing symptoms as well as a lack of skill in communicating with people at the end of their life (Brazil and Vohra, 2005; Wells *et al.*, 2001). As a consequence of this, there is a risk that people find themselves isolated at a time when they have a right to support, both personal and professional. The right to appropriate treatment therefore involves active measures that are focused on the management of distressing symptoms rather than attempts at sustaining life at all cost, and priorities that have been discussed and mutually agreed.

The right to information

Central to the right of autonomy is the need for information upon which to make informed choices. Health care professionals are expected to provide this information in a non-judgemental and balanced way while also maintaining a sense of compassion towards the individual and their family. There are ethical consequences to any incidence of communication between professionals and their clients.

As we have already identified, poor communication frequently has a detrimental effect on a person's sense of hopefulness. There is also a potential risk that the person who is dying has a different information agenda to their family members. You may want to reconsider Case study 9.2 - Sandra Shah: truth and hope to identify these differing agendas and the tensions surrounding the use of family members as conduits or channels for information exchange.

The right to choose where to die

In a situation in which people have very little control, being able to choose where to die is extremely important. Beyond simple location, the place in which people choose to die is a statement of 'how' they wish to die and with whom they choose to share their final moments. For some this will be in a hospital or hospice environment with ready access to professional carers. Many people, however, choose to die at home, in familiar surroundings and in the company of friends and/or family. Facilitating this and ensuring adequate support is available within a community setting can be extremely challenging.

The vast majority of people may not actually have a choice. Factors such as the speed of deterioration, availability of resources and support may combine to dictate where someone dies. It is, however, the responsibility of hospital and community teams to work with people and their families and coordinate their activities to respect the choices of individuals as far as possible.

The right to hope

The importance of hope has already been discussed in relation to loss and illness. At the end of someone's life, fostering hope allows people to live rather than focusing on the act of dying. As a concept, it is understood to have different meanings for each individual but it is agreed that living without hope increases both physical and emotional suffering (Moore, 2005).

The right to spiritual expression

As people approach the end of their lives, many seek to try and understand the meaning of their existence and their illness as well as to consider the journey ahead of them. Those with formalised beliefs may seek an enhanced understanding of their faith through the practice of their religious beliefs. Others may wish to discuss their spiritual experiences with people who will assist them to explore and develop their own insight. To facilitate this, health care professionals must demonstrate cultural and religious sensitivity and reflect this as a priority within their care, independent of their own world view (that may be different).

As with any form of rights, there is potential conflict. The rights of the dying person may clash with the rights of other people, including family members, others receiving care and health care professionals. Resolving this conflict is often difficult and in some circumstances may not be possible. The case study below serves to illustrate this point.

Activity

Read the case study and answer the question at the end.

Case study 9.4
Ashraf Khan and whose rights?

Ashraf Khan was diagnosed with a degenerative neurological condition a number of years ago. He has 'fought' the condition throughout and has refused to let it beat him, continuing with as many activities as he can. Gradually he has lost more and more motor function but has continued to work for the family's printing business. Ashraf's son, Jamil, took over running the business four years ago. His daughter Naira recently completed her law degree and began a new job 70 km away.

As Ashraf's condition deteriorates, he requires increasing support from his son and daughter. Ashraf wishes to be cared for and, ultimately, to die in his own home, a decision that will necessitate one of his children arranging a leave of absence from work. Both are, however, concerned that they do not have the skills or the constitution to watch their father die in the family home and would rather he spend his final days in hospital.

Question

➤ In this case study, all the parties involved have rights and responsibilities. Consider the scenario and identify the rights, responsibilities and possible actions needed to resolve this situation.

By respecting these rights and ensuring that they are achieved whenever possible, health care professionals are more able to provide a supportive structure for the individual and their family as they experience a fundamental and supremely challenging loss. Respecting rights must, however, occur within the wider context of ethical practice. The following section will consider some of the key ethical concepts relevant to those working with people experiencing loss through illness.

Doctrines of double effect and totality

In Chapter 8 you were introduced to the doctrine of double effect in relation to providing analgesia. It was said that the principle of double effect can be applied if the following criteria can be met (Ashley and O'Rourke, 1989):

- First, the intended object of the act must not be intrinsically contradictory to a person's fundamental commitment to God and neighbour (including self).

- Second, the intention of the health professional must be to achieve the beneficial effects and to avoid the harmful effects as far as possible. That is, the harmful effects should not be wanted, but only allowed.

- Third, the foreseeable beneficial effects must be equal to or greater than the foreseeable harmful effects.

- Fourth, the beneficial effects must follow from the action at least as immediately as do the harmful effects.

How much analgesia can be given in these circumstances? According to the third criterion, the beneficial effects must be equal to or greater than the foreseeable harmful effects. That is, if the effect of the opioid analgesia (beneficial effect) is greater or equal to drowsiness or lowered state of consciousness, and or respiratory depression (harmful effect), then the opioid analgesia can be given (Ashley and O'Rourke, 1989).

If in such a situation a dose and strength of opioid can be given that does not cause loss of consciousness or respiratory depression then that is the dose that needs to be given. However, if this is not possible, then the dose and strength that possibly might cause loss of consciousness or respiratory depression can be given provided this meets the fourth criterion (Ashley and O'Rourke, 1989).

According to the fourth criterion the beneficial effects must follow from the action at least as immediately as do the harmful effects. This means that the pain relief (beneficial effect) needs to occur before or at the same time as any loss of consciousness or respiratory depression (harmful effect) (Ashley and O'Rourke, 1989).

Pause and think

➤ Can you see that the amount allowed was proportionate between the good and bad effects?

When the normative theory of Natural Law was discussed in Chapter 5, the doctrine of totality was briefly mentioned. This doctrine allows a person to dispose of an organ when the whole body demands it. For example, a hysterectomy could be performed if menorrhagia was causing the woman to be debilitated, and the operation was therefore necessary for the whole body. Consequently, again the notion of proportions was used.

Doctrine of totality and integrity of the human person

The doctrine of totality and integrity of the human person states that all persons must develop, care for and preserve their natural physical and psychological functions. The doctrine comes from Roman Catholicism which considers the person to be a custodian of their body, created in the image of God, and therefore not to be sacrificed unnecessarily (Canadian Catholic Health, 1992).

Application of the doctrine of totality and integrity of the human person occurs in relation to therapeutic decisions concerning treatments that have a destructive effect on a part of the body. The doctrine requires not only that individuals maintain their physical, mental, emotional and spiritual wellbeing as an integrated part of the whole, but also that health professionals do the same when providing care and treatment. The modern interpretation of the doctrine includes the responsibility to maintain higher order functions such as intellect and conscience and to avoid activities that may impair these abilities (O'Rourke and Boyle, 1989).

Pause and think

➤ Many people are not of the Roman Catholic faith, be they clients, patients or health professionals, and so are these doctrines relevant for those people as well?

➤ Is there similarity between double effect and totality and other ethical beliefs?

Sanctity of life

Many ethical issues or concepts are based on underpinning the philosophical tradition; for example, the sanctity of life which arises from Western philosophy. The sanctity of life asserts that human life is a gift from God and is therefore sacred (Hawley, 1997f). The basis of the principle is that only God has the authority to give and take life.

People who support this view believe that the concept has the highest order of status in determining the morality of an action and can never be violated regardless of the circumstances. Inherent within the concept is the idea that no person's life is more precious than any other, because all lives are sacred irrespective of the actions of a person, their health or social status.

Those who have this belief (sanctity of life) usually also believe that all life has a purpose even though that person or others may not be aware of what that purpose may be. This is intrinsically bound up with faith and a belief that all experiences serve to teach us something about the whole and ourselves. This includes physical or emotional suffering.

However, such suffering cannot be ignored, and is it right?

Quality of life

Those who reject the principle of the sanctity of life often do so on the basis that distress and suffering are destructive rather than constructive. The notion of quality of life is based upon the belief that the value of life varies with quality (Hawley, 1997f). Philosophers and health professionals have argued and debated the issues of sanctity of life v. quality of life long and hard. In fact, it would be difficult to pick up an ethics book and not find a great deal written about them. Quality of life is often viewed as a tool or an endpoint to aid and justify decisions in a range of health care environments, including the extent of active treatment and the termination of supportive measures.

One might be forgiven for assuming that this happens through the application of a universally agreed definition and framework. However, close consideration of the notion of quality of life reveals it to be an immensely complex and difficult concept to define (Moons *et al.*, 2006; Jocham *et al.*, 2006).

On a macro level, quality of life often refers to issues of income, status, education and environment. These features are objective and relate to society as a whole. On a micro level, the concept of quality is very subjective and is dependent upon the values, beliefs and experiences of the individual. Central to the concept is the notion of a life that is not worth living. Extreme suffering, loss of dignity or loss of function may all serve as grounds for an individual to arrive at the decision that there is no quality in their lives and, therefore, it should not be sustained.

Activity

In your Ethics Portfolio, list the things that contribute to the quality of your life. Return to the types of loss identified earlier to ensure you consider the range of factors that are important for you.

The debate surrounding sanctity v. quality of life is intense and draws in cultural and religious perspectives. It also highlights the conflict between beliefs and rights. We have already considered autonomy and identified scenarios where exercising this right generates conflict. Here we have conflict between a right and a religious principle. Proponents of both view points are able to make strong cases for their own position.

Pause and think

➤ What is your standpoint on this issue? Does this affect the way in which you perceive or care for people who have a contrary view?

Euthanasia

The subject of euthanasia often generates polarised responses among the general population and health care professionals. The debate is complex and ongoing, and the following section is designed to assist the reader in considering their own position, the principles upon which it is based and comprehend the alternative arguments.

Activity

Spend a few minutes identifying what your personal and professional position is in relation to euthanasia.

➤ Do you consider it to be a morally justifiable action or not?

➤ Upon what principles or beliefs do you base this judgement?

The word euthanasia is a combination of classic Greek words for 'good' and 'death'. In modern language it refers to the practice of ending life with an intention of minimising pain and suffering when recovery is no longer possible.

Active and passive euthanasia

One of the key distinguishing features between passive and active euthanasia is whether an action or the omission of an action brings about the death of the individual (Hawley, 1997f). In cases of active euthanasia a deliberate action is taken to end life. This may be technical through the administration of a muscle relaxant designed to stop the heart beat after a coma has been induced or it may be simple, e.g. smothering. This is different from passive euthanasia, in which death is brought about through the deliberate omission of an action or the withdrawal of life-sustaining treatment (Hawley, 1997f). Withholding fluids and nutrition will ultimately resulting in the death of the individual through inaction. A similar result will occur if, for example, a person is dependent on a mechanical ventilator that is switched off. It is important, however, not to assume that the action defines euthanasia. In each of these examples, the intention is to kill. It is this intention that defines euthanasia and is morally distinct from the practice of letting someone die.

Voluntary, involuntary and non-voluntary euthanasia

Many countries and states have considered the legal status of euthanasia. Some European countries have legislated to bring tolerated practices within the law while others have rejected legislation or have yet to debate the issue formally. Where euthanasia is legal, a formal set of conditions must be met. These operate to ensure that both informed consent and competence are confirmed. As these are central concepts involved in distinguishing between voluntary, involuntary and non-voluntary euthanasia, it is appropriate that they be briefly considered here. They are also discussed in Chapter 16.

In a case of voluntary euthanasia, the person whose life is ended is an active participant in the decision-making process (Hawley 1997f). To do this, they must be competent to make decisions. The notion of competence refers to the person's ability to consider the options rationally and make a choice. To reach this decision, a person must be given the necessary information. Defining necessary information is often difficult; however, it is considered morally acceptable to ensure the information is balanced and presented in such a way that it is not interpreted as coercive. That is, it presents the advantages and disadvantages equally, without omissions. This will allow the individual to make an informed choice and give consent or agreement to the particular course of action.

Involuntary euthanasia occurs if the action to end life is carried out either without the consent of the individual or is contrary to the patient's expressed wishes (Hawley, 1997f). It is likely that this form of action was taken historically as a way of managing complex and challenging situations. A further form of euthanasia has been suggested to explain situations where the consent of the individual cannot be confirmed. Non-voluntary euthanasia occurs in situations in which the individual is unable to be an active part of the decision-making process. This may be because of immaturity in cases involving children, or incapacity when a person is in a coma. In each of these situations, it is not possible for the health care practitioner to be certain of the wishes of the individual. The common mechanism for managing such events is to seek the input of the family or next of kin. While this is a pragmatic approach to these situations, it is not without its problems. The next of kin often find themselves in a very difficult position, making decisions on someone else's behalf. The use of advanced directives and living wills is one way in which people are able to express their wishes at a point in time when they are able to be active in the decision-making process. Many people take this course of action explicitly to protect their family from these dilemmas. While the legal status of these documents varies throughout the world, it is a statement of autonomy in a situation in which people fear losing control. There are, however, drawbacks that need to be addressed before someone takes this course of action. Circumstances may change and it is essential that these documents be updated to reflect the individual's contemporary wishes.

Physician-assisted suicide

Distinct from voluntary euthanasia is the practice of physician-assisted suicide (PAS), which has a different legal and, some argue, moral status in certain countries. In these circumstances, it is the individual who carries out the final act in a situation that has been arranged by the medical practitioner.

This may be through the prescription of a lethal overdose (or by setting up an intravenous delivery system whereby a fatal dose can be triggered by the patient themselves) of barbiturates, narcotics, benzodiazepines, tricyclic antidepressants or a combination of these. Some countries/states which prohibit voluntary euthanasia have legislated to allow individuals the right to take their own life with the assistance of a medical practitioner provided the conditions of competence and informed consent have been achieved along with a confirmed life-limiting prognosis.

The debate concerning the ethics of euthanasia and PAS has increased, particularly in health care systems where medical technology has advanced to the point where life can be sustained almost indefinitely. It is a debate, however, that engages people across the opinion spectrum who are influenced by personal, professional, religious and ethical values. The pro and anti lobbies, made up of pressure groups, advisory bodies, religious organisations, patient and professional interest groups, all have well rehearsed arguments concerning the matter. The following section outlines some of the main arguments in this ongoing debate.

Arguments for euthanasia

The central feature of all pro-euthanasia arguments is the right of the individual to determine their own destiny by exercising autonomy. This is often regarded as the highest of ethical principles, and is only limited when an act impinges upon the autonomy of another person. People have the right to make choices about their treatment and to do this without coercion from health care personnel or society as a whole. Advocates of euthanasia suggest that this must also extend to the right to choose not to have treatment and ultimately to the right to die. The ethical principle of autonomy is recognised as one of the rights of all patients and is expressed in numerous codes of professional conduct throughout the world.

Another of these fundamental ethical principles used in support of euthanasia is that of justice. People have the right to be treated fairly and equally regardless of the nature or severity of their illness. A person experiencing intolerable pain with no option for relief will find themself in a different circumstance to others with a similar condition. If people's pain cannot be controlled then they are required to live with their suffering. The familiar phrase 'You wouldn't let an animal suffer like this!' suggests that differing standards are applied and therefore that this is a breach of natural justice.

In addition, without the right to end his or her own suffering, the individual is obliged to accept the values of others. If they are personally in favour of euthanasia and yet it is unacceptable to wider society they are forced to comply. To address this perceived injustice, increasing numbers of people with debilitating conditions are seeking to travel to countries where the euthanasia option is available to them.

Many people argue that the loss of control often experienced by those with chronic or life-threatening illnesses results in a corresponding loss of dignity. No longer being able to care for oneself and reliance on others for basic needs impacts negatively on a person's self-concept and self-respect. Experiencing intolerable distress and suffering has much the same effect.

Exercising control over when and how life is ended is viewed as a means of maintaining dignity. This argument is based on a particular interpretation of dignity, a concept that is culturally defined and that emphasises that the notion of suffering and dependence are 'undignified'. It may also be shaped by perceptions of other people's experiences (Kissane and Kelly, 2000). Interestingly, these witnessed perceptions may not reflect the true sense of dignity felt by the individual concerned and serve to highlight that the concept is essentially a personal construct.

The notions of dignity and suffering are often linked by those in favour of euthanasia; however, they also argue that minimising suffering is a morally justified act in its own right. As has been considered earlier, allowing someone to experience ongoing distress contravenes the moral principle of justice and equity. Those in favour of euthanasia suggest that health care professionals have a responsibility to minimise pain and suffering and that, when avenues of treatment have been exhausted, individuals should have the right to request to end their life. Clearly there is a twofold expectation associated with this line of argument. The first is that it is a just act to end a person's suffering and, second, that health care professionals have a moral responsibility to carry out such an act.

The final major pro-euthanasia argument is based upon the notion of altruism, the concern for others without regard to self. This ethical doctrine is found in various forms in both

Eastern and Western philosophy, and stresses the moral value of acts that are intended to serve others. Some philosophers argue that, when an individual becomes a burden to society through illness or physical deterioration, voluntary euthanasia is simply an act of altruism. This notion is not, however, restricted to pure philosophical consideration. Many people feel that this should be an option available to them to save family members from the responsibility of providing care or witnessing deterioration and decline.

Arguments against euthanasia

In many countries, the anti-euthanasia lobby strives to maintain the status quo by offering counterarguments to those outlined in the previous section. There is, however, a separate case which opposes euthanasia independent of the campaign for it.

Many health care professionals argue that the developments in life support technologies have been matched by developments in palliative care. Formally recognised as a clinical speciality, palliative care is intended to address issues of pain and symptom management actively with the express object of facilitating people to live to the end of their lives. Knowledge and skills associated with the control of pain and other distressing symptoms have improved significantly over the past 30 years. In addition, practitioners are better able to support people adjusting to living with long-term or life-threatening conditions. The assertion is that suffering is not an inevitable consequence of major illness when the appropriate care and treatment are provided. The argument is that, since suffering can be minimised in all but the most severe cases, euthanasia is no longer necessary. Indeed, it is the reduction of suffering that is the primary focus of health care practitioners rather than the ending of life.

In many ways, the minimal suffering argument opposing euthanasia is a result of consequence. A more fundamental attitude suggests that, rather than being unnecessary, euthanasia is morally unjustified. At the heart of this argument lies a basic belief in the sanctity of life, as discussed earlier. Killing someone, regardless of the circumstances, is unacceptable and can never be justified. Linked to this is the notion that euthanasia facilitates discrimination, setting conditions under which it is appropriate to end life. Euthanasia of a severely disabled newborn implies that the lives of healthy children are more valuable and suggests that some lives are not worth living. Proponents of the sanctity of life believe that only God has the authority to end life and that humans have a duty to protect and preserve it. This does not require action at all costs but prohibits any action specifically intended to kill.

The notion of discrimination and unfair treatment forms the basis for two other arguments proposed by the anti-euthanasia lobby. The first involves the potential for abuse, particularly affecting those vulnerable members of a society who are unable to advocate for themselves. It has been suggested that individuals with learning disabilities or mental health conditions as well as frail older people may find that their security is undermined. Voluntary euthanasia requires competency and informed consent on the part of the individual. Establishing or achieving these is not without its difficulties and it is this ambiguity that provides a foothold for abuse. Relatives expecting inheritance, struggling to provide ongoing care or organisations seeing growing long-term care costs may be inclined to exploit any legal act to end someone's life. The argument makes the point that a society is judged by the way in which it cares for its vulnerable population through its formal and informal care networks.

Many opponents of euthanasia do so on the grounds that a more permissive approach is the beginning of a 'slippery slope'. They suggest that accepting any relaxation of the current prohibition in the short term will result in a wholesale adoption of euthanasia as an accepted and acceptable health care measure in the longer term. They argue that arresting this development would be impossible as momentum builds. The question often asked is 'where will it stop?' Some fear that accepting voluntary euthanasia paves the way for some of the other forms identified earlier in this chapter. However, in those countries where it is available, it is only a very small proportion of people that ask and end their life in that way.

The final anti-euthanasia argument returns us to the principle with which we started, that of autonomy. While those in favour suggest they have a right to make a choice, opponents question the rationality of that choice. They contend that, when a person expresses a desire to end their own life, they are unable to be either rational or fully informed about the options available to them. It is suggested that such choices are made under stressful and desperate circumstances and do not reflect an objective consideration of the situation. In essence, the argument questions the capacity of individuals to make such decisions.

Each of the positions outlined above, both pro- and anti-euthanasia, are either a matter of philosophical controversy or the basis for a counterargument that results in a sustained and, at times, heated debate. It is essential that practitioners working in any health care environment are aware not only of the basis for their own standpoint but are also able to engage in the wider debate (Berghs *et al.*, 2005).

Activity

- Having reviewed these major arguments, take a few minutes to identify the limitations, inconsistencies or counterarguments for each. Use the notes made at the beginning of this section to inform and develop your own view point.

- Think about the availability of hospice beds in your country. Are there sufficient for everyone who would like that type of care?

- One of the States in Australia (Northern Territory) had a very short-lived active Euthanasia Bill, which some cynics said was a publicity stunt. In reality, at that time there were very few hospice beds, and many people were dying in pain and distress because staff outside of the hospice were ignorant of effective palliative care. Although the bill only lasted a few months and was highly publicised in the press, it did bring about improved care. That is, the Federal Government Department of Health (equivalent to the NHS office in Whitehall) quickly implemented sufficient hospice care in that State. The Federal Government then overruled the State Government's Active Euthanasia Bill.

Question

➤ If active euthanasia was made legal (in your country), what rights would you, as a professional, like? That is, would you like the right not to participate in providing care for a client or patient who wishes to die in this way?

Rights of professionals

In Chapter 4, the rights of health professionals were explained. These included the right to a safe work environment, the right to refuse to provide some treatment and care, and the right to support. In Chapter 8, requests for analgesia for euthanasia were also discussed, but primarily from the analgesic point of view. In the majority of situations, the rights of ill people and the duties of health care personnel match up to ensure an ethical service. There are, however, potential situations in which rights and duties may conflict and result in the loss of choice.

Activity

Read the following case study and answer the questions at the end.

Case study 9.5
Joseph Hsu

Joseph Hsu works as a pharmacist for a small, family-run business. He has a strong Catholic belief and has been increasingly concerned by the number of prescriptions he has dispensed for oral contraceptive. Feeling unable to ignore his personal beliefs any longer, Joseph refuses to supply a prescription for a 35-year-old woman despite the fact that she has a properly completed prescription.

Questions

➤ Consider the ethical implications of Joseph's actions.

➤ Do practitioners have the right to refuse in these circumstances?

➤ What might be the boundaries of the right to refuse?

In each of these cases, the expected duty of the practitioner conflicts with their right to individual moral choice and the client's right to receive care.

The right to refuse to provide specific treatments or care

It is generally accepted that no health professional is required by law to undertake care or treatment to which they consciously object. However, professionals cannot abdicate their responsibility to the client or patient until another professional is able to provide that care or treatment. Neither can an employer expect an employee to undertake an action that they belief is either unsafe or to which they consciously object. This means that when recruiting staff, health organisations need to consider the values and beliefs of those that they employ and ask if there are some aspects of care or treatment that the professional would refuse to undertake. When rostering staff the manager would need to take these into consideration.

In relation to the client or patient who is chronically ill and requiring palliative care, the autonomy of the patient cannot override that of the professional by demanding a treatment that the professional does not think is in the client's or patient's best interest. That is, the patient cannot demand active euthanasia or PAS, as such a request would impinge on the autonomy of the staff involved.

Returning again to the doctrine of totality and integrity for the human person; in relation to the care of the dying person, this doctrine would mean that people of the Roman Catholic faith may refuse to begin or to continue to use a medical procedure where the burdens, harm and risks of harm are out of proportion to any anticipated benefit. Likewise, there may be a wish to avoid the application of a medical procedure that is disproportionate to the expected benefit or that may impose excessive burden on the family or community (Canadian Catholic Health, 1992).

While the Roman Catholic Church's doctrine has been discussed here, members of other faiths will also have ethical or moral expectations not to perform certain treatments and care.

The right to support

In relation to the professional caring for the client or patient who is dying, the professional who is an employee has a right to support. This is particularly the case in a situation where individuals are exposed to the daily stress of caring for clients or patients who would be described as 'burdensome' and at the same time continue with their other workload as well. The common result of this is known as 'burnout' which is similar in presentation of signs and symptoms as depression.

The incidence of burnout among those working in health care settings is considerable (Maslach, 2003). Burnout is a physical, cognitive and affective state, and can present with a range of symptoms including depression, loss of energy and a sense of hopelessness. This stems from emotional exhaustion, a frequent consequence of sharing people's daily health traumas. Health care professionals have a right to work in a supportive environment. In some cases this refers to the structures of the organisation but in many situations is more about the supportive attitudes of colleagues and a commitment to be vigilant on behalf of others. Many health organisations are now making 'care services' available to employees where they too can be cared for (someone to talk to, and perhaps a massage).

Summary

Throughout the world, the concept of illness differs and is dependent upon the prevailing culture and people's health beliefs. In Western societies, nurses have begun to push for an ethics of care based on people's illness experiences. However, the medical model, with its focus on cure, remains the dominant perspective. This sometimes sits uneasily with the parallel notion of loss. Both are inextricably linked, and health care professionals are faced on a daily basis with clients who will have experienced a diverse range of loss.

These may result from the physical effects of the disease itself, the treatment or, most commonly, from both. Illness generates potential loss of psychological and emotional comfort, of familiar life style, of social support mechanisms and roles. It affects people on every level of their lives, particularly when it leads to bereavement following loss of life.

Professionals who are aware of the nature and extent of illness-induced loss are best placed to provide support for clients and their families. They are also in a position to understand the contrasting and, at times, conflicting ethical principles influencing this care. Issues of double effect and of sanctity v. quality of life are common considerations with which health care professionals should be familiar. The key points outlined in this chapter should help to inform, explain and justify practice. They are also intended to enhance debate within interprofessional teams.

This is also the case in terms of euthanasia and PAS. The lobbies for and against both have well developed cases but neither is without its controversies or counterarguments. Taking time to identify your own perspective and, more importantly, the ethical basis for this view point will enhance self-awareness and provide a foundation for clinical practice.

Professional development

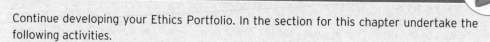

Continue developing your Ethics Portfolio. In the section for this chapter undertake the following activities.

1 Consider the different cultures that attend the health care organisation where you undertake clinical practice. Access the literature and other resources as to how their beliefs would or would not help them cope with illness and loss. Document this in your Ethics Portfolio.

2 How would these different cultural groups want to be cared for when dying? Document this also in your portfolio.

3 If there are team members from different cultures to you in the team, what rights would they want and need when caring for clients or patients experiencing illness and loss, and dying?

4 Revisit Case study 5.3 – Lorraine and Max (p. 83) and see if you can identify the losses they experienced. Also, now that you have acquired greater knowledge and understanding from this chapter, how would you provide care for them?

5 Read the following case study and answer the questions at the end.

Case study 9.6
Alphonse Martinez and Mark

Alphonse Martinez has been discharged from the coronary care unit (CCU) and placed in a step-down cardiac ward following his myocardial infarction (MI). While he had been in CCU the staff had felt that he had exaggerated his chest pain. That is, when they asked him to rate his pain from 0 to 10 he sometimes stated that it was 14 or 12. In response staff reacted in a rather disapproving manner.

During the first evening on the cardiac ward he asked Mark, one of the nursing students on clinical practice, to contact the hospital priest to come and see him and give him the last rites. Mark did so immediately and then went back to sit with Mr Alphonse.

Later Mark's mentor (clinical supervisor) called him to one side and asked why he was sitting with Mr Alphonse. Mark replied that Mr Alphonse was anxious and so he was sitting with him. The mentor asked Mark, 'do you think you could be making him more anxious by sitting with him?' Mark replied that he didn't think so, and he was only doing so until the priest came.

The mentor then asked why the priest was coming, and Mark said that Mr Alphonse had asked for the priest, and so he had contacted him to come. The mentor then said to Mark, 'did you not think you should have told me what you had done?' With that Mr Alphonse's buzzer went and, turning to go back into the room, the mentor and Mark saw Mr Alphonse have a cardiac arrest.

Despite vigorous and sustained effort Mr Alphonse could not be resuscitated.

Questions

If you are not a nurse or nursing student, imagine the case study from your discipline's perspective. That is, if you are a physiotherapy student, a patient could still ask you the same things as he asked Mark.

➤ What would be good quality care for a patient who had had an MI and was anxious?

➤ What is the relationship between body, mind and spirit?

➤ How far should a health professional go in obtaining spiritual or religious care for a patient?

➤ To what extent should spiritual or religious practices be encouraged while a patient is in hospital. For example, should staff provide privacy and encourage a person to pray or meditate, or have a shrine on their bedside table?

Critical reflection

Write a critical reflection for this chapter to place in your Ethics Portfolio about illness, loss, dying or death. The item or issue that you may want to work through or critically analyse could be something that you need to explore further from:

● One of the case studies.

● Reading that you have done.

● A different point of view that someone raised in discussion in class.

● A general feeling of disquiet about pain which you want to explore through reflection.

● Clinical practice:

  ○ such as your values and beliefs in relation to illness, loss, death or dying are different from some members of the team;

  ○ how you have realised that the care you have provided for a patient on clinical practice was incorrect and consequently, unethical; or

  ○ another member of the team on clinical practice is ignoring the client's or patient's rights and needs in relation to illness, loss, dying or death.

10

Making decisions that are ethical

Georgina Hawley

Why this chapter is important to me . . .

✔ There are all sorts and different types of problems in health care.

✔ There are various causes of ethical or moral problems.

✔ Different types of problems require different methods when making decisions.

✔ It is imperative to include vital data before making a decision.

✔ Decisions need to respect the integrity and dignity of the client or patient.

✔ Decisions need to be transparent and honest.

Many situations in health care need problem-solving skills. Some are financial and relate to waiting lists; others are management, security, food and nutrition, patient transport, scheduling of appointments and operations, and the delivery of test results from the various diagnostic units to the professionals. Consequently, there is no one way of making decisions that would be applicable to all problems. However, if we recap or revisit what ethics in health care is about, it is possible to identify how we can approach decision-making so that it is ethical.

First, we need to remember that ethics is not something that is separate from client or patient care that we only think about occasionally. Second, ethics is clinical practice that is regarded as quality care (Bishop and Scudder, 2001; Zanner, 1993). Third, the ethical ideal of caring requires us to be culturally sensitive and competent. Fourth, the very nature of the subject requires us to reflect systematically and critically on actions (or proposed actions), the rationales or reasons for those actions and outcomes (or anticipated outcomes), and the decisions made and consequences (Beauchamp and Childress, 1983). Consequently, for our decisions to be ethical we need to:

● assess the problem and consider what would be quality care for the proposed actions;

● systematically and critically analyse either:

  ○ the presenting problem,

  ○ the proposed action, or

  ○ the case that has occurred.

This chapter will highlight how decisions can be made so that you can be confident in your ability to make decisions that are ethical rationally and correctly. This involves:

- Assessment and setting out of the problem.
- Consideration of what would be regarded as quality care.
- A systematic work-through of the problem and proposed actions, checking for cultural sensitivity and competence.
- Critical analysis of all the collected information. This would include not only the views of the health care team but also the client's or patient's perspective of the problem and the available options.

To be able to do this we need to bring to mind all the factors that have been written about to date in this book; that is, values and beliefs, culture, the various ethical issues and problems, client's or patient's rights and protecting the vulnerable, the Western and Eastern philosophical traditions, working as part of a team, pain and resuscitation, and illness and loss.

The approach to decision-making has changed a great deal since the author first started teaching ethics in the middle of 1986 (Hawley, 1997b). At that time, I was combining quality care and philosophical theory to state the correct ethical decision. In this way, it was similar to many basic methods in books and journals by other lecturers in health care ethics. Over the years, I have experimented with adding some criteria and removing others. However, what has become increasingly essential is that the client or patient be fully involved (including his or her cultural and spiritual perspective), and working in a collaborative manner with the other members of the interprofessional team. In this way, it reflects Zanner's ethical requirements when making clinical decisions.

- There needs to be strict focus on the specific situation of the client or patient and any others involved.
- The moral issues that arise are presented solely within the context of the actual situation (that is, not something that is esoteric and divorced from the clinical situation).
- The participants (client or patient, family and health professionals) are the principal resources for resolving the ethical or moral problem.

This decision-making framework can be used in three ways:

- When health professionals are faced with a problem involving patient care, and they do not know which option (or treatment) to use.
- When a poor decision involving patient care has been made which the staff need to review so that learning can occur.
- When a decision needs to be made that does not involve patient care but will reflect on the integrity of the professional.

In this chapter the different stages of decision-making will first be explained (assessment, systematic analysis and critical analysis). Second, case studies will be used to demonstrate how to use the decision-making model. Finally, the Professional Development section will complete the chapter.

Assessment of the problem

Although assessment of a problem seems very basic, you would be amazed at the number of people who make decisions without fully assessing the situation. Consequently, the gathering of data is paramount, including the need to clarify the facts obtained and verification of these facts with others.

The facts you will need to obtain include:

- The client's or patient's diagnosis and prognosis, including their culture and health beliefs toward their illness and possible treatments.
- The opinions of the family or loved ones.
- The different clinicians' or teams' views regarding the diagnosis and prognosis, proposed treatments, the ethical issues and problem, the costs and availability of resources. If the clinician's culture is different from that of the client or patient, this also needs to be considered.

What would be regarded as quality care

Health care has greatly improved in the past 20 years, with the development of new knowledge and understanding of the human body and how it works, but also with different treatments that can remedy health problems when they occur. These developments have occurred through research studies by both national and international collaborations between professionals across many countries. For health care to be of high quality, not only does the care need to be undertaken with high standards of technicality, empathetically with due consideration of the respect and dignity of the client or patient, their culture, values and beliefs, and behaviours, but also the professional needs assurance that treatment is the best there is, and safe (and will not harm client or patient). This assurance is available to the professional by using evidence-based treatments or care, and adopting a model of cultural competence (see Chapter 2).

Evidence-based care

Evidence-based health care is a discipline centred upon evidence-based decision-making about groups of patients or populations. This may be manifest as evidence-based policy making, purchasing or management. There are two main reasons that the focus of evidence-based practice is on decision-making. According to Muir Gray, in the UK alone 40-50 million decisions are made about individual patients by clinicians, and thousands of decisions about groups of patients or populations are taken by managers. In addition, decision-making has a direct influence on the cost of delivery of a health service. Therefore, the driving factors in making decisions about quality care are evidence, values and resources (Muir Gray, 2001).

Each decision about quality care needs to be based on a systematic appraisal of the best evidence available at the time in relation to the prevailing values and the resources available.

Using evidence-based care will improve:

- client or patient choice (based on best current knowledge, patients need to be able to choose from treatment options);
- clinical practice; and
- health service management (policy, purchasing and management of resources).

Approaches to evidence-based decision-making include the development of clinical guidelines, the production of integrated care pathways and the introduction of managed care. Clinical guidelines are systematically developed statements to support professionals and patients when making decisions about the most appropriate treatment in a particular circumstance. These guidelines can be produced locally or nationally. It is advisable not to import such guidelines as they stand, but instead to adapt them to the local circumstances. Guidelines will have more effect on implementation if their adaptation has involved all of the relevant professions engaged in the care of a particular group of patients.

Integrated care pathways define the expected course of events in the care of a patient with a particular condition, within a set time scale. They are also known as critical care paths, care paths and anticipated recovery paths (for example, hip and knee replacements, and myocardial infarction). Managed care is a systematic approach whereby a predetermined care package is delivered to groups of patients who have common conditions.

Clinical governance

Dovetailed or intertwined with evidence-based practice is clinical governance. Clinical governance is quality management within the health service, and incorporates four distinct areas, which are:

- professional management (technical quality);
- resource use (efficiency);
- risk management (including the risk of injury or illness associated with the service provided); and
- satisfaction of patients with the service provided.

In this way, the clinical care provided by professionals is paramount throughout the organisation, the responsibility resting with the Chief Executive. Contained within the clinical governance processes are:

- clear guidelines of responsibility and accountability for the overall quality of care;
- a comprehensive programme for quality improvement activities;
- clear policies aimed at risk;
- procedures for all professional groups to identify and remedy poor performance.

Sourcing evidence-based resources

When sourcing evidenced-based care for decision-making, much will depend on the profession of the clinician, the diagnosis (or possible diagnosis) of the client or patient, and the context. Therefore, the clinician may use managed care, integrated care pathways or develop guidelines with colleagues. There are also many text and reference books, and articles in professional journals that stipulate that they are evidence-based, which the clinician could use.

For the undergraduate student who wants to know what would be regarded as quality care, they can access the latest texts and research journal articles. Many texts now state that care is based on evidence-based practice, and offer the assurance of quality care. Some even hint of this in the title, e.g. 'Medical–surgical nursing: clinical management for positive outcomes'.

Work through the problem systematically

To work through the problem systematically, you need to display (in a document or on a whiteboard) all the information (facts and data collected). Then, examine the options, the resources available and possible outcomes. For example, it would look something like this:

- Name of client or patient, diagnosis, and their understanding of the problem, needs and wishes.
- The client's or patient's culture and health beliefs of the illness and possible treatments.
- The perspective of the client's or patient's loved ones or family (this would not be included if the client or patient did not want their involvement).
- The various professional views of the team, including proposed treatment (which is evidence-based), alternative treatments, costs and available resources.

By setting this out and displaying it as hard copy or on computer, the professional can present this to the team, so that they can discuss the problem point by point. Once this open interprofessional discussion has taken place, the team can then analyse the problem critically.

Critical analysis of the problem

Critical analysis is about weighing up all the possibilities for action and being able to make a reasoned and rational choice. The professional needs to be able to make connections between disparate pieces of information, to develop ways of organising or re-organising thoughts, and to explore issues and structures to be able to gain new perspective(s) on the problem or situation. This will include discussion of the ethical issues and problems, the rationales for each of the treatment options, available resources, and consideration of the merits of each of these with how they may affect the patient and his or her family. The team may also need to discuss the effect on the organisation as a whole if the proposed care is controversial or expensive.

When the team has come to a decision about the choices they are able to offer the client or patient and/or family, they need to be able to sit down with them, discuss the problem, and allow the client or patient to make the decision.

Once the decision has been made, it is documented along with the reasons for taking it. This will then allow the team to evaluate the situation or problem accurately once the decision has been implemented.

Activity

Read the following case study and then follow the reasoning that follows.

Case study 10.1
Aminah and the ethical problem of confidentiality

Aminah is a young woman who has just graduated from university with a 2:1 in pharmacy. She has been offered a job in the local NHS hospital pharmacy, but she declines as she and her fiancé plan to live in Iran. She has not seen her fiancé for two months, since he finished his residency in medicine and went back to help his elderly father who is also a doctor in Iran.

Aminah is rushed by her parents to the emergency department of the local NHS with acute abdominal pain.

On examination she has an elevated temperature, rapid pulse, hypotension, rigid abdomen, bright pelvic loss and is sweating ++.

Analgesia is given and abdominal and pelvic ultrasound demonstrates a ruptured ectopic pregnancy. She is scheduled for emergency surgery.

The nurse goes to the waiting room to tell Aminah's parents that they can come and see her briefly before she has an operation. They ask the nurse what is wrong with their daughter; she replies that she is sorry but she cannot give them that information, and they need to ask Aminah.

When they go in to see Aminah, her father holds her hand and her mother wipes Aminah's brow tenderly and tries to comfort her as she is distressed. They ask her what is wrong with her, but she remains crying, sobbing and inconsolable. They leave when Aminah is taken to the operating department.

On the way out of the emergency department, they pass one of the doctors' rooms, where three young doctors are talking to each other. 'I noticed that Ahmed's fiancée Ami has come in, and gone up for an op'. Another asked 'Oh, what is wrong with her?' 'Ruptured ectopic, poor woman, and she is in a bad way,' was the reply.

'Ahmed is working in Iran now with his father, isn't he?' asked another doctor. 'Yes' replied the original doctor, 'I told him he should use something more reliable than condoms for contraception, and now look what has happened'. The doctors hear a cough and turn to look towards the sound, and see an elderly man and his wife standing outside the door.

'Hallo' said the woman to one of the doctors. 'I don't know if you remember me but I met you when my daughter's fiancé Ahmed introduced us at his farewell party.' The young doctors all look very embarrassed and quickly say, 'so sorry but we can't stay and talk as we have an emergency on' and with that rush out of the door and along the corridor.

Racing around further down the corridor, the young doctors nearly knock over one of the senior emergency department consultants. He said 'Okay, what is going on that you need to bowl me over in such a hurry? One of the young doctors replied 'Oh, it is alright we are just on our way to an emergency.'

The senior doctor replied, 'Funny that I have not been informed.' He looked at the three doctors and said 'by your demeanour, I think perhaps we need to have a talk' and, with that, led them into his office and said 'Okay, spill the beans and tell me what has happened.'

They tell him what has happened, and he says 'You don't know how much Aminah's parents heard of your conversation?' 'That's right, sir, and Aminah's parents' being Muslim, and not supposed to have sex before marriage.............'

An example of making an ethical decision

Case study 10.1 is an example of setting out a client or patient problem that needs to be resolved.

Setting out of the problem to work through the case systematically

Name of client or patient, diagnosis and his or her understanding of the problem, needs and wishes

Aminah, who has been given a diagnosis of ruptured ectopic pregnancy, and is now having an operation to repair the damage and stop the bleeding. She has not told her parents of her diagnosis, and her fiancé is in Iran. Aminah has just graduated in pharmacy, and would have some knowledge of the condition.

Culture and health beliefs of a person with illness and possible treatments

This section would normally be provided by the client or patient; however, in this case it is not possible until Aminah is well enough to do so. However, it is recorded on her patient records that she is by faith a Muslim. It is commonly known by hospital staff that the local Muslim community regard marriage and family as important. Also, as a young Muslim woman, Aminah would have been educated that sexual intercourse in the context of marriage is a legitimate and enjoyable activity.

The perspective of the client's or patient's loved ones or family

The young doctors do not know:

a. if Aminah told her parents of her diagnosis; or

b. if they overhead them talking about Aminah and the diagnosis.

Team views of patient diagnosis, prognosis, options, etc.

Views

The doctors are concerned that, if Aminah's parents overheard her diagnosis, there may be problems between Aminah and her parents, if they thought sexual intercourse should only occur within the context of marriage.

Diagnosis and prognosis

The priority of care with a ruptured ectopic is to control the internal haemorrhage and to repair or remove the damaged Fallopian tube (Pillitteri, 1999). The young doctors do not know how successful the operation will be in repairing the Fallopian tube that ruptured as a result of the ectopic pregnancy, and whether or not it will need to be removed as a result of the damage. Irrespective of whether or not the Fallopian tube did need to be removed there is no reason at this stage to indicate that Aminah would not be able to fall pregnant again. They do realise that Aminah will need time and help to recover from the blood loss and trauma. Also, she will need to grieve for the loss of the baby (Pillitteri, 1999).

The young doctors realise that they have possibly breached confidentiality and caused stress to Aminah's parents.

Available options open to the young doctors

- Ask Aminah's parents if they overheard them talking about her and apologise.
- Wait until Aminah recovers from the anaesthetic, and then ask her if she has told her parents. If she hasn't, tell her that her parents may have overheard them talking about her, and apologise.
- Phone Ahmed in Iran and ask him what they should do.
- Ask the hospital Imam to go and see both Aminah and her parents and explain the situation.
- Do nothing and wait and see if anything happens. Aminah's parents might tell her that they know of her condition and say how they found out. They may complain to the hospital authorities.

Facts in relation to cultural sensitivity

Islamic beliefs usually have a central role in the lives of Muslims. The belief system is divided into internal and external forms of worship. The internal worship (imaan) has seven facets which include:

- oneness with God (Allah);
- Allah's angels;
- Allah's books;
- Allah's messengers;
- the day of judgement (the hour of reckoning);
- destiny or fate (Al-Qadar); and
- life after death.

External worship consists of five basic duties or pillars, which include:

- Shahadah (deep understanding and acceptance of Allah and prophet Mohammed as the final messenger);
- Salah (five compulsory daily prayers);
- Zakah (giving charity to the poor);
- fasting (abstaining from eating during daylight hours in the month of Ramadan);
- Hajj (if a person can afford to do so, a pilgrimage to Mecca). Inherent within the philosophy or religion are the four noble truths.

Health beliefs

The usual health beliefs of Muslims were discussed in Chapter 6 (pp. 115-117); however, it would be more appropriate to ask the client or patient his or her beliefs in case they are different compared to perceived cultural or religious beliefs.

In Islamic culture, respect and esteem increase with age. Elderly parents are respected because of their life experiences and their hierarchial position within the family unit.

Ethical facts and issues

- Patient rights: as supported by ethical principles and rules (autonomy, beneficence, justice, non-maleficence, veracity and confidentiality).
- Pain and loss from the ectopic pregnancy and the accompanying resultant feelings.
- The doctors were disrespectful to Aminah's parents by not staying and talking with them at the time. Instead they lied and said there was an emergency.
- Fidelity (loyalty to their colleague Ahmed and his fiancée) has been breached.
- Values and beliefs: the doctors do not know how their behaviour may impact on the relationship Aminah has with her parents. Given Aminah's present condition, when she goes to a ward following the operation it is doubtful that she will be able to deal with any unnecessary aggravation or upset. Her parents may have heard their daughter's diagnosis from the doctors. Also, her parents may have heard the doctors talk about the contraception that Ahmed used. This could be understood by them that Ahmed, their future son-in-law, discussed the sexual relationship with his friends when it should have remained between Ahmed and Aminah. This, coupled with Ahmed having sexual relations with their daughter prior to marriage, may cause them to lose respect for Ahmed.

Critical analysis stage

Remember that critical analysis is about weighing up all the possibilities for action and being able to make a reasoned choice. The young doctor needs to be able to make connections between disparate pieces of information, to develop ways of organising or re-organising thoughts, and of exploring issues and structures to be able to gain new perspective(s) on the problem or situation.

In critically analysing the case, they will need to discuss all of the information that is provided during the systematic analysis, including the ethical issues. Once they have done this, they then need to identify the ethical issues and problems.

In this case study, the major *ethical issues* can be identified to be:

- the client's or patient's right to confidentiality;
- the client's or patient's right to be treated with respect and dignity according to her own values and beliefs;
- pain and loss of child and grandchild.

The ethical problem primarily is breach of Aminah's confidence and rights as a person. These two issues of confidentiality and patients' rights are mandatory if Aminah is to be able to trust the health professionals caring for her. (The issue of patients' rights was discussed in Chapter 4 and confidentiality in Chapter 5.) It is possibly too strong to say that the problem has been caused by the doctors' incompetence. However, they have displayed moral insensitivity by not making sure the door to their office was closed when discussing a patient. (The types of moral problems were discussed in Chapter 3.)

Application of views or opposing theories

As discussed in Chapter 5, when using ethical principles to help make a decision, then the ethically correct option is the one that fulfills the most principles. For example, if you had a problem and there were two ways of going about it, the option that fulfilled or met most of the ethical principles would be the one to use.

Then, if you wanted to use ethical theories, you needed to consider that:

- Teleological theories emphasise the outcome or end.

- Deontological theories emphasise the means or manner in which the action is performed.

- Feminist theories emphasise love, compassion, kindness, self-esteem and justice.

- Care ethics emphasises the individual nature of the client or patient, and the situation, and that those directly involved in the care will have a different perspective from others who are divorced from the situation. Also, that by the very nature of caring the professional will experience emotions related to the client or patient and the care. Consequently, this can cause moral or ethical problems.

- Virtue ethics emphasises the behaviour of the professional.

This means that there are four or five different possibilities of what is ethically correct using theories from the Western tradition alone.

Therefore, if faced with a complex decision, it is suggested that you use at least two different theories to gain a more balanced perspective of what would be ethically right.

To do this, you would work out the options that could be taken. Apply the first theory to the options and see which is the ethically correct option to use. Use another theory with the same options and see which option is ethically correct. If the same option is highlighted, then that is fine.

However, because the theories can be so different you will sometimes find that a different option is highlighted, so you end up not knowing which one to use. If this happens, try a third theory, and see what you find.

So, which theories would you use?

If you are going to use teleological theory, then this needs to be balanced with either deontology or feminist principles. Likewise, if you are going to use deontology, balance this with teleological or postmodernism (care ethics or virtue ethics).

So, back to the case study

Ethical principles and then the ethical theories of teleology (Utilitarianism) and deontology (Ross's prima facie duties) will be used here so that you can see how easy it can be. However, any of the other theories could be used.

In Table 10.1, the ethical principles are written across the top and the options 1-4 down the side. In the top right hand corner you will notice the column 'results' which is where how many ethical principles are upheld by that option is recorded. For example, with option 1, the ethical principles that are met or upheld are autonomy, justice and non-maleficence, therefore the digit 3 is placed in the results box, as two principles have been met and one other has possibly been met.

So far it would appear that option 1 would be the best thing to do in the circumstances.

Table 10.1 Application of ethical principles to the alternative options available to the team

	Autonomy	Beneficence	Justice	Non-maleficence	Results
Option 1 - the team could find Aminah's parents, apologise and find out how much of the conversation they overheard. If they did hear what was wrong, they could apologise and explain that they were not maliciously gossiping about Aminah, but had genuine concern for her wellbeing. They would also need to apologise to Aminah and tell her how her parents found out	Not met	This may be actively doing good for Aminah Met	Met	This action is in some ways trying to prevent harm to Aminah Possibly met	2 and possibly 3
Option 2 - wait until Aminah recovers from the anaesthetic, and then ask her if she has told her parents. If she hasn't, tell her they may have overheard them talking about her, and apologise	This is respecting her autonomy, but only if she recovers quickly and is able to deal with the situation May be met	This may be beneficial, but only if she can cope with the situation Given the loss of her baby, this is unlikely Not met	This is not just. It is abdicating responsibility to someone who is weak and vulnerable Not met	Giving Aminah the information immediately after the operation will possibly cause additional distress and pain Not met	?!
Option 3 - phone Ahmed in Iran and ask him what they should do	Given that Ahmed does not know of the situation, this is breaching Aminah's confidentiality further. While they can assume he is the father, only Aminah can tell them that Not met	If Ahmed is the father and he flew back to the bedside of his fiancée this may be beneficial to Aminah. However, the doctors would need to ask her if she wanted Ahmed phoned ?Met	This is not just and fair	If Ahmed is the not the father this could cause greater harm Not met	0 ?!
Option 4 - ask the hospital Imam to go and see both Aminah and her parents and explain the situation	While the ethical rule of confidentiality can be overruled in some circumstances, this is not one of them	While Aminah is grieving for the loss of her baby, she may need the Imam, but not in the way that the doctors propose Not met	This is neither just nor fair	This is not undertaking an action to prevent harm from occurring. In fact it may make the situation worse Not met	0
Option 5 - do nothing and wait and see if anything happens. Aminah's parents might tell her that they know and say how they found out. Or they may complain to the hospital authorities	This action would not uphold Aminah's autonomy	This is not actively doing good for her	This is not just and fair, unless the doctors were going to treat all patients this way	This is not preventing harm from occurring	0

However, normative ethical theory could also be used to try and work out which would be the best option. With Utilitarianism, it is the end or consequences that are important and dictate whether or not an action is ethical. This theory is measured in + or − in relation to good (+) or happiness (+), and pain (−) and unhappiness (−). The time factor is immaterial.

Table 10.2 Application of teleological theory

	Utilitarianism (teleology)	Results
Option 1	Shows respect to Aminah's parents (+) May help Aminah by finding out if her parents overheard or not (+)	+ +
Option 2	Ignores Aminah's parents (−) Places unhappiness and pain on Aminah (− −)	− − −
Option 3	Ignores Aminah at present (−). Informs Ahmed (+); this may be good if it was known for sure that the baby was his (−)	− + −
Option 4	If Aminah wanted reassurance of Allah's will then the Imam would be the person to give both this and spiritual help in grieving for her lost baby. However, to involve the Imam without giving her the choice would be wrong (−). Her parents too would feel that they were not worthy of respect (−)	− −
Option 5	There would be good gained if the parents had not overheard, and did not complain (+). However, if they had overheard and confronted Aminah for answers while she was recovering from anaesthetic and very vulnerable, this would cause pain and unhappiness (− −)	+ − −

By applying Utilitarianism to the options, option 1 appears to be the ethically correct way.

Finally, Ross's prima facie duties (deontology) will be applied to the five options. See Table 10.3.

Although the names of these duties might be the same as the ethical principles, Ross does ascribe slightly different meanings, therefore it would be prudent to return to Chapter 5 to re-read these.

Therefore, in the application of ethical principles and theories of Utilitarianism and Ross's prima facie duties, it is quite transparent that the option that the young doctors need to undertake is option 1. If, on going to see Aminah, they ask her if she wants them to phone Ahmed to come and be with her, this would be beneficial to both of them so that they could grieve for the baby together. However, given the amount of time it would take Ahmed to arrive from Iran, they would still need to undertake option 1. Also, although it is assumed that she will survive the operation, that also is not known.

Table 10.3 Application of Ross's prima facie duties (deontology)

	Fidelity	Gratitude	Justice	Beneficence	Self-improvement	Non-maleficence	Result
Option 1	Met. The doctors have dual obligations to both Ahmed and Aminah	Met. Not to lie, to be truthful	Met	Met	No	Not met	4
Option 2	Met	Met	Not met	Not met	Not met	Not met	2
Option 3	Met	Met? A husband has the role of providing for and protecting the wife and family. So if Ahmed flew back from Iran to be at his fiancée's bedside and if he was the father then it is met	Not met	Not met	If Ahmed flew back from Iran to be at his fiancée's bedside and if he was the father then it is met	If Ahmed is not the father of the baby this action will cause harm to Aminah	1 or 1 + ?!
Option 4	Not met	Not met	Not met	Not met	If Aminah requested the Imam, then this may help her, but not otherwise	Not met	0
Option 5	Not met	Not met	Not met	Not met	Not met	Not met	0

Different case study

If the case study had been different and needed a client or patient to make a treatment choice, then once the team had worked out which was the most ethical option, that information would need to be taken to the client or patient so that (s)he could make the decision.

When using opposing theories

When examining ethical issues that involve the Eastern philosophical tradition, it is quite acceptable to use the appropriate genre to work out which option to use. For example, Islamic philosophy could have been used; however, Western philosophy has been satisfactory in this case. Alternatively, feminist moral theory could have been used instead of one of the Western theories.

When using the method of decision-making discussed above (that is, assessing the situation, structuring the problem, seeking options of quality care, systematically analysing the collected data, then performing critical analysis), the advantage is that it allows for a holistic perspective to be gained, including the important cultural perspective.

Using the model to review past cases

Sometimes the team do not plan the care in the best way as a situation may have arisen very quickly, or the staff are inexperienced and not aware of the need to make reasoned decisions. Therefore, reviewing a case afterwards can be both a clinical governance measure and a professional learning exercise for the staff involved.

In the case study of Donny and the oncology team given in Chapter 8, the care has already been given, and the interprofessional team need to discuss critically and reflect on their actions to improve the quality of future patient care.

Activity

Re-read the following case study.

Case study 10.2 (previously Case study 8.7)
Donny and the oncology team

Donny is a 45-year-old Malaysian nurse living in Hong Kong. He starts to suffer severe chest pain along the lower border of the lower lobes of his lungs. He sees the staff doctor in the hospital in which he is working. Chest X-ray reveals shadows along the border of the lower lobes with the pleural cavity. Later that day a CT scan demonstrates cancer of the pleural cavity and lower lobes. Chemotherapy is instituted immediately. After a series of treatments, Donny recovers and is in remission. He values the time he has with his wife and family, and his friend, a Buddhist monk.

Five months later a repeat chest X-ray and CT scan reveals widespread cancer of the pleural cavity. Danny is breathless and suffers a respiratory arrest. He is successfully resuscitated – namely, he is intubated and placed on a ventilator to assist his breathing. Later that day he is taken to the operating department for a tracheotomy, which is then attached to the ventilator to take over his breathing for him. Chemotherapy is once again commenced.

Several days later Donny signals for pen and paper and asks why the tracheotomy and the chemotherapy?

The doctor replies that the team want to do everything they possibly can for him.

When his wife and children come to see him, he writes on the pad to his wife that he is ready to die and wants to see his friend the Buddhist monk. His wife tells this to the team. However, they become extremely concerned as Donny is such a well loved nurse that they cannot think of him dying. When they convey this to him, he writes that he knows he will not recover and wants to go to a better life, and they are not to resuscitate him if he should have another respiratory or cardiac arrest.

The Buddhist monk arrives, greets Donny and then commences chanting prayers for him to be released from this world into the next.

The staff interrupt and say that the monk must leave.

The monk goes outside the door with the staff and explains about the Buddhist religion and their way of dying.

He then slips back into Donny's room, locking the door after him so that no-one can enter and interfere. Once more he sits with Donny and, quietly meditating, watches as his friend dies in the company of his family.

When Donny dies, the monk takes a note of the time and, when he has finished the ritual, goes to the door, unlocks it and tells the doctor and nurses waiting outside the time of death.

The monk then asks permission from the staff to prepare the body for burial. Some members of the team ask the monk if they can help him prepare Donny's body for burial.

Setting out of the problem to work through the case systematically

Name of client or patient, diagnosis and his or her understanding of the problem, needs and wishes

Donny had pleural mesothelioma. He knew it was a type of cancer affecting the mesothelial cells (which cover the outer surface of the majority of internal organs). He had awareness that the disease is difficult to treat; the aim is usually to control the disease and keep the symptoms under control as long as possible. Donny understood about his chemotherapy, especially that the second round treatment would be palliative.

Culture and health beliefs of person with illness and possible treatments

Donny and his family are Buddhists from Malaysia, living in Hong Kong. Buddhists believe that since birth has occurred death will also happen, and that a Buddhist prepares for death from birth. There is also the belief in reincarnation and therefore Donny would not see the need for extraordinary treatments to keep himself alive.

Death is to be calm and peaceful surrounded by family and friends who chant prayers of comfort to the dying person. There is no wailing, nor pleas for the person to stay alive or crying as it is necessary for a peaceful death to occur to allow the spirit to ascend from the physical body to another life.

The perspective of the client's or patient's loved ones or family

Donny's wife and family are fully aware of his wishes, and contact his friend the Buddhist monk for him.

Team views of patient diagnosis, prognosis, options, etc.

Mesothelioma is invariably well advanced when initially diagnosed. Evidence-based care states that treatment at best can control the disease for a short time. Death will occur and so it is only a matter of time before palliative care is commenced. Therefore, quality care includes palliative chemotherapy if the patient wants it, analgesia and other comfort measures, and the rights of the dying person and their family (see Chapter 9).

However, the team 'can't think of Donny dying, as he is such a well loved nurse'. When a respiratory arrest occurs he is resuscitated, a tracheotomy is performed, and Donny is connected to a ventilator to assist his breathing. Donny tells the staff they are not to resuscitate him again should he arrest.

The staff appear to be unaware of his cultural needs, the ethical issues and problem. Consequently, there is no indication of how they will proceed in caring for Donny and his family other than to try and keep him alive.

Facts in relation to cultural sensitivity

- Buddhist philosophy and/or religion are based on the concepts of respecting human relationship of one-to-another, non-violence, meditation and karma.
- Inherent within the philosophy or religion are the four noble truths:
  1. All living things are characterised by suffering and unhappiness.
  2. It is the wrong desire and selfishness that has caused suffering.
  3. When a person gets rid of the wrong desires and selfishness then suffering and unhappiness will lessen.
  4. The means to remove wrong desires and selfishness is through the eightfold path to enlightenment.

Eightfold path to enlightenment:

The Buddhist person needs to have a complete understanding of life, involving:

- right outlook and motives;
- right speech, and not to lie or gossip;
- be good, by not doing evil things and have 'perfect conduct';
- earn a wage or salary according to Buddhist teaching;
- develop self-discipline to make the right efforts in life;
- undertake mental exercises in self-awareness and concentration in order to develop and attain right mindfulness.
- regularly meditate and undertake self-analysis, and Buddhist philosophy and teaching.

The Buddhist facing death

As previously stated, the Buddhist prepares for his or her death since birth. In this way, they are psychologically prepared for the event, and do so with dignity and calmness. He or she likes to be sufficiently aware of the surroundings and what is happening, and will therefore refuse doses or strengths of analgesia that would make him or her stuperose (a state of unconsciousness) or difficult to rouse.

Ethical facts and issues

- Staff do not appear to understand that resuscitation is an ethical issue.
- DNR was not discussed with Donny despite his diagnosis and deteriorating condition.
- Donny is mentally competent and aware of his condition, and has made an autonomous informed choice about not wanting to be resuscitated and is ready to die.
- Donny will die, irrespective of what the team attempt to do to keep him alive.
- The team have not asked Donny and his family what they need in relation to his dying.
- The team have lost sight of the therapeutic relationship, which is deteriorating rapidly. They are upset at the sight of the Buddhist monk and even ask him to leave!
- The Buddhist monk made Donny's need for care and compassion in dying with dignity a priority by respecting his integrity as a human.
- The Buddhist monk also collaborated with the team in explaining the Buddhist way of death, and then having them help him in caring for his body after death.

Critical analysis of the case

Remember that critical analysis is about weighing up all the possibilities for action and being able to make a reasoned choice. The team needs to be able to make connections between disparate pieces of information, to develop ways of organising or re-organising thoughts, and to explore issues and structures to be able to gain new perspective(s) of the problem or situation.

In critically analysing the case of Donny and his family, the team will need to discuss all of the information that is provided during the systematic analysis, including the ethical issues. Once they have done this, they need to identify the ethical issues and problem.

During critical analysis, the *ethical issues* can be identified as:

- The client's or patient's right to access health care and at the same time refuse specific treatments if they so desire.
- The client's or patient's right to die with dignity according to his own values and beliefs.

The ethical problem is primarily ignorance of Donny's rights as a person; he is entitled to be treated and cared for with dignity and respect of his human integrity.

The type of moral problem the team have is that of knowledge deficit* about ethics and cultural competence or adopted groupie moral behaviour,* in relation to Donny's rights (both as a patient and as someone who is dying, and resuscitation), and Buddhist culture and religion.

*These are both described in Chapter 3 (under causes and types of ethical or moral problems).

Options available to the staff or team before the resuscitation

1 The team could have made a decision about resuscitating Donny without consulting him. Remember this is what the team did do.
2 The team could have discussed with Donny his feelings about his condition, prognosis and resuscitation, which would then be documented and accepted.

3 The team could undertake the second option; in addition, when talking with Donny they could have discussed his Buddhist beliefs of life and death to be able to support him in dying with dignity and respect.

4 The last option would be for the team to do nothing. That is, not discuss the issues with him and also not attempt to resuscitate him.

Application of views or opposing theories

As with Case study 10.1, ethical principles, and then the ethical theories of teleology (utilitarianism) and deontology (Ross's prima facie duties) will be applied so that you can see how easy it can be. However, any of the other theories could be used.

Table 10.4 Application of ethical principles to the alternative options available to the team prior to the resuscitation

Ethical principles	Autonomy	Beneficence	Justice	Non-maleficence	Results
Option 1	Not met	Not met	Not met	Not met	0
Option 2	Donny's autonomy would be upheld	Fulfilled	Fair and equitable Met	Donny not harmed	3
Option 3	Met and Donny given greater autonomy	Met and greater beneficence supplied	Met ?more justice	Not harmed and safeguards put in place	4++
Option 4	Not met	Possible beneficence with no resuscitation taking place	If all patients were treated the same then this may be met?	Potential for harm to occur to Donny Not met	?+/−

Table 10.5 Application of teleological theory

	Utilitarianism (teleology)	Results
Option 1	There would be no good, only pain, and no happiness	−−
Option 2	Some good for Donny, as his wish for DNR respected. There will also be some pain, and no true happiness, as his Buddhist needs are not met	+/−
Option 3	Good for Donny as his wishes for resuscitation respected. No pain from resuscitation or through ignorance of his Buddhist needs. Happiness gained through Buddhist death	+++
Option 4	Some possible good if resuscitation does not take place. Pain if resuscitation does take place and pain if Buddhist needs not met	?+/−

Table 10.6 Ross's prima facie duties (deontology)

	Fidelity	Gratitude	Justice	Beneficence	Self-improvement	Non-maleficence	Result
Option 1	Not met	Not met Even though there was an existing relationship between staff and Donny, therapeutically they abandoned him, and were unable to provide his basic needs of respect and dignity (by caring for him through discussion and upholding patient rights), and cultural competence	Not met	Not met No benefit given to Donny	Not met As Buddhist needs not met nor patient's rights	Not met Donny harmed through resuscitation and Buddhist needs not met	0
Option 2	Met	Met	Met	Met	Met	Met	6
Option 3	Greatly met	Greatly met	Greatly met	Greatly met	Greatly met	Greatly met	6+
Option 4	Not met	Not met	Not met	Possibility of being partially met if resuscitation does not occur. Not met if resuscitation does occur	Not met as Buddhist needs ignored	Not met Harm done by not meeting Buddhist needs and if resuscitation occurs	Possible range of 4 to ?2

Therefore, in the application of ethical principles and the ethical theories of Utilitarianism and Ross's prima facie duties, it is quite transparent that the option that the team should have undertaken was option 3 (and then, in decreasing order, options 2, 4 and 1). Bearing in mind that it was option 1 that the team did undertake, it is anticipated that if they learn ethics and undertake critical analysis when examining or making decisions, they will discover this for themselves. Also, now that they have undertaken the decision-making process once, they will be able to use this framework when faced with problems again.

According to Freeman and McDonnell (2001, p. 222), 'Good decisions result from an inter-active, even symbiotic, relationship between patient and physician. The relationship also includes family members, friends, nurses, and other members of the health care team. All participants in the process must work within the limits of their own tolerance.'

Decision making when a client or patient is not involved

When a decision needs to be made that does not directly involve a client or patient, the same structure can still be used. That is, the problem situation is described instead of the patient's diagnosis; however, the decision-making steps remain the same. Some people think that in health care we only have to worry about ethics when clients and patients are involved, but this is erroneous. The type and structure of the organisation will influence the extent to which the decision can be made and implemented.

Cast your mind back to some of the ethical tragedies that have occurred in health care. The factors that blocked the early discovery and resolution of these included the type of organ-isation, the extent of the decision-making process and the authoritarian nature of one or more of the key professionals (see Types and causes of ethical and moral problems in Chapter 3).

In relation to the Bristol Royal Infirmary Inquiry (2001), a consultant anaesthetist, Dr Stephen Bolsin, spent 5 years trying to draw attention to the unsatisfactory standards of paediatric cardiac surgery. His efforts were persistently blocked by the organisational structure of the time. Since then changes such as those covered by Clinical Governance have been made in the NHS, and the new law to protect employees who 'blow the whistle' on substandard care or practice, named 'Public Interest Disclosure Act 1998, has come into effect. (Stephen Bolsin is now a professor in anaesthetics in Australia.)

Assessing and setting out the problem for systematic analysis

- Nature of the local problem, context and extent, influencing factors and constraints, available options for solving or resolving the problem.
- Stakeholder's perspectives or needs (including culture, environment, context and extent, influencing factors and constraints).
- User's or patient interest group's perspective of the problem or situation, including their preferred choice of solving or resolving, and alternative options (Clinical Governance states that every NHS trust and Primary Care Trust (PCT) in England must have an Independent Patients' Forum). This forum has powers to inspect all aspects of work in the trust and provide representatives as needed for committee work, etc. In Australia, the

name is different and the group is the Health Consumers' Network, but their function is similar in some respects.

- If it is a team decision (and most are), the various professional perspectives of the problem or situation and available options (including culture, environment, context and extent, influencing factors and constraints).

Activity

Read the following case study.

Case study 10.3
Angel of Delight Community Hospital

Angel of Delight Community Hospital faced a crisis. With declining patient numbers and health professionals not wanting to use the facilities, the government had stated that, unless a business plan for restructuring the hospital was presented within 90 days, it would withdraw funding and the hospital would close immediately.

The hospital, which was built in the 1970s, was now 'faded' not only in its façade, but many people in the community thought that its way of caring and treating patients was also faded and out of date. The wards were open bays and patients needed to use communal bathroom facilities and toilets. Many of the younger generation in the community preferred to travel 50 miles to a more modern health centre.

The hospital administrator and the matron were from 'old families' in the area and they told registered nurses that they would write the business plan by themselves, as 'we are the experts'. The nurses were concerned as they liked working locally as they had children at the local school and it was convenient for them. They also knew how hard it had been to get the matron to listen to their requests for changes in the past.

Realising that their future was at stake, they decided at a meeting to issue an ultimatum to the matron and administrator. This stated that the matron and administrator were to request outside expert help in writing the plan, and involve the staff and the unions. If this was not done the nurses stated that they would go to the national press. The matron was dismissive of the nurses' requests and told them she would not do as they asked, and if any of them went to the press they would be instantly dismissed.

Work through the problem systematically

Problem

- The pending closure of the hospital and the staff losing their jobs, in particular the nursing staff.

Context and extent

- A community hospital that has in the past been vital to town. If the hospital is closed the nursing staff will need to travel 50 miles to the nearest hospital to obtain employment (unless other work becomes available within the community).

- The nurses' children attend the local school and it would be difficult for them to travel the 50 miles and also look after their children.

Influencing factors

- The hospital is no longer attractive to the community as it is regarded as old-fashioned.
- The matron will not listen to the nurses' ideas for change, nor implement them.
- The authority is withdrawing funding from the hospital and therefore it will close if proposed changes are not incorporated into a business plan and presented to the authorities within 90 days.

Stakeholders' perspectives or needs

- The Department of Health providing the funding.
- Staff presently working at the hospital may need to find alternative employment if the hospital closes, or undertake retraining if it remains open and changes.
- Users or patient interest groups (Clinical Governance states that every NHS trust and PCT in England must have an Independent Patients' Forum). This forum has powers to inspect all aspects of work in the trust and provide representatives as needed for committee work, etc.
- The local borough or county council, as the closure or changes will affect services for the town.
- Other health services in the area, as whatever happens with Angel of Delight Community Hospital will have an effect on the services that they supply.
- The local Member of Parliament in whose constituency the hospital sits, as whatever the outcome is for the hospital will affect the voting at the next election. Likewise, the opposition party to the government.
- The community, who would use the hospital if it was more to their liking.
- The taxpayers, who indirectly support the hospital.
- The wider public, who would be involved if the hospital closed or changed, as this would make a difference to where or when they obtained health services.
- The Press, who feel that the 'public per se have a right to know what is happening'.

Options available to the team of nurses

When the group met after the threat from the matron they realised that they had the following options.

1 Go to the press and tell their story.
2 Contact their nursing union to ask advice, support and assistance.
3 Call a public meeting, and invite the local MP and local county or borough council members to gauge community support for the hospital.
4 Contact the Department of Health, and tell them they are concerned that the matron and administrator are writing the business plan themselves.
5 Contact other health services in the area (the other hospital 50 miles away, the local GP surgeries) and tell them about the situation, that they are concerned about the effect the closure might have on the existing facilities, and find out how the closure of the Angel of Delight Hospital would affect them.

Table 10.7 Application of ethical principles to the options

Ethical principles	Autonomy	Beneficence	Justice	Non-maleficence	Results
Option 1 – go to the press and tell their story	It is their choice what they do, therefore this option would support their autonomy. Also, telling the community would provide them with information which they need to act in their best interests	Would provide them with information which they need to act in their best interests	This would provide the community with the information that they need to act in whatever way they thought fit to influence or gain a fair and equitable health care service at the hospital	This action could be sufficient for the nurses to lose their jobs. Even if the union does step in and help them after they are dismissed they would be without employment and no immediate redress	3 ethical principles met
Option 2 – contact their nursing union to ask advice, support and assistance	It is their choice what they do, therefore this option would support their autonomy	The union would provide the necessary advice and give some protection. However, the community would not know the situation regarding their hospital, unless the union managed to get the matron and administrator to do something about it	This would be insurance of justice and fairness for the nurses. However, the community would still not know about the situation. If the union was worried about all the other jobs at the hospital they could visit the matron and administrator. They might also be able to advise the matron about asking for community input into the business plan, etc.	This would be actively protecting themselves from being harmed	4 ethical principles met

Option 3 – call a public meeting, and invite the local MP and local county or borough council members to gauge community support for the hospital	It is their choice what they do, therefore this option would support their autonomy	This would be doing good for the community by informing them of the situation, and then allowing the community to act in their own best interests	This would be in the community's best interest as they could discuss the issue there and then. In this way it would be fair and equitable for everyone	The nurses would be opening themselves to possible harm by giving the matron grounds to dismiss them	3 ethical principles met
Option 4 – Contact other health services in the area (the other hospital 50 miles away, the local GP surgeries) and tell them about the situation, that they are concerned about the effect the closure might have on the existing facilities, and find out how the closure of the Angel of Delight Hospital would affect them	It is their choice what they do, therefore this option would support their autonomy	It is now known how much, if anything, the other services know about the possible closure. Providing the other services with the information would allow them to act in their own best interests	This would only be partially just and fair as, although the other organisations are not the press per se, the nurses may not be dismissed if she found out. On the other hand, unless the other services tell the community the locals are still no wiser, therefore this may not be just and fair to them	This may partially prevent harm, in that it is hoped that the other services will try and do something so that the local community do not suffer. Likewise it is hoped that the nurses may not lose their jobs this way	3 ethical principles met
Option 5 – Contact the Department of Health, and tell them they are concerned that the matron and administrator are writing the business plan themselves	It is their choice what they do, therefore this option would support their autonomy	Informing the funding agents of the situation would allow them to act and intervene if they wish. However, it may be in their best interest at this stage not to act, and allow the matron and administrator to fail	This would be just and fair as the nurses are not going to the press and therefore they would not immediately lose their jobs. However, it may not be just and fair to the community if the department do not tell the community	If the department do not tell the community of the possible closure then the community could be hurt when and if it closes. The nurses would not to be hurt as they have not gone to the press	Only 1 ethical principle fully met; the other 3 principles only partially met. Therefore an overall result of 2.5 given

Ethical issues

- Paternalistic behaviour by the matron and administrator.
- Client and patient rights.
- Staff rights.
- Allocation of resources.

Critical analysis

Ethical or moral problem to be resolved

- The authoritarian manner of the matron who is blocking the nurses from telling the community of the problem that will affect the whole of the community.
- In addition, the matron along with the administrator not involving the staff and community in the writing of the business plan that represents their future.

Table 10.8 Application of teleological theory

	Utilitarianism (teleology)	Results
Option 1	Would not be met from the nurses' perspective, but would be from the community	−+
Option 2	Would be met from the nurses' perspective. No evidence that it would be met from the community's perspective	+−
Option 3	Would be met from the community's perspective and gives the nurses a chance to demonstrate their capability	++
Option 4	May be partially met if the agencies act on the information and assist the nurses and also inform the wider community	?+
Option 5	May be partially met if the Department of Health acts on the information and assist the nurses and also inform the wider community	?+

Therefore, in the application of ethical principles and ethical theories of Utilitarianism and Ross's prima facie duties, it appears that it would be in the nurses' best interests to contact the nurses' union, and follow advice to try and protect themselves and their jobs. Depending on the advice from the union and their obligations to the community and altruistic nature, they could decide whether to leak the information to the community or demonstrate their full concern for the situation by arranging a public meeting. However, it would be unwise to do either of these actions without the support of the union. The union is outside the remit of the matron and administrator, and it is they who would inform the other local health care agencies and also the health department of their concern. Consequently, the best option for the nurses is option 2, to get the union involved.

Table 10.9 Ross's prima facie duties (deontology)

	Fidelity	Gratitude	Justice	Beneficence	Self-improvement	Non-maleficence	Result
Option 1	Yes	Met, as the nurses do have a relationship with the community	Yes for the community but not for the nurses	Yes for the community, but not if the nurses lose their jobs	This would be self-improvement for the community but not for the nurses if they lose their jobs	This is leaving the nurses wide open to be harmed through being dismissed	2
Option 2	Yes	Yes. The nurses do have a prior relationship with the union and it allows them to provide protection	Yes for the nurses, possibly not for the community	Yes for the nurses, possibly not for the community	Yes for the nurses, possibly not for the community	Yes for the nurses, possibly not for the community	6
Option 3	Yes	Yes	Yes	May not be for the nurses if they are dismissed, but yes for the community	May not be for the nurses if they are dismissed, but yes for the community	May not be for the nurses if they are dismissed, but yes for the community	4.5
Option 4	No	No	No	No	No	No	0
Option 5	No	No	No	No	No	No	0

Summary

This chapter has shown how decisions can be made using a similar framework for three different types of situations or problems. The first was when a situation arose and the staff needed to make a decision about their plan of action. The second situation was when care had been given and the staff needed to review their actions so that they could learn from the experience for future patient care. The third type of situation was when a professional needed to make a decision not about patient care, but involving their professional integrity.

Professional development

Continue to develop your Ethics Portfolio. For this chapter you may wish to include other decision-making modules that appeal to you and that you think are useful.

Read the following two case studies and then answer the questions at the end.

Case study 10.4
Ruth and her possible dishonesty

Ruth is a second-year student studying health promotion. She needs to do the same psychology module that all the other second-year students have to do. You and your friends are studying another of the other disciplines required to take the module (for example, physiotherapy, nursing, occupational therapy, social work, paramedic or operating department practitioner). Ruth is nice and friendly and gets on well with everyone.

One day you are in the car park going home and, as you pass a car, you hear someone talking, saying 'The assignment is due now, so how much will that cost'. You do a double-take at what you are hearing, and accidentally drop one of the books you are carrying; as you bend down to pick up the book you hear the words 'Okay, that is fine, remember I don't need the assignment to look too good, just a high C will be fine'.

As you are picking up the book you overbalance and knock the car.

With that the person who had been talking looks at you and you realise that it is Ruth.

You notice then that she must have been talking on her mobile phone, making the arrangement for someone to do her assignment.

Ruth says hi to you and starts her car to drive off and you keep on walking to yours.

Question

➤ What are you going to do about what you have overheard?

➤ Use the decision-making framework to help you decide.

Care study 10.5
Is it child abuse? What should I do?

You are undertaking clinical practice on a children's ward. A baby of 9 months old is admitted from the emergency department with blood loss as a result of a circumcision performed earlier that day. As you help the staff prepare the baby to go to the operating department, you notice there are small lacerations on the baby's feet and bruises on his legs. You do not say anything as the priority is to get the baby to the operating room to stop the bleeding.

Later, you discuss the issue with the staff; one thinks the baby must be Jewish as the circumcision was performed at home. Another thinks the baby might be being abused.

Next day you return to clinical practice to find that the baby has been discharged. You ask what has happened, and are told that the baby recovered and was sent home with the parents.

You ask about the circumcision and the child's lacerations and bruises, and you are told that the parents are Jewish.

That evening at home you look up circumcision on the internet and discover that the Jewish faith circumcises the male baby in the first week or so after birth. Next day you discuss this with the staff, saying 'I don't think the family could have been Jewish as they circumcise when the baby is much younger, so perhaps it was abuse?'

You are told, 'Jew, Muslim, they all circumcise their babies, we can't be investigating child abuse for every child who comes in bleeding from one'. You then say, 'but this baby had other injuries as well'.

With that you are told, 'we haven't got time to investigate and report the little abuse cases, we only focus on the big ones'.

Six months later you read in the newspaper that a man and a woman have been charged with the manslaughter of their son, and you feel sick as you recognise the names as the parents of the young baby who had been bleeding from circumcision.

Question

➤ What are you going to do?

Critical reflection

Write a critical reflection for this chapter to place in your Ethics Portfolio. The item or issue that you may want to work through or critically analyse could be something that you need to explore further from:

● One of the case studies.

● Reading that you have done.

● A different point of view that someone raised in discussion in class.

● A general feeling of disquiet about decision making which you want to explore through reflection.

● Clinical practice:

○ such as your values and beliefs in relation to decision making are different from some members of the team;

○ how you have realised that the care you have provided for a patient on clinical practice was incorrect and consequently, unethical; or

○ another member of the team on clinical practice is ignoring the other team members and the client or patient in decision making.

Part 2

Different types of clinical practice or situations

Ethical issues in primary health care

Jill Barr

Why this chapter is important to me . . .

✔ Primary health care is recognised worldwide as the first stage or layer of health care; this is followed by secondary and tertiary care.

✔ The World Health Organization (1978) states that primary health care should be available to everyone. However, this should be in relation to what each country can afford.

✔ As a health professional you will find that all countries offer primary health care. In some it has more importance than secondary and/or tertiary care, because some countries are not able to afford and offer tertiary care.

✔ The health professional working in primary health care will face ethical issues and problems on a day-to-day basis just as in other practice areas.

✔ Consequently, there is a need for health professionals to be aware of some of the common ethical issues in primary health care.

Primary care is regarded as the first layer, step or stage of health care in society. Throughout the world, primary health care is structured differently dependent on which country the health care professional is in practice. However, irrespective of these differences worldwide, the aim of primary health care is the same; that is, to provide a service where a person, family or community can request help for their health problem.

This can be explained better by providing examples. In the UK the first point of call for the client wanting health treatment could be at the local medical centre where there is a practice nurse, general practitioner (GP) and health visitor. However, the UK primary care team might also be involved in developing and implementing a strategy for an 'out of hours' health service operating from a local community hospital. Likewise, in Australia the first port of call for a person wanting health care could be a local health centre or general practitioner. However, the health professionals in this primary health care team might also be involved in developing and implementing strategies for a safe water supply to prevent an outbreak of disease in a remote Aboriginal community. This means that primary health care, although being the point of access and first layer of health care, can function in slightly different ways depending on the country, context and culture.

Irrespective of where the primary health care is delivered it is governed by the World Health Organization's (1978) remit of 'essential care based on practical, scientifically and socially acceptable methods and technology, made universally acceptable to individuals and families in the community through their full participation and at a cost the community and country can afford...' If we unpick this definition we realise that the very words 'individuals and families' mean that ethically we need to consider clients' or patients' rights and protecting the vulnerable. Likewise, the words 'practical, scientifically and socially acceptable methods and technology' reminds us to think of the issues of values and beliefs, and culture, pain and resuscitation, illness and loss, and decision-making. Then, the words 'at a cost the community and country can afford' should alert us to think about the allocation of resources. These topics were covered in Part 1 (Chapters 1-10), and you are now ready to gain the knowledge and understanding of primary care. This chapter will address the common ethical issues and problems that can arise in primary care, such as the right to health care, the therapeutic relationship (including confidentiality and truthtelling), allocation of resources, the concept of primary intervention and paternalism. First, the concept of primary care is discussed; second, the right to health care; third, the therapeutic relationship between the person, family or community and the health professional; fourth, the political, economic and ethical involvement in the allocation of resources; fifth, primary intervention and paternalism; and finally, the Professional Development section is provided at the end of the chapter to increase your knowledge and understanding of primary health care.

Primary health care

Primary care is providing the first-line of health care provision within society. The second-line of provision is secondary care, which involves the intermediate range of care given by acute hospital treatment for common conditions and chronic diseases and associated rehabilitation. This includes the care of clients who have a fractured femur from a road traffic accident, those needing a bowel resection because of cancer, those who have suffered a myocardial infarction or a stroke. The third-line provision of care is tertiary care, which involves the highest level of available care given by large specialist hospitals for those conditions which do not affect all the population. This includes invasive cardiac surgery, neurosurgery, lung and heart transplants, clients with rare illness (in Western society), such as tetanus and diphtheria. Secondary and tertiary health care is medically driven, whereas primary health care needs to include the social understandings of health (Martini, 1997).

Who is the patient?

The health care professional working in primary health care can work with an individual, a family or a whole community of people. Irrespective of who the health professional is caring for, the term 'patient' is not used; the word 'client' is preferred. Therefore, in primary health care when you see the word 'client' you need to realise that this may not be just one person, but can mean a family or community (Blackie, 2000). Consequently, in this chapter the name 'client' will be used to mean all three (person, family or community).

What does primary health care involve?

What did you write?

Maybe you listed the GPs, the practice nurse, most likely the district nurse, the health visitor, the midwife, the child health nurse and the school nurse. It could be that you also recognised the pharmacist, occupational health nurse, mental health nurse or the learning disability nurse who work in industry or community settings, and you may also have recognised public health consultants or specialists.

These are all correct, but primary health care involves more than these, as it also emphasises curative, preventative, promotive and rehabilitative activities which are developed and implemented within a unique partnership with the community (Ebrahim and Rankin, 1993).

So who else do you think needs to be added to your list?

Involvement of professionals outside the medical model

According to Blackie (2000) primary health care is a concept, philosophy and a set of activities of how health care provision needs to be offered. That is, it also involves the planning and delivery of health services. This means that the care can involve health-related areas that you might not have thought of, such as safe water supply, nutrition, sanitation, housing and education.

Although these services are usually outside the medical model of health care, they are very much within the list of organisations responsible for primary health care. This means that health professionals could be working outside the normal health care environment. In Chapter 7, Hutchings and Reel listed the health care professionals belonging to the typical interprofessional and/or multidisciplinary team (see p. 138). However, in primary health care this may also include working in conjunction with housing, sanitation engineers, environmental scientists, teachers, planning authorities, health promotion psychologists, anthropologists and sociologists. However, irrespective of the composition of the team the same ethical protocols for behaviour remain.

Equitable, just, empowering and culturally sensitive services

Given the philosophy of primary health care, we can see that the ethics need to encompass equity and justice, empowerment, self-determination and culturally appropriate services (Martini, 1997). These will be addressed in the next section of the chapter on the right to health care.

Right to health care: greater equity in health care

In previous chapters it was stated that clients and patients have an ethical right to health care. Therefore we can accept this as a given, and then ask the question, what extra is required when we think of the right to health care in relation to primary health care. In primary health care, one of the aims is to reduce the inequalities of power and wealth in health provision (WHO, 1978).

You can probably think of many incidents in the world and in your own country where equity in health care does not occur; this will be written about later in the chapter (allocation of resources).

However, there are still ways that the health professional working in primary health care can address the issue of equity and the right to health care. The important thing to remember is that the client needs to be on an equal footing with the health professional (Martini, 1997); that is, the health professional works *with* and on behalf of the client to improve their health status (Martini, 1997). According to Blackie (2000), primary health care does this through:

● empowering the client (family or community);
● working in partnership with the client; and
● changing society's notion and that of a country's health care system from a medically driven acute care approach to one of health prevention and client-centred care.

When primary health care improves a client's health status through these strategies, social change occurs which will result in greater equity in health care (Blackie, 2000).

Activity

Read the following case study and answer the questions at the end.

Case study 11.1
Working in an isolated community and the pregnant woman

It is common practice in isolated communities that only offer primary health care (that is, no secondary care) to transfer women at 38 weeks' gestation to the nearest obstetric facility for full prenatal assessment before labour starts. In this way any risk factors can be identified and a birthing plan developed for implementation.

Imagine you are the only health professional working in that isolated community at the time. You could be a social worker or a physiotherapist or a mental health nurse, developing a health strategy to be implemented (it doesn't really matter who you are in this case study).

On the day the weekly plane arrives to bring in supplies and passengers, a woman comes to tell you that one of the other women from the village who is 38 weeks' pregnant does not want to get on the flight and go away to have her baby.

You go and see the woman and explain the importance of her leaving the community to give birth, and that there is no midwife to assist her. However, she is adamant that she wants her child born in the village.

Questions

➤ In considering the client's rights to equity in primary health care what are you going to do?
➤ What other person or people do you think have rights in this situation?

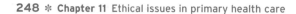

The obvious issues in the case study are those of the client's and patient's rights and allocation of resources. That is, that while the client has the right to access health care, she does not have the right to demand a resource which is not readily available. Given that the ethos of primary care is first-line or base provision of care, if there is no facility to provide additional support of any sort the clients or patients need to be referred and transferred to those services that can give the care and treatment.

This may sound a little strange to those of you who just need to jump into your car and go to your local doctor or hospital. Many people in the world live hundreds of miles or kilometres from the nearest district or secondary hospital. Consequently, people living in small remote communities that need centralised specialist and acute services such as midwifery or obstetrics have to rely on primary care resources more than those living in a town or city. They may be expected to travel away from homes and communities to gain access to secondary care. For example, in some parts of Canada, patients with cancer who live in rural areas may be expected to travel 300 miles for their chemotherapy sessions plus having to pay their own travel costs. In Australia, the government pays the travel costs for these patients (or a contribution towards the cost).

In the case study, the mother appears to have to comply with the health service arrangements to move her out of her own community, regardless of her social commitments to other children or family, concern for her own home and sometimes livelihood, or fear of the unknown risks of delivering a baby while on the flight or even managing to get her and her baby home together to their own home as quickly as possible. The anxiety of leaving her partner and family for an impending birth may be too much to take.

The health professional dealing with this situation may recognise the risks to the mother and baby of staying without a full midwifery/obstetric service but may also identify with the psychological needs of the mother. To whom do you have a 'duty of care'? You may see the problem for the mother but what about the unborn child? What is your assessment of the risks of supporting the autonomy of the woman and agreeing to her decision to stay and give birth within the village? With whom can you confer? Does the autonomy of one individual override the rights of the unborn child? These are not easy questions to answer. The way primary and secondary care is organised and delivered often suits the professionals rather than the needs of communities.

Therapeutic relationship

The culture within primary care is based on the importance of the therapeutic relationship between client and health professional. Building a therapeutic relationship with a client has been covered in other subjects and is not repeated here; however, think about the important components of how such a relationship is built. First, you need to respect the client and, second, the client needs to be able to trust you to work collaboratively with them. This is vital in primary health care if we are to achieve the aims of improving health. Therefore the giving of accurate information and communication become essential components of the therapeutic relationship.

Read the following case study and answer the questions.

Case study 11.2
Karin, the health visitor and truthtelling

Karin, a health visitor, has at 9.00 am just been notified through a copy of a letter sent to a GP from a paediatrician that a recent brain scan performed on baby Jon, who is 5 weeks old, indicates severe abnormalities of brain development. Karin realises that this accounts for Jon's constant crying, poor development, feeding issues and history of tremors.

Karin is due to see his mother later that morning when she is scheduled at 11 am to visit them at home.

Questions

➤ Karin has less than 2 hours to prepare for the home visit. What would you recommend that she does?

➤ What are the ethical issues in this case study?

➤ Should Karin go and do the home visit and pretend she does not know about the letter and the results of the brain scan?

➤ Is lying ever justified?

➤ What damage can occur when a health professional lies to a client?

➤ Who can support Karin in dealing with the family home visit?

➤ How should Karin deal with the contact with Jon and his family?

The importance of fidelity and veracity

Some philosophers and ethicists say that the ethical principles of autonomy, beneficence, justice and non-maleficence need to be expanded to include fidelity and veracity. Fidelity relates to the loyalty and obligations that we have with another person with whom we have a relationship (Hawley, 1997b). Similarly, veracity is also related to those with whom we have a relationship and this principle states that we will not tell lies or be deceitful. According to Bok (1978), there is a moral obligation against deception, lies and non-disclosure of information in therapeutic relationships, since trust can be destroyed by deception. However, professionals also need to be sensitive, as moral problems can be caused by a rigid attitude to truthtelling, and rushing in with information before a client or patient is ready to receive the news (remember that this was mentioned in Chapter 3, when the different types of moral problems and what causes them were described).

In relation to the case study, the timing of the family appointment means that it may be difficult to confer with the GP or paediatrician to agree an action plan to tell the family of the scan findings. In primary care, important information often reaches key people at different times and logistically there are difficulties in agreeing *how* the 'truth' should be conveyed to clients/families.

It could be that Karin is able to contact the GP and a joint home visit could be rearranged for that day to convey the news and look to future treatments and support plans for the family. This may be seen as 'best practice'. A worse case scenario is that primary health care professionals assume the 'truthtelling' has been conveyed by others and the family feel shocked by off-the-cuff disclosures by an individual health care worker, trained or untrained, and the family may thus feel betrayed by key professional people they thought they trusted or by the health service as a whole. They may well then communicate with the wider community and distrust in any primary health care professional will be a consequence.

The whole of the client (person, family or community)

In primary health care, professionals need to recognise clients as a whole, influenced by the society in which they live, and in which they have been. This recognition includes the cultural and local moral beliefs of society or community (Martini, 1997). Internationally, Western medicine, for example, has had little impact on improving the health of Aboriginal people in Australia. While an understanding of the environmental conditions impacting on health is common, the issues of power, equity and cultural sensitivity are often overlooked. Consequently, for optimal client care we must first know the client. The experience of the illness as lived by the client, the cultural characteristics, and beliefs and perceptions of spirituality are all important. Remember that the ethical principles do not change; it is the surrounding circumstances that lead to the various ethical problems (Martini, 1997).

It was mentioned previously that people's values and beliefs can change (see Chapter 2), and this is not only the case for an individual, but also for a family and even a society and/or culture. Consequently, there is a need for primary health professionals to reflect critically on their own practice, for team members to include situations and incidents that arise to prevent harm from occurring. Ethical issues and problems can readily arise from:

➤ What would be regarded as the best interest of the individual, be that an unborn child, a neonate, a child, adolescent, a middle-aged adult or an older person?

➤ What would be the best interests for diverse patient groups, e.g. antenatal or postnatal mothers, parents of young children, working population, those with certain medical conditions or those people who live in a residential establishment?

➤ What would be the best interests of the community as a whole?

Activity

Read the following case study and answer the questions.

Case study 11.3
The issue of immunisation, consent and coercion

Georgina Truelove, a second-year student in children's nursing has been allocated to health visiting and school nursing practice.

One day her mentor Lettie, a health visitor, takes Georgina to the local general practice for the busy weekly baby clinic. Georgina observes how the practice staff greet mothers and babies, and how the place soon fills up with prams and pushchairs.

Georgina stays with Lettie to see how she deals with weighing/measuring babies/children, discussing growth and development, giving anticipatory advice on safety, play and issues of maternal concerns, using a transcultural approach to care and record-keeping.

Georgina then spends some time with the Francis, the practice nurse, whose role in the clinic relates to maternal postnatal care and child immunisation.

Mrs Whelan, a mother of three teenage children, brought her baby Alexandra into the practice nurse. She had not seen Lettie at this point but wanted to say to Francis that she really was not keen on Alexandra being immunised with the MMR vaccine as none of her children had been affected by not having the vaccine. She had heard all kinds of stories where the MMR vaccination was linked to autism.

Francis was keen to hear Mrs Whelan's story and present the facts on MMR. Georgina felt, however, that the immunisation was given as the discussion was still taking place and wondered whether consent had actually taken place beforehand.

Georgina raised her concerns with Lettie later that afternoon when they were on their own.

Questions

➤ What are the rights of mother, child and society in this case?

➤ What ethical principles are not upheld or not fulfilled in the case study?

Culturally competent care

As with other knowledge and skills in the therapeutic relationship, the primary health care professional needs to develop cultural competence. However, before practitioners can become sensitive to, and accommodate, a client's beliefs and values, they must first understand about their own background. According to Blackie (2000), primary care practitioners need to be aware of how their own cultural origins have affected their personal beliefs before interacting with people from another culture at a professional level. Consequently, if you skipped the exercises in Chapter 2 in relation to your own uniqueness and value beliefs, it is important that you do these now, so that you can differentiate between your own perspective and that of the client (be that an individual, family or community).

Ignorance of clients' health care needs

It is not unusual for clients' cultural needs to be ignored when primary health care is planned and implemented. For example, Harper (2004) discovered that Afro-Caribbean clients with Type 2 diabetes were not attending a UK primary care trust because the health teaching and care was inappropriate for their cultural needs. That is, the health teaching literature and care did not recognise these clients' health beliefs and other aspects of their culture. Based on her research Harper was then able to plan and implement culturally appropriate care with the successful outcome of the Afro-Caribbean clients now attending and receiving appropriate treatment for diabetes.

Nazroo (1997) reported on a national British survey using a structured questionnaire. A commercial translation agency identified 8000 people of Caribbean, Asian or Chinese origins (as well as a 'white' population) and their health status was ascertained. In this study it was noted that Bangladeshis and Pakistanis, followed by those from the Caribbean, reported the worst health and that Chinese men reported the best health.

The Nazroo study also found that:

1 One-third of all people from ethnic minorities reported less than good health or a long-standing illness/registered disabled.

2 One in 25 reported a diagnosis of heart disease.

3 One in 20 reported a diagnosis of diabetes.

4 One in 10 reported a diagnosis of hypertension.

5 One in five reported symptoms suggestive of respiratory disease.

6 South Asian and Caribbean respondents were at least as likely as white people to consult their primary care GP, whereas Chinese people were less likely to see a GP.

7 In contrast, ethnic minority respondents were less likely than whites to be admitted to hospital.

8 Significant numbers of South Asian or Chinese people who had had a GP consultation noted that they did not understand GP language or felt they were not understood by the GP.

Pause and think

➤ If these problems have occurred, is primary health care equitable to all people irrespective of culture?

➤ Knowing this information, how does this influence the way in which you would like to provide care in your community?

➤ How could you help clients from ethnic minorities to access primary health care?

➤ How can health care professionals in primary care address the issues of language barriers between themselves and their clients?

Transcultural care model

Giger and Davidhizer (2005) maintained that transcultural care can be achieved by providing:

1 culturally diverse care;

2 health professionals who have knowledge and understanding of each of the cultures attending the service;

3 recognition of an individual's uniqueness within a culture;

4 an environment at the health centre which is sensitive to the different cultures; and

5 an understanding of health belief behaviours in relation to specific illnesses and treatments.

When providing and implementing a culturally competent assessment of clients, primary health care professionals should recognise the importance of the following six characteristics that affect each different cultural group:

1 Their method and style of communication.

2 Their use of personal space, touch and closeness, and what is regarded not only as acceptable but also what is inappropriate.

3 Social organisation of their community or culture group.

4 Their concept of time.

5 Their types and methods of environmental control.

6 Biological variations within the cultural group.

Microcosm of society in health care

It is generally accepted that any given health care population (that is, people who work in health care) is a representative mix of the wider society in which we live and work. This is usually so, except for some international aid work, etc. This leads to the emergence of a more culturally mixed health workforce attempting to offer more culturally sensitive primary health care. However, this in itself can create some challenges that need discussion, e.g. in terms of the cultural needs of individual staff members v. the need for a more culturally mixed workforce. Consider the Israeli Orthodox Jewish public health consultant who does not want to work after sun down on Friday nights?

Activity

During Ramadan, when fasting from food needs to take place between sun up and sun down, is it right for a health professional to fast even though it might put his/her clients in danger? This may be caused by the health professional having a low blood sugar level from insufficient food intake, causing headache, clouding of perception and lack of cognitive ability.

Read the following case study and answer the questions at the end.

Case study 11.3
Fatimah, the occupational therapy student and her mentor

Fatimah is a first-year occupational therapy student who has just commenced her primary health care placement, based in a mental health team linked to a local primary care organisation.

She is to be mentored by a registered occupational therapist, Peter Perinski. On the first morning, Peter discussed the purpose of the mental health team and the geographical areas it covered. He then explained that they would be visiting some clients in their own homes, and today they would be going to see a lady with Alzheimer's disease.

Fatimah was concerned about travelling unaccompanied in a car with Peter as he was a man and this was not right in her culture. She did not want to be seen to be making a fuss; however, on the other hand she did not want someone from the Muslim community to see her acting in an inappropriate manner.

Questions

➤ If you were Fatimah how would you handle the situation? Use either the philosophy of Islam or the ethical principles of autonomy, beneficence, justice and non-maleficence to support your argument.

➤ How do you think Peter could deal with the situation?

Allocation of resources

The allocation of primary health care resources can only be made within budget limits and what the particular health service wants to achieve. Williams (2005) notes that, generally, health services have two main purposes:

- To improve the health of the total population.
- To reduce inequalities in health within the population.

These issues, however, are often in conflict. That is, the first purpose gets more attention than the second, which involves the pursuit of *equity* in health care. Two questions concerning this are posed:

➤ Do some people deserve better health care than others?

➤ What is the difference between *inequality* and *inequity*? If you do not know the meaning of these words, you need to look them up in a dictionary.

Pause and think

➤ What are your thoughts on the difference between inequality and inequity?

➤ Do you think that some people in the community who are seen to lead healthy life styles deserve to receive better medical treatment than others?

➤ What about those who:

○ drink too much and have cirrhosis of the liver?

○ smoke heavily and are progressing towards peripheral vascular disease and chronic obstructive airways disease?

○ engage in illegal drug use?

When health resources are limited, some people might say that these should be available only to those who lead a healthy life style, as that is more cost-effective. On the other hand, we may feel more compassionate towards those people who may not have as many opportunities in life as others and engage in unhealthy behaviours to compensate, and feel that both groups have an equal right to health care.

Inequality

An *inequality* reflects differences between individuals. Some babies are born with good hearing and others are born deaf. This reflects inequality but not necessarily inequity. Inequity is an ethical issue and in this instance relates to the allocation of resources. It could be that there was little that could be foreseen in preventing the congenital condition of the deaf baby.

Inequitable

On the other hand, it could be that the mothers of the babies had a different and *unfair* quality of social situation or health care from each other. Perhaps the hearing loss could have in some way been prevented, such as by prenatal maternal rubella immunisation. This then becomes an inequitable situation.

It could be considered that certain health problems take precedence over another in primary care in relation to government policy. More resources may be put into heart disease and cancer whereas mental health and learning disability services may feel they are only a 'Cinderella' service. For the health professional working in primary health care, the distribution decision when allocating resources may have already been made by a government body and therefore the health professional can only implement orders set out in the budget policy.

This may cause ethical issues or problems when dealing with inequity. Having knowledge of our personal beliefs and values can help in understanding each perplexing inequitable situation. Sometimes when placed in these situations, professionals want to be creative with the budget and resources 'to make it right'. However, before they do so they need to clarify their own values and beliefs and this sometimes helps them to realise it is out of their control. If the creative urge still exists then they need to have very good reasons for any actions or decisions they make in manipulating the allocation of budget and resources, otherwise they risk disciplinary action from their superiors and even censure by their professional registration body.

Activity

Clarify your own values and beliefs in relation to the allocation of resources in primary care. That is, what are your values and beliefs in relation to:

➤ Immunisation programmes?

➤ Free dental care for children?

➤ Free medical care for children under the age of 18 years?

➤ What priorities should take precedence?

➤ Health prevention and health promotion?

There are also tensions between preventative care and working with well individuals and populations, and caring for those people and populations with established health problems. The importance of ethics in delivering health care in the primary health care setting is thus complex because of the many tensions in the needs of various client groups (see Chapter 9).

Primary intervention v. paternalism

Pause and think

➤ When and how much should a government or health professional interfere with the health status of a client?

The use of genomics

We have all seen images on television of outside aid being flown in to famine-stricken communities and we probably all think this is ethically correct. But what about intervention that involve genomics?

That is, if we can genetically test, say, a client population for stroke, do we then implement a health care strategy so that the stroke will not occur?

Do we also say that the client will have that treatment and care?

This is not as far fetched as you might think. In February 2006 there was a conference in London debating the ethics of genomics in relation to cardiovascular and other diseases.

So where does the client's best interests and paternalism start and stop?

Population screening

Screening is another such issue that is initiated in primary care and involves identifying those at risk of a health problem in the 'specific population' through a test or interview. Examples, include cervical screening for women (a form of mass screening), genetic screening for diseases such as sickle cell, selective screening of high-risk immigrant people for diseases such as tuberculosis or HIV, and screening in general practice to detect trends such as diabetes.

In this way screening may be seen as another form of paternalism and, although it may be seen by some as a positive consequence that people get earlier treatment if diagnosed, the cost to the client may be to cause more anxiety and more invasive treatments, causing more psychological harm than they really want or find acceptable (Naidoo and Wills, 2005).

Activity

Read the following case study and answer the questions at the end.

Case study 11.4
Libby v. paternalism and screening

Libby is 28 years old and has been sent six letters from her medical centre, requesting that she attend the practice for cervical screening (or smear test).

Libby's mother died of ovarian cancer when she was 8 years old.

Four years ago, when Libby went to the practice for her 'smear test', she waited about an hour past her appointment time to be seen. Then she found the procedure distressing as one of the practice nurses demonstrated to a student practice nurse how to insert the vaginal speculum. The manner in which this was done left Libby feeling as though they had no respect for her and certainly none for her dignity!

This episode made her wonder about her own mother's problems. Was this the type of care she received?

Libby feels that the health care system is the cause of her losing her own mother 20 years ago, and therefore blames 'them'.

She felt dehumanised on the last visit, with the nurse being more concerned with teaching the student and the task of getting the cervical screening completed to comply with GP targets and payments, rather than Libby's needs.

Questions

➤ Does paternalism override the respect for the need for an individual's autonomy?

➤ When Libby went for her smear test 4 years ago, how could the practice nurse have conveyed to Libby through verbal and non-verbal communication that (s)he respected her rights of integrity and dignity, even though (s)he wanted to teach the student?

➤ How could the practice nurse respond to Libby?

Summary

This chapter has focused on the issues of ethics within the concept of primary health care. The rights of individuals and families as well as the rights of society to health care have been discussed. The therapeutic relationship between primary health care professionals and their clients highlighted some of the ethical issues and problems that can readily occur. Underpinning the concept of primary care is the need for the professional to approach team working in a collaborative manner, and also create a service which is culturally sensitive.

The political and economic context has been raised in relation to ethics, resource allocation and rationing in primary care. Equality and equity have been explored in relation to these ideas. Finally, the nature of paternalism in primary care was seen in the context of screening and immunisation.

Professional development

1 Continue to develop your Ethics Portfolio. Do not forget to mention that this is now Part 2, and is thus building on the knowledge and understanding gained in Part 1.

2 Discuss the following two case studies and answer the questions in your Ethics Portfolio.

Case study 11.5
Harrison and his duty of care to children

Harrison, a newly qualified health visitor, has attempted to contact Ms Grasso to make an appointment to visit her new baby (Angelo) who is now 11 days old. Although Harrison has phoned several times and left messages on the answering machine for Ms Grasso to phone him with a suitable time to visit she has not replied.

Harrison is concerned that Ms Grasso might not be coping and decides to go and see her at the home address, even though he realises that she could be at work (even though he felt it was a bit early for her to return to work).

However, little information was available from the hospital where she had delivered Angelo, other than that Ms Grasso left the care facility after 24 hours.

On arriving at the address given, Harrison notices that it is a small, poorly kept house with a yard and a fence dividing it from a very large farm. In fact, in the distance Harrison can see a huge double storey farm house and quality farm outbuildings.

Harrison knocks at the door and the door is opened by a small boy around the age of 8, who appears somewhat unkempt and pale. As he opens the door, Harrison is able to see directly into the sitting area and sees the young baby lying on a settee supported by some old pillows.

Harrison asks the boy if his mother is at home. The little boy replies, 'she's not here at the moment – I'm looking after the house while she is doing some work on the farm'.

Harrison then asks the little boy, 'who is looking after baby Angelo?' to which the little boy replies, 'I am'. As if on cue the baby starts to cry. Harrison asks the boy if his mother is due back soon. 'I dunno', is the reply.

Concerned, Harrison asks the boy what he usually does when his baby brother cries. He receives the answer that sometimes he nurses the baby and if it cries too long he makes him a bottle. With that the little boy goes over and lifts the baby up. Harrison notices the nappy is sodden and soiled and is concerned what to do next.

Questions

➤ Who is the client in this case study?

➤ From what perspective are you going to examine the situation (that is, from Harrison's or the family's)?

➤ From that perspective, what are the ethical issues and/or problems?

Using the decision-making framework from Chapter 10, work out how you would resolve the ethical problem. Issues you may need to consider are:

➤ What are the laws in your country about the care of children? That is, what legal obligations do parents have in looking after their children?

➤ Under what circumstances can children be removed from their parents and placed 'in care' to be looked after?

➤ Would having the children (the new baby and the small boy) placed in care help the situation?

Case study 11.6
Mrs Bristol and her competence to participate in self-care

Mrs Bristol is a frail but competent 62-year-old black lady who lives at home with her friend and carer Mr Thomas. To all intents and purposes Mr Thomas (who is 65) seems fairly reliable in helping Mrs Bristol.

Mrs Bristol, who has no family of her own, has chronic respiratory and cardiovascular problems affecting vision, mobility and nutritional intake. Owing to refusal to use dentures, she lives on a semi-fluid diet supplemented with high-calorie drinks and prefers to lie on the settee during the day watching television, and smoking.

Mrs Bristol has a number of medications, including oxygen and nebuliser therapy. The couple live in a second floor flat that is in need of attention and repair.

The community nurse visits on a regular basis but is becoming concerned that Mr Thomas is becoming less reliable and is only offering Mrs Bristol something like soup around 11 am and then some milk pudding or scrambled egg around 4 pm, despite being advised to offer a nourishing diet of about four to five small meals a day. Occasionally, medication is also found in the bed or seen on the floor by the community nurse.

Questions

➤ What are your values and beliefs in relation to people with Mrs Bristol's condition?

➤ What ethical issues and problems are in the case study?

Using the decision-making framework from Chapter 10, work out what would be the ethically appropriate way to resolve the problem. Issues you will need to consider are:

- Mrs Bristol's health status, for example:
  - ➤ Do you think she is lazy – just lying on a settee each day and not helping herself?
  - ➤ Do you think she does not bother about herself since she does not wear dentures so that she can eat solid food?
  - ➤ If she is just lying on the settee and does not help herself, can she be classified as being competent to care for herself?
- Options for her care and treatment:
  - ➤ Do you think the allocation of resources in the local primary health care organisation (or trust) should allow for Mrs Bristol to be placed in a residential care facility?
  - ➤ Would it be in Mrs Bristol's best interests if she was placed in a residential care facility?
  - ➤ What other options would be open to you in providing health care to Mrs Bristol?

Write your documentation of the decision-making process in your Ethics Portfolio.

Critical reflection

Write a critical reflection for this chapter to place in your Ethics Portfolio. The item or issue that you may want to work through or critically analyse could be something that you need to explore further from:

- One of the case studies.
- Reading that you have done.
- A different point of view that someone raised in discussion.
- A general feeling of disquiet about clients or patients, or about your own values and beliefs which you want to explore through reflection.
- Clinical practice:
  - ○ how you have realised that the care you have provided for a patient on clinical practice was incorrect and consequently, unethical;
  - ○ another member of the team on clinical practice is ignoring the client's or patient's rights and needs; or
  - ○ that the care is substandard due to the allocation of resources, etc.

Ethical problems occurring in mental health and psychiatric care

Phil Maude

Why this chapter is important to me . . .

✔ The person suffering from a mental health problem or psychiatric illness is extremely vulnerable and open to mistreatment and abuse.

✔ The very nature of a diagnosis of a psychiatric illness can be an ethical issue and problem.

✔ The different treatments for these illnesses can raise serious ethical issues and problems.

✔ Patient violence can be a protest against the behaviour of the health professionals!

Psychiatric patients expect to be controlled, manipulated, used and derogated or belittled and in general are seen as worthless.

(Peplau, 1998, p. 91)

What better way to start a chapter that explores ethical consideration toward people with a mental illness than by a quote from Hildegard Peplau. Peplau became a mental health nurse because she saw so many people on the street with an obvious mental illness and no-one to care for them. In her book she later comments that staff working with the mentally ill can reinforce patients' self-disempowering beliefs by disregarding their opinion and not engaging with them in a therapeutic relationship.

People experiencing mental illness can be the most politically powerless and vulnerable group within society. This is a population of people who find the concepts of autonomy and self-advocacy difficult to achieve. The manifestations of mental illness often include low self-esteem, withdrawal, self-doubt and distortions in thinking. Taking into consideration these factors and the stigma attached to having a mental illness, it is not surprising that these people find it difficult to negotiate health care systems. Hence, it is probably no surprise that this chapter develops the knowledge and understanding gained in just about every chapter in Part 1. For example, in Chapter 1 you learnt about the dreadful tragedy at Chelmsford Hospital; later clients' and patients' rights and protection of the vulnerable and decision making were discussed.

This chapter has been written for all health professionals irrespective of their area of clinical practice. Why – you might be thinking. The reason is that a person with a mental health or psychiatric illness quite often requires physical care and therefore they need this care and treatment away from those who are familiar with them. For example, the young teenager who has a car accident and is admitted to hospital with a leg fracture may have schizophrenia. The middle aged woman who has just been diagnosed with cancer of the cervix has bipolar disorder. This means that if you are involved in health care you need to have the knowledge and understanding of this chapter to help this client or patient group.

Sometimes it is not the client or patient with whom we are working, but a family member or significant other who is visiting or making contact by telephone. Often people experiencing mental illness are our co-workers, and many of us may have experienced a troubled family member or even had a diagnosis ourselves. Therefore, we all need to raise our awareness of the needs of people with a mental illness.

In this chapter it becomes apparent that ethical clinical practice issues abound in the mental health area. The ethically aware professionals practising in this area will notice these occurring on a daily basis. First, the diagnosis of mental or psychiatric illness as an ethical problem will be discussed; second, the ethical issues involved in treatment are covered; third, patient violence and protest behaviours; fourth, the situations of suicide, involuntary committment and the deinstitutionalisation movement; and fifth, the issues arising within client therapy are discussed. Finally, the Professional Development section will conclude the chapter.

Activity

➤ What are your values and beliefs about mental health problems and psychiatric illnesses?

List them in your Ethics Portfolio.

Psychiatric diagnosis as an ethical issue

Psychiatric diagnosis should be the most fundamental aspect of mental health care delivery under ethical examination. The effects of such a diagnosis on an individual include loss of personal freedom, imposed treatment regimes and the possibility of lifelong labelling (Maude, 1997).

Diagnosis is a powerful tool. It has the capacity to explain behaviour that is odd or objectionable, but has also been used to explain behaviour that is illegal. In the latter case, the law recognises that mental illness compromises a person's free will and classifies them as not legally responsible for their own actions. So, a diagnosis of mental illness can in some cases benefit a person (Maude, 1997). However, the process of psychiatric diagnosis has also been reported as having poor or questionable reliability (Sealy, 2004).

In mental health, physical signs and symptoms are not always evident so it must be accepted that diagnosis is a difficult procedure. Clients do not always tell the full story or may tell a story that is based on fantasy or denial (Maude, 1997). Diagnosis is often made on subjective data and has been found to vary depending on the psychiatrist's own bias (Sealy, 2004), or the impression the client gives to the psychiatrist. Furthermore, diagnosis plays a powerful role within people's lives. We must accept that the process of diagnosis has its limitations, certainly in its ability to label people as deviant, its ability to misdiagnose behaviours relating to cultural beliefs and also in its inability always to protect clients from potential self-harm (Maude, 1997).

To diagnose someone with mental illness describes them as deviant from the normal population and results in predetermined behaviours in both the person diagnosed and those health care professionals caring for the client. Have you ever had a client handed over to you as 'the woman in room 4' and then gone to introduce yourself to your new client? If the handover was 'the schizophrenic in room 4' how might your initial introduction differ? There are strong messages in the words we use, especially when they become labels.

Pause and think

> Who has the right to decide what types of behaviour are considered to be mental illness rather than moral deviance?

> How do we classify people who show the following behaviours: verbally abusive when drunk, heavy substance use, antisocial behaviour, homosexuality, sadomasochism, religious beliefs or gambling?

Some of these you may see as mental illness, but other people would disagree with you. Local custom and societal norms have a lot to do with how we determine who is mentally ill or not.

Ethical aspects of psychotherapeutic treatment

Although the Mental Health Act (you may live in a country with a national Act or there may be Mental Health Acts that are only relevant to your region or state) provides guidelines as to the legalities of treatment methods used in mental health settings, treatment is often conducted against the person's will. Treatment can be prescribed in the form of a community treatment order (contract) that specifies where the person will live, provides agreement for clinical access and review, and imposes conditions (such as medication compliance) for the person to be able to continue living in the community. Treatment often consists of the control of one human's behaviour by another and the client's right of choice is deferred to a hospital board for decision-making.

Pause and think

> Is it justifiable to impose treatment upon people against their will? This is especially so when many clients with mental illness have experienced varied diagnoses and treatment regimes from differing hospitals.

> In this case, who made the correct diagnosis and who provided incorrect treatment?

Until the 1950s there were few treatment modalities available for mental illness. The advent of psychopharmacology has caused a decline in the number of people requiring hospitalisation;

however, these drugs are potent agents, causing major side effects and in some cases problems with toxicity (Maude, 1997). They have many interactions with other chemotherapeutic agents, so need to be monitored closely.

When the phenothiazines were first introduced in the 1950s, little was known of their properties, but side effects were quickly reported. Three complications of psychopharmacology have proved to be dangerous or at least disturbing to the client's self-image. These are neuroleptic malignant syndrome, serotonin syndrome and tardive dyskinesia (Maude, 1997). Neuroleptic malignant syndrome is, thankfully, rare but deadly. It manifests with high temperatures, muscle rigidity, loss of consciousness and a mortality rate of 20%, largely caused by renal failure (Bhanushali and Tuite, 2004). Several medications of the antidepressant genre have been reported to induce serotonin syndrome: these are monoamine oxidase inhibitors (MAOIs), L-tryptophan, fluoxetine, clomipramine, meperidine, dextromethorphan, pentazocine, fenfluramine (Mueller and Korey, 1998). Tardive dyskinesia is common among people who have been taking major tranquillisers. It is a progressive drug-induced disorder manifesting with choreoathetoid movements of the tongue, lips, mouth, trunk and limbs (Brown, 1999). It is marked and thus draws considerable attention to the person experiencing tardive dyskinesia (Maude, 1997). This is difficult to rationalise when the initial purpose of the drug therapy was to improve quality of life.

In recent years, the risk of dependence and drug withdrawal from minor tranquillisers has caused much debate in the literature, with dependence occurring in up to 40% of users (Galbraith *et al.*, 2004). Withdrawal symptoms may include insomnia, agitation, muscle twitching, headache, tremor, nausea, double vision and sweating (Gorman and Davis, 2005). These symptoms may persist for up to 6 months after withdrawal of the medication (Brown, 1999). The question that needs to be asked is, who watches for these serious complications when clients are in the community? General practitioners have the right to prescribe such treatment but are not always able to monitor the person closely (Maude, 1997). Sleath *et al.* (1998) suggest the importance of training GPs to probe and to provide patients with an opportunity to discuss their emotional symptoms.

In respect to drug treatment, what are a person's rights when placed on psychotherapeutic agents? These rights should include: access to effective professional treatment, information concerning the drug prescribed (desired effect, side effects, contraindications and complications), and the freedom to accept or refuse treatment (Maude, 1997). Of course, this form of negotiation is limited if the person is a non-voluntary patient under the Mental Health Act. All clients should have some voice and choice in the selection of drugs. If the side effects of a particular drug are difficult to live with, the person should be able to ask for a review and change of treatment. A goal of treatment should be to promote compliance through client education (Maude, 1997).

Other forms of psychotherapeutic treatment that are prescribed for the mentally ill include electroconvulsive therapy (ECT), side room management and psychosurgery (now banned in most countries throughout the world).

Electroconvulsive therapy

ECT is used mainly for psychotic depression. Compared with chemotherapy, ECT is proven to be more effective in the treatment of depression (Merskey, 1999). The major ethical problem occurs when the person refuses consent for the treatment but it is deemed the best treatment for that person. This creates problems because the client is required to have a general anaesthetic. The thought of having ECT can be traumatic to clients and may cause them to act on their suicidal thoughts to avoid the treatment. All treatments of this type need to be carefully negotiated with the client, who is often in a state of negativity and unwilling to see a solution to their depression (Maude, 1997). In the case of refusal, some mental health services require a second opinion and others have the power under the Mental Health Act to prescribe ECT without the client's consent. However, health professionals need to ensure that these clients have been informed of the nature of the procedure and why consent has been provided by another source. Furthermore, offering comfort through reassurance is important to support the client through the experience.

Side room management

Side room management, or seclusion, is prescribed to clients who become aggressive or are a danger to themselves or others. Restraint (e.g. straitjackets) is also used in extreme situations (on one occasion, a patient was so psychotic that he was peeling his fingernails back from his fingers). These forms of intervention should only be used when an emergency occurs. Seclusion should never be used as a form of punishment (Maude, 1997). It must also be noted that when a person is responding to psychotic phenomena they need stimulation to reorientate them back to reality. Seclusion in a side room isolates the patient and encourages hallucination. Observations of the client while in the side room are required to ensure client safety. These are conducted at least every 15 minutes. The client should also have comfortable bedding, clothing and toilet facilities. Nutritional input needs to be taken into consideration. If side rooms are used they need to be used for emergencies and for the least time possible (Maude, 1997). Clients placed in side rooms need debriefing afterwards. How would you feel if you were placed in a locked room the next time you become angry?

Psychosurgery

In the not-too-distant past, surgical procedures such as leucotomy for the control of depression and amygdalotomy for the control of aggression were performed (Merskey, 1999). These procedures removed or destroyed the nerve pathways between lobes of the brain. This in effect was surgery on healthy brain tissue in an attempt to control behaviours. With the advent of psychopharmacology such surgical procedures have become obsolete, but the practitioner may find some older patients who have undergone such procedures (Maude, 1997). Health care professionals need to be aware of psychosurgery as it is still provided as a treatment option in some Mental Health Acts.

Activity

Here are two things for you to do and write in your Ethics Portfolio.
1 Find out if psychosurgery is still allowed under the Mental Health Act.
2 Do an internet search to see if you can find out when psychosurgery was last conducted in your country.

Ethical aspects of patient violence and protest behaviours

People with mental illness have a false reputation for being superhumanly aggressive. Often aggression is caused by frustration or fear and manifests so strongly due to disinhibition. The very nature of hospitalisation creates situations that potentiate aggressive thoughts in clients (for example, loss of control) (Maude, 1997).

In the past two decades researchers have shown a growing interest in what appears to be the escalating problem of clients or patients and members of the public being violent towards health professionals and other staff. It has been speculated that poor public perceptions of hospital services, altered or disturbed mental states and exposure to prolonged physical or psychological discomforts are major factors contributing to patient-generated violence in hospitals. It is also likely that increasing rates of occupational violence in the health care industry are a function of rising levels of violence in the general population, and the increasing use of violence as a means of solving problems.

In systems such as emergency care and psychiatric settings, forced periods of detention and treatment being administered against a person's will may result in patient resistance to the system. Patients can engage in what Mason (2000) has described as protest behaviour to challenge authority, and this can manifest in acts of physical violence towards self or others, property or verbal abuse. Such behaviour is destabilising and interferes with the therapeutic relationship between the professional and patient (Maude, 1998).

Studies have indicated that occupations where cash is exchanged for service or which require face-to-face contact between workers and their clients are at a greater risk of experiencing workplace violence than other occupations. Health professionals work closely with patients and perform invasive acts and ask confronting questions.

Activity

➤ When thinking about an incident of violence, do you perceive this as patient aggression or protest?

➤ Whose side do we need to consider, that of the patient or the health professional?

If we apply the ethical principles to a situation of patient protest or aggression we can see that the system and also the professional or staff member need to be considered to gain a full understanding of the situation. In our Western health care system:

● Access to health care is seen as a human right (United Nations Declaration of Human Rights).

● The care of the client or patient is at the centre of health care delivery but must be viewed with the benefits of all in mind (beneficence).

● The health care system has a responsibility to prevent injury and violence (non-maleficence).

● All individuals have a responsibility to improve quality standards and care, including consumers (justice and beneficence).

- Professionals need to see working with violence as a clinical situation that can be de-escalated rather than a control issue (autonomy and respect for the dignity of the person).

Activity

Take a moment to reflect on your own experiences with anger.

➤ Have you ever become angry or had to face someone who becomes out of control with anger?

➤ How did this impact upon your ability to think and problem-solve?

As humans we experience anger and are also confronted by what to do with these feelings. What we need to do is consider that anger is a common human emotion that can be managed or prevented. Anger that leads to violent outbursts is anger that is out of control and needs intervention.

In mental health, anger can be a common occurrence owing to the frustration that patients experience. We need to focus on the problem and not the client or patient and see that it is a situation that requires care and health teaching. We also need to ensure that our colleagues and other patients are safe and that we are protected from harm.

Management of protest and angry behaviour

The first thing to do when confronted by an angry client or patient is to ask the question, 'what is the reason behind the person's behaviour?'

Mason (2000) describes that most aggression arises from four different causes and each may require an adjustment to your approach.

1 Criminal behaviour occurs when the use of a weapon is involved or there is deliberate harm to others or property. This is a non-clinical situation and should be considered as a police matter. It is important and moral to ensure that all patients are aware that this behaviour is not acceptable and what the consequences may be. It is also important to ensure that other patients are protected.

2 Aggrieved behaviour will occur when the person feels let down by the health care system or their family. They could feel disregarded; waiting time is often voiced by patients as the leading cause of distress leading to anger. Health professionals are often in the front line of patient aggression.

3 Behaviour arising from feeling estranged or detached from society through grief, loss or even psychosis can manifest as aggression towards others.

4 Manifestations of mental illness, which can arise from mistrust, voices, confusion or feelings of self-doubt can lead people to lash out in an attempt to find a solution. Mental illness is not a rationale that excuses a person from aggressive behaviour. Everyone can become angry but there are many options for the person experiencing anger - resolve the situation, withdraw or seek help are positive options. Anger that leads to aggression is anger that is out of control.

When a person becomes aggressive for any of the above reasons, the power relationships that exist within psychiatric settings must be considered. Health professionals need to ensure that everyone is safe (including the person who is being aggressive) and de-escalate the situation rather then overcontrol it. You have to consider that many patients want to save face and will be confused, feeling guilty and even exhausted after an outburst. Keep your distance and engage in conversation that requires the person to reflect on their options. Ensure you have up-to-date training in the management of patient/family aggression.

Ethical aspects of suicidal behaviour

Care of the potentially suicidal client is possibly the most challenging clinical situation a mental health professional must face (Maude, 1997). The problem of suicide within the developed world is well documented, but few realise that the number of unsuccessful attempts at suicide is eight to ten times higher than the figures for actual suicide (Heyd and Bloch, 1999). This widespread incidence of suicide renders it hard to ignore but it remains a confronting issue to humanity. The prospect of many members of our community considering whether they wish to live at all destroys our image of life as a cherished and worthwhile commodity. Suicide is confronting as it poses a threat to our convictions as to the sanctity of life and makes us face the reality of our own mortality. Because of this, our society is unable to see any worth or rationale in thinking that a person may wish to end his or her life (Maude, 1997).

Suicide is often referred to as a 'cry for help', 'acting out' or 'being out of control'. Because of these labels many people who have made suicide attempts are treated as problems. There is a feeling that they must be punished for their 'bad behaviour' by being ignored and are often dealt with quickly in the emergency department and left alone by staff or treated roughly with no thought to pain, anguish or suffering. This is probably largely because health care workers, who work to save life, find the act of attempted suicide confronting (Maude, 1997).

The ethics of involuntary commitment

Institutions providing care for the mentally ill have often been criticised for demeaning psychiatric patients. Although the manifest function of mental health hospitals is to care for the mentally ill, it can also be argued that a latent function exists to control and socially isolate people (Maude, 1996; 2001). Control of behaviour by using ECT, psychoanalysis, chemotherapy, behavioural modification and psychosurgery are all controversial when prescribed against a person's will.

When a person is committed to a mental health hospital the major ethical debate centres on legal v. moral rights. When should a person be admitted as an involuntary patient under the Mental Health Act? The answer is simple, 'when the person is a danger to themselves or others'. However, consider if the person we are talking about is a member of your family or a close friend. Would you feel comfortable committing this person to a mental health hospital? I remember talking to a group of students about what to expect when they were in the psychiatric setting for practice. We discussed their feelings when interacting with a withdrawn and depressed client. After the lecture, a student came to me in tears. Her sister was out of control and suicidal. Her parents were distraught. Here was an excellent student who was capable of effective decision-making in the clinical setting but unable to problem-solve when it came to a family member. I am certain that all health care workers would have empathy with what this student was living through.

A voluntary patient seeking treatment for a mental illness should be treated as fully competent and retain the right to give or withhold consent to treatment (Wallace, 1995). An involuntary patient is admitted to hospital under the enforcement of the local Mental Health Act. The involuntary patient has no legal capacity to refuse or consent to treatment (Staunton and Whyburn, 1997). Ethical principles in providing treatment to such a client against their will involve beneficence and non-maleficence. This requires that the committed person is kept from harm. But is this paternalistic? Utilitarianism asserts that paternalistic actions are justified when the person is being protected from harm and does not have the capacity to make decisions by themselves (Mappes and Zembaty, 1997). It is not hard to see how such an argument is left open to personal interpretation and how abuse occurs within the health care system. A simple rule of thumb would be to ensure that all patients are treated with the same degree of respect that you would require and, whenever practicable, the person's autonomy is maintained. This would ensure that the person would maintain some of their integrity and not feel so vulnerable and powerless (Maude, 1997).

The ethics of the deinstitutionalisation movement

Deinstitutionalisation of the mentally ill has occurred since the early 1950s. The history of the movement and the reasons for it occurring raise a number of ethical issues. While many people are discharged from mental health hospitals to supportive settings, and the illnesses of other people require no follow up, thousands of patients have been discharged to inadequate housing or even to the streets (Peele, 1999). Reasons for deinstitutionalisation are many: overcrowding of institutions, reduction of government expenditure, greater community awareness of the needs of the mentally ill, the availability of treatment modalities such as psychopharmacology, and sociopolitical movements such as the mental hygiene movement (Maude, 2001).

In Australia until the 1950s, both state and federal governments placed strong emphasis on building larger institutions to house the 'insane'. Over the past 30 years Australian governments have strived to close down these asylums (Maude, 2001). This has been welcomed by many members of the public, as people incarcerated in asylums have been seen to have no political power and therefore unable to empower themselves. Taking into consideration the effect of incarceration, the stigma attached to mental illness and the debilitating nature of psychiatric disorders, it is little wonder that there are so many inequalities between the mentally ill and the general public. It could be argued that the community has been ill prepared for the shift to deinstitutionalisation, that prejudice abounds and resources within the community for services such as community mental health nursing are scarce.

Governments are often criticised for not addressing the needs of the individual experiencing mental illness. This is largely because issues arising in mental health care delivery do not fit easily within a health care system that is tailored to the needs of the physically unwell

(Ovadia and Owen, 1992). People experiencing the often debilitating nature of mental illness face the same economic challenges as all citizens, but have the added burden of stigma and the personal cost of their illness. Issues such as equity in access to health care, affordable accommodation, adequate income and meaningful work are all made so much harder with the complication of mental illness (Maude, 1997). Although these fundamental needs may be tenets of primary health care delivery, they are not often under the control of the health care system.

The major impact of the changes in health care policy should be seen in the community setting. The Mental Health Acts commonly aim to reduce the incidence of stigma of mental illness by, wherever possible, treating the person in the community or in general hospital settings rather than in specialised psychiatric settings (the least restrictive environment). The breakdown of institutional services should not be replaced by private hostel and board-ing house care (Maude, 1997). This in effect is replacing one socially unacceptable institution with another.

Ethical consideration and client therapy

In general the ethical guidelines for one-to-one therapy or group work are threefold: first, to protect the client from exploitation, incompetence and pressure to perform; second, to uphold the right of the client to be provided with information and make informed decisions concerning their life; and third, to foster personal growth and wellness (Bancroft, 1999). The first two goals protect the client and the promotion of the client's rights. The third goal out-lines the true goal of therapy. It is often taken for granted that therapy is always beneficial to the client. After all, to look at oneself or share beliefs during group work should help us to grow and understand why our lives have evolved as they have. Unfortunately, this is not true when the therapy is not client-centred, but rather outcomes are based on the needs of the institution or the therapist who is unprofessional in conduct, e.g. sexual exploitation of the client.

There are problems with the process of therapy of which the clinician needs to be constantly aware. These are transference and countertransference as well as the 'saviour' persona the clinician takes on for many clients (Maude, 1997). Transference refers to when the therapist/client relationship has developed, resulting in the client holding strong feelings towards the therapist. Freud believes this is an inevitable occurrence in therapy because the client sees the therapist as a saviour and facilitator of problem resolution. It is important for the therapist to scrutinise all feelings towards the client as the client is easily exploited during transference.

Countertransference refers to the therapist's feelings and responses to the client in therapy. The therapeutic relationship is a privileged state for both the client and the clinician. The clinician should be self-analytical and use a co-therapist to discuss client care confidentially and debrief. When you are working closely with a client, you may have feelings of impend-ing friendship, wanting to save the client from reckless behaviour, boredom with their lack of progress or a sense of knowing what the client needs. These are all signs of counter-transference (Maude, 1997). The clinician needs to be reflective and aware of the boundaries needed to keep the therapy sessions therapeutic and client-centred. A trainee psychiatrist once showed me a book of poetry that a client had written and dedicated to him. The client had been sexually abused and was now often suicidal and unable to trust the opposite sex. The problem with the presentation of this gift was that the client was exposing transference, and the clinician was proud that the client had grown because of him not because of the client's personal work through therapy. In this story the level of esteem the therapist was held in by the client is obvious, but the risks of this would emerge on that inevitable day when the therapist lets the client down.

Psychotherapy

Contemporary society often refers to psychotherapy as the talking therapy. Psychotherapy is based on the work of Sigmund Freud. The goal of psychotherapy is to assist clients to modify or overcome feelings, behaviours or thoughts that are hindering their life. For this to occur the client places his or her trust in the therapist, expecting that the therapist will not exploit that trust. When this trust occurs, a therapeutic relationship starts and can be maintained.

The therapeutic relationship between therapist and client is psychotherapy's strength and weakness. The therapist gains notoriety for his or her work and also power within the relationship (Barker and Kerr, 2001). The ethical issue is how to use this power. Does the power remain egalitarian or become authoritarian? To what extent does transference within the relationship hinder the therapeutics? The therapist may become the most important person in the client's life and runs the risk of assuming priority over all others. Therapists need to remain client-centred at all times.

Behavioural modification

The major ethical issue when considering behaviour modification is power, control and the potential dehumanisation of the client (Maude, 1997). Behavioural therapy is often questioned because, unlike psychotherapy, it does not expand the client's awareness. For many it fosters a machine model of man and portrays the therapist as a technician who manipulates the patient (Bancroft, 1999). Behavioural modification is often conducted against the person's will and, in the case of the involuntary client, methods have often been applied in the absence of consent (Maude, 1997).

Coercive controls of behaviour manifest in seclusion of the client or restraint. If the client is out of control and a danger to himself or herself, behavioural control is justified on the principles of beneficence over client autonomy. Restraints are not always mechanical. Chemical restraint is achieved when the client is sedated and unable to act on violent thoughts towards self or others. This may appear to be less coercive but in actual fact involves the same ethical issues (Carson and Arnold, 2004).

Behavioural controls can manifest in the form of positive reinforcement by rewarding desirable behaviour and negative reinforcement for undesirable behaviour. This form of behavioural manipulation of clients often manifests in the form of token economies within mental health/psychiatric units. The health professional holds the cigarettes and the client may have one on the half hour but only if there has been no disturbing behaviour (Maude, 1997).

When considering behavioural modification, the questions that should be asked are:

➤ Who sets the standard of behaviour?

➤ How will reward and punishment be carried out?

➤ Has this decision been made with consideration of the client's needs and benefit?

Sex therapy

Sexual expression involves a whole gambit of human emotions, joys and risks. Needless to say it is not unusual for a client to be in therapy because of sexual issues; for example, a married couple who feel they have lost the 'spark' in their romance. When these situations arise the therapist may place themselves, in the eyes of the client, as being in the position of being an expert in sexuality. In such a situation it is not unlikely for the client to divulge that sexual feelings are emerging towards the therapist.

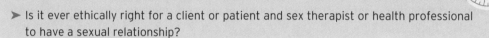

Pause and think

➤ Is it ever ethically right for a client or patient and sex therapist or health professional to have a sexual relationship?

The answer is quite simply *no*.

This is especially important because the client tends to role-model the therapist's behaviour. Sexual relationships between client and therapist must be considered the quintessence of misuse and exploitation of the transference that occurs within a relationship (Maude, 1997).

Human sexuality is expressed in many ways and we each have our own beliefs concerning the boundaries of this expression. What does the therapist do if a client reveals sexual feelings or acts of expression that conflict with the therapist's own beliefs? The answer to this is within the concept of unconditional positive regard. That is, the therapist sees the client as an individual and respects the client no matter what. If the therapist is not able to keep the therapeutic relationship separate from one of friendship or indeed a sexual relationship, then (s)he needs to hand over the treatment and care to another therapist or professional. This is because the client or patient relationship with the therapist is no longer therapeutic.

One of the most debated issues of this kind is the treatment of homosexual and transsexual clients. In the past, because homosexuality was (and still is in some countries) regarded as a psychiatric disorder, treatments involved behavioural modification and aversion therapy (Maude, 1997); e.g. the use of electrical shocks to the genitalia when confronted with pictures of members of the same sex.

These practices are now contraindicated as homosexuality has been removed from the ICD 10 and DSM IV (note revisions are being made for a DSM V during 2006–2007) as classified illnesses. However, beliefs concerning homosexuality as deviant behaviour still persist. A recent review of the literature concerning this topic revealed that many therapists still regard homosexuality as undesirable, if not pathogenic (Bancroft, 1999).

Confidentiality within group work

Clients or patients often give health professionals information and at the same time ask that it is kept secret. Confidentiality is a primary principle of the therapeutic relationship, but how can it be upheld if the client reveals information that must be shared with the rest of the team? Never promise to keep a secret; these are appropriate within a friendship but never within a therapeutic relationship (Maude, 1997). Previously, in Chapter 5, when ethical principles and rules were discussed, it was mentioned that the rule of confidentiality was allowed to be broken in certain circumstances. This is an example of such a situation. Consequently, it is probably paramount that the client or patient is made aware that all necessary information will be shared with the team and that this information will remain within the team. So too, when commencing a discussion during group therapy it is always an excellent idea to remind people that what they share with the group is for the group alone and not to be taken out of the room.

Summary

This chapter has attempted to raise several issues that may arise within the mental health area of health care. The major objective is to assist you to think about your own beliefs concerning mental health and how these would impact on your delivery of care to people with mental illness.

The legal restrictions placed upon involuntary admission of a client may place restrictions on an already compromised therapeutic health professional/client relationship. In these situations it is the health professional who holds the social control of the client. It is the nurse who initiates *pro re nata* (to be given or taken when necessary) medication and restraint of the client. Mental health is not an area where the nurse can refer the client to the doctor for the answers, because it is often the nurse's actions that the client or patient is questioning.

In many instances the client is unable to make autonomous decisions and the health professionals may be called on to intervene in situations ranging from areas of daily activity and hygiene to the decision to conduct invasive treatments. How to care for a client must be decided after careful consideration of client autonomy and the ethical principles of beneficence and non-maleficence within health care delivery.

Professional development

1 Continue to develop your Ethics Portfolio.

2 Read Case studies 12.1 and 12.2 and answer the questions.

Case study 12.1
Four people who want to die (Maude, 1997)

The ethical debate of suicide largely centres on the moral justification of limiting a person's choice to live or die. Health care workers have a duty to intervene by preventing the suicidal act or treating the person who has made an attempt on their own life. Let us now consider some cases:

Minnie Tsing

Minnie Tsing is a 33-year-old Chinese woman who tells you she wants to die as she cannot get over the death of her husband and 6-year-old son in a motor vehicle accident 11 months ago. She has no family and has lost her home as she is on unemployment benefits and was unable to pay the mortgage. She feels the pain is too great and just wants it to end.

Sanjeev Singh

Sanjeev Singh is a 59-year-old widower who has been diagnosed with liver and bowel cancer, and presents in considerable pain and distress. He advises the health professionals that he has always believed in euthanasia and has decided that his time is now up. He does not want to be a burden on his daughter and wishes to die with dignity. He is open about his wish to die and has planned his suicide. All his affairs are in order. He believes that he will carry this out sooner rather than later, as the pain is now too great and he just wants it to end.

Augusta Armouries

Augusta Armouries is a 15-year-old girl who arrives at the emergency department after ingesting 24 Panadol tablets. She has been struggling with anorexia nervosa since she was 11 and now feels that her life is heading nowhere. She is transferred as an involuntary patient to the local mental health hospital and is prescribed a course of electroconvulsive therapy, which is given without her consent. She remains suicidal 21 days later and is now being tube-fed. She wants to be left alone as she cannot face the pain of life any more.

Film star X

Film star X, an 84-year-old famous actress, has refused food and drink for 6 days as she does not want to live any more. She has right-sided paralysis following a cerebrovascular accident. She wants to be remembered as young and beautiful. She feels her life has been full and now wants it to end as she feels her future prospects are hopeless.

Questions

➤ Which of the above four people is making a rational choice to die?

➤ What are our responsibilities in each case as health professionals?

➤ Do we have the right to stop people when they wish to die?

Case study 12.2
Dame Johnston-Hawleton and the cultural aspects of suicide (Maude, 1997)

Dame Johnston-Hawleton is a 58-year-old Roman Catholic woman who has been admitted to a secure ward with a diagnosis of endogenous depression. Her family state she has deteriorated over the past 10 days and now will not shower or speak.

On admission her belongings are searched and razor blades are found in the battery compartment of her portable radio. When the staff supervise her in the shower they find a rope with multiple knots tied around her waist. When this is taken from her she becomes hysterical and needs to be restrained by four staff and taken to a side room. While here Dame Johnston-Hawleton is held down and given 5 mg intramuscular Haloperidol.

The family are distraught as to what has happened and advise that their mother likes using the knotted rope during prayer as she keeps losing her rosary beads. The staff on the ward feel it is not safe to provide the patient with a knotted rope and keep it in storage.

Questions

➤ Using the decision-making framework in Chapter 10, document in your Ethics Portfolio how you could resolve the issue. Issues you may need to consider are:

  a. Were the staff correct in taking the knotted rope from Dame Johnston-Hawleton?

  b. Dame Johnston-Hawleton has been prescribed electroconvulsive therapy. As she has refused to sign the consent form the Superintendent of the hospital has consented for her, using the power of the Mental Health Act.

  c. You are one of the professionals who has responsibility to escort her for her general anaesthetic and treatment. How will you undertake this? Consider the legal and ethical issues involved.

➤ What types of people or patients do you believe should be involuntary patients (under the Mental Health Act)? Do you think this only need to apply to psychotic people (for example, people living with schizophrenia)?

➤ Have we gone too far in controlling people when clients or patients with eating disorders can also be detained and treated against their will?

Critical reflection

Write your critical reflection for this chapter. Issues you might like to consider include:

➤ What mental health illnesses and psychiatric disorders are acceptable by your professional body or council? Do you think this ethically correct?

➤ How do you think it would be if you were a professional who developed one of these illnesses or disorders, and was informed that you can no longer practise? Would you be tempted to keep quiet about it, and not tell your employer and professional body or council?

➤ Is paedophilia a psychiatric disorder?

13

Complex care: ethical problems in the emergency department, perioperative, intensive and coronary care units

Louise M. Terry

Why this chapter is important to me . . .

✔ Professionals practising in complex care often need to make rapid ethical decisions about patient care. When only some team members are involved in making decisions this can cause problems.

✔ Sometimes the outcome of these quick ethical decisions may mean that one or more patients will die.

✔ These decisions may have to be made without knowing what the patient wishes.

✔ Complex care is financially expensive.

✔ Team members can quite easily become physically, mentally and emotionally tired owing to the complexity of care required.

Complex care involves the care of clients or patients that need specialised, multifaceted and difficult procedures and care. This term is usually used to define the care within the different hospital departments or units such as emergency, perioperative, intensive care unit (ICU), coronary care unit (CCU) and high dependency unit (HDU). Consequently, this chapter adds on to just about everything covered in Part 1 of this book. This includes people's values and beliefs, ethical issues and problems, clients' or patients' rights and protecting the vulnerable, working in a team, pain and resuscitation, illness and loss, and decision-making. Consequently, it is not surprising that some of the most demanding and complex challenges faced by health care professionals arise with critically ill patients. The chain begins with the emergency services being called upon to provide immediate care to patients who often have life-threatening injuries, illnesses or diseases.

Different countries take different approaches as to whether the patient will be stabilised at the scene and then transferred to hospital or if transfer will be carried out as fast as possible. The critically ill patients are received in emergency departments (emergency rooms (ER) in some countries, accident and emergency (A&E) in the UK). Urgent surgery or resuscitation may be required. Patients are often then transferred to ICUs, also called intensive therapy units (ITUs) or CCUs if they have cardiac (heart) problems. These units can provide highly technological care with usually only one or two patients per nurse. Once a patient is more stable, he or she may be moved to an HDU where care of a technological and complex nature can still be provided before transfer to a normal ward. ICUs also provide care for patients who have undergone planned surgery where close observation and technological support are required afterward to ensure the best possible patient outcome.

Activity

Take a moment to think about the system where you live or undertake clinical practice.

➤ What happens with the transfer of patients to hospital: are they stabilised at the scene or are they sent immediately to the emergency department?

➤ What happens next?

Find out, as once you know what happens at the hospital you are at you will be able to understand this chapter much better.

Advances in medicine mean that patients who would not have survived devastating trauma, disease or illness do so. Sometimes survival comes at huge physical and psychological, if not financial, cost to patient, family or health care provider. The impact of suddenly requiring emergency care, or needing surgery (planned or unplanned) and admission to an ICU/CCU or HDU for patients, families and significant others must never be underestimated. Understanding this potential impact, and exploring some of the ethical or moral problems that may be faced is important for the professional who wishes to provide care within an appropriate ethical framework.

Although the ethical issues and problems associated with complex care are interrelated, this chapter has been divided into three parts to make it clearer to read and understand.

● Part A is concerned with the care of patients in an emergency department.

● Part B is concerned with the care of patients in a perioperative suite, unit or department. This involves the care of patients requiring operations. Sometimes these departments are known as operating departments or, as some English hospitals say, theatre.

Pause and think

Stop and think about your values and beliefs in relation to complex care. These might include:

● The value you place on human life.

● Whether life-saving procedures should be performed on all people, irrespective of a person's age or financial position.

● Whether a person should be maintained on life-support machinery if the relatives are unable to accept that brain death has occurred.

● People who are brain-dead and use of organs for transplants.

- Part C discusses patients who are in an ICU/CCU/HDU, with the aim of helping you to think about issues around patient or family values and the appropriateness of treatment decisions.

Finally, at the end of the chapter you will find some learning exercises to help you further develop your understanding of ethical issues in complex care situations.

Part A Emergency care

The care of a patient in an emergency department raises the ethical issues of:

- The use of appropriate resources.
- Triage; that is, in what order should patients be treated (those most critically injured or the first person waiting)?
- Confidentiality and the balancing of the best interests of the patient.

At the end of Part A a brief summary will be given.

Appropriate use of emergency services

Inappropriate use of the emergency department is a huge challenge. It is easy to condemn the person who presents with a sore thumb 3 days after hitting it with a hammer, but not every patient is registered with a GP (primary care physician). Other people may come into the emergency department with a complaint hoping that they will be sufficiently ill to warrant a warm bed on a cold wet night. However, the real work of the emergency department must continue so, while the staff need to pay some attention to those they would rather go elsewhere, they also need to concern themselves with emergencies that constantly come through the door. This may on occasion be someone who dies shortly after arrival, and the staff rightly need to spend time with the relatives after the event when it is desperately hard to accept. At other times there are stabbings or motor vehicle accidents. In particular, the issue of resuscitation is a challenge to the emergency department staff and ambulance paramedics and technicians.

Activity

Read the following case study and the reasoning that follows.

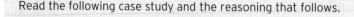

Case study 13.1
Mohammed and resuscitation in the terminal stages of cancer

Mohammed is a 69-year-old man in the terminal stages of cancer. A do not resuscitate (DNR) order was placed in his hospital notes. He has been cared for at home for the last 2 weeks since he wishes to die in his own bed with his family around him. When his condition deteriorated, his daughter panicked and called for an ambulance. When the ambulance crew arrived, they commenced resuscitation and took him to the emergency department where resuscitation continued for a time while information was sought about Mohammed's medical history. Eventually, Mohammed was declared dead and the family informed.

In this case, there was no challenge over whether the DNR order was appropriate. The difficulties arose because of a lack of continuity regarding how Mohammed was to be cared for in the community. In some regions, protocols have been implemented to allow ambulance personnel some discretion over withholding or limiting resuscitation attempts where they are likely to be futile (Marsden *et al.*, 1995). Even if the resuscitation were to succeed, Mohammed would almost certainly need to be transferred to a ward or unit for ongoing care, possibly with some brain damage from lack of oxygen, and end up dying there against his wishes.

Clearly the ethical principles of autonomy, beneficence and non-maleficence are breached in such a situation. That is, his daughter removed his autonomy by calling emergency services to take him to the hospital. Beneficence was breached because Mohammed needed to die peacefully, and non-maleficence was breached because, by resuscitating Mohammed, the staff have caused him pain and harm.

The ethical principle of fidelity is also important. Mohammed had stated his wishes clearly and expected his family and the health care system to respect them. The lack of continuity of approach between hospital and ambulance betrayed him, thereby breaching the principle of fidelity. Good systems management could have avoided the problem.

However, the daughter, as a person with her own values and needs, reacted as many would when faced with the imminent death of a loved one. It would be too harsh to judge her as having betrayed her father's trust. Perhaps she was too unprepared when the moment came. Perhaps she had not come to terms with his illness. Perhaps she was afraid of what would happen to her when he died. She could feel betrayed and abandoned. She needs care, compassion and support, not condemnation.

Triage: choosing which patients to treat first

When patients present in an emergency department the 'triage nurse' allocates the patients to different areas for full assessment, diagnostic tests and treatment. For example, the person with a broken arm will probably be sent to minor injuries or the treatment room to wait his or her turn in having the arm X-rayed and plaster applied. In another case, the ambulance crew will have radioed ahead and notified the staff that they are perhaps bringing in two patients from a motor vehicle accident, both with head injuries. The ambulance crew would be told to take the patients to the resuscitation area on arrival, and the nursing and medical staff would in the mean time prepare the resuscitation area for the new patients. In this way the person with a critical condition is seen before someone with a minor injury.

A different challenge faced by the emergency department and neurosurgical teams (those who look after patients with brain and neurological injuries such as damage to the spinal cord) is that of the patient with devastating brain trauma. The emergency department team taking over from the ambulance personnel will work to assess and stabilise the patient before deciding upon surgery. While triage means that the most seriously ill patients are treated first, sometimes choices that make the difference between life and death have to be made between patients. The surgeon who is called to see the injured patient has the power to decide whether to carry out surgery or not.

Read the following case study and then follow the ethical reasoning given.

Case study 13.2
The motor cyclist and his pillion passenger

A motor cyclist and his pillion passenger are brought into the emergency department. Both have head injuries with subdural bleeding into the brain. The motor cyclist also has severe injuries to his right leg. The pillion passenger has a C2/3 cervical fracture of the spine. The motor cyclist starts fitting, confirming major cerebral irritation. The neurosurgeon assesses both patients, reviewing their scans and other injuries. He knows he can only operate on one patient and any delay in operating may have devastating, if not fatal, implications for the other patient. Neither patient is stable enough to move to another hospital.

In this situation, the neurosurgeon literally holds the life of both patients in his hands. He must either choose to try to save one patient or decide that no surgery should be attempted for either. Since both patients lack autonomy, and there is no other evidence of what their wishes would be in such a situation, the neurosurgeon must consider what is in the patients' best interests. In so doing, he has to consider the principles of beneficence and non-maleficence, and weigh the benefits and burdens (risks and likely outcomes) of surgery against each other.

The motor cyclist's injuries have become more immediately life-threatening since the onset of epileptic fits, which means that the bleed may have damaged a greater area of the brain than indicated on the initial scans. If the motor cyclist survives neurosurgery (with or without his leg which the vascular surgical team may not be able to save), he could spend months in a coma or end up in a persistent unconsciousness state.

Burden on family and health system v. other possible outcomes

These injuries would place a huge burden on the family as well as the health care system. However, it is ethically debatable whether the potential burden on the family or health care system should be weighed as part of the decision-making process. It can be argued that the doctor's decision should concentrate only on the best interests of the patient, not the best interests of others. The potential outcome of surgery with both patients is that they could die during the operation. Death during surgery has an impact upon the surgeon's mortality figures. This can affect the way that his skills are perceived. If the surgeon has a lot of patients die during surgery, the public may think he is less good than another neurosurgeon or specialist, or a bad surgeon. The level of trust the public is likely to put in him and in the hospital could be reduced.

Choosing which patient to treat and/or operating or not operating

If the neurosurgeon operates on the pillion passenger, he is likely to be left completely paralysed from the neck down and totally dependent upon others for the rest of his life because of the spinal fracture. In addition, he may also have other neurological deficits such as memory or speech problems. Some patients can adapt to such a situation but others do not. Much depends upon the patient's own value system, their beliefs, religious or otherwise, their culture and their family or community as well as the availability of continuing aftercare and support.

The patient's right to refuse treatment

In 2002, an English patient, Ms B, was told that she had a brain aneurysm (a weak point in the wall of a blood vessel which could burst). She made an advance statement of wishes saying that she did not want surgery if the aneurysm burst. However, when that happened, emergency department doctors and neurosurgeons treated her even though she had refused treatment. She was left ventilator-dependent, paralysed from the neck down and needing 24-hour care. Eventually, Ms B went to court to ask that her ventilator be turned off so that she could die (*Re B v. NHS Hospital Trust* [2002] 2 All ER 449). She saw death as preferable to life in this situation. Her doctors refused to remove the ventilator since they believed strongly that their role was to save life not take it. The court did not believe that the sanctity of life argument should prevail over the patient's wishes. Nor did the court feel that her wish to have the ventilator turned off was the same as wanting to commit suicide. Since Ms B was fully autonomous, under English law she had the right to refuse life-saving treatment.

Ms B was transferred to another hospital and the ventilator was removed, allowing her to die. High profile cases like this one, which was widely discussed in the media, are likely to have an impact upon the way people think. The more people who say that in the same situation as Ms B they too would prefer death over life, the less support there is likely to be for a view that life in itself is something good to be treasured. Society may become less tolerant of money or resources being spent on patients like Ms B. Yet to many, however difficult life or living might be, it is seen as valuable.

A spiritual person may feel that the problems of life are part of the journey we all must take. However, society might not want to spend money or resources on patients like Ms B. In those societies that focus on gaining immediate pleasure, there is a danger that professionals who have the power to decide who lives and who dies may have values and beliefs that only clients or patients who are likely to have a good quality of life or no cognitive impairment should live.

Activity

Take time out to think about whether those patients who already carry the burden of impaired autonomy are less likely to be given treatment opportunities that are offered to others.

➤ What if the pillion passenger were known to have Down's syndrome?

➤ How would that affect the neurosurgeon's decision?

➤ What if the person was someone with a criminal record?

➤ Would it make any difference if the person was the son of another doctor?

This author, when researching how consultants within the British NHS make decisions about who to treat or not treat, was told by one neurosurgeon that his role was to ensure that patients did not survive with devastating neurological deficits such that they became a burden upon society (Terry, 2001). He felt it was obvious given resource limitations such as NHS finances and the lack of ITU beds and nursing staff. He admitted that some patients might have unexpectedly survived with good outcomes had he agreed to operate but said he had to protect himself from such thoughts. The emotional and long-term psychological toll must be hard to handle even if, as he said, he had the full support of his emergency department colleagues.

Conflict within the team about resuscitation

What if there is disagreement within the emergency department team over the decision? All members of the team have to be able to work together in enclosed spaces, providing rapid, high-quality care to ensure the best possible outcomes for their patients. There needs to be a high level of trust within the team and any perceived betrayals of trust, or inappropriate decision-making, need to be dealt with fast. It is useful to hold regular debriefing sessions as well as to develop the ethical understanding of the complex and challenging situations that may arise.

Confidentiality and the balancing of issues

Emergency department staff also have to act as an interface between patients and society. The usual rules of patient confidentiality may have to be set aside in cases of serious crime, terrorism or serious threat to public health. Emergency department staff frequently have to act as an interface between patients and families.

Activity

Read the following case study and then follow the reasoning.

Case study 13.3
Jani, a 12-year-old girl and possible pregnancy

A 12-year-old girl, Jani, accompanied by both parents, is admitted to the emergency department with severe abdominal pains and PV bleeding (bleeding from the vagina). One of the possible diagnoses is ectopic pregnancy (where the baby is growing inside the abdomen instead of inside the uterus). A pregnancy test needs to be carried out. It is considered ethically necessary to obtain consent before doing this. The emergency department team need to consider from whom to gain consent and also how to handle the request. Ectopic pregnancies are life-threatening.

The case raises several issues. Jani is under the age for lawful sexual activity so if she is pregnant the background will need to be investigated. Who made her pregnant? Was it a 'consensual' relationship with a peer even though she is a minor? Or has she been abused? For example, she may have been 'groomed' by a paedophile prior to having sex so she is likely to feel guilty at betraying her abuser. If the abuser is a family member or family friend she will probably feel even more confused.

Depending on the criminal law of a country, the police may need to be informed. In England, the Sexual Offences Act 2003 makes it a very serious offence to have sex with someone under 13 years of age, punishable by up to 14 years in prison.

Activity

➤ Is it mandatory for health professionals to report sexual abuse in your country?

➤ If so, who on the team has that responsibility?

Patient's trust v. angry parents

Emergency department staff need to try to gain Jani's trust to provide the most appropriate care. If staff are completely open with Jani and her parents about the possible diagnosis of ectopic pregnancy, strong parental passions may be aroused. Parents may feel outraged at the suggestion that their daughter is no longer innocent (a virgin). They can become very angry about underage pregnancies. They might also become violent towards Jani.

Strategies for raising the issue of pregnancy testing can be prepared in advance by the health professionals. For example, they may indicate that a pregnancy test is simply a routine procedure which has to be carried out along with a variety of other tests as part of carrying out a competent diagnosis. In other words, it would be negligent for the emergency department staff not to do all the tests that they would normally do, just because of Jani's age. Therefore the staff have the choice of either asking Jani for consent to perform the pregnancy test (providing the staff think she is competent to do so) or ask one or both of her parents for permission.

Application of ethical principles

Since the question of possible pregnancy is so sensitive, some emergency department staff prefer to try to speak with young female patients without their parents being present. The ethical principles of beneficence and non-maleficence can support this idea. It may be hard to find an opportunity when Jani is alone because worried parents will often want to stay with their child. Regardless of the issue about possible pregnancy, Jani is likely to be very distressed as she is in pain. She will need a lot of reassurance. However, to move beyond calming and reassuring Jani to actually asking her permission to do a pregnancy test takes time to build the therapeutic relationship and, hence, trust.

Legal issue of consent

Jani can only give consent to the pregnancy test if she has sufficient autonomy. In other words, is she competent to make her own decisions? In the UK and Australia, Jani would need to be able to demonstrate sufficient understanding about what the proposed treatment or test entails, possible side effects and outcomes (Hendrick, 2000).

The requirements of the law and child abuse regulations place restrictions upon confidentiality. Regardless of Jani's expressed wishes, her age means that she must be protected from abuse, if this has occurred. This means that the emergency department staff need to be able to gain her trust to have the information that they need to first ascertain if she is pregnant, and with whom she has had sexual intercourse. Then, the staff can make a decision as to whether or not they need to encourage Jani to tell her parents (if consensual); however, if the sex was a result of abuse or was with someone much older, the staff may need to tell the parents on Jani's behalf. Of course, if it is a family member or close family friend who has done the abusing then the first priority is Jani's safety and protection in hospital.

Possible complications

If Jani does have an ectopic pregnancy, which can be a life-threatening condition (if a laparoscopic operation is not performed), the emergency department staff will need to persuade her that it would be wise for her parents to know. Hopefully, Jani's parents could give emotional and psychological support. However, that depends on the sort of relationship Jani has with her parents. In some cases, the emergency department team might agree simply to tell the parents that Jani needs an operation to stop the PV bleeding. The principles of beneficence and non-maleficence will be paramount and Jani's privacy will be maintained. The emergency department staff may feel as if they are lying if Jani's parents ask them 'Is she pregnant?' The ethical rule of veracity does not always need to be upheld. In such a situation they could reply, 'I think you need to ask Jani that after she has recovered from the operation.'

Stereotyping and labelling

Pregnant teenagers can be labelled as irresponsible or promiscuous. Health care professionals have to set aside their own beliefs about 'proper' sexual conduct. The deontological perspective, which underpins professional codes of conduct, holds that it is not for them to judge her. Jani must be treated as well and as compassionately as any other patient.

Summary of emergency department care

You have read about the appropriate use of resources and which clients and patients to treat, including the concept of surviving patients who may be a burden on their family and the health care system. Also discussed were when should resuscitation be performed and what happens when team members do not agree? Finally, the issue of balancing confidentiality with gaining the trust of a child who does not want her parents to know she could be pregnant was covered.

There is a lot of information to absorb in Part A, and therefore if you are dyslexic or have spLD and have had difficulty understanding Part A of this chapter, I would suggest you go back and re-read it again before commencing Part B. Why? Because although Parts A and B are related, the issues raised in Part A are different from those in Parts B and C. Therefore, it makes sense to be clear in your own mind before trying to gain additional knowledge and understanding.

Part B Perioperative care

Perioperative care is a worldwide term that describes the health concept of providing care to patients having operations. The concept of 'peri', meaning 'around' an operation, includes preoperative, intraoperative and immediate postoperative care of patients. This part of the chapter, on perioperative care, includes the ethical issues of possible incompetence of a team member and patients refusing an operation (that is, having surgery).

Interprofessional care and possible incompetence

Well planned and executed surgical care is unproblematic – all parties are satisfied with the outcome. However, difficulties may arise through unchecked incompetence or through disagreement between some of the parties (patient, relatives, surgical team, health care provider) as to what treatment options are acceptable and the standard of care.

Activity

Take time out and think about incompetence. That is, read the following case study and answer the questions at the end.

Case study 13.4
Mr Consultant and Ms Scrub nurse and handling of suspicions

An orthopaedic consultant employed by a large hospital to undertake knee operations frequently performs knee operations on young men who have injured cartilage while playing football.

A very experienced orthopaedic scrub nurse (the nurse handing the consultant the instruments during the operation) is concerned that each time this consultant does these operations, he uses a slightly different technique.

Also, she fears that he is damaging the articulating surface (the end of the bone) unnecessarily.

This means that, within a few years, these young men will have serious problems with the joint.

When the scrub nurse asks the consultant to explain his technique, he is unable to answer her questions to her satisfaction and eventually implies that she is only a nurse and should not question his authority.

Questions
➤ What ethical rights and responsibilities do members of a multiprofessional team have towards each other?
➤ What rights and responsibilities do members of a team have to ensure that patient care meets set standards?

Doing no harm (non-maleficence) and possible legal negligence

Few health care professionals wish to harm their patients deliberately. The Hippocratic Oath has as its starting point, *primum non nocere* – first, do no harm. The principle of non-maleficence is seen as a stronger obligation than the principle of beneficence (Beauchamp and Childress, 2001, p. 114). You must always try to avoid harming your patient. However, some doctors are cavalier and do not take their responsibility to providing care to patients seriously. In the UK this year two doctors were charged with criminal negligence, and the Medical Board deregistered them for life. Their subsequent appeal was unsuccessful.

In perioperative care, trust is essential between all members of the team. Even in routine operations, unexpected events such as haemorrhage or a sudden physiological change in the status of the patient can arise, and the patient's life may hang upon the skills of the team working as one.

In this scenario, there may be some misunderstanding or communication problems. The surgeon may be acting competently. His technique may be of a standard that would be accepted as competent by his peers. The nurse may not know what the patient's goals are. The surgeon may have discussed several different operative approaches with the patient and the patient has selected the one that (s)he considered preferable. It may be that the patient is prepared to take the risk of future problems. For example, if the patient is a professional footballer, he may wish to start playing again as fast as possible. The probability of early-onset arthritis may be a risk he is prepared to take. His professional footballing career would be over before then. If he does not have this operation, he may not be able to play professionally again. However, the surgeon should be able to explain his actions. After all, if the patient is unhappy with the outcome of the operation, the surgeon may one day have to explain his actions in a court of law.

Reporting another member of the team

The nurse is ethically obliged to report her concerns to management. There should be mechanisms for the nurse to do this without fear of personal sanctions or being treated as a troublemaker. A culture of openness is essential for health care organisations to reduce the potential for mistakes and negligence occurring (Kennedy, 2001). If the surgeon lacks the proper skills, the management must have the courage to deal with this and prevent harm to future patients. In the tragic case of babies and children undergoing cardiac surgery at Bristol Royal Infirmary (as described in earlier chapters), an anaesthetist was worried about the surgical technique of two surgeons. Babies were dying or being left brain-damaged. The anaesthetist tried to alert senior management to his concerns but no-one listened to him.

Allocation of resources in relation to perioperative care

There is the possibility that the surgeon's technique varies from time to time because of the lack of certain equipment. Financial constraints can lead to restrictions and an organisational culture where 'getting by is prized as success' (Kennedy, 2001, Chapter 22, paragraph 5). The often utilitarian nature of state-funded or charitable health care delivery (as opposed to privately funded health care) means that sometimes the most suitable techniques, procedures or drugs cannot be used.

Patients may receive less than the best care when inexperienced staff are expected to perform tasks they are not fully competent to do simply because there is no-one else available to perform them. This means that they may make mistakes and harm patients even though that was never their intention.

Activity

Read the following case study and follow the ethical reasoning.

Case study 13.5
Aimee Lee, an 83-year-old, refuses surgery

Aimee Lee is an 83-year-old woman who is diabetic and has no close relatives. Although she came to the UK as an illegal immigrant many years ago, it does not appear that she has been assimilated into the local Chinese community as no friends visit her in hospital. She has already had a below-knee amputation (after amputation of her heel about a year earlier), but gangrene has returned and surgeons have recommended further amputation. Aimee seems a bit confused at times. She agreed to the further amputation but then told the nurse that she just wanted to be left alone and withdrew her consent.

A few days later, after discussion with her surgeon, she signed another consent form, but later changed her mind again. At one handover, comments were made that she is just wasting people's time and should make her mind up.

When asked again Aimee agreed, and has now been brought to the perioperating department. She has become very distressed and says she is an old lady and asks why do the doctors want to keep doing these awful things to her?

Questions
➤ What ethical principles are involved?
➤ Which principles and rules are upheld and which are not?

Health beliefs and values

- It would be very easy simply to say that Aimee is an old lady and there is no point attempting any life-saving heroic measures on her.
- However, is amputation of a diseased limb heroic? This will often depend upon the surrounding circumstances.
- Are there the resources (money, staff, equipment) to provide aftercare or social care to help her after the operation.
- Aimee may be a poor anaesthetic risk and may die during surgery or have a very bad chest infection afterwards.
- After surgery it may be hard to get Aimee to mobilise sufficiently. How independently mobile she will be also remains uncertain – she may survive longer with the operation but not recover sufficiently to be discharged.

Is age an issue?

Aimee's age is relevant in that she is probably of the generation that was raised to believe that 'doctor knows best'.

The 'fair innings' argument considers that people over 70 years of age have lesser rights to health care than younger patients (Harris, 1985). This implies that Aimee has already had a 'fair innings' and has lived long enough. By not treating her, she may die sooner and the hospital bed will be available for someone else.

Aimee may feel that she is being rude to the surgeon if she tells him that she does not want surgery. As she has no close friends or relatives to support her when she is seen by the surgical team it may make it very hard for her to express her feelings, fears, hopes and wishes. Usually patients from an Eastern background are supported by their community but, as yet, this has not occurred. At the moment, Aimee seems abandoned and alone. The notion of an extended family might ensure that she is still seen as 'belonging' to someone and so she might have visitors and people to support her. As an elder person, she would probably be venerated as a link with the past. Cultures that value an oral tradition of history, such as the Australian Aboriginal and the New Zealand Maori, would consider it important that she is at least given the opportunity to have treatment since she holds the history of the tribe in her head. This history must be protected and passed on to the next generation.

The key questions are not just what treatment is clinically appropriate, but what is appropriate for the patient and who decides? If the surgery represents sound clinical practice, is Aimee able to decide for herself if she wants it? The presumption is that adult patients can make their own decisions, but Aimee seems to be confused at times. Does that confusion impair her decision-making capacity? Is it a treatable confusion? Possible causes of confusion in the older person are dehydration and malnutrition. Her diabetes may not being properly controlled or she may have developed a urine infection.

The ethical ideal of care by health professionals

In the chapter on clients' or patients' rights we stated that the ethical ideal included being caring and compassionate, being accountable, advocacy and collaboration. To be caring involves being alert to changes in the patient and being prepared to think about the reasons why they might be behaving as they are.

Patients should never be labelled 'difficult' or 'uncooperative'. They are just the same as the health care professional – there is no power difference! Perhaps the situation in which a patient finds himself or herself is intolerable, and so anger is expressed in inappropriate ways. It is the health professional who has the knowledge and skills to explore these situations and remedy the situation; the patient cannot do this as (s)he is sick and ill.

If Aimee has the capacity to make her own treatment decisions, the principle of autonomy requires that her decision be respected. Although it will mean that the time slot is wasted, Aimee can change her mind at the operating room door and it must be respected. In fact, her refusal at this point could have been predicted. Duress to make her agree to the surgery is inappropriate, even if the surgical team are completely convinced that it is in her best interests. The principle of autonomy accepts that we are all capable of acting in ways that conflict with what is best for us. For example, you might want a night at home but your friends want you to come out with them.

Does Aimee lack the capacity to consent?

If Aimee lacks the capacity to make her own decision, this must be assessed in accordance with accepted good practice. This can include legal guidelines, hospital policies or professional codes of conduct depending upon the country in which treatment is being provided. In England and Wales, Aimee's doctor would be the person who had to decide what was in her best interests. It is important to remember that laws and rules can change.

In other countries, the person to decide could be someone Aimee has appointed herself. The decision-maker may be someone that is appointed to act for her. Again, depending upon the legal framework, the proxy decision-maker may be able to make the decision about amputation as if he or she were Aimee. In other words, the proxy may not have to act in Aimee's best interests. Accepting the potentially life-prolonging option of amputation may be in Aimee's best interests but, like Aimee, the proxy could refuse the operation.

Aimee's 'best interests'

In contrast, decisions on patient best interests are underpinned by the ethical principles of beneficence and non-maleficence. However, the rules for patient decision-making generally only reflect the values of the dominant cultural (westernised) group. Within Chinese culture the family would be living with each other or in close contact and so it would be the family that would know the mother's or sister's wishes and make the decision with the team as to whether or not the operation would be performed (see Chapter 6).

In cases like Aimee's, it is important for health care providers to think about her psycho-social needs as well as her physical needs. She is alone and probably lonely. She may be missing her home, her pets, her routines, her favourite television programmes and food, all the things that have made life valuable or interesting to her. She may be grieving for her lost mobility and her increasing loss of independence. She may be frightened about what the future holds for her if she lives as well as if she dies. She may be afraid of death or she may have no such fears. This often depends on someone's cultural background as well as their religious or spiritual views.

Activity

If you have not already done so, it is time to explore the health beliefs of Chinese people.

Also, if you live in a country where Chinese culture is the result of immigration, find out the names of the various organisations that provide that cultural link, newspapers, social events, and any other resources. For example, is there an organisation that does hospital visiting and provides home care?

Activity

Read the following case study.

Case study 13.6
Ben, a 15-year-old refusing life-saving surgery

Ben is a 15-year-old who had a shunt fitted soon after he was born with hydrocephalus (excess fluid on the brain). Occasionally, the shunt will block and has to be replaced as an emergency. If left untreated, pressure builds up on the brain, causing headaches, and eventually leads to collapse. Permanent brain damage could result. Ben has been admitted to the neurosurgical ward as an emergency admission. He had not told his parents about his worsening headaches and is still refusing to have surgery to replace the shunt. His parents consent to the surgery.

Ben's case has some similarities to Aimee's. Both are reluctant to face surgery. However, Aimee has provided reasons for her refusal (her age, the uncertainty of outcome). Ben has not – he appears to be in denial about his condition. In addition, Ben's youth means that if surgery is successful, and there is little reason to doubt that it will not be, he will probably have many years of life ahead of him. His youth also raises questions about his capacity to make his own decisions about something so critical. Unlike Jani, whose refusal of a pregnancy test or to allow her parents to be told about her condition, death or severe brain damage is imminent for Ben.

When a child refuses an operation

In the UK and Australia where children have tried to refuse life-saving surgery, the courts have always, to date, allowed surgery to proceed if the parents and medical team thought it was in the child's best interests. However, in Australia there is an age limit as to when the child's wishes will be overturned.

Pause and think

Take time out and think about:

➤ What is the legal position for young adults in your country?

➤ If you were Ben how might you be feeling?

➤ If you were Ben's parents how might you be feeling?

➤ How might you as a health professional handle this situation?

Morally what can be done?

Ethically, the professionals need to work with Ben to try to understand his thinking and help him understand the need for surgery. A named nurse should be appointed to Ben. That way, there will be one person in particular who is working to establish a relationship of trust and empathy. There may be a particular doctor or a nurse or occupational therapist that Ben already knows and trusts. It might help if that person could be identified and asked to listen to what he has to say and discuss issues with him. Even a telephone conversation with that person might be sufficient to allow Ben to explain his refusal of surgery, his fears and why he had not told his parents about his headaches. Encouraging Ben to express himself shows respect for his autonomy.

Summary of perioperative care

The concept and ownership of interdisciplinary care is very strong in perioperative care owing to the nature of the patient's condition. When one health professional does something wrong the other members of the team have not only a legal but also an ethical obligation to ask questions. If the scrub nurse and others in the operation room at the time do not question, it can be seen as though they were agreeing with what the consultant surgeon was doing! The ethical issue of allocation of resources is no less important in this department as any other within a hospital.

The legal and ethical issue of a patient's right to refuse treatment also concerns perioperative staff, and what should be done in relation to Aimee's best interests and how to provide ongoing care has been discussed. Likewise the case of Ben; although similar to Aimee, this was different in that Ben is younger and the health worker's professional obligation to providing ongoing continuing care for this troubled teenager is paramount.

Part C Intensive, coronary care and high dependency units

The development of ICUs (including CCUs and HDUs) is a modern phenomenon. The care of patients in these hospital units is 'high-tech', with all the latest equipment (or the latest the hospital can afford), a high patient-to-staff ratio, rapidly changing conditions, and an element of differentness to the rest of the hospital environment. That is, the patients are critically ill or unstable and require constant monitoring via state-of-the-art equipment, visitors are restricted to enable staff easy access at all times to the patient should something go wrong, and there is no place for patients' personal belongings or gifts, flowers, etc. In fact, flowers and pot plants are not allowed because they can cause irritation to and inflammation of the respiratory system (from the smell and pollen of flowers) and possible infections (through soil-borne bacteria in pot plants). Hence these wards or units look different, and this in itself can cause anxiety to both patients and relatives (sometimes described as 'sort of artificial' or 'unnatural' or 'not at all homely'). This part of the chapter discusses the ethical issues of the health professional's obligations in relation to trying to meet various and very different families' needs, the cost of caring, and also responsibilities when relatives ask for futile treatment to be performed.

Trying to meet the various and many different families' needs

The Western biomedical model tends to see death as an enemy to be defeated. Since the development of the 'iron lung', medicine has become increasingly adept at saving people who would otherwise have died. A whole new science of intensive care medicine, including cardiac and high dependency care, has arisen. This new medicine has created new ethical considerations for care givers. Deciding who and how much to treat in ICU/CCU/HDU is difficult. Freeman and McDonnell (2001, p. 222) say 'the technological power of modern medicine easily can convert beneficence to arrogance. With growing confidence in their abilities to help patients, physicians sometimes help them to live or die in ways those individuals disapprove'.

Facilitating spiritual beliefs

The family in Case study 13.7 have indicated a belief in the healing power of prayer. Although the scenario does not say which religious or spiritual faith the family has, this situation is not unusual. The difficulty comes in trying to accommodate spiritual or cultural values in an environment devoted to clinical wellbeing.

Activity

Read this case study and answer the questions at the end.

Case study 13.7
Maya and her family's wish to stay and pray with her

Maya is 50 years old. She has undergone extensive abdominal resection for cancer and has now been admitted to an ITU. Her prognosis is expected to be good in the long term, as surgeons believe they have caught her cancer early enough. Her family wish to be with her, praying and supporting her emotionally day and night. The ITU policy is to restrict the number of visitors and is reluctant to allow a continuous family presence.

Questions

Here you have an ethical problem: on one hand you have Maya's best interests in relation to her physical care; on the other you have her best interests in relation to spiritual care.

➤ Are the ethical principles of autonomy, beneficence, justice and non-malificence being upheld?

➤ As a health professional, how would you approach the situation?

➤ As a health professional, how would you resolve the situation?

With patients and families from Eastern and Aboriginal cultures, the underpinning philosophy of ICUs, CCUs and HDUs may be strongly in conflict with their beliefs. Patients such as those of Native American and similar Aboriginal cultures, view death 'as part of life that one prepares for by being in harmony with one's surroundings' (Burkhardt and Nathaniel, 2002, p. 244). The surroundings of the ICU, CCU or HDU may be so alien that they actively contribute to patient and family 'disease'. The traditional approaches to serious illness of 'touching, praying and presence' (p. 348) or the creating of a 'sacred space' (p. 351) are difficult to accommodate within high-tech, sterile environments.

Pause and think

Take time out to think about the following questions:

➤ If Maya was from your culture, what spiritual care would need to be provided?

➤ If Maya was ethnically different from you, would this make a difference as to how you would facilitate the spiritual care?

➤ Do you sometimes think that other people's spiritual beliefs are silly and not worth bothering about?

If you answered yes to the previous question and display or voice these opinions you are being culturally incompetent and you could be breaking the law (religious tolerance). You need to find out what your professional code of practice asks of you. Most codes of conduct state that respecting clients' or patients' culture (including their spiritual beliefs) is necessary and not to do so is unprofessional and/or unethical.

➤ So, are you being unethical?

Read this case study and follow the ethical reasoning that is given.

Case study 13.8
Lee, a young father, and whether to keep treating him

Lee, a 34-year-old man, was admitted to intensive care 3 weeks ago with a diagnosis of viral encephalitis. Lee is married, with three children under the age of 6, and was working towards a doctorate (PhD) in his spare time. It seems certain that he has suffered significant brain damage but it is impossible to tell what impact this will have if he survives. The question of how aggressively to continue treating him has now been raised at the weekly ITU team meeting.

One of the biggest challenges for critical care units is a shortage of beds or staff to support patients admitted to those beds. Consequently, there may be pressure to justify the continued occupancy of each bed. For example, if the patient is not going to recover, should (s)he still be in the ITU? Is this an appropriate use of a scarce resource? Sometimes an ICU continues to treat patients for longer than they should because the family, or one member of the interprofessional team, is not ready to stop. In this scenario, the question that is really being asked is whether it is now time to withdraw treatment. In other words, should the team allow Lee to die?

Quality of life v. quantity of life

The decision means looking not just at Lee's clinical condition but also at his expected quality of life. Hidden in the discussion will be the idea that perhaps continued life would hold little quality or meaning for Lee. Perhaps, if Lee could tell the team what he wanted, he might prefer death. 'In medical ethics life is not the ultimate good nor death the ultimate evil' (Handley, 1990, p. 152).

Lee was obviously a highly intelligent person before his illness. The difficulty is knowing the extent to which he has been robbed of his intellect. Scans may help identify the damaged areas of the brain but still cannot definitively answer what effect these will have on him. Lee is clearly not brain stem dead so does not meet the legal criteria for declaring him dead and stopping treatment. When making decisions about his care, so much depends on the values and beliefs of the patient and the relatives. In this case study, Lee's wife may want to uphold what she believes would be his wishes.

Legal frameworks

Some countries have enacted legislation such as a Medical Treatment Act (Victoria, Australia) that provides a framework for how to proceed in cases like Lee's. In England and Wales, the Mental Capacity Act 2005, expected to come into force in 2007, sets out a new framework. In countries where there is no specific Act, common law can be used to justify actions.

In an English case on withholding and withdrawing life-prolonging medical treatment (*Airedale NHS Trust v. Bland* [1993] AC 789) it was decided that treatment could be withdrawn so a patient could die. The Bland case involved a British patient (Tony Bland) left in a persistent vegetative state following the Hillsborough football stadium tragedy. Many people were crushed and some died. Tony was resuscitated but was left in a persistent vegetative state. The House of Lords ruled by three to two that life-prolonging artificial nutrition and hydration could be withdrawn from Tony to allow him to die. Medical associations such as the British General Medical Council and British Medical Association have published guidance on withholding and withdrawing life-prolonging treatment (GMC, 2002; BMA, 2001).

Patients may have enacted advance statements of wishes to cover such situations but there is no evidence that Lee had done this. These advanced directives or living wills were discussed in Chapters 8 and 9. (Also the use of Clinical Ethics committees was discussed in Chapter 4 in relation to clients' or patients' rights.) Withdrawing treatment would only occur if it was considered both legal and ethical. If it were ethical to withdraw treatment but not lawful, treatment would have to continue. In this way the professionals involved would not face legal sanctions or professional censure by acting outside the law even if their conduct is believed to be ethically correct (as they have a right to maintain their personal integrity).

A useful ethical framework for discussing cases like Lee's is the Jonsen model (Jonsen *et al.*, 1998). This sets out a series of questions for professionals to ask. The questions fall into four sections: medical indicators, patient preferences, quality of life and contextual features.

- The medical indicator questions extract information such as the diagnosis, prognosis, treatment plans and likely outcomes.

- The patient preferences questions explore what is known about the patient's competence, views and value systems, and whether an advanced directive exists.

- The quality of life questions consider the likelihood of the patient returning to his or her previous quality of life, the extent of the deficits the patient is likely to experience, and whether these are such that continued life would be considered unbearable by the patient.

- The contextual features ask whether there are family or health care provider issues that might affect the decision, financial, religious or cultural considerations, and the legal implications of the treatment/non-treatment decision.

- The Jonsen model (Jonsen *et al.*, 1998, p. 13) can also be modified to include the issues surrounding social care so that these are also taken into consideration (Terry, 2007). These would include: what are the person's social problems (infirmity, paralysis, learning difficulties, mental illness, dementia); how do these affect the medical problem; what is the possibility of meeting the necessary required social care interventions; and what would occur if the planned health care (medical) did not work?

Withdrawing treatment does not mean withdrawing care!

If the decision to discontinue aggressive treatment is made, this does not mean that Lee should not receive the best possible care for his other needs. Neither he nor his wife and other significant persons should be abandoned by the professionals involved in his care. While their time and attention might be of greater benefit to other patients, the principle of fidelity means that Lee is still their patient. His dying should be handled just as considerately as when everyone was still trying to save his life. Nursing staff who act as coordinators of care may have to ensure that this occurs. The team will need to demonstrate good communication skills, empathy and compassion towards Lee's wife.

The impact of caring upon health care professionals

Working in environments like ICUs, HDUs and CCUs inevitably places health care professionals under immense strain. The problems of 'burnout' and stress are recognised as a major cause of staff leaving to work in less pressurised environments. This condition was explained and discussed in Chapter 4.

Activity

Read this case study and answer the questions at the end.

Case study 13.9
Esther, the 'heart-sink' patient

Esther is a young woman of 28 years who has the condition congenital ichthyosis. Repeated bacterial and fungal infections of the skin folds have left her blind and virtually completely deaf. She communicates using a form of sign language that requires her to touch the hand of the person to whom she is talking. She is prone to septicaemia.

The chronically infected skin folds mean that she smells. Her condition is so disfiguring that if she leaves home she travels under a blanket. She is fully competent. Her mother is her main carer.

The HDU specialist who has cared for her for several years describes her, in private, as a 'heart-sink patient' and he has grown to dread her admissions even though Esther and her mother are devoted to him. Esther has been readmitted with a treatable septicaemia.

However, the doctor has suggested to Esther's mother that this should be considered as a terminal event and antibiotics withheld. He proposes to give analgesia to ensure Esther is in no discomfort.

Questions

Imagine what it would be like caring for Esther. Describe how this would be for you.

➤ Would you feel nauseous each time you went near her owing to the smell?

➤ Would you dry retch as you provided care for her?

Imagine that you were Esther and your own olfactory nerve was no longer stimulated by your smell, but you could feel what the health professionals thought by their non-verbal communication.

➤ How does that make you feel?

➤ How can a health professional control their non-verbal communication in the 'best interest' of the patient?

All-important communication between patient and health professional

In the chapter on decision making, it was stressed that communication and gaining the perspective of the client or patient (including their health beliefs) was important, as were those of the team. However, in the case study, even though it states that Esther has treatable septicaemia the doctor has said that the hospital admission should be treated as a 'terminal event' and that Esther should be given analgesia so that she feels no pain or discomfort.

- Why?
- If the health problem is treatable, why not provide the care and treatment needed?
- Has Esther said that next time she is in this condition she wants it to be the last?
- Has her mother said something similar?
- Has there previously been a discussion between all three of them?
- Is this a decision the doctor has made on his own?
- Could it be that the doctor is no longer able to cope? That is, his good care of Esther in the past has clearly ensured her survival, but now this doctor has reached the limits of his own tolerance. The stress the doctor is under is affecting his judgement.

An otherwise good doctor is suddenly at risk of an action that could jeopardise his career as well as cost a patient her life. Likewise, some carers also reach their limits and end up carrying out so-called 'mercy killings'. These carers may even be people that others admire and respect for their ability to cope. Carrying out a mercy killing does not mean that the carer never loved the person for whom they were caring. It is often a tragic result of carrying too heavy a burden.

Sanctity of life v. quality of life

Just because the patient's life is, or would be, a burden to her, this does not, in law, mean that treatment can be withheld. Deliberately failing to treat a patient that should be treated can result in murder charges for Esther's doctor (*R v. Arthur* (1981) 12 BMLR 1). The underpinning ethical concept is that of the sanctity of human life. In the UK, disagreements between patients, families and health care providers may fall to the courts to resolve.

Doctrines of double effect and totality and integrity for the person

Even if treatment is commenced, it may be unsuccessful. It is possible that the septicaemia could trigger organ failure. Then there is the issue of pain relief; Esther will need analgesia to make her comfortable and pain-free. Enough pain relief could be given to make Esther comfortable. In Chapter 8, the doctrines of double effect and totality and integrity for the person were discussed in relation to the administration of analgesia. If these doctrines are applied to Esther's case then it is possible that, if she suffers severe pain and needs high doses of analgesia to make her comfortable and pain-free, the analgesia may shorten her life. That is, it would be ethical to give Esther as much analgesia as was necessary to control the pain; however, it would not be ethical to give her more than was needed and could bring about her death. You may wish to go back to Chapter 8 and refresh your memory about the criteria that need to be met when adhering to the two doctrines.

Possible outcomes for Esther

In discussing the idea of not treating the septicaemia with Esther's mother, the HDU doctor may think that he is being open and genuinely acting in Esther's best interests. However, the doctor may also be seeking approval or absolution from her mother. Esther's mother may feel that she is being asked to let her daughter die – and is she?

If she is tired by the constant caring she may be relieved that the end is in sight. However, she may be distressed and upset by the doctor she trusts talking in this way. However, the doctor may have become 'burnt out' and not be able to engage with the ethical ideal or standard when caring for vulnerable patients (as discussed in Chapter 4; caring, advocacy, accountability and collaboration). The ideal includes:

- For a health professional to be caring in the moral sense, his/her actions need to demonstrate or manifest respect of dignity, compassion and kindness, and the preservation of health.

- With advocacy, the health professional assists in the self-determination of clients or patients like Esther. This can greatly influence the standard and quality of care.

- Within advocacy are the two concepts of fidelity (being honest and truthful) and respect for human dignity.

- Respecting the human dignity of clients or patients also extends to privacy and choice. This includes making sure that professionals and the information that they provide is accurate and honest so that clients or patients can make their own choice.

- Making sure that others respect the self-worth of the client or patient.

- To be morally accountable, the health professional is responsible for his or her behaviour; (s)he is answerable to client or patient, employer and professional body.

- Collaboration is twofold: the first is with clients or patients as equal partners in their care (to facilitate and negotiate the delivery of their care); the second is participation with other professionals to achieve the best possible outcome for the client or patient.

- Collaborative caring is going beyond multiprofessional care to achieve the gold standard of interprofessional practice (or provision of care). It certainly does not mean participating in moral problems caused by groupie behaviour or authority (as described in Chapter 3).

So how would the situation with Esther need to be resolved. First, the doctor needs to recognise his 'burnout' and ask someone else to be in charge of her care so that he can recover his perspective. Second, if the doctor cannot recognise this, then someone on the team needs to mention this to him sensitively. Support from others is imperative when we can no longer care. Third, if the doctor is unable to hear (and this is not uncommon in cases of extreme burnout), the team need to notify his superiors so that he can be ordered to take sick leave before he does any professional damage to himself or his patients.

Emotional and psychological burden

The emotional and psychological burden that some patients present to the health care team, not just their families, should never be forgotten. An organisational culture within ITUs, CCUs and HDUs needs to be developed whereby health care providers can unburden themselves freely without fear of condemnation. Acknowledging that the 'limits of tolerance' have been reached, and seeking support, should never be seen as weakness; nor should requesting that another person takes over the care of a particular patient be seen as unprofessional. Caring for the carers, including all professional staff, is vital to avoid burnout and loss of valuable employees to the organisation.

Ethical professional conduct requires being alert to the difficulties others may be facing. Johns (2000) describes how undertaking critical reflection can be transformative and can help the professional work through these difficult times. Also, some organisational structures and management and leadership styles can be more stressful to workers than others, which can lead to burnout of staff. Johns suggests that managers and leaders change from a hierarchical and authoritarian style to a more collaborative and transformative approach. When this is successful, holistic care is evident with staff being available to clients or patients and each other (Johns, 2000).

Requests for futile or inappropriate treatment

Sometimes staff receive requests for treatment to continue, even when it is clinically futile, from both the patient and family. Often, such requests are because of a failure to come to terms with the inevitability of death, or the client or patient or relative is scared of death.

Summary of ethical issues in intensive care units

The need for health professionals to balance the best interests of the patient with those of relatives has been considered. The balance between meeting the patient's physical needs with those of the spiritual nature is an issue for all staff in ICU. This is because one moment a patient can be alive and minutes later dead. There are also the patients who, to all intents and purposes, are not alive, but are being kept alive by technological machines and other equipment; when the machines and equipment are removed they will die a recordable death (that is, the time of death is stated in the hospital records). These are not easy situations for the health professionals; consequently, the carers need caring provided for them as well.

Summary

This chapter has examined the three main areas of complex care: emergency department, perioperative care, and ICUs, CCUs and HDUs. While providing the care and treatment that these clients or patients require, each of these areas also requires specific knowledge, understanding and skills.

The main ethical issues and problems are those concerned with patients' rights, the vulnerable client or patient, the use of resources, resuscitation, illness and loss, and making ethical decisions.

Professional development

1 Continue to develop your Ethics Portfolio.

2 Answer the following questions:
   ➤ If you found that your values and beliefs were in conflict with someone else in the complex team, how would you resolve the situation?
   ➤ If you thought you were experiencing burnout, what would you do?
   ➤ When should health professionals be able to withhold treatment?

3 For the following two case studies identify the ethical issues and problems, and work out how to resolve the situation (using the method of decision-making from Chapter 10).

Case study 13.11
Farah refuses a life-saving Caesarian section because of her dream

Farah is 24 years old, married to Joe and 38 weeks pregnant with their first baby. She has developed pre-eclampsia, a pregnancy-related life-threatening condition. She needs to have a Caesarian section to save both her life and that of her baby. Farah is afraid of surgery because she had a dream that told her that she would die during an operation. She refuses to have the Caesarian section. Joe desperately pleads with her and with the doctors, asking them to operate without her consent.

Case study 13.12
Tommy's family wants doctors to operate to try to save his life

Tommy is 22 years old. He has Down's syndrome which significantly affects his intellectual abilities. He was born with a congenital heart defect which was not corrected. Tommy's heart condition has worsened. It has damaged his lungs and he can only walk a few steps. Tommy has now been admitted to the coronary care unit. He is not suitable for a heart–lung transplant. Tommy probably only has a few weeks to live. Tommy's family want the cardiac surgeons to operate to try to cure the heart defect. The doctors have told the family that Tommy's lungs will not cope and he will probably die during surgery.

Critical reflection

Write your critical reflection for this chapter. Issues you may want to consider include:

- A heart-sink patient that for whom you have cared.
- DNR orders.
- A patient in an ICU or CCU that was scared of dying.
- A case study in this chapter that raises issues for you that you want to explore more fully.
- A complex care issue that occurred in clinical practice or in discussion with your peers.

Who gets what? In other words, the allocation of resources

Angelica Orb

Why this chapter is important to me . . .

✔ There is a close relationship between moral, clinical and economic factors involved in allocation of resources.

✔ Health care, at home or in business, needs to establish priorities about how monies will be expended, especially when resources are limited.

✔ There are difficult moral choices to be made when resources are limited.

✔ Resources must be allocated and there will be competition between the various social demands.

✔ Health and social care demands require a budget, which determines the allocation of resources.

You only need to watch the television news, listen to the radio, or read a newspaper to know the relevance and importance that your government places on the expenditure of health care. Often the government says: 'beds will be lost at Merrysad and Cooper's Meadow Hospitals because of overruns in budget'.

The definition of health resources is broad and refers to any good or services that have a positive effect on health. However, you will find that cost, quality and access to services are some of the most common problems faced by health services. For example, while African health care professionals are concerned by the lack of resources allocated to the care of patients dying of AIDS, Australian health professionals are concerned by long waiting lists. In some countries governments only state how much they are going to spend on health and social care when they want to be voted into office. You will also find that health and social care are allocated funds along with other services and commodities such as education, pensions, housing, defence and immigration. In other words, health funds are competing with other needs. Moreover, you also know that the health system has experienced dramatic changes. So, how do we reconcile the limitless health needs with the limited health resources?

The purpose of this chapter is to help you to understand the issues related to allocation of resources, implications to professional practice, and how this causes ethical issues and problems.

The chapter will first examine the ethical, economical and political issues associated with allocation of resources; second, we will identify the different theoretical frameworks applicable to allocation of resources; and third, we will discuss different models used to allocate scarce resources. Finally, issues of Professional Development will conclude the chapter.

Activity

Read the local newspapers and identify issues related to funding of health care services. List them in your Ethics Portfolio and state your point of view regarding each case. What did you find?

Demand for resources within health care

In recent years, health systems around the world have been under significant pressure trying to balance the demand for services with spending and allocation of resources. It is important that you differentiate between needs and demands. While needs are expressed by the actual requirements of the population (e.g. to reduce alcohol consumption among young people), demands refers to what the community wishes to be provided (e.g. every community hospital should have a cardiorespiratory unit) (Downie and Calman, 1994). Other aspects that will influence the demand for allocation of resources are the health beliefs of a community. You need to remember that allocation of resources reflects values.

Activity

➤ What negative and positive effects will the values and beliefs of a culture or a society have on the way in which the health budget is allocated?

You may need to review Chapter 2, which discusses values and beliefs, to answer this question.

Factors influencing a government's budget spending

Governments have the task to find what resources are available to achieve expected health outcomes. The wealth of a country is measured by its gross national product (GNP) per capita. In other words, how much a country earns in exports and how much it pays in imports. This income marks the differences between richer and poor countries, just like you may have a different income to spend compared with someone else. The World Bank (2001) reported in 1998 that countries that had a GNP of $9361 or more were described as high income, those between $761 and $9360 as middle income and those with less than $760 as low income. Consequently, when making decisions about patient care, health, economics and ethics are directly correlated because these decisions always involve resources and difficult moral choices (Hawley, 1997e).

Pause and think

➤ What are the different aspects in your country's health care budget?

1 Primary care and health promotion?

2 Secondary care?

3 Tertiary care?

4 Education for new professionals to enter the workforce?

5 Staff development for those already in the system?

6 Research?

7 Other areas?

Within the present and future developments of health care, the increasing demands will not decline. Therefore, governments will be faced with difficulties in the distribution of resources because of:

1 Elevated costs.

2 Increased numbers of the elderly population.

3 Rapid technological developments.

4 Consumers will be better informed and will demand better access and quality care.

In every aspect of care that health professionals provide, there is a cost attached. Technological advances have enabled us to save and prolong the lives of clients and patients. Recent debates have included whether babies born at approximately the 24th week of pregnancy should be saved and sustained. These decisions are not new, but on-going. In the past, babies weighing less than 1000 g were not kept alive. As health science progressed, it was felt that babies born weighing less than 500 g should not be kept alive, and so new guidelines were set up. Consequently, as advances are made, the boundaries that stipulate who might survive and who might live have changed. This situation occurs not only with premature babies, but in all sorts of treatments and care. For example, recently, a lady of nearly 100 years had a total hip operation in the UK. Previously, such treatment for an older person would not have been contemplated, let alone performed.

Activity

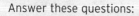

Answer these questions:

➤ As discussed above, at what gestation/week of pregnancy should a baby be treated, if born, and to what extent?

➤ What are the clinical guidelines in your country regarding the treatment of elderly patients with terminal illness? For example, is excessive expenditure on health care an issue?

➤ What is the cost per day of a patient in an acute hospital bed? A pacemaker? A hip replacement? A kidney dialysis?

Specific demands in different countries

Given that health plays a significant part in the life of everyone, professionals working in any health care system in the world will be confronted daily with issues evolving from the allocation of resources. It has implications at an international, national and regional level. For example, as a professional you could work in the UK, Africa, Thailand, Japan or Australia, but all or some practitioners may feel occasionally, in one way or another, frustrated because they cannot deliver 'the best care'.

It is also necessary to add that the increasing number of elderly people and the advances in technology are issues that are compounded by resource availabilities.

Macro- and micro-allocation of resources

Macro- and micro-allocation can be understood as the distribution of the country's wealth to provide services for the population. The difference between macro- and micro-allocation is determined by the level of decision-making authority. The macro-allocation of resources refers to the health care expenditure and the distribution of health care resources. The macro-allocation decisions are usually made by state legislatures, health organisations, private foundations, health insurance companies, federal, state and local agencies. Micro-allocation refers to how these specific amounts of money will be spent within various organisations or institutions. The micro-allocation decisions are made by the hospital staff and individual physicians (Buchanan, 1989; 1991).

Macro-allocation

At present:

- The Netherlands spends 8% of its GNP on its health system.
- The USA spends 13% (van Delven *et al.*, 2004).
- Other countries, such as Germany, Japan, Canada and Australia spend less than 9% of their GNP on health care (van Gelder, 2005).

In each of these countries the amount budgeted reflects the values and beliefs of the government of the day in relation to governmental policies and election promises to voters.

Pause and think

➤ If these differences are so remarkable, can we propose that a small amount of money spent on weapons be redirected to provide minimal levels of health care?

Who should decide how resources are allocated?
As previously stated, the macro-allocation of resources refers to the amount of money or kind of goods that are available to a particular society, as well as how they will be distributed. In spite of this, there is the contentious issue of who should make these decisions

(van Delven *et al.*, 2004). It is clear that, in a climate of scarcity of resources, there are hard choices to make, involving the macro level of government policy-making, as well as the micro patient/doctor level (NHMRC, 1999).

Pause and think

➤ Have the politicians in your country promised something in relation to health as part of their election campaign to be voted into office? (Hawley, 1997a)

Activity

➤ At the level of macro-allocation, who should make the decision as to how much is spent on health care – the politicians in government, the clinicians, the community, or all three together?

➤ Should the responsibility be shared between governments and clinicians?

Factors and processes to be considered when resources are allocated

According to Bryant (2002) there are five factors determining how resources are spent:

1 The type of service that a society or culture wishes to offer.

2 Who will receive the service and on what basis.

3 Who will be involved in the delivery.

4 How the financial load for the cost will be distributed.

5 How the power and control of the services will be distributed.

To illustrate these points let us compare Scotland and India. According to Munro (2000), in 1999 the Scottish National Services (NHS) had a total health budget of £4934 million for a population of 920 000. The Scottish NHS applied selection criteria to the allocation of resources. This was a formula based on equal access to health care, regardless of individuals' economic status or whether they were living in metropolitan or rural areas. In this example, you can identify the values held by those that made the decision, those of the community and their affordability. In the same year in India, despite the wealth of the top strata of society and their GNP, the government felt that they did not have the financial resources to provide health care for all people. In fact, there were severe constraints for those in rural and poor areas in relation to access to care and especially lack of drugs, equipment and technical support (WHO, 2003).

Activity

In your country:

➤ Who makes the decision as to how resources are allocated?

➤ What criteria are used to decide how the money is spent?

➤ Do you agree with how this is done?

Micro-allocation

As previously stated, micro-allocation refers to how specific amounts of money will be spent within various health organisations or institutions (Hawley, 1997e). This is when health professionals have greater power and say in the allocation of funds. The issue is now a highly ethical one as it is directly related to how to spend or allocate these resources, especially so when there is a limited amount of resources available (Gillette, 2000).

Who makes the decisions?

Health authorities, boards or trusts, including hospital staff, often make the micro-allocation decision. These allocation decisions involve not only department or unit budgets, but also bed allocation, and the decisions of whether to treat or not to treat. For example, in emergency departments priority is given to one patient over another. Another example is organ procurement. Who will receive the organ and who will miss out?

Pause and think

In 2005-2006 the UK Health Care Commission introduced annual health care checks for workers in health care organisations (hospitals of all types, primary care, etc.). The criteria included quality of services and use of resources. While some organisations were able to achieve acceptable standards for both criteria, many were found wanting in relation to the use of resources.

Think about how the inefficient use of resources would affect not only patient care but also impact on the health care budget.

Factors that need to be considered in micro-allocation

The committees responsible for allocation of resources in various countries focus on expected health outcomes and evidence-based practice. Thus, the services and treatments which are resourced are those that are more effective. This is important considering that the funds available for health care are diminishing quickly; the question to ask is how will these resources be distributed equitably?

In light of this evidence health agencies and health care professionals have to look for certain criteria and ethical principles that can guide their decision-making processes. A number of philosophical choices can also guide us on how to distribute what is available. Several criteria have emerged to assist in this deliberation: equity, rationalisation, the right to health care and individual responsibility for health, and these are discussed in the next section of this chapter.

Ethical frameworks for use in allocation

Questions about the rights and costs of health care are closely correlated to the notions of availability and competition for resources and services. The manner in which services are determined and who should benefit involves difficult moral choices. Since you cannot offer everything that people need or want, you have to resort to some guidelines to focus your thinking process. In the preceding chapters we have discovered that it is not possible to have a rigid set of rules to dictate ethical decisions. Consequently, we will discuss opposing ethical view points, which reflect the moral philosophies of their writers. These include the principle of justice, and the moral philosophies of Utilitarianism, liberal-welfare state, and libertarianism.

Ethical principle of justice

A brief overview of the theory behind the principle of justice can assist health professionals' understanding of the competing goals in the allocation of resources. According to Staunton and Chiarella (2004), justice has two meanings:

- The first refers to the concept of fairness: the idea of treating people equally and giving them what they deserve. It means that all people, irrespective of wealth, status or religion, should have fair access to services.
- The second concept refers to the notion of equal distribution of burdens and benefits.

Whether the principle of justice is defined as equity of opportunities, equity of access or distribution of benefits or burdens, it is central to public health and policy. However, when matters of distribution justice are discussed, a number of choices come to the surface. Some may indicate that all people should receive equally despite their needs. Others would consider:

- merits;
- social contribution;
- rights;
- individual effort; or
- the greatest good to the greatest number (Burkhardt and Nathaniel, 2001).

Moral philosophies in which the principle of justice is embedded

The distribution of justice is significant since it involves equitable and appropriate distribution of limited resources. Based on this rationale sensible policy-makers would certainly be able to argue that some models and theories may help with the decision-making process. There are three main theories that have implications in the decision-making process of allocation of resources (Buchanan, 1991). These are:

- Utilitarian;
- Liberal-Welfare State; and
- Libertarian theory.

Utilitarian theory
Utilitarianism is concerned with the principle of doing good for the greatest number (Hawley, 1997c). The theory of utility defines 'good' as happiness and rights which maximize the good (Buchanan, 1991). Jeremy Bentham considered that an action was right if it promoted

happiness. This happiness meant pleasure and absence of pain. Utilitarianism, according to Bentham, follows the principle of utility, which has two great virtues: it is universal and can be measured (Grassian, 1992).

In the case of maximum utility, it is necessary to add utilities and disutilities. In other words, the principle is measured considering its costs and benefits (Buchanan, 1989). In this way Utilitarianism favours social programmes that support the principle of utility.

Liberal–welfare state theory: justice as fairness

The liberal-welfare state theory is supported by Rawls, who describes the principles of justice as follows:

- The principle of greatest equal liberty.
- The principle of equality of fair opportunity.
- The difference principle, which refers benefit maximally to the worst off (Hawley, 1997c).

According to Rawls (1971), justice refers to the distribution of what he calls 'primary goods', such as income, property and freedom to political participation. He bases his theory in the Kantian principles of autonomy and rationality. Social Welfare Liberals claim that people have the right to adequate food, shelter, medical care and to a job. So, applying Rawls's principles, the first two refer to equality and the third allows inequalities, as long as the worst off or the least advantaged are supported. Hence, Rawls, as a Social Welfare Liberal, supports the notion of redistribution of wealth to reduce the barriers of unfair social inequalities. He claims that if the veil of people's ignorance of their physical and mental attributes were lifted, they would accept the principles that they have equal rights and that the social inequalities could be rearranged (Grassian, 1992).

According to Rawls, the inequalities of power, wealth and resources are justifiable if they act in support of the worst-off members of society. This theory is also known as egalitarian theory, which promotes the notion of a positive social duty to reduce the barriers that prevent fair equality of opportunities and equal distribution of resources (Burkhardt and Nathaniel, 2002). Consistent with this view are the terms 'fair share' and 'fair opportunities', which are applied in allocation of resources. According to Buchanan (1991), Rawls's theory is the most influential deontological theory.

The Libertarian theory: the right to health care

Conversely, Libertarian conservatives like Nozick claim that these inequalities are not unfair. For Nozick, justice implies an absolute respect for certain basic human rights (Grassian, 1992). Thus, if inequalities exist because of acquisition of goods, justice stresses that we bear the consequences and pay the price. For Nozick, people are entitled to the material things they have accumulated; they are entitled to their wealth.

According to Nozick, when people are left to make these decisions they cannot demand that the state provides for them to pursue their ends. Consequently, Nozick claims that 'a state is not justified in redistributing the wealth of its citizens' (Grassian, 1992, p. 104) or having a paternalistic legislation. Following Nozick's argument then, these people are entitled to purchase private health insurance and request the services that they can afford, such as cosmetic surgery or IVF. Health care is perceived as a commodity and not a right.

Activity

➤ In relation to your own values and beliefs, which of the theories discussed in this chapter supports your view?

➤ Do you think that it is morally wrong that some members of the community have the right to access to specialist services that they can afford?

Answer the following question in your Ethics Portfolio:

➤ Which of the justice theories supports your values and beliefs about the allocation of resources?

Ethical issues and problems

There are a number of ethical choices to be made under the principle of justice. For example, if you believe that the basic principle of distribution of justice is to treat similar people equally, one alternative to achieve this aim is to offer less expensive treatment. Another alternative could be that you may find a justification for excluding certain people from treatment. So, in deciding how to distribute what is available you are making an ethical decision. Therefore, being aware of these ethical issues will allow you to be better prepared to participate actively in reaching resolutions. There is no doubt that the right to health care is an obvious ethical issue, as well as inequity and rationing of health treatments.

Pause and think

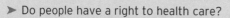

➤ Do people have a right to health care?

➤ Are they entitled to health care?

➤ Is health care a privilege?

Models used by different countries to overcome inequity

The challenge remains for policy-makers to find an allocation model that benefits those who are facing health inequity, particularly when there are increasing health care needs of an aging population.

Care provided related to diagnosis

During the early 1980s, in an effort to contain the escalating cost of health care in the USA, the diagnostic-related group (DRG) was introduced; this originated from empirical findings. The DRG is a system of payments by the government to public and private hospitals. Hospitals are paid for Medicare patients, placing responsibilities for efficiency and cost saving on hospitals and medical doctors. Burkhardt and Nathaniel (2002) indicate that, after a decade in use, the system was in a state of disequilibrium. However, DRGs are currently used internationally. For example, Australia redefined the DRG (AR-DRG) and its development is ongoing; Germany introduced the DRG using the Australian AR-DRG in 2001.

The payment of a DRG is based on a complex formula of benchmark price and cost weight. Australia uses the following criteria to pay for the DRG:

- A fixed payment for each DRG episode.
- Payment on an average DRG length of stay.
- Request hospitals to conduct quality assurance programmes to examine length of stay and avoid readmissions.
- Encourage early discharge.

This model of allocating the resources has been supported by the paying agencies because they can control the monies reimbursed to the hospitals. Insurance agencies also have a more direct control. The downfall is that in Australia small hospitals cannot produce the DRG product, and so some small hospitals have closed down (TC Health Administration Pty. Ltd, 2001).

Casemix

Australia has proposed the use of the 'casemix' system in hospitals, which is based on DRGs and is similar to the type of managed care used in the USA. The term 'casemix' refers to the process of application of DRG financing but also considers the range of DRG in any one hospital. For example, a paediatric hospital may have a reduced range of DRG types while a general hospital may have a large range. So, the comparison of hospitals corresponds to the difference in the mix of cases between hospitals (TC Health Administration Pty. Ltd, 2001).

Casemix groups patients into a large number of DRGs. Thus, hospitals are paid a fixed amount for all patients under a particular DRG. If patients need to be kept in the hospital for longer than the expected time, the hospital will have to carry the extra cost (Kerridge et al., 1998). This system has resulted in shorter hospital stays for patients, thus decreasing waiting lists, as hospitals are encouraged to have greater 'through traffic' of patients. The system also allows providers to use the funds in the services that they want to offer.

Managed care

In the USA, although there are a variety of managed care models, there is not a clear definition of it. However, their purposes are to manage the quality and the cost of health care. According to Maddox (2001) the term 'managed care' describes a continuum of managed care organisations which provide insurance and health care services. Unfortunately, the increase of managed care systems has diminished individual choice. Some of the most common models of managed care are the health maintenance organisations (HMOs) and preferred provider organisations (PPO).

Cost-benefit, cost-effectiveness and quality-adjusted life year

Policy analysts have developed some tools to measure efficiency. These are:

- Cost-benefit analysis (CBA), which values all outcomes in dollars, considering years of life and morbidity rates. Resources are allocated to those uses that have the highest health benefits, therefore this approach is considered Utilitarian.
- Cost-effectiveness analysis (CEA) compares different alternatives to achieve specific outcomes. All health benefits are measured by a common unit called QALY.

In 1968, the quality-adjusted life year or QALY was created as an economic measure. It combines quantity and quality of life. To determine QALY any state of health or disability is assigned to a utility measure on a scale from 1.00 (being healthy) to 0.00 (being death). The outcome is then calculated in years of life, giving an estimate of the extra quantity and quality of life provided by an intervention. This measure is not associated with financial outcome (Downie and Calman, 1994). It is a common unit used to carry out CEA. Consequently, it provides information to make efficient decisions. However, QALY must be used with caution, as there are limitations because QALY, like any other measure, needs to be meaningful, valid, relevant and reliable (McGregor, 2003).

Potential risks

Searching for a model that can reduce the cost and maintain the quality of care can compromise health care professionals' integrity, in particular those who use advanced technology. Therefore, bearing in mind this potential risk, it seems important to protect health care professionals from excessive cost containment pressures by strengthening the need for continuing ethical scrutiny of health care plans and costs.

Activity

Read the following case study, think about the actions of the nurse, and answer the questions at the end.

Case study 14.1
The community nurse and allocation of resources

A community nurse manager noticed that patients with congestive heart failure who were discharged home from acute hospital care were at high risk of being readmitted and dying because of the shortage of nurses to attend home-based care. She requested that nurses be employed to cope with the demand of these patients. The nurse manager was advised that this request could not be considered since these needs were not part of the priorities of the budget. She had some options. She could continue attending to the needs of the clients with the current staff and face the consequences of this shortage, or look for other strategies that could convince the authorities that having these extra nurses would improve the quality of life of these patients as well as reducing the cost of the readmissions. She carried out a research project that demonstrated that high-risk patients with congestive heart failure who had home-based care had lower numbers of unplanned readmissions and out-of-hospital deaths, which consequently reduced the cost of readmissions.

Questions

In this scenario we see how the nurse produced evidence that demonstrated to those in charge that a small research project could be a positive tool in support of actions that could meet the needs of the most vulnerable members of the community.

Identify a similar problem in your profession.

➤ Could it be resolved in the same way the nurse did?

➤ If not, how could it be resolved?

Organ transplants

The ethical issues related to organ transplants are the same as those of allocation of resources. This is because organs for transplant need to be allocated just the same as any other resource in health care. Consequently, these ethical issues are the right to health care, inequity and rationing. For example, should organ transplants be available to everyone who needs a new organ? If only some clients and patients are given a new organ why is this not the case for others and, if organs are rationed, how and who makes this decision. Organ transplantation has been one of the big medical successes of recent times, which has subsequently increased the demand for the treatment. The first successful renal transplantation was done in Boston in 1950 (Cobley, 1995). In the 1960s the kidney was the most frequent organ used in transplantation. Organ donation will be discussed first and then transplantation.

Activity

1 Identify your values and beliefs in relation to organ and tissue donation.
2 Likewise, identify your values and beliefs towards transplantation.

Organ donation

Donor organs come from a deceased donor, a living donor or an animal.

Regarding organ donation, individuals have a legal right over their body as personal property. Consequently, they have the right to control its disposition before and after death. It is also important in the case of deceased donors that the grieving family can pay respect to the body of the loved one.

Activity

➤ What is the legal position in your country about organ and tissue donation and transplantation?

You will find that the legal system stipulates those organs and tissues that can be used from a live donor; likewise, those that can be used from someone who has died. List the types of organs and tissues that can be transplanted.

● Organs and tissues that can be obtained from a living person, e.g. blood.
● Organs and tissues that can be obtained from someone who has died, e.g. cornea.
● Organs and tissues that can be obtained from an animal to be transplanted into a person, e.g. pig's heart.

How organs are procured from live donors

How organs and tissues are obtained for donation depends on what tissue or organ is involved. For example, giving blood for donation is a relatively simple procedure. However, when an organ such as a kidney is involved, careful consideration needs to be taken. To be precise, the donor needs to understand the task fully and the reason why (s)he is doing so. In countries such as the USA, Canada, the UK and those in the EU, the live donor is usually a close relative to the person needing a kidney (e.g. a parent or sibling).

Other tissues that can be used from live donors are bone marrow and stem cells. As with blood transfusion the donation of bone marrow does not have to come from a relative but needs to be from the same specific blood type. The matching of stem cells between donor and recipient is more specific, and so it is usually only a sibling that can donate (usually a baby or young child). This raises serious ethical concerns as the baby or young child cannot give consent to the procedure, which is usually needed to save the life of an older sibling who is dying or will die without the donation. However, in recent years, with the advances in science, autologous transplantation of bone marrow and haematopoietic stem cell transplantation are occurring more frequently. These procedures are conducted in patients with blood or bone disease and in certain types of cancer. Some parents are now requesting that stem cells from the umbilical cord of a newborn baby are saved and stored in case the child needs them at a later date.

The shortage of organ donors has increased the use of organs from people who are living as a feasible alternative to organs from someone who has died. Living donors are usually family members, friends or people willing to donate an organ to a stranger. Some of the drawbacks of becoming living donors are consequences of the removal of the organ or tissue, such as pain, bleeding and the potential for infection. It can also create psychosocial consequences such as family pressure, guilt and resentment. While the transplant surgeon or the team becomes the advocate of the patient, living donors do not always have advocates to turn to for advice or guidance (University of Minnesota's Center for Bioethics, 2004). Consequently, many hospitals now provide separate teams of staff to care for the potential donor and the possible recipient.

In the USA, a few non-profit organisations have lists of people willing to donate bone marrow or kidneys to strangers. However, another source for donor organs is the internet, where patients needing transplants seek partners willing to donate organs other than their hearts. The United Network for Organ Sharing (UNOS) has condemned this direct soliciting of organs.

The UNOS is the national organisation responsible for the distribution of transplant organs in the USA. According to Lott (2005), organ donation initiatives need to improve, since there are approximately 90 000 Americans on the waiting list for kidney and liver organ transplants.

How organs are procured from dying or dead donors

Some organs can be harvested hours after the donor has died. For example, the cornea of the eye and the long bones can be obtained hours after death and stored with no negative effects on the transplantation. Other organs need to be procured while there is still some oxygenated blood within the tissues of the organ (e.g. heart, kidneys, liver and lungs), so that they do not die. This means that these organs need to be obtained at death, under specific conditions, and transported in a way in which the organ can be successfully transplanted.

Often emergency department and intensive care clinicians and donor coordinators seek permission from the relatives of the dying person to donate one or more organ when brain death has been established. This means that there is no brain activity and that the person would be dead if it were not for the respirator or ventilator and other equipment, or medications keeping the person alive. Once brain death has been established and the decision is taken to remove the ventilator which is sustaining the lungs and heart, death will occur shortly (within minutes) after the respirator or ventilator is removed.

Activity

Answer these questions.

In normal circumstances (that is, when organ donation is not involved) the dying person and their significant others or loved ones have rights.

➤ Does the patient whose organs are going to be used have rights? If so, what are these rights?

➤ Do the patient's significant others or loved ones have rights?

➤ What kind of dilemmas can occur in these cases?

➤ How can a loved one say goodbye to the person whose heart, lungs, liver or kidneys will be used for transplantation? Do they do it while the person is still attached to the ventilator, or after the organs have been removed?

➤ If the organ needs to have oxygenated blood by perfusing the tissues at the time of removal, can the loved ones say goodbye in some other way than in the four points above?

Pause and think

➤ What are the causes of death of organ donors in your country? Cerebrovascular accident, brain haemorrhage, motor vehicle accident?

➤ What are the criteria for kidney transplantation in your country?

➤ Are there moral distinctions between the use of cornea, kidney or heart for transplantation?

➤ Are the moral grounds the same for the use of live donors and cadaveric donors in transplantation?

Given the shortage of kidney, heart and lung donors, transplantation of these organs raises the same issues as the allocation of resources. Likewise, the principle of justice is applied in relation to access, equity and rationing. To overcome the acute shortage of organs, different countries have tried and continue to use different mechanisms that are acceptable to the people as a whole. The common element in all of these countries is the use of advertising and health promotion to change people's health beliefs about organ donation. Additionally, this encourages people to talk with their loved ones about the issue, and for people to carry an organ donation card or similar, so that hospital staff are aware that the person could be a potential donor.

UK

Although advertising and health promotion has been used and people are encouraged to carry a donor card, there is still a greater demand for organs than availability. However, it is hoped that this will change and improve now that a new Human Tissue Act (2004) has come into effect. This new Act states that if a client or patient is on the donor register, the relatives of the dead or dying person cannot overrule that person's wishes.

Some other European countries, Singapore and Brazil

In Austria, Demark, Finland, Norway, France, Singapore and Brazil, organ procurement is based on a system of presumed consent. Under this system, any person in the event of his or her death is presumed to consent to organ donation, unless they have given notification to an authority that they wish not to donate their organs. In these countries organ procurement has increased. However, although there is public acceptance of the system, it has been criticised on the grounds that people who have not formerly refused are likely to be poor, uneducated or disenfranchised (Kerridge *et al.*, 1998). Singapore has promoted financial incentives such as tax relief, fixed grants and subsidisation of medical expenses (Teo, 1991, cited in Kerridge *et al.*, 1998).

Australia

In Australia, the person's consent to organ donation is documented on the driver's licence or organ donor card (Staunton and Chiarella, 2004).

In Australia, consent for organ donation is based on the principles of autonomy and altruism. In some Australian states the law states that, if the person has died in hospital, tissue can be removed if oral or written consent has been given by the person willing to donate, or the next of kin has agreed and the potential donor has not expressed objection.

In 2004, in Australia, the major cause of donor death was cerebrovascular accident (53%), followed by road trauma in 15% of cases (ANZDATA, 2004).

Commercial procurement of organs

In Australia, Western Europe, the UK, the USA and Canada, as in some other countries, commercialisation of organs is not legal. However, health care has its rogues just as in any other profession or occupation. Consequently, there is a black market in the sale of organs throughout the world.

There are some countries in which individuals can legally sell certain body tissues such as plasma, semen or hair, and also receive payment for body services like renting a womb. It is also well known that some countries can provide organs for transplantation or that people can travel to receive a transplant. For example, India, China and some of the former Eastern European countries.

'Hotspot' areas for the trade of organs are China, India, the Philippines and Thailand (Scheper-Hughes, 2005). Similarly, new data has been obtained that there is trafficking of children's organs in Africa (Episcopal Conference of Mozambique, 2004).

Cultural and religious issues in relation to transplantation

In the Western world, it is morally correct to remove organs with the consent of the donor or the family if someone has died. Johnsen (1989) asks if people have the right to mutilate their bodies, that is, to separate from themselves a part or organ. According to him, Roman Catholicism and Judaism forbid self-mutilation. This action is only acceptable if the person will benefit from the mutilation. For example, the amputation of a leg of a diabetic person will save his or her life. However, in both faiths, removal of an organ or tissue for benefit of another person is not considered as mutilation but as an act of charity. Consequently, it is important to recognise that culture and religion frequently have a close association to both donation and receiving of organs and tissues. However, the topic remains controversial with certain individuals and cultural or religious groups. It is well known that people of the Jehovah Witness faith do not accept blood or blood products from another person.

In Buddhist and most Christian denominations organ donation is considered a gift, an act of charity, and individuals will therefore donate and receive organs. Muslim beliefs are more controversial. Although the Qur'an does not forbid tissue donation, various Muslim religious leaders have different interpretations. According to Nather (2004), there is a common misconception that organ and tissue donation are not permitted by Islamic law. This is because some Muslims believe that God created them whole, their body is a gift by God, and they cannot give away what does not belong to them. Therefore, there is a big shortage of organs in countries such as Pakistan, Bangladesh, Malaysia and Indonesia.

Activity

Read the following case study and follow the ethical reasoning that follows.

Case study 14.2
Mrs Jeffery's daughter

Mrs Jeffery is a 72-year-old woman who has a progressive dementia. She recognises her family occasionally and does not respond to questions from the members of the health team. She had chronic glomerulonephritis, which has progressed to end-stage renal failure. While competent, she never expressed a preference for a kidney transplant. Her treating doctor does not recommend that a transplant be performed. However, her daughter has offered to be a donor, insisting that, as long as her mother recognises her, her life should be prolonged.

Ethical reasoning

In this scenario, the daughter, who seems to be well informed about her mother's condition, has based her decision to donate one of her kidneys on what she considers to be her mother's best interest. A kidney transplant would prolong her life at a quality the daughter believes is acceptable. On the other hand, the treating doctor considers that Mrs Jeffery's condition is poor and cannot justify the cost of transplant. To add to this, the hospital has announced the closure of some beds because of a budget deficit. Since the hospital does not have a policy to limit care, costs could be completely uncontrollable. In this case, rationing of health resources is permissible and even obligatory if other patients will be harmed.

Summary

The subject of the allocation of resources involves both ethics and economics, and neither can be discussed without the other coming into the conversation. With the ethical side of the discussion the issues of justice are paramount. That is, is the distribution of the resource (including an organ for transplantation) fair and equal for everyone? In relation to the economic side, is the amount of GNP used for health care fair and equal in relation to the other demands on the budget? Also, is the way the budget for health care is allocated fair and equitable? Who makes these decisions and is the process open and transparent to be fair and equitable?

The allocation and efficient use of resources is not something new, as the amount available is finite, and that there are definite parameters. For health care professionals the availability of adequate resources to undertake quality clinical practice proficiently can affect our job satisfaction.

Professional development

1 Continue to develop your Ethics Portfolio.

2 If you have not already done so, include in your Ethics Portfolio what your values and beliefs are in relation to the allocation of resources and organ donation.

3 If you have not already done so, find out the health care budget of your country, the manner in which it is allocated and the different areas.

4 Likewise, have a look at the annual health care checks and see if the hospitals or health care organisations are efficient in their use of their allocated budget. For example, has the hospital met the basic core requirements for patient care?

5 Read Case studies 14.3 and 14.4 and answer the questions at the end of each.

Case study 14.3
The health budget purse is empty

Imagine that you are a professional working in clinical practice. Over the past 12 months you have become more and more concerned about the shortage of qualified staff and not being able to deliver quality care. You recognise that you cannot continue working in this manner indefinitely, and realise that you need to do something.

Question

Using the decision-making framework in Chapter 10, work through the problem and decide how you are going to resolve it. Options you might like to consider include:

- Ignore the problem and carry on working.
- Raise the problem at the next team meeting.
- Discuss the problem with management.

- Confront your superior and discuss your views.
- Write an anonymous letter to the management.
- Write a letter to the local newspaper.
- Resign.

Case study 14.4
Mr Blake and his pillion passenger Ms Stewart

Mr Blake is a 60-year-old from the USA touring your country on his motor cycle. Ms Stewart is his pillion passenger. They have an accident when Mr Blake drives around a bend too fast, losing control of the vehicle and crashing, with both of them landing on rocks below the road.

On admission to hospital, Ms Stewart is found to have extensive brain damage as well as fractures to the legs and arms. However, Mr Blake only has fractures to pelvis, legs and arms.

The staff consider that Ms Stewart would possibly be a good donor (for kidneys, heart and lung). They ask Mr Blake if Ms Stewart has ever spoken to him about being an organ donor.

Mr Blake replies, 'Well, she is just a little bit of fancy I picked up to keep me company, so to speak, on my travels. I know nothing about her'.

The staff then ask Mr Blake for next of kin details of Ms Stewart, to which he replies: 'I don't know'.

The staff keep Ms Stewart alive by life support while they try to contact her next of kin. Unable to do so, they then speak with Mr Blake once again, explaining the situation, and ask if he would consent to Ms Stewart's organs being donated.

Mr Blake replies, 'Well, as I said before she is just a little bit of fancy I picked up to keep me company on my travels. But since I paid her some money before we started and she was going to get some more when the trip finished, I guess you could say I have rights to her body. So, I don't mind donating some parts to people in your beautiful country that need them'.

Questions

➤ Do you think the staff made the right decision by asking Mr Blake to give consent for Ms Stewart's organs?

➤ Do you agree with Mr Blake's way of thinking about rights?

➤ If not, in which way do your values and beliefs differ?

➤ In your country, what is the role of the donor coordinator?

➤ What criteria are used in identifying suitability for organ donation?

➤ What is the process for requesting organs and tissues for donation (including who asks the client or patient or significant other)?

➤ How might the lack of organs or tissues affect client and patient care in relation to your profession?

Critical reflection

Write your critical reflection for this chapter to place in your Ethics Portfolio. The item or issue that you may want to work through or critically analyse could be something that you need to explore further from:

- One of the case studies.
- Reading that you have done.
- A different point of view that someone raised in discussion in class.
- A general feeling of disquiet about pain which you want to explore through reflection.
- Clinical practice:
  - such as your values and beliefs in relation to the allocation and use of resources are different from some members of the team;
  - how you have realised that the care you have provided for a patient on clinical practice was incorrect and consequently, unethical; or
  - another member of the team on clinical practice is being wasteful when using different resources.

15

Sexuality: masculine and feminine ethical issues

Brenton Lewis and Catherine Ward

Why this chapter is important to me . . .

✔ Sexuality is different from what you might regard as sex.

✔ Social, cultural and religious influences discussed in earlier chapters have reminded us of the importance in exploring our own values and beliefs. This becomes essential when we need to both understand and deal with issues of sexual orientation, dysfunction and reproduction in clinical practice.

Everyone has their own values and beliefs about sexuality. Some of these reflect their culture, while others have arisen during primary and secondary socialisation. That is, consider that the values and beliefs you hold are the product of your culture, religion and family dynamics, and can influence your perception of sexuality and sexual behaviour.

So, before reading this chapter list your values and beliefs about sexuality.

Activity

In your Ethics Portfolio list your values and beliefs in relation to sexuality. You may like to use the following questions as a guide.

Do you believe:

➤ men and women are equal?

➤ homosexuality is a disease or illness, and people can, or need to, be cured of the condition?

➤ sexual intercourse is a natural expression of love towards another person?

➤ sexual intercourse is only something young people should engage in?

➤ should middle-aged and older people still engage in sex?

➤ the use of protection during sexual activities is unnecessary or wrong?

➤ human life begins at conception?

- ➤ abortion or termination of pregnancy is wrong?
- ➤ male babies are more important than females?
- ➤ only married people should be allowed to have and rear children?

The answers to these ten questions or statements will reveal some of the values and beliefs you have about sexuality. It is important that you reflect on these questions because of the values and beliefs you have about sexuality. List your values and beliefs in your Ethics Portfolio to refer to later.

Why it is important to list my values

We want to raise your awareness of the ethical issues related to sexuality, and therefore, depending on your background, values and beliefs, you may find this chapter challenging and thought-provoking. Our intention is to enhance your thinking as a health care professional because you will provide care to people from different cultural backgrounds. Some people may be confronted by the spectrum of illnesses related to reproduction and sexuality dysfunction. To behave ethically when providing that care, we must be able to accept a client or patient independently of our own values and beliefs.

Activity

Read the following case study and then answer the questions.

Case study 15.1
Age and parenting

A 66-year-old Rumanian woman gave birth to a baby girl on 16 January after years of fertility treatment, becoming the world's oldest mother ever. Adriana Iliescu, a university professor, had been pregnant with twin girls. One died *in utero* and doctors decided to perform a Caesarean section in the 33rd week of pregnancy to save the other.

The doctor stated that both mother and baby (who weighed 1.4 kg at birth) were in a stable condition, but that the baby would have to remain in hospital until she reaches 2 kg in weight. Iliescu, who will be 67 in May, became pregnant via IVF, and this was her third attempt at carrying a pregnancy to term. The eggs and sperm used had come from 'healthy young people'.

chinadaily.com.cn/star

Questions
- ➤ Is the use of IVF justified in this case?
- ➤ Should health care resources be employed to allow this woman to have a baby?
- ➤ Do these questions raise ethical dilemmas for the health care practitioner?
- ➤ What do your answers indicate about your values and beliefs?

Some of the situations we confront involve a young teenager who requests contraceptive advice, a same sex couple who want to be parents through *in vitro* fertilisation (IVF), the diabetic man who wants to have sexual relations with his partner and, because of his condition, cannot, the male or female rape victim with injuries both physical and psychological, the middle-aged woman who asks for a termination of pregnancy at 18 weeks gestation as the ultrasound scan shows the fetus to have serious congenital physical abnormalities. These are possible ethical issues and/or ethical problems which can occur for health professionals in their clinical practice.

Sex and sexuality

Sex is defined as the characteristics which distinguish a person to be either male or female (Mosby's Dictionary, 2006, p. 1570). Sexuality, according to Mosby (2006), relates to the 'sum of the physical, functional that are expressed by one's gender identity and sexual behaviour', that is, distinguish who is male or female.

According to Edelman and Mandle (2002) a person's sexuality is the behavioural expression of his or her sexual identity and functioning. In other words, it encompasses more than just a person's sex. In fact, a person's sexuality is very important in relation to health as it is closely connected to self-perception, self-concept, role, gender identity, body image and the psychological self. The manner in which a person's sexuality develops also has an effect on his or her reproductive capacity, ego identity and family life cycles, including the aging process.

Sexuality and ethics

The concepts of morality and ethics surrounding sexuality become intertwined, sometimes confused and often compromising. Previous chapters on culture (Chapter 2), clients' or patients' rights and the vulnerable (Chapter 4), emotional and mental pain (Chapter 7), illness and loss (Chapter 8), and mental and psychiatric health (Chapter 11) have included the knowledge and understanding required to develop your professional code of ethics. This requires of you the responsibility to accept the values and beliefs of others (which will include their views on sexuality) even though you may not agree with them.

This chapter is in two parts. Part A discusses masculinity and femininity in relation to parenting, and the ethical issues related to sexuality before birth. Part B discusses ethical issues related to sexuality, including childhood and adolescence, heterosexuality, homosexuality, HIV/AIDS, sex in later years, and then specific men's health problems such as erectile dysfunction, and rape and sexual assault.

Part A   Sexuality, reproduction and parenting

This section provides an overview of the issues and views related to sexuality and concepts of masculinity and femininity, which will be followed by ethical issues that become important in the debate on conception and pregnancy. At all times the reader needs to be aware of the principle of autonomy, and just whose autonomy as health professionals we need to protect.

There is then discussion of termination of pregnancy or abortion, assisted conception and pregnancy (through IVF, sperm and ovum donation, and surrogacy). Finally, infertility and the implications of the woman's perspective of her sexuality and feminine role are explored.

Masculine and feminine

Being feminine or masculine is pivotal to who we are, how we perceive who we are, and how we act. Through biological differences we are identified as male or female. On the other hand, gender is 'understood as a social construction organized around biological sex' (Laurie *et al.*, 1999, p. 3). Although born either male or female, as we grow and interact with society we develop a gender identity, and from this we understand what it is to be a man or woman (Berger, 2005). Chapter 2 discussed that the differences evolve through socialisation and male and female ethical frameworks have actually been produced (Gilligan's ethics of care and Kohlberg's ethics of fairness). Hence the construct of male and female can influence the very perspective that individuals adopt when discussing morality.

Gender roles

Society invests gender roles by conferring prescribed behaviours on males and females to enable identification of that construct. For example, women are discouraged from acting like men, and are considered to be 'the weaker sex', thus enforcing the feminine role.

Motherhood is the expectation of females and endorses being feminine. Similarly, to be masculine is to adhere to a construct of society; namely, the expectation that men will be physically stronger and risk-takers. Being masculine means that men cannot transgress the social norms and can be sanctioned if they do so.

The impact of masculine and feminine traits has the effect on society's expectations that people should become mothers and fathers. It needs to be remembered that not all women are 'mother earth' and not all experience a smooth transition to mothering. Some women do not warm to the mothering role, or indeed bond to their newborn. Although motherhood is the central focus of many women's lives, some women do not choose to be a mother.

Pause and think

➤ Does a choice of childlessness make women less feminine?
➤ Do women feel comfortable expressing that they do not want children, perhaps inviting censure or suspicion about their sexuality?

According to Laurie *et al.* (1999) 'motherhood is a complex social phenomenon: it varies over time and space, and is intimately bound up with normative ideas about femininity' (p. 91). The complexity of life in Western society involves women in many different roles. Career is the most important focus for some women, therefore some may not want to stay at home and 'bring up baby'. In contrast, some women delay motherhood until the time is right for them, and reproductive technology has allowed this choice. Some women want a baby without the 'encumbrance' of a male partner, and some women in a same sex relationship can express a desire to have children.

Recent studies have shown that men also enjoy early and continued interaction with their children (Boback *et al.*, 2005). The conflicting roles, however, between that of care giver and breadwinner remain pivotal to the diminishment of the nurturing role of the father (Lupton and Barclay, 1997).

The male sense of identity is often drawn from the female's affirmation; could this also be true of fathering? Men are also able to care for children, therefore caring for them need not be regarded as solely the female's job. Indeed, gay men in stable partnerships have proven to provide children with secure and loving homes. The fusion of male and female sexuality, and perspectives on femininity and masculinity, need to remain a focus in any discussion of the broader ethical issues that evolve from a discussion on sexuality.

Autonomy

Chapters 5 and 6 indicated that there was a divergence of moral and philosophical perspectives. It is accepted that some moral philosophies and religious beliefs (Christian, Jewish, Muslim) have different views and constraints surrounding sexuality. These different views are evident in the moral philosophies of deontology and natural law theory, and the religious beliefs of Christianity, Judaism and Islam, who all value the sanctity of life (that is, all life is sacred, even the unborn). The feminist moral theorists and libertarian philosophers, however, maintain that, since the blastocyst/embryo or fetus cannot survive independently from the mother, it does not have equal 'value' and rights. This fundamental issue raises very different perspectives. That is, do we regard the blastocyst/embryo/fetus as an autonomous human being from conception irrespective of the issue of independence from the mother? Whose autonomy should we as health professionals protect – the mother or the unborn? To answer this we need to explore the following questions.

Pause and think

➤ At what stage does the blastocyst or a cluster of cells become a human being?
➤ At what stage does that blastocyst or a cluster of cells have independent rights?
➤ When does human life begin?
➤ When does a human being become a person?
➤ When does a human being or person have legal and ethical rights?

Your responses to these questions will depend on your values and beliefs in relation to the development of human life. In fact, even to believe that a question exists, or not, indicates your moral beliefs.

As health has become more of a global issue and is hence multicultural, there is the potential for conflict in values and beliefs in relation to sexuality and ethics. As health professionals we learn that we should not impose our cultural values upon another, nor be confronted when differences occur. This, however, is difficult to do unless we are aware of our values and beliefs and are therefore guarded in our expression of them. Also, ethical issues in relation to genetic testing, sex selection, and abortion, or termination of pregnancy, need to be explored as they can cause immense distress to health professionals.

Pause and think

➤ How do we, as health professionals, maintain our values and beliefs and yet allow for the autonomy of those who seek our care?

Prenatal screening

There are many genetic disorders; most are debilitating and lead to an early death, e.g. Tay–Sachs. In contrast, many disorders do not prevent children from leading a full and happy life, e.g. Down's syndrome. To monitor genetic disorders in the population would be to mass test to determine carriers. According to Davis (2001) a mass test was undertaken in Montreal to identify the incidence of Tay–Sachs disorder in Jewish children. This data could also be used to screen for other genetic disorders. The ethical dilemma this poses is whether or not it is right to eliminate genetic disorders from any specific population?

Such action could be perceived as valuable intervention; however, if undertaken without parental consent, or indeed made mandatory, would it be seen as a form of eugenics? To ensure the appropriate ethical standards are met and that such interventions are not merely a reflection of cultural and political norms, health professionals must be aware that all actions should be guided by the ethical principles of autonomy, beneficence, justice and non-maleficence (Beauchamp and Childress, 2005), and by the ethical rules of confidentiality and veracity, as discussed in earlier chapters.

Activity

Read the following case study and use the decision-making model in Chapter 10 to work out what would be the most appropriate action for Meredith to undertake to resolve the situation.

Case study 15.2
Midwife Meredith Merry and the doctors

Midwife Meredith Merry is currently assigned to work on a postnatal ward. One day she observes that two junior doctors (also assigned to that area) enter the nursery and begin to examine the babies. She observes that one of the doctors begins to collect blood samples from each baby.

Sue approaches the doctor and states, 'I wasn't aware that any of these babies needed blood tests. Which consultant ordered them, and when?' The doctor replies that he is collecting blood to determine the proportion of HIV within the community.

Termination of pregnancy or abortion

No other issue creates as much passionate debate as abortion; however, abortion is not a new phenomenon. Throughout history women have sought ways to terminate an unwanted pregnancy. Philosophers, religious groups, health professionals, lay people and women's groups have wrestled with the complex issues inherent in the debate.

Abortion, however, continues to be a highly political, extremely sensitive and complex ethical issue. Attempts to resolve this ethical issue through discussion and law have reached an impasse because of the two mutually exclusive positions: those who support women's choice and those who support the fetus (pro-life groups). Abortion on demand (either surgical or the 'abortion pill') at whatever stage of pregnancy perceives the fetus to be part of the mother, not a person in itself (Steinberg, 2003). The ethical issues raised earlier in the chapter (p. 323) are again pivotal here.

Pause and think

➤ At what stage does a mass of cells become a human life?

➤ Is life inherently sacred and to be preserved?

Global perspective of abortion

Abortions occur worldwide, in countries with or without family planning programmes. In Western societies the most common reasons for an abortion are that the parent or parents cannot afford a child, the timing is wrong or the woman does not want to rear the child alone (Sanger, 2004). In total, 50 million abortions (equal to the population of the UK) are performed each year. Of these, 30 million occur in developing countries and 20 million of these are undertaken in unsafe conditions (WHO, 1999).

Not all women have an abortion because having a baby is inconvenient. In developing countries and those torn by war, poverty, hardship, rape and non-marital sexual relationships or incidents are some of the reasons why women want an abortion. Not all women have the convenience of planning a family (WHO, 1999).

Points of view inherent in abortion

1 A woman who is pregnant as a result of rape might request an abortion since keeping the baby would be a constant reminder of the rape. You may, however, believe that a baby should not be denied a chance of life because of this incident; thus, the baby should not be perceived to be at fault.

2 Some individuals may believe that the current number of abortions assists to lower the global population, with the result that major environmental issues are contained.

3 Alternatively, some may mourn the loss of potential intellectuals, artists, leaders, mothers and fathers, and what these individuals could have contributed to our world and our lives.

4 Would family planning be a viable alternative?

5 Discuss the ethical reasons for people to attend, or not attend, family planning and contraception clinics.

Prenatal sex selection

According to Sanger (2004), sex selection abortion is a social disaster. Historically, male
children have always been favoured by many cultures and continue to be so, e.g. India, South
Korea and China; in contrast, the Japanese prefer girls (Davis, 2001). Sex selection abortion
is not a permitted practice in the UK, the USA, Australia and Europe. However, the availability of early prenatal tests to ascertain the desired sex of the fetus can in effect mean the
demise of the female species.

Pause and think

➤ Why should a fetus be aborted when its sex does not fit the expectation of the parent(s)?

➤ In today's enlightened world should females have an equal chance of life?

➤ Justice is an ethical issue that forms, and informs, the expectations of, and for, the male.

➤ What resources would be deemed appropriate to determine if justice is done?

➤ If all life is sacred does this then make this discussion redundant?

Activity

The following two case studies present a different perspective on the issue of abortion.
Answer the questions related to each case study.

Case study 15.3
Heir to the throne

Susan is 25 years old and having her first baby. At her first visit to the midwife she asks about an early
ultrasound scan to ensure the baby is healthy. During their conversation Susan talked about having a
boy and how happy the family would be as it would be the first boy for four generations. If the baby was
a boy, he would inherit the very profitable family business. The midwife is suspicious.

Question

Using the ethical decision-making model in Chapter 10 work out the correct action(s) that
you think the midwife needs to take. Issues you might like to consider when doing this are:

➤ if the fetus is female do you think Susan might consider a termination of pregnancy?

➤ should the midwife alert the doctor of her suspicion or preserve the woman's right to
choose?

Case study 15.4
Anjali in India

Anjali is a 19-year-old married woman. She lives in a northern part of India with her husband and two daughters. Anjali realises she is pregnant; however, her husband and in-laws do not.

Her in-laws are angry and cross because she has failed to provide them with a grandson. Anjali knows that boys are valued as they will look after the parents in their old age and carry on the family name. Girls are only chattels. Anjali is afraid, as her friend Suki was killed because she did not produce sons. Another woman died of burns, and a woman in the same village was battered to death when washing clothes in the river.

In such cases the village police do not investigate, as these women had only produced girls and it was regarded as their fault.

If Anjali does not produce a son from this pregnancy, she will bring about her own demise. She secretly borrows money from her parents and travels to the nearby city to a clinic that performs ultrasounds. Anjali is informed that she is having a third daughter and realises the terrible consequences that will befall her and her baby daughter. The clinic offers her a termination, and she accepts the offer.

Questions

➤ What are the fundamental differences between Case studies 15.3 and 15.4?

➤ In Chapter 6 you learnt that autonomy, beneficence, justice and non-maleficence may not be compatible with Eastern philosophy so, using the Indian system, what can you interpret?

Shunning the way of nature

Historically, human nature, gods or spirits have provided an almost equal chance of having a male or female baby, thus sustaining a balance of the sexes. Globally, however, nature is not allowed to manage such matters: sex selection, abortion and infanticide are among the extreme measures to ensure the 'right sex' is achieved (Sanger, 2004).

China's male babies

China's cultural preference for male babies, one child policy and prenatal sex selection abortion has resulted in a potentially catastrophic imbalance of males and females in the population. In China abortion is allowed as a contraceptive measure (Bergland, 1998) and late term abortion is supported.

As a consequence, in the next decade it is estimated that 30–40 million Chinese men will be unable to find a bride. According to Sanger (2004) this dire shortage of females may cause families to organise early arranged marriages or kidnap girls from neighbouring villages for marriage.

Activity

➤ If you are of Chinese origin or live in Asia, China or Japan, do you think this will happen?

Long-term effect of sex selection

Sex selection abortion has far reaching implications and is undoubtedly a complicated ethical issue. It is often guided by short-term economics, with little thought given to the possible long-term social and psychological impact of this imbalance.

Health problems related to illegal abortions

Unsafe abortion procedures cause major health problems in countries where abortion is illegal and poverty prevents safe practice. The health problems include infertility and death, caused by the complications of haemorrhage, trauma (lacerations and perforation) and infection (Ber, 2000). It is known that, in European and Mediterranean countries where abortion is illegal, the ensuing costs arising from the complications of illegal abortions are far more than those involved from legal abortion. This of course then causes problems in the allocation of resources in those countries.

Non-trained workers

In some African states and parts of India and Bangladesh, abortions are carried out by inexperienced people, using unsafe procedures in unhygienic conditions. It is estimated that 80 000 deaths result from abortion in developing countries (WHO, 1999).

India
In India, complications as a result of unskilled people performing abortions account for 23-30% of maternal deaths in hospitals (Santhya and Verma, 2004).

Africa
A woman having an unsafe abortion in Africa is 700 times more likely to die than a woman in a developed country (Ber, 2000). If the woman survives the procedure she has a significant risk of infertility and permanent physical trauma (WHO, 1999). It is inconceivable to consider that having an abortion in such atrocious conditions seems a better option than having another mouth to feed.

Pause and think

Consider the following questions in relation to the mother, fetus, baby and society.

➤ What would happen if countries in the developed world decided to change the law and made access to abortion illegal?

➤ Would this signal the return of the 'back street abortionist'?

➤ Would prohibition change the ethical or moral perspectives of pro- or anti-abortion lobbyists?

➤ How are your answers influenced by your values, religious beliefs and the culture to which you belong?

Religious perspectives of abortion and patients' rights

All recognised mainstream Western religions (Jewish, Muslim and Christian) are opposed to abortion on demand. However, some believe that it is morally acceptable under certain conditions and leave the decision to the woman to make. The Roman Catholic tradition is possibly the strictest and opposes abortion in all situations even when the mother's life is at risk (although efforts should be made to preserve both lives). However, interpretation of this varies from country to country.

For Muslims, abortion is permitted before 120 days gestation, when the woman's health is in danger, or if it means she needs to cease breast-feeding another child, or rape. Western Jews advocate screening before marriage to avoid congenital disorders such as Tay-Sachs, cystic fibrosis and other prevalent genetic disorders. The Jewish religion permits abortion when the mother is in danger both physically and psychologically (Steinberg, 2003).

By law, health professionals need to provide the woman concerned with accurate information about her condition and the options available to her, along with the appropriate care and treatment. If the health professional does not believe in abortion and the woman requests such treatment, the health professional must refer the client or patient on to another professional who will offer the appropriate care and treatment. To do otherwise is in breach of the law and the professional body's standard of practice and ethics.

It is important that health professionals providing care for a woman who is pregnant do not assume that she will have the same values and beliefs as the religious group to which she may belong. Many women, when faced with a pregnancy (although their religion might say that abortion is not right), will want to explore the option of having a termination. Consequently, when undertaking an assessment or during ongoing assessment, exploration of the woman's personal values and beliefs is more important than noting her religion.

The rights of the father in relation to abortion

There is abundant literature discussing the rights of women and abortion; however, there is little research related to male partners and abortion. In the UK, Australia, Hong Kong and New Zealand, when discussing the issue of termination of pregnancy with a woman, it is she who has the autonomy to make the decision. This is because the male partner or father is not recognised in law as having legal rights to the unborn child. Neither can a husband or partner stop their wife or partner from having an abortion. However, in some countries, certain cultures and religions might expect the male to be involved in the decision. For example, the Roman Catholic Church would expect the husband to be involved in the decision (or even counsel against the abortion). Similarly, in an Islamic country, the husband would be expected to be involved in the decision. This means that when people migrate from these countries to the UK, Australia, Hong Kong and New Zealand, they will assume that similar male involvement will apply unless they are informed otherwise.

Activity

Consider the following case study and answer the questions.

Case study 15.5
Nick and Jane: intimacy without contraception

Nick and Jane engage in sexual intimacy without contraception. After some months, Jane discovers she is pregnant. After a week of morning sickness Jane decides she does not want to continue the pregnancy and tells Nick that she wants an abortion. Nick is shocked and states that Jane should not have the abortion. They did not use contraception, therefore both knew there was a risk of pregnancy. Nick believes that he should be included in the decision-making process since the baby is his.

Questions

➤ Do you agree that Nick should have equal rights in the decision to have an abortion? If so, why?

➤ Others would argue that the decision is the woman's alone. Do you agree? If so, why?

Infertility

Infertility is not a new phenomenon. There have always been non-fertile couples; according to Butler (2003), over 180 million couples globally (excluding China) are affected by infertility and over 25% of couples may never have a baby. For some women infertility can mean disaster. For women living in countries such as India, Bangladesh, the Middle East and Africa, infertility can result in divorce, being ostracised from the family, or in more severe cases they can be subject to violence or death.

According to Warnock (2002), women aged 40 and over have less chance of success with IVF and artificial insemination. In Western societies this observation is especially poignant as more women are delaying motherhood until they are over 35 years of age.

Assisted reproductive technology

Assisted reproductive technology (ART) is the name given to various treatments which assist a woman to become pregnant when she cannot conceive in the normal or natural way (Pillitteri, 1999).

ART includes:

- artificial insemination;
- IVF and embryo transfer;
- gamete intrafallopian transfer (GIFT);
- zygote intrafallopian transfer (ZIFT); and
- surrogate embryo transfer.

Artificial insemination

This treatment involves the instillation of sperm into the female reproductive tract to aid conception. The sperm can be instilled into the cervix (intracervical insemination or ICI) or into the uterus (intrauterine insemination or IUI). Either the husband's sperm (artificial insemination by husband or AIH) or donor sperm (AID) can be used (Pillitteri, 1999). When donor sperm are used there are legal issues to consider, depending on which country the woman is living in.

Activity

Identify the law in your country about the collection and use of sperm from the husband and also from donors.

Artificial insemination by husband (AIH)

In AIH, the semen is collected and concentrated in the laboratory and is then transferred into the woman's reproductive tract (either ICI or IUI). This method is used when there is a low sperm count, or when the vagina is not able to facilitate the sperm's progress into the cervix and uterus (Pillitteri, 1999).

Another method of collecting sperm, which has raised ethical concerns, is harvesting sperm from an unconscious or newly deceased male who has suffered an unanticipated sudden and fatal illness or severe accidental trauma (Schwartz, 2004).

Activity

Read the following true case and answer the questions at the end.

Case study 15.6
Diane Blood and her need for her husband's sperm

Diane Blood asked that semen be harvested from her husband in the UK and frozen while he was in a coma. Following the death of her husband she applied for AIH but was refused. The reason for refusal was that there was no written permission from both parents for the baby to be born posthumously. Diane went to Belgium for the treatment where the laws are not so stringent; the AIH was successful and she had a son. She repeated the procedure and birthed a second boy (Warnock, 2002).

Questions
➤ Is it ethical to retrieve sperm from a man who is dead or in a vegetative state without prior consent?
➤ If the sperm is frozen, who then owns the sperm?
➤ How long should sperm remain frozen?
➤ Should only the patient's wife/partner be allowed insemination?
➤ Should the man's parents be involved in the decision-making process?
➤ Should frozen embryos be available for scientific research?

Artificial insemination by donor (AID)

Donated sperm can be sourced from legitimate sperm banks or friends or relatives. AID is not something new, and is something that families have practised for generations with the 'secret' being kept within the family. That is, if a couple had not been able to get pregnant (e.g. if the male had had mumps as a child) it has not been unusual for a male (brother or father) within the family to be asked to donate some semen. The husband and wife would then use a pipette to place the semen high in the vagina as close as possible to the cervix. The family doctor could advocate that sexual intercourse take place at the same time so that the couple would not be aware who the father really was. It was the father's name that appeared on the birth certificate.

For many years AID was illegal in many countries, and still today many religions oppose the use of this treatment. However, as AID became more accepted in developed countries, issues related to legal, social, psychological and moral considerations emerged (Daniels, 1998; Murphy and White, 2005).

Before 1990 the child born by AID was deemed illegitimate, and there was also the issue of the identity of the donor. However, before 1990 many couples named the husband on the birth certificate as the father. In a 5-month period in 1991 over 4000 women in the UK received donor insemination (Daniels, 1998). Legal and ethical problems can occur with AID in relation to the identity of the donor and what information is given to the child as they grow up. For example, in some countries the identity of the donor is not available to the woman or couple, whereas it is in other countries.

Activity

Read and think about this case and then answer the questions.

Case study 15.7
Lucy, Sally and Ian

Lucy and Sally have lived happily in a same sex relationship for 5 years. To fulfil their relationship Lucy wanted a baby, and she asks her long-time friend Ian to be a donor. Ian has no desire for children but wants to help his friends. He agrees on condition that he would remain anonymous and no financial support was expected. All agree to this contract.

Two years after the birth of the baby, Sally ends the relationship. Lucy has no social support and is unable to work, and she applies to social services for financial assistance; unfortunately Lucy is refused financial help. Social services state that she must contact the father of the child. Lucy is very reluctant to provide Ian's details; however, she is desperate for money. Social services then inform Ian that he must pay an allowance to Lucy until the child is 16 years of age.

[This case occurred in Australia.]

Questions

➤ Do you agree, or not, that Ian should support the baby financially? Why?

➤ Should Ian be allowed to maintain his anonymity since he donated his sperm in good faith?

➤ Do you think Sally should be responsible for financial assistance since she and Lucy decided to have a child?

➤ What ethical principles should guide the decision to act as donor?

AID using a sperm bank

Donating sperm in the early days was relatively easy. The donor went to the clinic, provided a sample in a cup, received his small reward and anonymity was preserved. Today it is a quite different scenario and, since most individuals are conversant with the super techno highway, selling sperm via the internet has become a very profitable business (Dwyer, 2005).

Selecting donors has become complex, as modern clinics only want the crème de la crème of sperm. Donors must be prepared to undergo stringent screening tests before being accepted as a donor (Daniels and Lewis, 1996). The donor provides the sample, which is tested for HIV; however, the sperm is frozen for 6 months before the test is done, and therefore the donor has to wait this time before payment is made. Changes in the law also mean that a subsequent child can, in the future, seek his or her biological father (Dwyer, 2005). According to Kirkman (2005), when the law in the Netherlands and Sweden changed to allow the donor-conceived adult to find his or her genetic father, the number of donors declined significantly.

Surfing the techno highway

It is estimated that $20 million is made in the USA from selling sperm on the internet. Women can shop on line for the ideal father for their child, selecting a donor from the USA, the UK or Denmark. A woman can choose the characteristics she prefers, such as hair colour, race, religion, height, shoe size, occupation and medical profile. With a click of the mouse she can select the perfect match for the perfect baby (Dwyer, 2005). Buying from a US sperm bank will cost between $135 and $420 and for this she receives a dose with a standard of '20 million good swimmers per milliliter' which she can charge to her Mastercard or Visa (Dwyer, 2005, p. 19). This process gives a novel perspective to 'looking for the right man'. It also highlights the role that men play, or do not play, in the reproduction arena.

Sperm recipient parents often do not disclose to their offspring the circumstances of their birth. These parents believe that disclosure would cause confusion for children when they discover that their social father was not genetically linked to them. Maintaining this secret not only protects the child but also the social father; after all, he proved himself a man because he sired a child and thus his masculinity remains intact (Kirkman, 2005). This secrecy could bring with it unforeseen problems such as:

- The child/adult could by chance meet a biological sibling.
- A generation of children seeking their biological father and in effect their identity.

Other fertilisation techniques

These treatments for infertility involve four different procedures which at this time are:

- IVF and embryo transfer;
- gamete intrafallopian transfer (GIFT);
- zygote intrafallopian transfer (ZIFT); and
- surrogate embryo transfer.

IVF and embryo transfer

IVF involves removing mature oocytes from a woman's ovary during a laparoscopic operation and then fertilising them by exposing them to sperm under laboratory conditions. Embryo transfer refers to the insertion of the laboratory-grown fertilised ova into the woman's uterus approximately 40 hours after fertilisation. It is used when the Fallopian tubes are not patent or when the sperm count is low or the sperm are not functioning efficiently, when the cervical mucus is not conducive to the sperm, or sperm antibodies have developed. The ova and sperm do not need to be from the couple; that is, the oocyte and/or the sperm can be donated (Pillitteri, 1999).

Gamete intrafallopian transfer

GIFT is similar to IVF and embryo transfer except that, instead of fertilisation occurring in the laboratory, both oocyte and sperm are instilled in the open end of a patent Fallopian tube. Fertilisation occurs within the Fallopian tube before moving into the uterus for implantation (Pillitteri, 1999).

Zygote intrafallopian transfer

In ZIFT the oocyte is retrieved by transvaginal aspiration and fertilised in the laboratory. Within 24 hours of fertilisation the fertilised ova are transferred laparoscopically into the open end of the patent Fallopian tube (Pillitteri, 1999).

Surrogate embryo transfer

Surrogate embryo transfer is used when no ova are produced by the woman. The donated oocyte is fertilised with sperm from the recipient's husband or partner, and is then transferred into the recipient woman. Alternatively, the oocyte and partner's sperm are instilled into the patent open end of the Fallopian tube (GIFT) (Pillitteri, 1999).

Activity

➤ What is the law in your country about ART?

Ethical issues related to assisted reproductive technology

During the past 30 years ART has advanced significantly to provide other more powerful means to conceive a child. This advancement has brought hope to the many women and men who have suffered the anguish and sorrow of infertility. ART is available in more and more countries (Butler, 2003) and has become a very profitable arm of health care provision. ART has allowed many women to conceive and birth a normal baby; however, not all individuals have been successful and many have suffered physically and psychologically from the intense medical procedures (Alesi, 2005). Add to this the persisting inequality of availability, and the lack of financial resources suggests that ART is not available to all women.

According to Schwartz (2003), reproductive technologies have helped infertile couples or single individuals to become parents; however, this technology has created 'fearsome ethical dilemmas' (p. 229) and solving these dilemmas is a challenge. Since 'technology' and 'science' are perceived as doing 'good', initially the general community and health professionals did not grasp the enormity and ethical impact of this new technology.

Those women who are successful have a significantly increased chance of multiple births than women who conceive naturally (Reynolds and Schieve, 2003). Consequently, ART has spawned a myriad of ethical issues related to sex selection, selective termination of abnormal fetuses, eliminated the possibility of passing on genetic diseases and multifetal pregnancy reduction (Pector, 2005; Warnock, 2002). It has also raised the dilemma of how and when to use scarce resources.

Pause and think

➤ What are your values and beliefs in relation to ART?
➤ Who do you think should have access to treatment?

Alternatives to childbirth

For some couples treatment for infertility will not be successful and these consider other options such as surrogacy, adoption and child-free living.

Surrogacy

Surrogacy is when a couple commissions a woman to carry their baby to birth so that they can become parents. There are three types of surrogacy:

- Traditional or gestational surrogacy permits the biological parents to donate the ova and sperm and, following IVF, the embryo is transferred into the uterus of the surrogate. In this case the surrogate does not have any genetic link to the fetus and at birth the baby is handed to the biological parents. This is used when a woman does not have a patent uterus in which the embryo fetus can develop and grow (Pillitteri, 1999).

- The surrogate's ova is used with the husband's sperm to result in a pregnancy which the surrogate carries to term. This is what was referred to earlier in this chapter as surrogate embryo transfer. That is, it is used when no ova are produced by the woman. The donated oocyte is fertilised with sperm from the recipient's husband or partner, and then transferred into the recipient woman. Alternatively, the oocyte and partner's sperm are instilled into the patent open end of the Fallopian tube (GIFT) (Pillitteri, 1999).

- The third type is when the surrogate receives oocytes donated from another woman and donated sperm or a donated fertilised ovum to carry on behalf of a couple. The only reason for this to occur appears to be the creation of a 'designer baby' which a couple own.

Society's attitudes to surrogacy are changing, and as a consequence the law governing this procedure is also changing. However, what might be regarded as legal in one country might not be regarded as such in another. For example, the laws for the UK, Australia, New Zealand and Hong Kong are different from the USA (and these differ from state to state). Therefore, the health professional providing treatment or care for the surrogate mother and the non-birth or adoptive mother and father needs to be thoroughly conversant with surrogacy law in their country. For example, a single man in the UK wanted to become a father by surrogacy. This was not permitted in the UK at the time, and so the man made arrangements with a surrogate in the USA. When the babies were born in the USA he brought them back to the UK.

Activity

Find out what the law is in your country about surrogacy.

Ber (2000) questions how much autonomy the surrogate possesses throughout the pregnancy. Since the surrogate is commissioned by the 'parents' to carry the baby to term, certain conditions may be imposed in relation to life style, diet, smoking, alcohol and drug use, and regular health checks. Some religious groups accept surrogacy while others do not.

Summary

We are now at the end of Part A, which focused on the concepts of masculinity and femininity related to reproductive ethical issues. Many of the issues raised in this discussion have a direct impact on the debate of allocation of resources. In Western countries most people believe that access to health care treatment is their right. Health care budgets are not a bottomless pit, and therefore not everyone can have every available treatment that they may want or desire. In Part B the emphasis is on the ethical issues after birth, which are related to sexuality.

Part B Ethical issues related to development and gender roles

In this section we discuss the issues of sexuality in relation to children, adolescents and aging, and then specific male health problems. Again, gender roles of masculinity and femininity are included.

Stereotyping of gender roles

Research indicates that pressure is exerted on young men and women to conform to stereotypical gender roles. These gender ideal roles vary across culture and societies and, importantly, within culture and societies. Cultural differences exist in the perception of sexuality and sexual behaviour. Sexual activity for many men in south Asia is what they do outside of the marriage. In marriage, sex is a 'duty' for men, while for women it is 'work' (Khan, 1999). Penetration and discharge is the focus of sex and the defining feature of manliness. Hence, a man penetrating another man is not perceived as homosexual. Sexuality, then, is conferred by the role, not the sex of the partner (Khan, 1999).

According to Sabo (1999), studies have indicated that an adherence to traditional notions of masculinity could increase physical risk-taking by males and result in emotional impoverishment. Although men have been economically and politically more powerful than women in the traditional notions of masculinity, they are often dependent on women to validate that masculinity. In the traditional view, 'real men' are heterosexual and sexually very active. If men adopt this construct of masculinity, this can lead to physical and emotional health problems; for example 'score keeping' of multiple partners, and the advent of oral erection stimulating drugs might increase the risk of STIs and HIV/AIDS.

Sexuality in children and adolescents

Sex education is pivotal in the process of understanding sexuality for children. Children are invariably confronted by self-doubt both in terms of gender identity and sexual orientation, particularly in later childhood as they grow towards adolescence. The issue of sexual orientation takes on more significant psychological features when sex education is limited, acceptance of orientation by society is muted and when consistency of information about their sexual orientation is value-laden.

Transition from childhood to adulthood is a road towards greater freedom and responsibility. However, this transition is influenced by culture, socioeconomic factors, and the teenager's physical, mental and emotional wellbeing (Sculenberg et al., 1999). To assist teenagers through this transition they need instruction about the physical, mental and emotional changes. In addition, they need teaching about etiquette and responsibilities in relation to sexual activities, contraception, sexually transmitted diseases, alcohol, smoking and illicit drug use.

Sexuality cannot be denied, thus the emphasis needs to be to teach children and adolescents about healthy sex, avoidance of STIs and that condoms do not provide 100% protection. The USA has allotted $50 million to the 'Say No' campaign to encourage sexual abstinence; one may ask the question, is this a logical educational path?

Pause and think

➤ At what age do you think sex education needs to commence?

➤ What do you think children should be told and when?

➤ Whose responsibility should it be to provide that education?

➤ Is there a moral responsibility to educate (or not to) and what, as health professionals, do we have to offer this debate?

➤ Given the spread of STIs can we afford to (financially and morally) ignore it?

Sexuality and disabilities

Disability, whether physical, psychological or intellectual, can be present at birth or occur at any time throughout life as a result of disease or accident. Sexuality remains important to both men and women throughout their lives (Morley, 2004), and intimacy can bring happiness and contentment (Kuhn, 2002). The following case studies present disability from a congenital and accidental perspective.

The adolescent with disabilities should also receive appropriate sex education. According to Lofgren-Martenson (2004) there is limited research in relation to the sexual development of these individuals. This is compounded by the possibility that these adolescents have difficulties in forming friendships and intimate relationships. This can lead to young adults with intellectual disability having problems expressing sexuality and love (Lofgren-Martenson, 2004). Are there any groups we should not educate in relation to sexuality?

Activity

Read the following two case studies which provide different perspectives on sexuality and disability. Answer the questions related to each case study.

Case study 15.8
Tina and Karl

Tina is a 20-year-old with high-functioning Down's syndrome. She lives in supervised accommodation and is able to shop, keep house and hold down a job. At her place of work she met Karl, who also has Down's syndrome. They formed a good friendship and over time their relationship became closer and intimate. Karl lives with his parents and Tina suggested that he move in with her. Karl's parents are against this but Karl and Tina tell them they love each other and would like to get married.

Questions

➤ Should these two adults be allowed to live together?

➤ Given your values and beliefs, what might be the ethical constraints in such a relationship?

Sexuality and dysfunctional problems

As people age they may suffer cardiovascular or neurological disease, which makes intimacy difficult. People may age but their desire for human closeness, intimacy and sexual expression does not fade (Kuhn, 2002). According to Gibson (1997), some individuals find it difficult to express their feelings about sexuality and therefore do not seek help. This observation not only applies to the patient, it can also apply to the health carers. The media constantly reminds us that society is aging and this is evident today with the increase in 'aging diseases', the most prevalent being Alzheimer's disease. Kuhn (2002) notes that little research has been done exploring the sexuality of residents with dementia living in care facilities.

Is this an area of sexuality that is too difficult or confronting to ponder?

Physical health

In male sexuality, any inability to perform sexual intercourse will be perceived by the male according to their own values and beliefs and those of the society in which they live. For example, erectile dysfunction (when the male is unable to have an erection or sustain the erection during sexual intercourse) may cause one male to go to the doctor for treatment whereas another might not. There are now several devices (such as penile implants) and medications which can assist the male in maintaining an erection to have sexual intercourse.

Society's attitudes towards aging have changed; whereas previously it might not have been acceptable for an older male to want to have sexual intercourse, this is no longer the situation. According to Potts (2005), thanks to the 'magic bullet' (a medication that a male can take to cause arousal), men can be elevated to the status of 'cyborg masculinity'.

Such assistance with erectile dysfunction has both positive and negative outcomes. The capacity for sexual intimacy is obviously a benefit in many relationships and, indeed, could be seen as pivotal to the maintenance of those relationships. Also, given the construction of maleness, the capacity to perform is pivotal for self-esteem. If, however, the outcome is a disassociation between the capacity to perform and sensuality or emotion, it may well have negative consequences in a relationship. If a woman has no commensurate desire to have sexual intercourse with the male who has taken medication (such as Viagra) so he can perform, then this can cause tension and/or conflict within the relationship. However, if there is mutual desire, then to deny this could undermine the relationship.

This yet again focuses on the stereotypical male role of penetrative performance with the possibility of undermining the broader central sensitive communicative dimensions of the relationship. It is an example of what Marshall and Katz (2002) describe as the 21st-century cyborg culture questing youthfulness and enhancement in all areas of life, including this reinvigoration of sexual activity.

Pause and think

➤ What are the ethical consequences of denying male sexual performance medication in a relationship?

➤ Should all who seek this medication be given it?

➤ Should there also be a similar drug for women?

Vulnerable groups

Culture and family norms determine the expression of sexuality in combination with other factors and priorities within the culture. Although sexual maturation is a key determinant of sexual behaviour, various other influences (including ethnicity and religion) influence how sexual activity begins and sexuality develops.

There appears to be no evidence that shows different psychological pathology between homosexuals and heterosexuals. Potential catalysts for dysfunction may be socially constructed and include increased stress on young gay men 'coming out'. The gay rights movement advocating equality has attempted to address the issues confronting gay youth and has done so with considerable success.

Until recent times, male homosexuality in particular was met with disapproval. Homosexuality was considered a mental disorder, the consequence of which was to pressure men into psychiatric therapy to change their sexual preference and orientation.

Anyone following the history of cinema can see the categorisation of the homosexual. The gay male was the victim or villain, the child molester or lecher, but he was most often stereotypically cast as effeminate. The furore that has surrounded the movie Brokeback Mountain is partly in response to the 'normalising' of the characters, and emphasis on the relationship, and hence the transgression to the 'maleness' of cowboys.

Despite increasing awareness in the Western world there are still those cultures and religions that cannot, or will not, accept this expression of male sexuality. In contrast, lesbianism has not been regarded with such open censure. According to Buunck (1983) women place a higher emphasis on emotional sharing and intimacy within friendships, and this may help to explain how lesbian relationships are perceived or generally accepted.

Examples of different countries attitudes to sexuality include:

- Singapore, where male homosexual behaviour can incur imprisonment under section 377A (obscene practices). Also, oral sex (between male and female) is prohibited as it is regarded as 'against nature' unless it is followed by vaginal sex.
- Fiji, where homosexual behaviour is illegal. Section 377 of the penal code addresses 'unnatural offences' while section 377A prohibits gross indecency with another male.
- China, where prohibitions also exist. There are moves in Eastern Europe to recriminalise homosexuality.

In these countries and others, where homosexuality is closeted, sexual behaviour is very often anonymous and furtive, with homosexual clients or patients reluctant to seek health care for any illness or diseases they may acquire, sexual or otherwise.

Consequently, attitudes towards homosexuality need to be understood by health professionals, and every effort should be made to be open and accepting. The danger is that, if health professionals do not exhibit appropriate behaviour, the homosexual person will not seek advice and treatment for health problems. This would potentially cause an increase in physical, mental and emotional health risks.

Disclosure of homosexuality

Making a disclosure about homosexuality raises many issues for the person concerned. Who should they tell? Do all health care practitioners need to know? If not, which ones? And why? The homosexual person will need guidance and advice on how to disclose and to whom so that he/they are offered and receive appropriate care.

Similarly, should the health professional who is homosexual disclose this to his clients or patients? Today, many segments of society are scared about HIV/AIDS and worry that they will catch the disease. For some, if they knew their health professional was homosexual they could be anxious about contracting HIV/AIDS from him. Strict hospital and practice protocols and universal precautions make this highly unlikely.

In this regard HIV/AIDS is most injurious for a person and for society as it raises ethical dilemmas arising from prejudice and bigotry. This in turn may create the social environment that leads to behaviours infused with fear and which are expressed anonymously. Anonymous sexual behaviour is the perfect environment in which to contract sexually transmitted infections, including HIV/AIDS (Kanuaha, 2000).

Activity

➤ What are your values and beliefs towards homosexuality?

➤ Have you ever considered that one of your colleagues may be homosexual?

➤ If you display negative attitudes towards the notion or concept of homosexuality, how do you think this may affect your homosexual colleague?

Sexually transmitted infections

STIs and HIV inevitably raise issues of morality in terms of transmission and prevention. Morality is essentially a set of norms to which all societies adhere. These norms, however, are unique to culture, history and context. Both the Vatican and fundamentalist Christians condemn the use of condoms. In parts of Africa beliefs about condom use are more important than the risk of disease (Pfeiffer, 2004). For many health care providers, this is a very real dilemma, particularly to those professionals representing or working with religious organisations. Condoms are also shunned in marriage in many cultures (e.g. Nigeria) where they are seen as indicators of mistrust and infidelity.

Women in these cultures, who are often powerless to demand their use, are open to more discrimination if they acquire an STI or HIV. This is evidenced in several Asian countries where discrimination occurs primarily within health care (Paxton et al., 2005). Similarly, legal and moral prohibitions are placed on the adoption of clean needle-sharing programmes given that there are few societies that have legalised drug use. There exist ethical considerations, non-maleficence and the legality of clean needles v. the law of the land.

This is particularly true of prison populations where they are adopted often by exception rather than by any systematic programme. In poorer countries, financial constraints prohibit the availability of either condoms or needles (WHO, 2005). In prisons, condoms are also needed but are most often denied. Distributing clean needles given the illegality of drug use, or the moral prohibition of condom use, poses ethical dilemmas for health care workers.

HIV/AIDS

HIV/AIDS is not a 'gay disease', nor the domain of any specific group. Societies, however, have marginalised the most at-risk groups, which has led to the rapid spread of the disease. Many countries do not, and have no plans to, address the issue. Clearly we can see the result of this folly and inaction as the disease continues unabated. The reality is, that for much of the time, the progression of the disease has been influenced by bigotry, fear and discrimination, based on religious or cultural views of sexuality, often perpetrated by health care professionals adhering to the predominant cultural values. The consequence of this prejudice and bigotry has accelerated the spread of HIV in populations in Eastern Europe, Africa and parts of Asia.

Activity

Think about the following:

➤ How are people with HIV/AIDS regarded in your country?

➤ What ethical principles and ethical rules are being met, or not met, because of this situation. For example, to uphold the autonomy of a person, are health prevention programmes in place? Can condoms be purchased?

➤ Does the macro- and micro-allocation of resources in your country reflect ethical considerations?

The primary mode of transition of the virus remains sexual contact. There are horror stories of contaminated blood sold in China (Farmer, 2005) spreading the virus but these are isolated to a few countries. HIV has rendered over 100 0000 children in sub-Saharan Africa orphans, and 41% of Swaziland is HIV-positive (WHO, 2005). The prominent mode of current transmission is in heterosexuals, and in the aforementioned parts of the world it is a catastrophe for individuals, socially and economically. For example, in Zimbabwe the United Nations (UN) notes that the life span has declined to 37 years of age as a result of HIV/AIDS. The disease is exacerbated by hunger, malnutrition, poor infrastructure, including an overburdened health system. In a population where one in 13 people are HIV-positive and facing economic failure (estimated at 8000/1.6 million), few can afford treatment (Thornycroft, 2006).

This also raises the issue of the equitable and appropriate allocation of resources to those individuals and countries that cannot afford treatment. In countries that can afford treatments and that can establish appropriate educational programmes, the human rights of the individuals must be acknowledged and balanced against the greater good of the community. There must be for these individuals the protection of informed consent and confidentiality, the safeguard that comes with autonomy and the justice that comes with respect. Should confidentiality be extended to those aware of their health status? When do we step in to protect individuals?

These measures are effective in containing the virus and yet could be in conflict with religious, moral and cultural imperatives in many countries. Given the health care code of ethics, legal and religious implications, when can health care workers override these three factors in the hope of saving lives? What are the legal constraints for the health care workforce?

(Chapter 1 discussed the increasing issue of the law in health care provision.) What are the moral/ethical dilemmas?

Read the following case study and answer the questions.

Case study 15.10
Mr Allcock and Mr Wright

Mr Allcock is a first year medical student who has been assigned to a medical ward to practise communication with patients and learn about the hospital environment. The senior nurse allocates him two patients to go and talk with. One of these is Mr Wright, who is HIV-positive and contracted the disease from his long-term partner who recently died from AIDS.

The medical student states a reluctance to communicate with the patient (as he is a confirmed heterosexual). The senior nurse asks him what he means. The student repeats his statement. Appearing extremely embarrassed, he blushes and states, 'well, it's to do with sex'. The nurse then asks the student, 'how will that affect your ability to talk with the patient?' The student replies that since the patient is homosexual and he is heterosexual he will not have anything to talk with the patient about.

Dr Ng, who has been listening to the conversation, cannot believe what he is hearing and seeks to clarify this with the student. He asks, 'Do homosexuals and heterosexuals talk about different things?' 'Yes', replies the student.

The nurse shakes her head and states, 'you really do not know much about communication, do you - the English talk about the weather, the Australians talk about sport. You might like to ask Mr Wright what he likes watching on TV or reading or what sort of music he likes. The last thing people talk about is their sexuality!'

Dr Ng says 'If you are going to be a health professional you must realise that all patients, regardless of their sexuality, have rights to non-judgemental care'.

The senior nurse and Dr Ng then discuss the benefit of Mr Allcock going to the hospital library to learn more about homosexuality and patients' legal and ethical rights.

Questions

➤ Clearly Mr Allcock has a knowledge deficit or learning needs that should be resolved. How do you think this would be best done?

➤ What will the student need to reflect on in relation to autonomy, beneficence, justice, nonmaleficence, informed consent and confidentiality and communicating with a patient who is homosexual?

Male rape and sexual assault

Sexual assault by males on males is not as well documented as sexual assault by males on females. It is estimated that 50 000 men are raped in USA prisons on any given day (Donaldson, 1990). The focus research on male rape and sexual assault has been primarily on childhood experiences, and little has been done on adolescents and adults. Since the 1980s, with the disclosure of sexual assaults by Catholic clergy, the severity, extent and implications have become known. Sexual assault and rape can be used to punish, humiliate and undermine the masculinity of the victim.

Rape is a feature of war, as seen in Abu Grabe where sexual assault was a method of 'softening' the victim for interrogation. Health professionals must be aware of the potential for this when dealing with refugees and asylum seekers (Jones, 2000). Sex is one acceptable way for men to express themselves emotionally; however, this can become a medium for anger, feelings of fear, hatred and loss (Scott, 2001). The expression of power can be a resolution to their feelings and rape can be the behaviour used for that resolution. Men who have been raped can become disoriented in terms of their own sexuality and identity.

To be raped represents a loss of masculinity or perhaps a sign of a lack of masculinity to begin with (Scott, 2001). Men can also feel shame and guilt if they have an erection during the rape despite the erection being the result of fear. The severity of the assault has links to the severity of the outcome (King et al., 2000). Men rarely report the incidence to the police or seek medical consultation (Kassing et al., 2005) and in the case of assault most often seek help only when injury has occurred and not for any psychological trauma (Scott, 2001).

Victims are the most vulnerable either physically or through intoxication or because they trusted the perpetrators. Hodge and Canter (1998) suggest that rape occurs for different reasons. These researchers found that homosexual men rape for sex, whereas heterosexual men were motivated by power and the desire to dominate. Heterosexual rape involves men of all ages who can operate in gangs. Homosexuals are more likely to have an acquaintance with the victim, aged between 16 and 25 years of age, and act alone (Hodge and Canter, 1998, cited in Vearnelo and Campbell, 2001).

Somehow rape occurring in prisons or the gay community is 'rationalised' because they are managed groups and pose no threat to mainstream notions of masculinity. Consequences of this ignorance and misunderstanding can lead to prolonged psychological and physical trauma for the victim. The lack of reporting, the negative long-term effects and the consequence of this can be directly linked to the construction of maleness. This one reason is why the discussion is important. Together with the potential physical damage, the psychological trauma is substantial for these men. For health care professionals, the ethical treatment of these victims is paramount. This is because the concept of distribution justice demands equal access to health care without fear of judgement or unfavourable treatment.

Male peer pressure and sexuality

Male peer group pressure emphasises the 'doing' not the 'being', and thus reinforces stereotypical behaviour that can objectify women and seek dominance over the female. Sporting teams, which tend to emphasise the group over the individual, can be abusive, sexually adhering to the prevailing male culture of physicality (Carlyon and Davies, 2004). This can be compounded by co-morbidity with drug and alcohol consumption. Sport and work are often the common ground for the development of male friendships. Both are characterised by competition and often ambition. To be emotionally vulnerable or to expose vulnerability in such environments could be perceived as threatening.

Emotional health problems

Courtney (1998) notes that males in the USA who display traditional beliefs about manhood are more likely to develop poor health habits than those who do not adhere to these beliefs. Eisler and Blalock (1991) found that these men are also more likely to suffer from degrees of mental health problems, including depression and anxiety. This is compounded by physical strength and competitiveness, which elicits distancing from their emotional self.

In many Western countries this focus is sport, while in Japan the focus is often on educational or financial success. If the demands cannot be met the male sense of failure is profound. The incidence of suicide is an extreme example of this sense of failure.

Often men have sex for the wrong reasons and disconnect their psychological selves and emotion from that sex act. Men and women have emotions underpinning their sense of self and, if denied opportunities to express that emotion in anything other than anger or aggression, they may fail to process or express other emotions adequately.

Suicide

The suicide rate among young men is a challenge for health professionals, as is the need to deconstruct the stereotypes without removing the man from his 'past'. To ask men to be passive and compliant is essentially removing men from the prevailing view of masculinity. In the same way the expectation of behavioural change from risky behaviours is to ask men to withdraw from their male culture. The medicalisation of male sexuality 'can deny, obscure and ignore social causes . . . helps men to conform to the script' (Tiefer, 1987, p. 165) and that script continues to focus on erection and/or inadequacy.

Allocation of resources in sexual health

The health status of men, as with women, has ethical implications if it is to be used to influence resource allocation, including the prioritisation of services and interventions (Murray, 1994; Hanson, 1999). Often the discussion of men's health is considered sufficient if the focus is either about prostate or testicular cancer. This, however, cannot account for the myriad of other conditions that affect men's health, nor does it account for the complexity of social and psychological pressures on men in families and society in general. To understand the issue of men's health fully the discourse must take into account the social barriers to health, including cultural influences, income and socioeconomic status, sexual identity and occupation. For women, health problems such as menopause or breast cancer are broader health issues related to aging which respond to effective management supported by appropriate resource allocation.

Summary

This chapter has provided an overview of some of the most important issues related to sexuality issues which have ethical implications in health care. Throughout the chapter you have explored your values and beliefs in relation to sexuality. The concepts of masculinity and femininity are pivotal to reproductive health, including termination of pregnancy (or abortion), infertility and assistance to achieve parenthood, and these have been explored and discussed in relation to ethics and the impact on resource allocation.

In any ethical debate related to sexuality, education about sexuality is seen as necessary. Gender roles imposed by society which can give rise to unhealthy behaviours which might result in suicide also act as a catalyst to render some groups more vulnerable. Health issues related to masculinity include rape, sexual assault of the male and sexual dysfunction. What we determine to be a vulnerable group is based on our own values and beliefs.

Professional development

1 Continue to develop your Ethics Portfolio.

2 Consider and answer the following questions.
   a. What is the legal situation in your country in relation to the following.
      i. At what gestational age or weight will neonates be resuscitated and given intensive care?
      ii. Age of consent for sexual activities.
      iii. Abortion and termination of pregnancy.
   b. How do we achieve balance between the rights of the patient and the need of others to know? This includes health professionals.
   c. If a health professional is HIV-positive do patients have the right to know?
   d. The case of the dentist passing on HIV to a patient (in the USA in 1991) highlights the risk; does it also highlight the ethical dilemma of full disclosure and the patient's right to know?

3 Answer the questions to the following two case studies and write the answers in your Ethics Portfolio.

Case study 15.11
Danny's sexual needs

Danny is 18 years old, 6 foot tall, good looking and very athletic. He is sexually active and has a steady girlfriend. He does weight-training four times a week and is a talented member of the basketball team. His trainer believes Danny has a brilliant future ahead of him. At the weekend Danny and his mates went to the beach; they had a great time diving off the rocks into the sea.

Unfortunately, Danny landed on his head, which resulted in him becoming an incomplete tetraplegic.

Danny has spent 12 months in rehabilitation. His mates visit him often; however, his girlfriend has stopped visiting. Danny confides to his best friend that he misses intimacy and sexual contact with women. His friend suggests to the staff that he ask a prostitute to visit him.

Questions

➤ Do you think Danny's friends should be allowed to ask a prostitute to visit him?

➤ The team meet to discuss Danny's ongoing care, and you raise the issue that his friends think he needs a prostitute. Using the ethical framework in Chapter 10, work out what would be the appropriate thing to do.

Case study 15.12
Kate, a mother of three children and expecting triplets

Kate is 28 years old and has three children: Anna, 6 years old; Clare, 4 years old; and Tom, 2 years old. This pregnancy was unplanned and initially Kate and her husband were happy; however, since being informed that she is having triplets, she is devastated. Kate cannot bear the thought of having three more babies to rear and asks the doctor if two fetuses can be aborted. The doctor explains to Kate and her husband that such a procedure would put all three fetuses at risk. Kate then asks that all three be aborted or she will find another way.

Questions

➤ The doctor is faced with a serious ethical problem – what is it?

➤ Using the decision-making process in Chapter 10, work out how to resolve the issue.

Critical reflection

Write a critical reflection for this chapter to place in your Ethics Portfolio. The item or issue that you may want to work through or critically analyse could be something that you need to explore further from:

● One of the case studies.

● Reading that you have done.

● A different point of view that someone raised in discussion in class.

● A general feeling of disquiet about sexuality which you want to explore through reflection.

● Clinical practice:

○ such as your values and beliefs in relation to sexuality or homosexuality are different from some members of the team;

○ how you have realised that the care you have provided for a patient on clinical practice was incorrect and consequently, unethical; or

○ another member of the team on clinical practice is ignoring the client's or patient's rights and needs in respect to their femininity, masculinity or sexuality.

How to do ethical health care research

Helen Aveyard and Georgina Hawley

Why this chapter is important to me . . .

✔ Research in health care is what allows advances to be made, providing new treatments and care.

✔ Some health professionals are not interested in research *per se*, and this is fine as long as they can identify when to protect clients and patients. This includes the following:

- There is no obligation on any patient to participate in research of any kind.
- Some groups of people require extra protection so that they are not misused.
- Projects or studies that have inherent risks should not be performed.

✔ To carry out a thorough research study, health professionals need to allow for an ample time frame to make sure their results or findings are robust and legitimate.

Research in health care can occur in any discipline, type of care, and client or patient condition. That is, a physiotherapist can undertake research, as can a nurse, doctor, occupational therapist or social worker. The study or project can be related to primary, secondary or tertiary care. Any type of client or patient condition means that the research could involve neonates with a specific type of heart defect, or a new type of medication for people with Alzheimer's disease.

History has demonstrated to us that health professionals can be as unscrupulous as any other professionals by disregarding the ethical rights of participants. Previously patients who were involved in research studies were referred to as 'subjects', then 'human subjects', and now the term 'participant' is used to differentiate the importance of the client's or patient's involvement. For, without clients or patients volunteering to be participants there would be no research studies!

In this chapter, first, the importance of ethics in health care research will be discussed. Second, the concepts of informed consent and confidentiality will be explored, followed by safekeeping for potentially vulnerable research participants who need extra protection. Third, the research process will be outlined, illustrating the steps that are used to protect the participants. Fourth, safeguards to protect clients or patients from unethical research, research governance and government control will be discussed. Finally, the chapter will conclude with Professional Development for you to undertake.

The importance of ethics in health care research

History has taught us that people are capable of extreme cruelty when conducting research. The most notable examples come from the research experiments carried out on Allied Forces prisoners of war (POW), Jews and Romanies (including their children) during the Nazi Holocaust in Germany (1933–1945). Full accounts of the atrocities are well documented (Grodin, 1992). During these experiments people were used as 'subjects' in the most degrading and cruel research to determine the limits of human tolerance to extreme cold and heat, psychiatric surgery, hereditary tendencies, etc. For some children their lives were spared simply because they were twins and therefore offered an opportunity for doctors to study differences and similarities.

Development of the Nuremberg code and Declaration of Helsinki

As a result of the experiments conducted on POWs, the Nuremberg code of ethics in medical research was developed by the Allies (UK, USA, Canada, Australia and New Zealand armed forces) after the Second World War. It was during the war crime trials in Germany that the code provided the standard against which the practices of doctors and nurses in the German (Nazis) armed forces involved in human experimentation were judged. The Nuremberg code set principles for good practice in the undertaking of research. These principles were then developed in the Declaration of Helsinki (1964 and 1975), which requires that all research should be of generally accepted scientific standard, should not cause harm, and should be carried out with the full consent of the participant. Since that time the Declaration of Helsinki has been upgraded, with the fifth version now in operation (produced by the World Medical Association in 2000).

Continuation of unethical experimentation on vulnerable people

It is unfortunate that such unethical experiments have by no means been confined to the Second World War. A useful commentary of recent unethical experimentation is given by Hornblum (1997), in which he describes the use of civil prisoners for research purposes against their will throughout the last century. Other atrocities are also documented, for example the research carried out in Tuskegee in which patients with syphilis were, unbeknown to themselves, left untreated so that physicians could chart the natural course of the disease. While there are now many safeguards in place to prevent such atrocities happening again, which will be discussed later in the chapter, all health professionals (including students) should be aware of the potential for the abuse of research participants and should not assume that research conducted in their area of work will be carried out to the highest possible ethical standards. A mandate for both registered health professionals and students is that they need to be alert to the possibilities of unethical research in any and every health care setting, be that any discipline, type of care, and client or patient condition.

Using and not using people in research

There are many ways to conduct research in health care.

● Sometimes people are needed as participants (participative research).
● At other times people are not needed (non-participative research).

Participative research

The previous horrible examples we have written about are examples of participative research. However, it would be wrong to think that unethical research can only occur when participants are involved for this is not the case.

Non-participative health research

This is when clients, patients or staff members are not needed as participants. For example, a research study could examine previously published research studies to determine the most effective treatment to be given in a specific illness or condition. Alternatively, a researcher may want to conduct an additional study on previously collected blood samples. Both of these are examples of non-participative health care research. Although these do not carry the same risks as studies that involve direct people contact, they can sometimes be unethical. This happens if the methodology is not performed accurately and the results are therefore incorrect. Imagine acting on someone's results only to be told later on that the design was flawed and therefore inaccurate! This mistake can and does occur; however, this chapter is primarily concerned with research when people are needed as participants.

The recruitment of clients and patients as research participants

Patients will often be invited to participate in a research study when they go to a primary health care centre or a hospital as either an inpatient or outpatient. That is, when to all intents and purposes they go expecting to be given care or treatments for their health complaint, but somehow or other they are informed of a research project or study taking place and are invited to take part.

Participative research: therapeutic and non-therapeutic

While it can be recognised that the aim of research within health care is to make or create advances in health care, sometimes there may not be any health benefit to the participant taking part. This type of research is termed non-therapeutic. It is only when a research intervention can directly benefit a participant that the term therapeutic can be used. For example, a non-therapeutic research study might be a cardiologist wanting to know and record average pressures within the ventricles and atrium chambers of the heart in people who have no cardiac problems. This is because the measurements will not benefit the client or patient in anyway. In fact such a procedure would carry significant risk to the participant, as it would need to be performed by cardiac catheterisation, which in itself is not risk-free. However, sometimes what is termed non-therapeutic research may by chance benefit a patient. For example, early studies into a new drug to determine safety, patient tolerance and so on (Phase I studies) would be classed as non-therapeutic research. While patients involved in these studies need to know that there is no expected benefit for them, in some instances the only treatment option open to them is the new drug. For example, in the 1970s when various chemotherapies were being trialled as Phase I studies, some adults with leukaemia would volunteer to take part when their disease was unresponsive to other medications and treatments.

The concepts of informed consent and confidentiality

Whether the participative research be therapeutic or non-therapeutic the concepts of informed consent and confidentiality are vital to protect the participants. In the Nuremberg code, mentioned earlier in this chapter, the absolute requirement that a patient should give his or her consent prior to involvement in clinical research was laid down.

> The person involved should have the legal capacity to give consent; should be so situated as to be able to exercise free power of choice, without the intervention of any element of force, fraud, deceit, duress, overreaching . . . and should have sufficient knowledge and comprehension of the subject matter involved as to enable him to make an understanding and enlightened decision.
>
> (Nuremberg Code Rule 1)

Faden and Beauchamp (1986), who replicate the requirements for consent as outlined in the Nuremberg Code, define informed consent as being:

- informed (that is, ample information is given, including the risks and benefits);
- voluntary (no persuasion, duress or coercion); and
- can only be given by mentally competent clients or patients.

It is generally agreed that the purpose of informed consent is to protect patient autonomy or self-determination. Kirby (1983) argues:

> The fundamental principle underlying consent is said to be the right to self-determination: the principle or value choice of autonomy of the person (p. 70).

O'Neill (2003) describes the purpose of informed consent as to prevent deceit or coercion on the part of the researcher towards those researched. Thus, prior to participation in any research project, it is vitally important that the research participant is fully informed about the study, does not feel under any pressure to participate, and has the ability to understand the research and so give a meaningful consent. In these conditions, the participant can be said to have given his or her informed consent.

The participants being fully informed

Irrespective of whether the study or project is therapeutic or non-therapeutic, the client or patient should be fully informed about the research study and be placed under no obligation to participate. (S)he should not feel any pressure to participate, even when (s)he is invited to do so by his or her health care provider. That is, participation in research is entirely optional and should only be done following full disclosure about the study and the participant's fully informed consent. It is most important that the information provided to the volunteer is accurate and also that it can be readily understood.

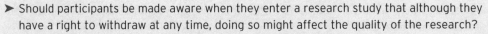

Activity

Answer these questions.

➤ Should participants be made aware when they enter a research study that although they have a right to withdraw at any time, doing so might affect the quality of the research?
➤ Would patients perceive such information to be coercive?

Confidentiality

The concept of informed consent is linked to the requirement for confidentiality within the research process. Students should be aware that the patient's right that their personal data and information is not passed on to a third party is not affected by their participation in research (Department of Health, 2001a). This means that health care professionals cannot pass information about a patient to a researcher without the consent of the patient. The implication of this is that researchers should not have direct access to the patient – the confidentiality between the patient and health care professional would be breached if the identity of a patient with a certain condition were revealed to researchers. Instead, the patient should be approached and invited to participate by the health care professional that is already involved in the patient's care. The same principle also applies to access to medical records, which cannot be shown to a researcher unless the permission of the patient has been obtained or the notes are anonymous.

It is important to note that the laws surrounding confidentiality are different in different countries and the student should be familiar with local policy. To facilitate patient consent to research, the researcher has the duty to give information necessary for the participant to decide whether (s)he would like to enter the research. Normally, because researchers from outside the institution cannot have access to patients for reasons of confidentiality, those recruiting for the trial will be the patient's usual care givers, e.g. doctors and nurses (Department of Health, 2001b).

When a client or patient declines to be a participant

Care must therefore be taken that the patient is not coerced into participation and is not under the impression that, if he or she does not wish to participate, this will affect the standard delivery of care.

Activity

Answer these questions.

➤ A drug company approaches a hospital and asks for a list of patients who have asthma so that they can be invited to participate in the trial of a new drug. How should the hospital respond?

➤ Would *confidentiality* be breached by giving this information to the drug company without the consent of the patient?

Protection of participants

Participants may be harmed in many ways by entering research. They may be inconvenienced by the research which has no direct benefit to them, they might be distressed by the content of an interview or questionnaire schedule, or they might react badly to a new trial drug.

Thus, while every effort is made to minimise the potential for harm to ensue following participation in research, this can never be guaranteed. In general, the concept of minimal risk is employed when considering ensuing harm following participation in research.

A risk is acceptable if it falls into the category of what would be encountered in everyday life, e.g. crossing the road or travelling by car (Hendrick, 2000). Health professionals and students need to remember that, if people will not benefit directly from the research, then harm must be minimal or non-existent. This is especially important when *non-therapeutic* research is considered. Importantly, they need to be vigilant of the possibility for harm and give their consent to participate.

Benefit v. risk

Research studies that will not be of any benefit to the client or patient and carry significant risk to the health of the volunteer should never be performed. That is, no ethics research committee should allow permission for the study to be performed in the first place, and should therefore dismiss the researcher's application.

Sometimes when a new drug is in short supply, it is used in a clinical trial to measure its effectiveness; it is also a means of rationing who can have the drug.

Horrible accidents or neglect?

In 2006 in the UK, six healthy volunteers had to be admitted to an intensive care unit following injections in a Phase 1 trial of a new type of monoclonal antibody known as TGN1412.

The men involved in the trial were paid £2000 for their participation. However, the tissue and organ damage caused by the drug has been extensive and will be long term. The subsequent investigations as to why this accident occurred and how has highlighted some serious concerns. If we start at the beginning and work through some of the issues.

- The information sheet given to the prospective participants or volunteers was written in a style that was difficult for an ordinary person to understand (Bulletin of Medical Ethics, March 2006).
- The definition of autoimmunity on the information sheet was incorrect.
- The description of the effects or side effects of cytokine release on the information sheet and consent form was incorrect (Bulletin of Medical Ethics, March 2006).
- All the volunteers were given their injections of TGN1412 at 10-minute intervals one after another. It has been reported in the press that the last injections were given even though the first volunteers were already in distress from the effects of the drug.
- The first two volunteers, who showed no ill effects, were allowed to go home before it was checked whether they had received a placebo (Bulletin of Medical Ethics, March 2006).
- The statement and report on the investigation issued by the Medicines and Healthcare products Regulatory Agency (MHRA) to the government (Hansard, 16.03.06 Col. 105-6WS) has been criticised and questioned by health care scientists and ethicists both in the UK (Bulletin of Medical Ethics, March 2006) and overseas.
- The men involved have complained in the press that they are not receiving follow up care and compensation for the injuries sustained by the administration of the drug.

Given the above information, questions such as the following need to be raised:

- ➤ If the information sheet had been clearly written, and accurately listed the possible effects of the drug, would the participants still have volunteered?
- ➤ Did the proposal and protocol list how and when the injections were to be given. For example, was the first dose administered the most diluted form of the drug? Did the protocol state that if the volunteer suffered ill effects no further injections would be given until the volunteer was treated and the cause was investigated?
- ➤ Since the drug had not been used in humans before, what medical staff and equipment were available to treat a participant for ill effects? For example, was it an ordinary office, or was it in a clinic with an emergency trolley (also known as crash cart) of resuscitation drugs and equipment so that prompt care could be given.
- ➤ Did the fact that there were six volunteers who became simultaneously seriously ill cause problems in obtaining adequate medical care?
- ➤ Did the consent form that the volunteers signed state who would take responsibility for ensuring and paying for long-term medical care should damage occur to the volunteer? In addition, was compensation and the amount that the volunteers could claim listed on the consent form.
- ➤ How did the research ethics committee check the proposal, including the information sheet and consent form? Was it not their job (the same as every other research ethics committee in the UK has the responsibility) to check the proposal for the risks involved in the study, the information sheet to ensure it is accurate and readable, and that the consent

form protected the volunteers. What training and education had they received in checking proposals? Does more hands-on education need to be given to research ethics committees of working through proposals and checking minute details?

➤ Should this checking in Phase 1 trials be the responsibility of research ethics committees?

The investigation and inquiries into this situation will be ongoing (long after this book has been published) and you will be able to read about them in various journals, both scientific and ethical. However, changes will need to be made, including more safeguards and robust checking to protect the volunteers.

Safekeeping of vulnerable participants

Some groups are at risk of possible exploitation when research is carried out in the clinical area. These include those that do not have the ability to understand the risks involved in a particular project (for example, those with specific learning difficulties or some mental health problems), babies and children. When the potential research participant does not have the ability to consent (is not competent) they cannot give that consent prior to participation in the research. This does not mean that they cannot participate in research, although extra measures need to be taken to protect the welfare of these participants. In most countries, when a patient does not have the ability to consent, he or she should be treated in his or her best interests (Aveyard, 2002).

Normally this principle is applied prior to the administration of care for non-research purposes. However, when the research poses minimal risk to those involved, it is generally agreed that entering a research study might be in the 'best interests' of the patient – or at least not against the patient's best interests. Thus it becomes ethically acceptable to enter participants who cannot consent in a therapeutic research project. In these circumstances the protector of the client or patient gives consent on his or her behalf (assent). However, it remains questionable as to whether participation in a non-therapeutic research project can ever be in the best interests of a patient who cannot consent.

The use of prisoners as research participants

There are other vulnerable groups whose consent we need to consider prior to their involvement in research. Prisoners, for example, can only participate if they give their consent; however, it can be questioned how freely or voluntarily this consent is given, given the living environment. Many people would argue that the environment in which prisoners live precludes voluntary consent, and that the nature of total institution is such that inmates can never be free from undue influence and duress.

Socioeconomically impaired or indigent people

Other socially and economically deprived patients might also be invited to participate in research projects, and studies have shown that such groups have previously been exploited in research prior to which the real risks were not adequately disclosed, e.g. the Tuskegee experiment.

Researchers also need to ensure that the design of research is just and that individual groups or participants are in no way disadvantaged. For example, research should not be targeted at disadvantaged groups who might be less assertive or less willing to refuse to participate (Hendrick, 2000).

The older person and the very ill

Other vulnerable groups might include the very ill or dying – if they are unable to consent, can the research be considered to be in their best interests? Health care professionals and students need to ensure that, when they observe participants entering a research study, they have given their consent to participate and, where this is not possible, that their participation can be considered to be in the participant's best interests and assent given by their protector. For example, with an older person who has Alzheimer's disease, the spouse or offspring may give permission on the patient's behalf. This assent form is similar to an ordinary consent form and has the same ethical power.

Activity

Answer these questions.

➤ Mrs Mphatso has a 3-year-old son who has been born with a rare genetic disease. There is no cure. There is an experimental treatment, which doctors are examining. A trial has been set up to compare this treatment with the standard treatment. Full effects of the new treatment are unknown. Is it reasonable to ask Mrs Mphatso whether her son may participate?

➤ Is it in the child's *best interests* to participate?

The research process

Ethical issues can occur at any point in the research process. Consequently, a brief overview of the research process will be given so that you can understand the various stages before describing and exploring ethical issues and problems in relation to health care research. The stages of the research process in relation to clinical practice are:

1 Questioning an area or incident in practice.

2 Consulting the literature to discern the best way to undertake that care or treatment (evidence-based practice). If many research articles have already published the researcher could decide to do a systematic review to discern which is the most appropriate care or treatment. Therefore there would be no need for participants.

3 If no evidence exists, then identify the gap in knowledge and understanding in the topic, which is called the research problem.

4 Formulate the research question to answer the research problem.

5 Find the most appropriate way of carrying out the study to answer the research question. This part is known as the methodology and/or method. Basically there are two types:

- *QuaNtitative* - *this uses statistics.* (A way to remember is that quantitative has an *N* in the name and therefore uses Numbers; that is, statistics.) A common use of quan-titative research is with medications or drugs using a randomised control trial. That is, randomisation is a process similar to a lottery, thereby ensuring that everyone involved has the same chance as all the others (that is, it is equal). This can be done by each participant's name being coded as a number. Participant numbers 2, 5, 8, 11, 14 and 17 are allocated to group 1; numbers 3, 6, 9, 12, 15 and 18 form group 2; and num-bers 1, 4, 7, 10, 13, 16 and 19 would become group 3. Then, say, 50 mg of the new drug X is given per day to group 1. Group 2 might only receive 25 mg of new drug X, while group 3 would receive the standard medication (that is, not the new drug).
- *QuaLitative* - this uses life experiences (that is, a story in the life of the participant). This may be how they coped with developing a chronic illness or caring for a child who is ill. Qualitative has an L in the name and therefore uses Language as the data (that is, the words that the participant has spoken). You could say that L is for Life experi-ences or narratives.

Irrespective of whether the research will be quantitative or qualitative, there needs to be design, data collection and data analysis.

6 Ethical considerations. Researchers need to make sure that the research proposal is eth-ical in both the methodology and the care of the participants. That is, the methodo-logy needs to be appropriate and effective, and to provide statistically correct and true results. If the methodology were going to give incorrect or false results then the study would be unethical! For a drug trial to be ethical, it is important that the treatment arms are equal and that there is no known benefit of one treatment over another. This is called equipoise.

The ethical considerations of the participants need to cover volunteering in an ethically correct manner. Health care professionals involved in the research must not directly approach possible participants and ask them to be involved in the study. An advertise-ment poster could be used. When people respond they are given both oral and written information about the study, time to think and talk about it with friends, relatives, etc. They can then decide either to volunteer or decline to take part.

If someone decided to become a participant, they are issued with a participant's informa-tion sheet/letter, which must be in readable English (that is, no medical jargon), and lists all the benefits and risks associated with the study. This also includes the information that they can withdraw at any time without the risk of losing ongoing correct treatment or care, and the names, addresses and contact telephone numbers of the researchers.

7 The researchers take the research proposal to a research ethics committee. In the UK and Australia these committees are geographically located and attached to tertiary hospitals and/or universities. The role of the research ethics committee is to examine the proposal and, after discussing its merits, do one of three things:
- Grant permission for the research study to proceed.
- Grant conditional permission if certain amendments are made.
- Refuse permission of the proposal in its present form.

When permission is granted then the research can continue. That is, the stage of the research which involves the participants can now go ahead.

8 Recruitment of participants. Patients are asked to volunteer by letter, posters, or advertisements in newspapers.

9 Consent must be given by participants. All patients who participate need to give their informed consent to take part.

10 Data is collected from participants. Once the data is collected the participant's role is complete.

11 Data analysis. The data collected is analysed using either:

○ Statistics (for quantitative research) – if the sample size was statistically correct and the appropriate statistics are performed on the data, then it can be said that the results will be ethical.

Or

○ The identification of exemplars and/or themes (for qualitative research) – these exemplars and themes illustrate the participant's life experience that the researcher is exploring.

12 Results or findings are obtained – in quantitative research these are called results, in qualitative research they are called findings.

13 Dissemination of the results or findings. The researchers now have the professional obligation to publish the results in a journal and/or present at a conference so that other health professionals will know of the research.

Activity

Read the following case study and answer the questions at the end. This is an example of a therapeutic study (that is, when a participant receives benefit from the research study).

Case study 16.1
Drs Alu Barth, Gujati Khatt, Guy Limberg and Stewart Taylor

Drs Barth, Khatt, Limberg and Taylor are interested in the use of antidepressant drugs, so they define the clinical question, 'Do patients receiving antidepressant X feel better more quickly than those receiving antidepressant Y?'

They then go to the health care journals and search for existing research to answer their problem. They find none, so they write a research proposal stating how they will conduct the research, including the following.

1 Background knowledge about depression and the use of antidepressant drugs.

2 Research question or research hypothesis.

3 The methodology and method – the method or design they decide to use is a randomised control trial. They state in the research proposal that they will have three identical groups of patients from ByBrook Health Centre, all of whom have depression and are in need of antidepressant medication. They state that the groups will be matched for size and other factors so that any differences in the rates of depression between the three groups who are treated differently can be attributed to the drug rather than to anything else. They decided that if all patients who received drug Y also lived

in a certain area of town, these living factors might hide the real effect of the drug. Yet if all those living in a certain area of town are allocated at random to any of the three groups, this will not be a problem. Therefore they state that they will do the following:

First, each participant will be randomly allocated to receive drug X, drug Y or no drug. To group 1 participants, the researchers plan to give drug X; to group 2 they plan to give drug Y; they plan to use group 3 as the control group. The researchers do not want to give any drug to the third group, but just observe them and see how they get on without any medication for their depression. Therefore this group is called the control group.

Next the researchers apply to the research ethics committee by submitting their proposal. The research ethics committee advises the researchers that it would be unethical to withhold the antidepressant medication from one of the groups involved in the study as they are in need of this drug. Therefore the researchers need to go away and think again about how to do the study. The researchers then revise their planned study according to the advice from the research ethics committee. They now plan to have two groups: one group of patients will receive drug Y and the other will receive drug X.

On resubmission of the proposal to the research ethics committee, the researchers are given permission for the study to go ahead. A poster is placed on the Patients' Notice Board. Some patients respond and are informed that one group will receive the prescribed drug Y and that the second group will receive drug X.

The participants give their informed consent to take part. Data is collected from patients concerning how they are feeling on the two different drugs. The data collected is analysed to see which antidepressant drug was more effective for these participants.

Results are obtained, and the researchers are able to prove with statistical significance (that is, the results were not due to chance) that patients who took drug X felt better more quickly than those who took drug Y.

Questions

➤ Why did the research ethics committee want the study to be changed from a three-arm to a two- or double-arm study?

➤ What ethical principles (autonomy, beneficence, justice and non-malificence) would not have been fulfilled if the study were not changed from a three-arm to a two-arm study?

➤ Now that the study has been changed and implemented were the ethical principles all fulfilled?

➤ Can you think of any ethical issues?

Application of ethical principles to Case study 16.1

There are various ethical issues arising from Case study 16.1. The following four ethical principles will help us explain them:

1 autonomy;

2 beneficence;

3 justice; and

4 non-maleficence.

Autonomy

The principle of autonomy refers to the right of the patient to determine what is done to him or her and principally concerns his or her right to consent prior to any involvement in research. Participants should be aware that they are under no obligation to participate and may withdraw their consent and hence their participation at any time with no impact on their standard clinical care.

To facilitate the consent of the patient to the research, the researcher has the duty to give information necessary for the participant to decide whether he or she would like to enter the research. Normally, because researchers from outside the institution cannot have access to patients for reasons of confidentiality, those recruiting for the trial will be the patient's usual care givers (e.g. doctors and nurses). Because of confidentiality, the researchers do not have access to a patient's records that state that (s)he has a diagnosis of depression. Placing a poster on the notice board is the correct method to gain volunteers.

Beneficence

The principle of beneficence refers to the duty of the researcher to bring benefit to the patient. In general, participation in research brings benefit to future patients rather than those who participate; however there is growing evidence that patients who enter research studies do fare better than those who do not (Braunholz et al., 2001). This is believed to be because they receive more attention from research staff. It is often difficult to establish what the benefits to participants will be when entering a trial. For example, in the research involving the antidepressant medication, it is unknown whether drug X or Y brings greatest benefit to those who participated.

Justice

The principle of justice refers to the duty of researchers to make sure that the research will be conducted in a manner that is fair and equal to all participants. Consequently, the researchers need to ensure that the design of research is just and that individual groups or participants are in no way disadvantaged.

Non-maleficence

The principle of non-maleficence refers to the duty of the researcher not to harm the patient. It has already been illustrated how research in recent history, even outside the context of the Second World War, has caused serious harm to participants. Safeguards, such as ethics committees, are now in place to protect participants from such atrocities. These are discussed in greater detail below.

Health care professionals and students should be aware of the possibility for harm if a participant enters a research project. In this case study, the research ethics committee advised that it would be unethical to withhold antidepressants from patients who were depressed and needed drugs. To withhold medication in these conditions would be to cause harm to the patient, therefore the principle of non-malificence would not be fulfilled. That is, participants must never be denied treatment, nor have it withdrawn, nor receive no treatment at all when their health problem clearly indicates that it is needed.

Research governance and government control

In 2001 in the UK, the Department of Health instituted a process whereby there were mechanisms to make sure that research was properly conducted, and that the various organisations and people involved had clear responsibilities. This development has strengthened the protection of patients and clients who are potential participants in human research projects. This has occurred through the mandatory introduction of monitoring strategies by research ethics committees and research governance management. This means that, if a health professional wants to undertake a research study involving an NHS hospital or primary care trust, (s)he must seek permission from both these committees (ethics and research governance) prior to seeking any research participants.

Activity

➤ In your country, what organisations and committees do you need permission from before research is undertaken?

Research ethics committee

In the UK the government ordered that research committees be set up within all geographical regions or counties. These research committees are charged with the responsibility to appraise all research applications critically (DOH, 2004). The head office of these committees is the Central Office of Research Ethics Committee (COREC), which is part of the Department of Health and National Health Service.

The aim of the COREC is to safeguard potential research participants and ensure that the applicant researchers have thoroughly addressed all potential ethical issues and concerns. At present, a health researcher can ask permission from any of the research ethics committees scattered throughout the country. While most researchers will apply to their local committee, it means that researchers who have a conflict of interest can apply to another committee. For example, say a member of a research ethics committee wishes to undertake a project, there would be a conflict of interest if they applied to their own committee, so they submit their application to another committee for approval. While most ethics committees meet monthly to review applications, there is nothing stopping a researcher from Northern Ireland from applying to the research ethics committee in north Wiltshire, if that meeting date was before another committee.

A common mistake made by health researchers when submitting ethics applications to research committees is not realising that if the research methodology is not sufficiently rigorous and sound then the study will not be ethically right or correct (as it could potentially result in incorrect findings, and be a waste or inefficient use of the participant's time).

Sometimes, the researcher is so eager to do the research that they do not think seriously of the risks they are asking the participant to undertake. That is, they underestimate the amount of emotional discomfort or distress, or physical and mental pain that the research project may cause the participant(s). Consequently, it is the duty of the research committee to point this out and refuse to let the study commence, until it has been changed.

Another factor that can be overlooked is that the health professional cannot directly ask a potential participant to be involved in the project; rather it needs to be done through a third party. This way the potential participant is more able to say no, and does not feel undue pressure or duress from the health professional.

Research governance management committees

Each of the NHS hospitals and Primary Care Trusts in the UK has a research governance management committee to provide an overview of the way an individual project is undertaken or carried out once it has been approved by a research ethics committee. If the health professional is not employed by that hospital or trust then they need to apply for a temporary licence to have access. This means that the researcher is vetted by the hospital or trust before they can have access to potential participants. The research management committees monitor the research process and make sure that it is undertaken according to the proposal and that the participants are protected (DOH, 2005).

Activity

➤ In your country, what process do you need to follow?

Steps in seeking approval

At present in the UK the approval steps for undertaking a research project are (in chronological order):

1　If the researcher is a university student, they first apply to the university or faculty research ethics committee for approval. This then gives the researcher insurance indemnity.

2　The potential researcher needs to ask for written permission from the Head of Department to undertake the research in their area. For example, if you want to do a research project as part of a Masters in Physiotherapy and want to undertake the research in the hospital in which you work, you would need to ask permission from the Head of Physiotherapy and submit that written permission with your research application to the local research ethics committee.

3　Applying for approval from the research ethics committee. This is a specific government form asking for information on all aspects of the proposed project. It is extremely comprehensive, covering several parts and currently runs to approximately 54 pages.

4　When this approval has been given, the researcher seeks permission from the research governance and management committee to undertake the project.

5. It is only when this series of approvals has occurred that the researcher can advertise for volunteer participants and commence data collection.

6. Given that each committee meets approximately monthly, the researcher needs to make adequate time lines. For example, most researchers would like their project to be approved first time by each of the committees. However, each of the committees may want changes made to the proposal or application. This means that, if a committee requests changes, the application would probably not be approved until the following month. For example, a student applying to the university may need to allow 4-6 weeks from when they first apply before they receive their letter of approval. Applying for permission from the research ethics committee can take another 4-10 weeks (if changes need to be made), and then applying for a licence and research governance approval can take another 4-8 weeks. This results in a time frame of approximately 12-24 weeks (3-6 months) to gain permission before potential research participants can be sought and data collection commenced.

Difficulties experienced by researchers

Some researchers underestimate the amount of time this whole process takes, and therefore become disillusioned at not being able to get on and do the research project quickly. Some become angry with the committees and cannot see that such committees have been charged with the duty to protect patients and clients from misuse and potential abuse in research. They forget that all the mechanisms are there to protect the research participant, who is the most important person of all, for without patients and clients willing to be participants these research projects and studies could not be done.

Summary

You have entered the world of health care research and discovered that research studies can be done with and without participants. When using participants there is therapeutic and non-therapeutic research using either quantitative or qualitative methodologies. However, irrespective of which type of research or methodology is used, the research process is basically the same, starting with a clinical query or problem all the way through to disseminating the results or findings. Through this maze of processes, although the aim of research is to determine new knowledge and understanding, the credibility of the research relies on:

- The ability to develop a sound ethical proposal, which clearly gives sufficient information to prospective participants and that the vulnerable in society are protected.

- The presentation of this proposal to be approved by the appropriate research ethics and research governance management committees.

- The understanding that benefits of the research outweigh any risks involved.

- That if any health problem arises as a result of the research, that the necessary care to the participant is covered by indemnity insurance.

Professional development

1 Continue to develop your Ethics Portfolio.

2 Write the answers to the following questions in your portfolio.

   a. Could a patient request that he or she enter a specific arm of a trial to receive a certain treatment or drug?

   b. How would this affect the randomisation process?

   c. A scientist is investigating a new treatment for hepatitis C infection that involves injecting live virus into the patient with a potential risk of infection. Should this study be allowed to go ahead?

   d. Would harm be caused to those who participate?

   e. Should informed consent prior to clinical research be taken more seriously than informed consent prior to routine clinical care given that participation in research does not benefit the patient whereas routine care procedures are carried out in the direct interests of the patient.

   f. Does the patient have a right to be free from all unwanted procedures, whether for clinical care or research purposes?

   g. Should patients who participate in a research project expect any direct benefit from their participation in the study?

   h. Is research undertaken for the benefit of the participation group or for *future* patient groups? How would you approach a patient who anticipated receiving some benefit from his or her participation in research.

3 Read the following case study and answer the questions at the end.

Case study 16.2
Willy Wilful and Prudence Carefulness

Willy is a research scientist working at ByBrook Hospital. This is a splendid tertiary hospital with a name for good research of high ethical standards. Willy reads in the Lancet medical journal of a new blood test that can test for carriers of various muscular dystrophies. He is aware that he has a number of blood samples left over from orders of routine full blood pictures. He knows he should have discarded these some time ago, but he kept them to 'play around with at a later date'.

Willy asks Prudence Carefulness, the hospital's clinical governance research and development manager, if he can use these old blood samples to do the test.

Prudence replies that he can but only after he submits a proposal to the research ethics committee to get permission, bearing in mind that he would have to write to the people whose samples he had, asking for consent before he could do the test. Willy finds out how long it would take to get the proposal through the two committees.

Willy has the adult form of ADHD (attention deficit and hyperactivity disorder) and this gives rise to him taking risks and being impatient at times; consequently, he dislikes the idea of waiting for some months. Secretly, he tests the blood samples for the muscular dystrophy carrier status.

No-one in the hospital laboratory is aware of what he is doing. After doing several of the tests he discovers some samples that prove positive; that is, the patients to whom the blood belongs are carriers of muscular dystrophy. Knowing their patient numbers Willy looks up their patient records and finds the recipients to be male and female 20–40-year-olds. He wonders if he should tell them that they are carriers of the disease and may be likely to have children affected with this incurable disease.

Willy then realises his dreadful predicament. He can throw away the samples and results and tell nobody, or he can tell his boss and risk disciplinary action for carrying out the tests without permission. However, his boss would have the authority to inform the patients of the additional testing and the results. He had thought of secretly going and telling the patients what he has found, but he knew that this would get him into worse trouble with the hospital authorities.

Prudence Carefulness notices that Willy's demeanour is anxious and asks him what the problem is. Willy is so relieved to tell someone about his troubles that he blurts out the whole story to Prudence.

Questions

➤ What are the ethical issues?

➤ What ethical principles are at present not being fulfilled?

➤ What should Prudence advise Willy to do?

➤ What ethical principles would then be fulfilled and how?

Critical reflection

Write your critical reflection for this chapter. Issues that you may want to consider include:

- Some research being performed where you do not think that the participant had the full information or it was given in a manner that he or she could understand.

- Another type of unethical research where the risks far outweighed the benefits.

- A research study that you have read about which raised issues for you and therefore you want to work through these.

- You would like to do some research but other members of the team are not interested, saying they are too busy already.

It isn't easy, but it is essential!

Georgina Hawley

Why this is chapter important to me . . .

✔ It would be so easy to think that ethics is just about following a few simple rules.

✔ However, no two ethical problems are the same, as there will be different actors in every problem. For example:

a. The client or patient will be different from the last because their culture, their health beliefs and their values and beliefs may also be different.

b. The health care team will be different.

c. The condition or illness of the client or patient may be different, with different health outcomes.

d. The setting or environment may well be different.

✔ The subject of ethics is dynamic and constantly evolving, and there is a need to commit to lifelong professional learning. But how?

So, you have nearly reached the end of the book! You may have thought that this was going to be the end of learning about ethics in health and social care. Although I do not want to give you bad news, you need to know that this will not be the end of your learning. Why? Because ethics in health and social care is a relatively new subject and is constantly evolving and progressing.

In the Preface, the history of ethics in health care was listed, with the subject developing in response to people's demands for their sociological rights and needs to be met. Therefore, as people demand greater or different rights, so too will the subject of ethics need to change and reflect these.

Today, ethics in health care requires practitioners to undertake critical reflection, provide quality care that is evidence-based, interprofessional and culturally sensitive.

In addition, no two ethical problems are ever the same: the clients or patients will be different, the other health professionals with whom you work will be different, it could be a different health service, or even a different country. Consequently, the purpose of this chapter is to dispel the idea that once a person learns the necessary rules of ethics, including moral philosophy, that finding answers will be a straightforward practice. While knowledge and understanding can assist us in reaching an ethical resolution for the issues and problems that we face in clinical practice, no two problems are ever the same. This is because the people involved or the context is always different. First, the same problem set in different contexts will be discussed; second, different countries and cultures will have different ways of providing health care; third, different clients or patients; and then how resolving one ethical or moral problem can give rise to creating another. The Professional Development section follows, and, after this, there is a further Professional Development section which includes making an Action Plan for lifelong professional development.

No two ethical problems are ever the same

Consider the following: one type of ethical issue but five different ethical problems!

Let us take the example of the ethical issue of a Jehovah Witness woman who, after giving birth, needs a blood transfusion due to postpartum haemorrhage, without which she could die. Let us image you are student midwife Judith Harrison.

1   The first time this ethical problem occurs you are a student midwife on clinical placement in a large teaching women's hospital, which is also the main tertiary referral centre. When the mother whose baby you have just delivered starts haemorrhaging, one of the senior obstetric consultants along with a clinical midwife specialist organises the care. Owing to timely specialised and expert treatment (non-blood volume expanders, etc.) the mother and baby survive.

2   The second time the ethical problem occurs, you are now a registered midwife. The proud mother has just delivered the baby at home, when she commences haemorrhaging. You inform the mother of the need to be transferred to hospital. The ambulance arrives and you accompany the woman, baby and husband to hospital. However, this time it is not a large tertiary hospital. The hospital is different, the team are different, there are no specialist consultants or midwives, and the staff do not have the knowledge and expertise. Consequently, without the blood transfusion or volume expanders the mother dies.

3   The third time you experience the same ethical problem, you are now a senior midwife in a secondary health centre (district hospital). The mother has just given birth and haemor-rhaging starts. There is no consultant obstetrician in the hospital, but after having lost one mother previously, you are not going to let it happen again. The obstetric registrar is in the operating department doing a Caesarean on another woman, and so you quickly tell the resident doctor what needs to be done. The mother notices your concern and asks if it is possible that she might die if she does not stop haemorrhaging. You believe she is entitled to an honest answer and so you say to her that, depending on how much blood she loses, this is a possibility. The wife and husband then say to you that, if it means that her life will be saved by a blood transfusion, they will renounce their religious beliefs, and consent. The woman does need the transfusion of blood and she survives.

4   The fourth time you experience the same ethical problem, it is the same hospital a year later. The mother has given birth and starts to haemorrhage. The consultant obstetrician

is in the hospital and comes immediately you page. The mother is given intravenous fluids and volume expanders. She is offered a blood transfusion and she and her husband refuse. Her best chance of survival is to be taken to the operating department and the bleeding blood vessel (*in utero*) surgically tied to cease the haemorrhage. The wife and husband give consent. The haemorrhage ceases, but the anaesthetist has difficulty reversing the anaesthetic as the woman's haemoglobin is so low. The situation is explained to the husband, and he is asked to consent to his wife having a blood transfusion. He refuses. The anaesthetist cannot reverse the anaesthetic. If he removes her from the anaesthetic machine, the mother will not be able to sustain her own respirations and she will die. He phones you on the ward, and asks you to bring the baby to the operating department. There the consultant and you explain to the father that if his wife does not have a blood transfusion now, she will die and the baby will not have a mother. The husband again refuses. The woman is transferred on a ventilator to an intensive care unit, where she dies 4 days later not having regained consciousness.

Pause and think

We did not get to example 5, but can you think what or where this may have been to make the ethical problem different.

If you thought of a different culture or country this is one of the correct answers.

By now you can see that even though the ethical issue is the same, the circumstances can be very different each time a problem arising from the issue occurs. Consequently, each time a similar ethical problem occurs, you cannot think that just because you have experienced this before, you can apply ethical principles, rules and moral theories in the same way.

The remainder of this chapter will work through some of these differences. First, an ethical problem of drug abuse will be used to illustrate how the context of a problem can change the way that health care professionals respond. Second, how people with similar health problems (dying from cancer) and their carers can respond differently to an ethical problem (that of needing to relocate from home care to hospital care) owing to the shortage of financial resources. Third, how the team, on resolving one ethical problem, can cause another to emerge.

An ethical problem involving drug abuse

The ethical responsibilities of health professionals are not something static. Indeed, they will change from country to country depending on the culture, the allocation of resources, and the availability of other health professionals to help at the time, and equipment.

Activity

Read the following case study and answer the questions at the end.

Case study 17.1
Xavier in England

Xavier is a 17-year-old male from a newly arrived family to the UK from Vietnam. His parents and younger brothers and sisters have settled in well. However, Xavier is experiencing problems at school. He starts taking drugs to help with the feelings of despair he is experiencing. One day his parents receive a phone call from the school to say that he has been found unconscious in the toilets and taken by ambulance to hospital.

When Xavier's parents arrive at the hospital, the doctor explains that Xavier had injected himself with heroin, which had caused his loss of consciousness. However, on receiving Narcan at the emergency department he is now well enough to be taken home.

His parents ask about treatment for the drug problem. However, they are told that there is a 12-month waiting list for young people to be admitted into a drug rehabilitation programme.

The school nurse who accompanied Xavier in the ambulance knows this and, on returning to the school, informs the Principal, who decides that Xavier must be expelled until he is drug-free.

Questions

➤ What are the ethical issues?

➤ What ethical principles and rules are upheld, and which are not met?

➤ How do you think the situation could have been handled?

The obvious ethical issue is the allocation of resources in relation to drug abuse for, while emergency treatment can be given to Xavier, there are no additional resources to enable him to access a drug rehabilitation programme immediately. There is also the issue of breach of confidentiality (ethical rule) by the school nurse on reporting the situation to the Principal. However, a health professional's obligation to confidentiality can be discharged in certain circumstances – is this one of them?

Explore and discuss the questions in detail.

Different environment and different responses

Activity

Read the following case study and answer the questions at the end.

Case study 17.2
Xavier in Vietnam and Thailand

Xavier's parents send him back to Vietnam to live with his aunt and uncle to continue his education and have drug rehabilitation. Xavier is miserable without his parents and younger brothers and sister and, although being part of a drug rehabilitation programme, is able to access heroin at the local market on the way home from school to help meet his needs.

To gain money to feed his habit he commences prostitution. One day a new client recognises him. The client is a successful German businessman who has done business transactions with the family. He accompanies Xavier back to the uncle and aunt's home and says that he wants to take Xavier on a business trip with him to Thailand for Xavier to gain work experience in the business world. The uncle and aunt are delighted and tell Xavier to pack his suitcase and go with the man.

Once in Thailand, the once considerate German homosexual starts sexually assaulting Xavier; however, he supplies him with ample heroin so Xavier does not mind.

One night the German invites other men back to the hotel room and Xavier is brutally raped. Left alone in the bedroom afterwards, bleeding and in pain, Xavier reaches for a syringe and heroin.

When the German checks on Xavier a couple of hours later he finds him unconscious and cyanosed. He and his friends wrap Xavier up and take him down the fire escape stairs to the alleyway behind the hotel. There they phone for an ambulance but, before it arrives, Xavier stops breathing. The men discuss whether to try to resuscitate him, and then decide not to in case he has HIV/AIDS.

With that, the ambulance arrives. While the paramedics institute CPR, the men tell the paramedics that they had 'found this young chap unconscious in the alleyway on their way back to the hotel from a nearby night club'.

The paramedics notice the old injection sites on Xavier's arms and surmise it is a drug overdose and stop CPR. The paramedics call the police to remove the body as the ambulance is needed for another call.

When the police arrive, the men have gone.

Questions

➤ What are the legal issues?

➤ What are the ethical issues?

The legal issues are those of sexual assault, rape and manslaughter. However, check whether male-to-male sexual assault and rape is a legal offence in Thailand. (Using the resources available on the internet will assist you.)

The obvious ethical issues are those of sexuality and the relationship to drug abuse and the allocation of resources. A different country means that there is a different priority to allocation of resources. First, in Vietnam Xavier had access to drug rehabilitation. However, in Thailand the need for heroin increased because of the sexual assaults, and ultimately rape. There the paramedics made the decision not to continue with CPR because of the evidence of drug overdose. Whether or not this was their personal choice or whether it was policy not to undertake resuscitation on those with drug problems because of reduced health resources is unclear. Again, the allocation of resources is an ethical issue, as the ambulance and paramedics were needed elsewhere and it was necessary to phone the police to take care of the body.

Explore and discuss the case study in detail. Both case studies raise ethical issues surrounding and including:

● patient rights and vulnerable people;

● pain and resuscitation;

- allocation of resources;
- sexuality and associated health problems (sexual assault, male rape, HIV/AIDS);
- illness and loss;
- the dying person; and
- death.

However, even though one ethical issue was the allocation of resources due to a drug over-dose, the context was different; not only that, but the participants were different. That is, in the first case study it was Xavier, the school nurse, hospital doctor and his parents; in the second it was Xavier, the paramedics and the German businessman and associates.

Different clients or patients

Sometimes decisions need to be made by health professionals that will be of advantage to some patients but not others, even though the patients have the same conditions, similar age and dependencies.

Activity

Read Case studies 17.3 and 17.4 and answer the questions at the end.

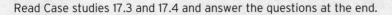

Case study 17.3
Denzil, Milly, Sybil, Tsu, Mol and the primary care trust

Denzil, Milly, Sybil, Tsu and Mol are an experienced team of health and social care professionals employed by a primary care trust (PCT) to care for patients receiving palliative care in their own homes. Their interprofessional care (physiotherapist, palliative care nurse, occupational therapist, social worker and part-time GP) is exemplary and is recognised nationally.

The PCT has found itself in severe financial circumstances and has decided to cease home care for these patients. Instead, there is a nearby acute hospital that has needed to close some wards (also because of financial constraints) and the PCT will transfer the home patients into the vacant wards. The PCT tells Denzil, Milly, Sybil, Tsu and Mol that they will be able to look after more patients in hospital as there will be no travelling involved between patients, etc.

Questions

➤ What are the ethical issues involved?

➤ What do you think might be the consequences of the PCT's decision?

Case study 17.4
Denzil, Milly, Sybil, Tsu and Mol telling the patients

The PCT has told Denzil, Milly, Sybil, Tsu and Mol that the patients need to be transferred into the hospital wards by the end of the month. The team's patients at the time include:

1 Mrs Bath, who is 55 years old and dying from breast cancer. She is married with no children. Although the main care falls to Mr Bath, the team have noticed a change in his attitude towards his wife.

2 Mr Pashigni, who is 60 years old and dying from lung cancer. He is married with seven children and twelve grandchildren. His wife, sons and daughters all help in his care; even the grandchildren come and read to him.

3 Miss Ngaire, who is also 60 years old and is dying from ovarian cancer. She is supported by her partner Ms Toglini.

4 Mrs Grantly-Smith, who is dying of throat cancer. She lives on her own, with her friends and neighbours dropping by to see her on a regular basis. However, the team think that, as Mrs Grantly-Smith's condition is deteriorating, the friends and neighbours are coming less.

The team decide how they are going to tell the patients and their carers about the transfer to hospital. The first patient they visit is Mrs Grantly-Smith. She welcomes the news and states, 'I was going to ask you to transfer me into hospital as I get scared here on my own, and my friends and neighbours are coming less and less as they have their own families to look after'.

The second patient is Mrs Bath, who cries when she is told and explains that she wants to die in the home in which she was born. Her husband, although appearing to be sympathetic, tells Milly outside the home that he 'can now get my own life back; I am not old so I can go down the pub and look around for the next wife'.

Miss Ngaire and Ms Toglini are informed next. Both are shattered by the news. They tell Mol that they are concerned that in the hospital they will not be able to kiss and cuddle each other as they do at home. Miss Ngaire says 'it is months since we had sex together, but I find the hugs, cuddles and kisses we share give me so much comfort'.

The last patient the team visit is Mr Pashigni, in the early evening. When Denzil and Milly come to see him, his family are all there. There are some little children playing in the front garden supervised by one of the sons, the daughters are cooking in the kitchen, the other sons are supervising the older children doing their homework. Denzil and Milly speak to Mr and Mrs Pashigni and tell them the news about the transfer. Mrs Pashigni does not want her husband to leave the family and states that it is his right to be able to die in his own home. Mr Pashigni, a retired dentist, knows that the hospital will not allow the whole family to visit him together, and the grandchildren will be excluded from visiting him. Mr and Mrs Pashigni cry together, then Mr Pashigni starts coughing, breathless and cyanosed. Milly gives him Morphine in the dose that usually settles him. However, it does not have sufficient effect (although he stops coughing), and his pulse is thready, his breathing very shallow and he nods when Milly asks him if the pain is crushing and going up into his neck. Milly and Denzil recognise the signs and symptoms of myocardial infarction, so Milly gives him another dose of morphine to ease the pain. As she does so Mrs Pashigni leaves the room to collect the sons and daughters to be with their father as he dies. When they silently enter the room and touch his body so that he is aware of their presence, he opens his eyes, smiles and then closes his eyes again and dies.

Questions

In Case study 17.4, we see different responses to one event that needs to occur: the cessation of home care and the transfer of patients to hospital.

➤ List the different types of responses.

➤ What do you think may have caused these responses?

➤ What types of other responses do you think could have occurred?

➤ What are the ethical issues?

Resolution of one problem causing another

While it can be assumed that resolving one ethical problem will remedy a situation, this does not always occur. For example, if the parents of a severely physically deformed newborn baby refuse to give consent to an operation to save its life, and the hospital applies to the courts for permission, what happens if the baby lives but is so severely impaired both physically and mentally that the parents feel that they cannot look after the baby, and place him or her with a government adoption agency? Then, no prospective adoptive parents want such a severely physically impaired baby and so a placement is found in long-term institutional care.

In such a situation, the health professionals feel that they are resolving the ethical situation of keeping the baby alive by requesting the Court's permission to operate. When the baby recovers from the life-saving operation and the parents relinquish him or her, has the ethical problem really been resolved?

1　Yes, in one sense it has because the baby is alive. However, now an ethical problem involving parent and child rights has occurred, with the baby and parents going separate ways.

2　While placing the baby for adoption may appear to resolve the ethical problem of the parents not being able to look after the child and therefore offer this opportunity to other people, the problem is not resolved.

3　Now that the baby has physical deformities/impairments, he or she may not to be chosen by prospective parent(s).

4　This means that in the end the baby is placed in long-term institutional care.

So, has the original option of saving the baby's life been successful?

In such circumstances, the outcomes of options of resolving an ethical problem must be seriously and extensively discussed. In such cases, if the health professionals had extended their discussions with the parents they could have found out that the parents did not have the social economic ability or lacked education and the ability to look after the child. Once they were in receipt of all the facts then, in consultation with the Coroner's Court, it may have been wise not to attempt the operation and allow the baby to die.

Activity

Consider the following questions and write the answers in your Ethics Portfolio.

➤ How do you feel about allowing a baby with severe physical impairments to die?

➤ What about a baby with severe mental and physical impairments?

➤ What are the other ethical issues in the example?

Summary

Clearly, there is no single rule, guideline or framework that can be used to resolve all ethical problems, for an ethical problem will be embedded in its own situation, involving different variations. This is because each client or patient is different from the last, with different relationships (significant others – husband, wife, partner, lover, friends or family) and different health professionals.

However, if health care professionals learn ethics from an interprofessional or disciplinary perspective then, with good communication skills, understanding and respect for each other's roles, ethical problems that arise in clinical practice can be discussed with the client or family (and, if necessary, significant others) and resolved.

Professional development

1 Continue to develop your Ethics Portfolio.

2 Read the following two case studies and answer the questions at the end.

Case study 17.5
The missing drugs

You are working in a closely knit team where everyone gets on well with each other. Jokes are shared and you frequently party together after work. One day an audit is conducted on the class A drugs/Schedule 8/dangerous drugs stored in the department, and it is reported that four ampoules of morphine are missing. The hospital solicitor and security are alerted.

You are perplexed as to how this could happen and even more so when you think that you know everyone so well. So well, in fact, that you could not imagine anyone stealing the morphine.

Questions

➤ What is the penalty in your profession for illegally obtaining Class A drugs, or Schedule 8 or dangerous drugs from your place of employment?

➤ What do think might cause a health professional to take drugs such as morphine?

➤ What might make you suspicious of a person taking the drugs?

Case study 17.6
No-one knew the other drugs were missing

A couple of months pass with no further drugs going missing from the unit. At a team meeting one day, Eve Adams (a consultant) says 'Did you know that our incidence of respiratory arrest is higher than the national average for a department of this size and population?'

The staff discuss how this could occur and what the reasons might be. None of the staff, when questioned by Eve, know how these respiratory arrests could have occurred, other than the patients' respiratory systems being compromised by their illness at the time.

Next day another unexplained respiratory arrest occurs. Eve is suspicious and asks for a *full* medication audit to be performed (the one previously performed was only concerned with pain analgesia).

When the more complete audit is performed it is found that other drugs are missing; these include muscle relaxants and sedatives used in anaesthesia.

The hospital solicitor is called to the department once again to investigate.

By examining the staff roster and comparing this with the dates and times of the respiratory arrests, it is discovered that only two staff members were always on duty. Extra surveillance cameras are installed in the department, and department heads agree that whenever either of these two staff are on duty an extra senior person must be in the department to watch them and handle any respiratory arrests that might occur.

They did not have to wait long, because the very next day another respiratory arrest occurred, and one of the two staff members was found to have an empty ampoule of an anesthetic drug in his pocket.

Questions

➤ None of the codes of ethics or standards of practice for any health or social care professional group would condone such behaviour, so why would a person think it was acceptable?

➤ Think how you might feel by being let down by a colleague in such a way?

➤ How are you going to be able to trust others in the future?

➤ It may be helpful to construct the problem using the decision-making framework in Chapter 10 so that you can work through the issue and make recommendations so that a similar problem could not occur again.

Critical reflection

Write your critical reflection for this chapter. Things you might want to consider are any of the questions arising from the chapter or discussions with peers and colleagues, or clinical practice. Topics might include Jehovah Witness patients, drug abuse, waiting lists, prostitution or severely impaired infants being allowed to die.

Further professional development

We would like to pose one further question to you. 'How are you going to demonstrate to your professional body or council that you are ethically competent?'

If you are wondering how to do this, we suggest the following activities.

1 Read your reflective journal from beginning to end, and as you do so take note of the following.

➤ How have your values and beliefs changed?

➤ When and how did you experience 'dissonance'? What did you do about that (did you talk to your tutor or lecturer, friends or peers, or ignore it)?

➤ Can you now respect your client's or patient's decisions even when they differ from yours?

➤ What do you think has been the catalyst for this to occur?

➤ Which person(s) do you find it most beneficial to discuss these with and why?

You will find it beneficial to document your answers.

2 An important question to ask yourself is, 'Can I now readily recognise ethical issues and problems in clinical practice?' If you are still having some difficulties it will be worth including steps to help you improve in the action plan referred to next.

3 Decide how you are going to sustain this professional learning and development. You may like to write an action plan to include in your Ethics or Professional portfolio (the name of this folio of documentation differs from one profession to another as do the requirements of one university to another). Irrespective of the style of the portfolio, you will be able to use it to demonstrate to future employers and your professional body your commitment to:

● continued learning of ethics in health and social care;

● your commitment to quality interprofessional care;

● your respect for holistic care that includes cultural and religious sensitivity;

● sustained use of professional reflection to increase your therapeutic availability to clients or patients; and

● your ability to think critically and problem-solve.

References

A

Alderson, P. (1992). 'Defining ethics in nursing practice'. *Nursing Standard* **6**: 33-35.

Alesi, R. (2005). 'Infertility and its treatment: an emotional roller coaster'. *Australian Family Physician* **34**: 135-138.

Allmark, P. (2000). 'Can there be an ethics of care?'. In: K. Fulfood, K. Dickinson and D. L. Murray (eds). *Health Care Ethics and Human Values: An Introductory Text With Readings and Case Studies*. Oxford: Blackwell Publishing.

AMA (2003). American Medical Association Continuing Medical Education Online. Pain management module. Retrieved 24/02/2006 from http://ama-cmeonline.com/pain_mgmt/module01/03paho/index.htm

American College of Obstetricians and Gynecologists (2001). Management of recurrent early pregnancy loss. *ACOG Practice Bulletin*.

Ames, R. T. (1998). 'East Asian philosophy'. In: E. Craig (ed.). *Routledge Encyclopaedia of Philosophy*. London: Routledge. Retrieved 19/01/2006.

ANZDATA (2004). Australia and New Zealand organ donation registry: 2005 report (p. 1). Retrieved 11/10/2005 from www.anzdata.org.au

Ashley, B. M. and O'Rourke, K. D. (1989). *Healthcare Ethics: A Theological Analysis*. 3rd edn. St Louis: Catholic Health Association of United States of America.

Atwal, A. and Caldwell, K. (2003). 'Ethics, occupational therapy and discharge planning: four broken principles'. *Australian Occupational Therapy Journal* **50**: 244-251.

Aveyard, H. (2002). 'Implied consent prior to nursing care procedures'. *Journal of Advanced Nursing* **39**: 201-207.

B

Bancroft, J. (1999). 'Ethical aspects of sexuality and sex therapy'. In: S. Bloch and P. Chodoff (eds). *Psychiatric Ethics*, 4th edn. Oxford: Oxford University Press, pp. 215-242.

Bandman, E. L. and Bandman, B. (1990). *Nursing Ethics Through the Life Span*, 2nd edn. Norwalk, Connecticut: Appleton and Lange.

Bandman, E. L. and Bandman, B. (1997). *Nursing Ethics Through the Life Span*, 3rd edn. Norwalk, Connecticut: Appleton and Lange.

Banks, J. A. (2004). 'Multicultural education: characteristics and goals'. In: J. A. Banks and C. A. McGee Banks (eds). *Multicultural Education: Issues and Perspectives*. Hoboken, NJ: John Wiley, pp. 20-25.

Barker, P. and Kerr, B. (2001). *The Process of Psychotherapy: A Journey of Discovery*. Oxford: Butterworth.

Barrett, G. and Keeping, C. (2005). 'The process required for effective interprofessional working'. In: G. Barrett, D. Sellman and J. Thomas (eds). *Interprofessional Working in Health and Social Care*, Chapter 2. Basingstoke: Palgrave Macmillan.

Barry, V. (1982). *Moral Aspects in Health Care*. Norwalk, Connecticut: Appleton Century Crofts.

Bartel, J., Besley, J. and Berry, P. H. *et al.* (2003). *Approaches to Pain Management*. Oakbrook Terrace, IL: Joint Commission on the Accreditation of Health Care Organisations.

Bayley, J. (1999). *Elegy for Iris*. New York: Picador.

BBC (2006). http://www.bbc.co.uk/religions/shinto. Retrieved 19/01/2006.

Beauchamp, T. L. and Childress, J. G. (1983). *Principles of Biomedical Ethics*. New York: Oxford University Press.

Beauchamp, T. L. and Childress, J. G. (1994). *Principles of Biomedical Ethics*, 4th edn. Oxford: Oxford University Press.

Beauchamp, T. L. and Childress, J. G. (2001). *Principles of Biomedical Ethics*, 5th edn. New York: Oxford University Press.

Beauchamp, T. L. and Childress, J. G. (2005). *Principles of Biomedical Ethics*, 6th edn. New York: Oxford University Press.

Ber, R. (2000). 'Ethical issues in gestational surrogacy'. *Theoretical Medicine and Bioethics* **21**: 153-169.

Berger, K. (2005). *The Developing Person*, 6th edn. Bronx Community College: City University of New York.

Berghs, M., Dierckx de Casterlé, B. and Gastmans, C. (2005). 'The complexity of nurses' attitudes toward euthanasia: a review of the literature'. *Journal of Medical Ethics* **31**: 441-446.

Bergland, C. A. (1998). *Ethics for Health Care*. Oxford: Oxford University Press.

Berney, L., Kelly, M., Doyal, L., Feder, G., Griffiths, C. and Jones, I. R. (2005). 'Ethical principles and the rationing of health care: a qualitative study in general practice'. *British Journal of General Practice*, August 2005, 620-625.

Bhanushali, M., and Tuite, P. (2004). 'The evaluation and management of patients with neuroleptic malignant syndrome'. *Neurologic Clinics* **22**: 389-411.

Bieri, D., Reeve, R. A., Champion, G. D. *et al.* (1990). 'The faces pain scale for the self-assessment of the severity of the pain experienced by children: development, initial validation, and preliminary investigations for ratio scale properties'. *Journal of Pain* **41**: 139-150.

Bishop, A. and Scudder, J. (2001). *Nursing Ethics: Holistic Caring Practice*, 2nd edn. National League for Nurses, Massachusetts: Jones and Bartlett Publishers.

Blackie, C. (ed.) (2000). *Community Health Care Nursing*. London: Churchill Livingstone.

Blum, L. (1980). *Friendship, Altruism and Morality*. London: Routledge.

Blum, L. (1988). 'Gilligan and Kohlberg: implications for moral theory'. *Ethics* **98**: 472-491.

Boback, I. M., Laudermilk, D. L. and Jensen, M. D. (2005). *Maternity and Child Care*. St Louis: Mosby.

Boivie, J. (1996). 'Central pain syndromes'. In: J. N. Campell (ed.). *Pain 1996: An Updated Review*. Seattle, WA: IASP Press.

Bounstein, M. (2002). *Communicating Effectively for Dummies*, New York: Wiley.

Bowlby, J. (1980). *Attachment and Loss, Vol. 3. Loss, Sadness and Depression*. London: Penguin.

Bok, S. (1978). *Lying: Moral Choice in Public and Private Life*. New York: Pantheon Books.

Bramley, S. and Cockshutt, G. (2005). 'Listening, not just talking'. *Occupational Therapy News* **13**: 24-25.

Braunholz, D. A., Edwards, S. J. L. and Lilford, R. J. (2001). 'Are clinical trials good for us (in the short term)? Evidence for a "trial effect"'. *Journal of Clinical Epidemiology* **54**: 217-224.

Brazil, K. and Vohra, J. U. (2005). 'Identifying the educational needs in end-of-life care for staff and families of residents in care facilities'. *International Journal of Palliative Nursing* 11: 475–480.

Breton, R., Isajiw, W., Kalbach, W. and Reitz, J. (1990). *Ethnic Identity and Equality: Varieties of Experience in a Canadian City*. Toronto: University of Toronto Press.

Bristol Royal Infirmary Inquiry (2001). 'Final Report on The Bristol Royal Infirmary Inquiry, 2001'. London: Ministry of the Crown Publishing. Retrieved 08/09/2006 from http://www.Bristol-inquiry.org.uk/

British Association of Social Workers (2003). *Social Work Code of Ethics*. London: BASW. Retrieved 27/10/2005 from http://www.basw.co.uk/articles.php?articled=2

British Medical Association (2001). *Withholding and Withdrawing Life-Prolonging Medical Treatment: Guidance for Decision Making*, 2nd edn. London: BMA.

Bromberger, B. and Fife-Yeomans, J. (1991). *Deep Sleep: Harry Bailey and the Scandal at Chelmsford*. Sydney: Simon & Schuster.

Brown, P. (1999). 'Ethical aspects of drug treatment'. In S. Bloch and P. Chodoff (eds). *Psychiatric Ethics*, 4th edn. Oxford: Oxford University Press, pp. 167–184.

Bryant, J. H. (2002). *Equity and Resource Allocation*. The Gale Group Inc. Retrieved 11/10/2005 from www.encyclopedias.families.com

Buchanan, A. (1989). 'Health-care delivery and resource allocation'. In: R. M. Veatch (ed.). *Medical Ethics*. Boston: Jones & Bartlett Publishers, pp. 293–327.

Buchanan, A. (1991). 'Justice: a philosophical review'. In: T. A. Mappes and J. S. Zembaty (eds). *Biomedical Ethics*, 3rd edn. New York: McGraw-Hill, pp. 552–562.

Bulletin of Medical Ethics, March 2006. News, no. 213. London: Bioethics Publications.

Burkhardt, M. A. and Nathaniel, A. K. (2001). *Ethics and Issues in Contemporary Nursing*, 2nd edn. New York: Delmar Thompson Learning.

Butler, P. A. (2003). 'WHO: progress in reproductive health research'. http://www.who.int/reproductive-health/hrp/progress/63/63.pdf

Buunck, J. (1983). 'Sex differences in friendship'. *Gedrag: Tjdschchrift Voor Psychologie* 11: 111–121.

C

Canadian Catholic Health (1992). *Health Care Ethics Guide*. Ottawa: Catholic Health Association of Canada.

Carlyon, P. and Davies, J.-A. (2004). *The Shame Game*. The Bulletin, pp. 17–20.

Carrithers, M. (2001). *Buddha: A Very Short Introduction*. Oxford: Oxford University Press.

Carson, V. and Arnold, E. (2004). *Mental Health Nursing. The Health Professionals/Patient Journey*. Philadelphia: W. B. Saunders.

Chartered Society of Physiotherapy (2001). *Rules of Professional Conduct*, 2nd edn. London: CSP.

Clear, E. H. (1998). 'Hindu philosophy, Indian'. In: E. Craig (ed.). *Routledge Encyclopaedia of Philosophy*. London: Routledge. Retrieved 19/01/2006.

Cobley, R. (1995). 'A history of transplantation'. *International History of Nursing Journal* 1: 32–42.

College of Occupational Therapists (2005). *Code of Ethics and Professional Conduct*. London: COT.

Coney, S. (1988). *The Unfortunate Experiment*. Auckland: Penguin Books.

Cook, G., Gerrish, K. and Clarke, C. (2001). 'Decision making in teams: issues arising from two UK evaluations'. *Journal of Interprofessional Care* 15: 141–151.

Courtney, W. (1998). 'College men's health: An overview and a call to action'. Journal of American College Health **46**(6): 279–298.

Covey, S. R. (1989). *The Seven Habits of Highly Effective People*. New York: Free Press.

Covington, E. C. (2000). 'Psychogenic pain – what it means, why it does not exist, and how to diagnose it'. *Journal of Pain Medicine* 1: 287-294.

Craig, E. (ed.) (1998). *Routledge Encyclopaedia of Philosophy*. London: Routledge. Retrieved 13/03/2006 from http://wwww.rep.routledge.com/article/G100SECT8

Cranston, M. (1973). *What are Human Rights?* New York: Taplinger, p. 68.

D

Daniels, K. R. (1998). 'Artificial insemination, using donor sperm as an issue of secrecy: the views of donors and recipient couples'. *Social Science Medicine* **27**: 377-383.

Daniels, K. R. and Lewis, G. M. (1996). 'Donor insemination: the gifting and selling of sperm'. *Social Science Medicine* **42**: 1521-1536.

Daut, R. L., Cleeland, C. S. and Flanery, R. C. (1983). 'Development of the Wisconsin Brief Pain Questionnaire to assess pain in cancer and other diseases'. *Journal of Pain* **17**: 197-210.

Davis, D. S. (2001). *Genetic Dilemmas: Reproductive Technology, Parental Choices and Children's Futures*. New York: Routledge.

Department of Health (2001a). *Building the information core, protecting and using confidential information: a strategy for the NHS*. London: Department of Health. Retrieved 30/12/2005 from www.corec.nhs.uk

Department of Health (2001b). *Research Governance Framework for Health and Social Care*. London: Department of Health.

Department of Health (2004). *NHS Central Office for Research Ethics Committees*. London: Department of Health. Retrieved 30/12/2005 from www.corec.nhs.uk

Department of Health (2005). *NHS Research and Development Forum*. London: Department of Health. Retrieved 30/12/2005 from www.rdforum.nhs.uk

Donaldson, S. (1990). 'Rape of males'. In: W. R. Dynes (ed.) *Encyclopedia of Homosexuality*. New York: Garland Publishing.

Downie, R. S. and Calman, K. C. (1994). *Health Respect. Ethics in Health Care*, 2nd edn. Oxford: Oxford University Press.

Dwyer, C. (2005). 'Selling sperm: the internal trade in sperm'. In: H. G. Jones and M. Kirkman (eds). *Sperm Wars*. Australia: ABC Books, pp. 18-30.

E

Ebrahim, G. J. and Rankin, J. P. (1993). *Primary Health Care: Reorientating Organisational Support*. London: Macmillan.

Edelman, C. L. and Mandle, C. L. (2002). *Health Promotion Through the Lifespan*. St Louis: Mosby.

Edwards, S. (1996). *Nursing Ethics: A Principle Approach*. Basingstoke, Hampshire: Macmillan Press.

Edwards, S., Lilford, R. J. and Hewison, J. (1998). 'The ethics of randomised controlled trials from the perspectives of patients, the public and the health care professionals'. *British Medical Journal* **317**: 1209-1212.

Eisler, R. M. and Blalock, J. A. (1991). 'Masculine gender role stress: implications for the assessment of men'. *Clinical Psychology Review* **11**: 45-60.

Episcopal Conference of Mozambique (2004). *Comunicado da Conferencie Episcopal de Mocambique*. 5 August 2005. Retrieved 01/12/2005 from meninosdenampula.0catch.com/document.htm

F

Faden, R. R. and Beauchamp, T. L. (1986). *A History and Theory of Informed Consent*. New York: Oxford University Press.

Farmer, P. (2005). 'Champion of the poor'. *Time Magazine*, 7 November, p. 48.

Firsher, R. and Ury, W. (1991). *Getting to Yes*. 2nd edn. Boston: Houghton-Mifflin.

Fishman, B., Pasternak, S., Wallenstein, S. L., Houde, R. W., Holland, J. C. and Foley, K. M. (1987). 'The memorial pain assessment card. A valid instrument for the evaluation of cancer pain'. *Journal of Cancer* **60**: 1151-1158.

Frank, C. (2003). 'Determining resuscitation preferences of elderly patients: a review of the literature'. *Journal of Canadian Medical Association*. 14 October 2003.

Freeman, J. M. and McDonnell, K. (2001). *Tough Decisions: Cases in Medical Ethics*, 2nd edn. New York: Oxford University Press.

G

Galbraith, A., Bullock, S. and Manias, E. (2004). *Fundamentals of Pharmacology*, 4th edn. South Melbourne: Addison Wesley.

Galer, B. S. and Jensen, M. P. (1997). 'Development and preliminary validation of a pain measure specific to neuropathic pain: the neuropathic pain scale'. *Journal of Neurology* **48**: 332-338.

Gamsa, A. (1994). 'The role of psychological factors in chronic pain in half a century of study'. *Journal of Pain* **57**: 5-15.

Gbadegesin, S. (2001). 'Bioethics and cultural diversity'. In: H. Kuhse and P. Singer, *A Companion to Bioethics*. Oxford: Blackwell Publishing.

General Medical Council (2001). *Good Medical Practice*. London: GMC.

General Medical Council (2002). *Withholding and Withdrawing Life-Prolonging Treatments: Good Practice in Decision Making*. London: GMC.

General Osteopathic Council (2005). *Code of Practice*. London: GOsC.

General Social Care Council (2002). *Code of Practice for Social Care Workers and Code of Practice for Employers of Social Care Workers*. London: GSCC.

Gibbs, G. (1988). *Learning by Doing: A Guide to Teaching and Learning Methods*. Oxford: Further Education Unit, Oxford Polytechnic.

Gibson, H. B. (1997). 'Emotional and sexual adjustment in later life'. In: S. Arber and M. Evandrou (eds). *Aging, Independence, and the Life Course*. London: Jennifer Kingsley Publishers.

Giger, J. N. and Davidhiser, R. E. (2004). *Transcultural Nursing: Assessment and Intervention*, 4th edn. Philadelphia: Mosby, Elsevier Science.

Gillette, M. A. (2000). *Introduction to Micro-allocation*. Virginia: Bioethical Services of Virginia, Inc. Retrieved 17/10/2005 from http://www.bsvinc.com/articles/allocation/micro-allocation.htm

Gilligan, C. (1982). *In a Different Voice: Psychological Theory and Women's Development*. Cambridge, MA: Harvard University Press.

Gorman, J. and Davis, J. (2005). 'Antianxiety drugs'. In: H. Kaplan and B. Saddock (eds). *Comprehensive Textbook of Psychiatry*, 5th edn. Baltimore: Williams & Wilkins, pp. 209-231.

Grassian, V. (1992). *Moral Reasoning. Ethical Theory and Some Contemporary Moral Problems*, 2nd edn. New Jersey: Prentice Hall.

Grodin, M. A. (1992). 'Historical origins of the Nuremberg Code'. In: G. Annas and M. A. Grodin (eds). *The Nazi Doctors and the Nuremberg Code*. Oxford: Oxford University Press.

H

Hall, D. L. and Ames, R. T. (2006). *Chinese Philosophy*. In: E. Craig (ed.). *Routledge Encyclopadia of Philosophy*. London: Routledge. Retrieved 19/01/2006.

Handley, A. (1990). 'Should we resuscitate?'. *Care of the Critically Ill* **6**: 152–153.

Handy, C. (2001). *Gods of Management: The Changing Work of Organisations*. London: Arrow Buiness Books.

Hansard (2006) Column 1184. Lord Joffe. Assisted Dying for the Terminally ill Bill, House of Lords. Retrieved 18/09/2006 from http://www.publications.parliment.uk./pa/ld200506/ldhansard/vo060512/text/60512-0htm

Hanson, K. (1999). 'Measuring up: gender, burden of disease and priority setting techniques in the health sector'. http://www.hsph.harvard.edu/grh/HUpapers/gender/hanson.html

Hare, R. M. (1981). *Moral Thinking: Its Levels, Methods and Point*. Oxford: Clarendon Press.

Harper, A. (2004). 'The barriers to self-management of type 2 diabetes for people from Asian and Afro-Caribbean communities'. Unpublished MSc dissertation. Oxford: School of Health and Social Care Oxford Brookes University.

Harris, J. (1985). *The Value of Life*. London: Routledge & Kegan Paul.

Hawley, G. (1997a). 'Introduction to moral aspects of nursing practice'. In: G. Hawley (ed.). *Ethics Workbook for Nurses: Issues, Problems and Resolutions*, Chapter 1. Sydney: Social Science Press.

Hawley, G. (1997b). *Ethics Workbook for Nurses: Issues, Problems and Resolutions. Teacher's Resource*. Sydney: Social Science Press.

Hawley, G. (1997c). 'Ethical issues, principles, and theories'. In: G. Hawley (ed.). *Ethics Workbook for Nurses: Issues, Problems and Resolutions*, Chapter 3. Sydney: Social Science Press.

Hawley, G. (1997d). 'Client's rights'. In: G. Hawley (ed.). *Ethics Workbook for Nurses: Issues, Problems and Resolutions*, Chapter 5. Sydney: Social Science Press.   P82

Hawley, G. (1997e). 'Allocation of resources'. In: G. Hawley (ed.). *Ethics Workbook for Nurses: Issues, Problems and Resolutions*, Chapter 8. Sydney: Social Science Press.

Hawley, G. (1997f). 'The dying person'. In: G. Hawley (ed.). *Ethics Workbook for Nurses: Issues, Problems and Resolutions*, Chapter 6. Sydney: Social Science Press.

Hayes, R. P. (1998). 'Indian and Tibetan philosophy'. In: E. Craig (ed.). *Routledge Encyclopaedia of Philosophy*. London. Routledge. Retrieved 19/01/2006.

Health Professions Council (2004). *Standards of Conduct, Performance and Ethics*. London: Health Professions Council.

Helman, C. G. (2000). *Culture, Health and Illness*, 4th edn. Pain and culture, Chapter 7. Oxford: Butterworth–Heinemann.

Hendrick, J. (2000). *Law and Ethics in Nursing and Health Care*. Cheltenham: Nelson Thornes.

Henley, A. and Schott, J. (2002). *Culture, Religion and Patient Care in a Multi-ethnic Society: A Handbook for Professionals*. London: Age Concern.

Heyd, D. and Bloch, S. (1999). 'The ethics of suicide'. In: S. Bloch and P. Chodoff (eds). *Psychiatric Ethics*, 4th edn. Oxford: Oxford University Press, pp. 243–264.

Hodge, S. and Canter, D. (1998). 'Victims and perpetrators of male sexual assault'. *Journal of International Violence* **13**: 222–239.

Hoff Sommers, C. (2000). 'The war against boys'. The Atlantic Online. Retrieved 20/09/2006 from http://www.theatlantic.co/doc/prem/200005

Hopkins, J. and His Holiness the Dalai Lama (2002). *Advice on Dying: And Living a Better Life*. London: Random House.

Hornblum, A. M. (1997). 'They were cheap and available: prisoners as research subjects in twentieth-century America'. *British Medical Journal* **315**: 1437-1441.

Hulsey, T. (2005). 'Prenatal drug use: the ethics of testing and incarcerating pregnant women'. *Newborn Infant Nursing Review* **5**: 93-96.

Hunt, G. (ed.) (1994). *Ethical Issues in Nursing*. London: Routledge.

Hursthouse, R. (1991). 'Virtue theory and abortion'. *Philosophy and Public Affairs* **20**: 223-246.

Hursthouse, R. (1999). *On Virtue Ethics*. Oxford: Oxford University Press.

Huszczo, G. (2004). *Tools for Team Leadership*. Palo Alto, CA: Davies Black.

I

Irvine, R., Kerridge, I., McPhee, J. and Freeman, S. (2002). 'Interprofessionalism and ethics: consensus or clash of cultures?'. *Journal of Interprofessional Care* **16**: 199-210.

J

James, W. (1948). Cited by Bishop, A. and Scudder, J. (2001). *Nursing Ethics: Holistic Caring Practice*. National League of Nurses. 2nd edn. Massachusetts: Jones and Bartlett Publishers.

Jensen, T. S. (1996). 'Mechanisms of neuropathic pain'. In: J. N. Campell (ed.). *Pain 1996: An Updated Review*. Seattle, WA: IASP Press.

Jocham, H. R., Dassen, T., Widdershoven, G. and Halfens, R. (2006). 'Quality of life in palliative care cancer patients: a literature review'. *Journal of Clinical Nursing* **15**: 1188-1195.

Johns, C. (2000). *Becoming a Reflective Practitioner*. Oxford: Blackwell Science.

Johnsen, A. R. (1989). 'Ethical issues in organ transplantation'. In: R. M. Veatch (ed.). *Medical Ethics*. Boston: Jones & Bartlett Publishers, pp. 229-252.

Johnstone, M.-J. (1996). *Bioethics: A Nursing Perspective*, 2nd edn. Sydney: W. B. Saunders Bailliere Tindall.

Johnstone, M.-J. (2004). *Bioethics: A Nursing Perspective*, 3rd edn. Sydney: Churchill Livingstone.

Jones, R. (2000). 'Untapped potential: adolescents affected by armed conflict'. New York: Women's Commission for Refugee Women. Retrieved from http://www.womenscommission.org/pdf.adol2.pdf

Jonsen, A. R., Siegler, M. and Winslade, W. J. (1998). *Clinical Ethics: A Practical Approach to Ethical Decisions in Clinical Medicine*, 4th edn. New York: McGraw-Hill.

K

Kadushin, G. and Egan, M. (2001). 'Ethical dilemmas in home health care: a social work perspective'. *Health and Social Work*, **26**: 136-149.

Kalichman, S. C. (1998). *Understanding AIDS: Advances in Research and Treatment*, 2nd edn. Washington: American Psychological Association.

Kanuaha, V. (2000). 'The impact of sexuality and race/ethnicity on HIV/AIDS risk among Asian and Pacific Island American (A/PIA) gay and bisexual men in Hawaii'. *AIDS Education and Prevention* **12**: 505-518.

Kassing, L. R., Beeslay, D. and Frey, L. L. (2005). 'Gender role conflict. Homophobia, age and education as predictors of male rape myth acceptance'. *Journal of Mental Health Counseling*, October 27(4).

Kasulis, T. P. (1998). 'Japanese philosophy'. In: E. Craig (ed.). *Routledge Encyclopaedia of Philosophy*. London: Routledge. Retrieved 13/03/2006 from http://www.rep.routledge.com/article/G100SECT8

Keene, M. (2002). *World Religions*. Oxford: Lion Press.

Kemp, C. (2006). 'Brief assessment of patient/family perceptions of health problems'. University of Baylor. Retrieved 26/09/2006 from Kennedy I. and Grubb A. (2000). *Medical Law: Text and Materials*, 3rd edn. London: Butterworths.

Kennedy, Professor Ian (Chair) (2001). *Final Report: Learning from Bristol: the report of the public inquiry into children's heart surgery at Bristol Royal Infirmary 1984-1995*. CM5207. London: Department of Health.

Kerridge, I., Lowe, M. and McPhee, J. (1998). *Ethics and Law for the Health Professions*. NSW: Social Science Press.

Khan, S. (1999). 'Men and HIV: Sociocultural constructions of male sexual behaviours in South Asia'. Paper presented at the Naz Foundation, 5th International Congress on AIDS in Asia and the Pacific, Kuala Lumpur, Malaysia.

King, M., Coxell, A. and Mezey, G. (2000). 'The prevalence and characteristics of male sexual assessment. In: G. Mezey and M. King (eds). *Male Victims of Sexual Assault*. Oxford: Oxford University Press.

Kirkman, M. (2005). 'Going home and forgetting about it: donor insemination and the secrecy debate'. In: H. G. Jones and M. Kirkman (eds). *Sperm Wars*. Australia: ABC Books, pp. 153-169.

Kissane, D. W. and Kelly, B. J. (2000). 'Demoralisation, depression and desire for death: problems with the Dutch guidelines for euthanasia of the mentally ill'. *Australian and New Zealand Journal of Psychiatry* **34**: 325-333.

Knott, K. (2000). *Hinduism: A Very Short Introduction*. Oxford: Oxford University Press.

Kohlberg, L. (1980). *The Philosophy of Moral Development*. San Francisco: Harper Row.

Kohlberg, L. (1984). *Essays on Moral Development: The Psychology of Moral Development. The Nature and Validity of Moral Stages*. San Francisco, CA: Harper and Row Publishers.

Kuhn D. (2002). 'Intimacy, sexuality, and residents with dementia'. *Alzheimer's Care Quarterly* **3**: 165-176.

Kylma, J. (2005). 'Dynamics of hope in adults living with HIV/AIDS: a substantive theory'. *Journal of Advanced Nursing* **52**: 620-630. http://www3.baylor.edu/~Charles_Kemp/beliefs_assessment.html

L

Laurie, N., Dwyer, C., Holloway, S. and Smith, F. (1999). *Geographies of New Femininities*. Harlow: Longman.

Lawton, J. (2003). 'Lay experiences of health and illness: past research and future agendas'. *Sociology of Health and Illness* **25**: 23-40.

Leaman, O. (1998). 'Islamic philosophy'. In: E. Craig (ed.). *Routledge Encyclopaedia of Philosophy*. London: Routledge. Retrieved 19/01/2006.

Leininger, M. (1998). 'Culture care: diversity and universality theory'. In: A. M. Tomey and M. R. Alligood (eds). *Nursing Theorists and their Work*, 4th edn. St Louis: Mosby.

Leininger, M. and McFarland, J. (2002). *Transcultural Nursing*. 3rd edn. New York: McGraw Hill.

Lofgren-Martenson, L. (2004). '"May I?" About sexuality and love in the new generation with intellectual disabilities'. *Sexuality and Disability* **22**: 197-207.

Lott, J. P. (2005). 'Direct organ solicitation deserves reconsideration'. *Journal of Medical Ethics* **31**: 1136. Retrieved 09/11/2005 from www.jme.bmijournals.com

Lupton, D. and Barclay, L. (1997). *Constructing Fatherhood: Discourse and Experiences*. London: Sage Publications.

Lusthaus, D. (1998). 'Buddhist philosophy, Chinese'. In: E. Craig (ed.). *Routledge Encyclopaedia of Philosophy*. London: Routledge. Retrieved 19/01/2006.

M

McCray, J. (2002). 'Nursing practice in an interprofessional context'. In: Hogston, R. and Simpson, P. M. (eds). *Foundations of Nursing Practice: Making the Difference*, 2nd edn. Basingstoke: Palgrave Macmillan, pp. 449-469.

McGregor, M. (2003). 'Cost-utility analysis: use QALYs only with great caution'. *Canadian Medical Association Journal* **168**(11): 1394-1396. Retrieved from www.QALYs.

MacIntyre, A. (1985). *After Virtue: A Study of Moral Theory*. London: Duckworth.

MacLachlan, M. (1997). 'Culture and physical health'. In: *Culture and Health*. Chichester: John Wiley.

Maddox, J. (2001). 'Managed care, prospective payment and reimbursement trends. Impact and implications for nursing'. In: J. McCloskey Dochterman and H. Kennedy Grace. (eds). *Current Issues in Nursing*, 6th edn. St. Louis: Mosby, pp. 387-400.

Mandelstam, M. (2003). 'Disabled people, manual handling and human rights'. *British Journal of Occupational Therapy* **66**: 528-530.

Mappes, T. A. and Zembaty, J. S. (1991). 'Biomedical ethics and ethical theory'. In: Mappes, T. A. and Zembaty, J. S. (eds). *Biomedical Ethics*. New York: McGraw Hill.

Mappes, T. and Zembaty, J. (1997). *Biomedical Ethics*, 5th edn. New York: McGraw Hill.

Marsden, A. K., Ng, A., Dalziel, K. and Cobbe, S. M. (1995). 'When is it futile for ambulance personnel to initiate cardiopulmonary resuscitation?'. *British Medical Journal* **311**: 49-51.

Marshall, B. and Katz, S. (2002). 'Forever functional: sexual fitness and the ageing male body'. *Body and Society* **8**: 43-70.

Martin, R. S. (1989). 'Mortal values: healing pain and suffering'. In: C. S. Hill and W. S. Fields (eds). *Advances in Pain Research and Therapy*, Vol. 11. New York: Raven, pp. 19-26.

Martini, A. (1997). 'Community health nursing'. In: G. Hawley (ed.). *Ethics Workbook for Nurses: Issues, Problems and Resolutions*, Chapter 16. Sydney: Social Science Press.

Marx, W. (1992). Cited by Bishop, A. and Scudder, J. (2001). *Nursing Ethics: Holistic Caring Practice*. National League of Nurses. 2nd edn. Massachusetts: Jones and Bartlett Publishers.

Maslach, C. (2003). 'Job burnout: new direction in research and intervention'. *Current Directions in Psychological Science* **12**: 189-192.

Mason, T. (2000). 'Managing protest behaviour: from coercion to compassion'. *Journal of Psychiatric and Mental Health Nursing* **7**(3): 269-275.

Maude, P. (1996). 'The development of community mental health nursing services in Western Australia: a history (1950 to 1995) and population profile'. Unpublished Masters thesis, Edith Cowan University, Perth, Western Australia, Australia.

Maude, P. (1997). 'The person who is experiencing mental illness'. In: G. Hawley (ed.). *Ethics Workbook for Nurses: Issues, Problems and Resolutions*. Sydney: Social Science Press.

Maude, P. (1998). 'De-escalating client aggression: control or negotiation?'. In: J. Horsfall (ed.). *Violence in Nursing*. Canberra: Royal College of Health Professionals, Australia.

Maude, P. (2001). 'From lunatic to client: A history/nursing oral history of the treatment of Western Australians who experienced a mental illness: 1852 to 1989'. Doctor of Philosophy thesis, The University of Melbourne, Melbourne, Australia.

Melzack, R. (1975). 'The McGill pain questionnaire: major properties and scoring methods'. *Journal of Pain* **1**: 277-299.

Mense, S., Hohesisel, V., Kaske, A. and Reinert, A. (1997). 'Muscle pain: basic mechanisms and clinical correlates'. In: J. S. Jensen, J. A. Turner and Z. Wiesenfiled-Hallin (eds). *Proceedings of the 8th World Congress in Pain Research and Management* **8**: 479–496.

Merskey, H. (1999). 'Ethical aspects of the physical manipulation of the brain'. In: S. Bloch and P. Chodoff (eds). *Psychiatric Ethics*, 4th edn. Oxford: Oxford University Press, pp. 185-214.

Merskey, H. M. and Bogduk, N. (1994). *Classification of Chronic Pain*, 2nd edn. Seattle, WA: IASP Press.

Mezirow, J. (1991). 'Transformative dimensions of adult learning'. San Francisco, CA: Jossey-Bass Publishers.

Milner, A. (1991). *Contemporary Cultural Theory: An Introduction*. Sydney: Allen & Unwin.

Misuse of Drugs Regulations (2001). In: British Formularly (2006). *Controlled Drugs and Drug Dependence*. Oxford: Pharmaceutical Press.

Mitchell, K., Kerridge, I. H. and Lovat, T. J. (1996) *Bioethics and Clinical Ethics for Health Care Professionals*, 2nd edn. Sydney: Social Science Press.

Moons, P., Budts, W. and De Geest, S. (2006). 'Critique on the conceptualisation of quality of life: a review and evaluation of different conceptual approaches'. *International Journal of Nursing Studies* **43**: 891–901.

Moore, S. L. (2005). 'Hope makes a difference'. *Journal of Psychiatric and Mental Health Nursing* **12**: 100-105.

Mosby's Dictionary (2006). *Medical, Nursing and Allied Health*. St Louis: Mosby Elsevier.

Morley, J. (2004). 'The aging man and woman: are the differences important?'. *Journal of Men's Health and Gender* 1: 224-226.

Mueller, P. and Korey, W. (1998). 'Death by "ecstasy": the serotonin syndrome?'. *Annals of Emergency Medicine* September, 377-380.

Muir Gray, J. A. (2001). *Evidence-Based Healthcare*. 2nd edn. Edinburgh: Churchill Livingstone.

Munro, A. (2000). 'The allocation of health services resources'. In: Scottish economic report. Edinburgh: Scottish NHS. Retrieved 11/10/2005 from www.Scotland.gov.uk/library

Murphy, T. F. and White, G. B. (2005). 'Dead sperm donors or world hunger: are bioethicists studying the right stuff?'. *The Hastings Center Report* **35**: 2.

Murray, C. J. L. (1994). 'Qualifying the global burden of disease: the technical basis for disability-adjusted life years'. *Bulletin of the World Health Organisation* **72**: 495-501.

N

Naidoo, J. and Wills, J. (2005). *Public Health and Health Promotion: Developing Practice*. London: Bailliere Tindall.

Narayanasamy, A. (2001). *Spiritual Care: A Practical Guide for Nurses and Health Care Practitioners*. 2nd edn. Dinton, Wiltshire: Quay Books.

Nather, A. (2004). *Legal, Religious and other Regulatory Aspects of Tissue Transplantation in Asia Pacific Region*. National University Hospital, Korea. National training course 1-3 December 2004. Retrieved 04/12/2005 from www.admin.koreahospital.com/user/katb/databbs/5-Aziz.pdf

Nazroo, J. Y. (1997). *The Health of Britain's Ethnic Minority*. London: Policy Studies Institute.

NHMRC (1999). 'Ethical considerations regulating to health care resources allocation decisions'. Canberra: NHMRC. Retrieved 11/10/2005 from www.nhmrc.gov.au/publications/synopsis/files/e24pdf

Nieto, S. (2004). *Affirming Diversity: The Sociopolitical Context of Multicultural Education*. Boston: Pearson/Allen & Bacon.

Nietzche, F. (1972). *Beyond Good and Evil*. Middlesex: Penguin Books.

Nigam, M. (1997). 'Culture and care'. In: G. Hawley (ed.). *Ethics Workbook for Nurses: Issues, Problems and Resolutions*, Chapter 2. Sydney: Social Science Press.

Nigam, M. and Hawley, G. (1997). 'Culture and care'. In: G. Hawley (ed.). *Ethics Workbook for Nurses: Issues, Problems and Resolutions*. Teacher's Resource, Section 2. Sydney: Social Science Press.

Noddings, N. (1984). *Caring: A Feminist Approach to Ethics and Morality of Education*. Los Angeles: University of California Press.

Nursing and Midwifery Council (2004). *The NMC Code of Professional Conduct: Standards for Conduct Performance and Ethics*. London: NMC.

O

Oberle, K. and Hughes, D. (2001). 'Doctors' and nurses' perceptions of ethical problems in end-of-life decisions'. *Journal of Advanced Nursing* **33**: 705-715.

Okin, S. (1987). 'Justice and gender'. *Philosophy and Public Affairs* **16**: 42-72.

O'Rourke, K. D. and Boyle, P. (1989). *Medical Ethics: Sources of Catholic Teachings*. St Louis: Catholic Health Association of United States of America.

Ovadia, F. and Owen, A. (1992). 'Mental health and primary care'. In: F. Baum, D. Fry and I. Lennie (eds). *Community Health: Policy and Practice in Australia*. Bondi Junction: Pluto Press, pp. 182-188.

P

Papadopoulos, I. (ed.) (2006). *Transcultural Health and Social Care: Development of Culturally Competent Practitioners*. Oxford: Churchill Livingstone-Elsevier.

Papadopoulos, I., Tilki, M. and Taylor, G. (1998). *Transcultural Care: A Guide for Health Professionals*. Dinton: Quay Books.

Parkes, C. M. (1986). *Bereavement*. London: Penguin.

Paxton, S., Gonzales, G., Uppahew, K., Abraham, K., Okta, S., Green, C., Thephthien, B., Maria, M. and Quisada, A. (2005). *Aids Care* **17**: 413-424.

Payne, M. (2000). *Teamwork in Multiprofessional Care*. Basingstoke: Palgrave.

Pector, E. A. (2005). 'Ethical issues of high order multiple births'. *Newborn Infant Nurses Review* **5**: 69-76.

Peele, R. (1999). 'The ethics of deinstitutionalisation'. In: S. Bloch and P. Chodoff (eds). *Psychiatric Ethics*, 4th edn. Oxford: Oxford University Press, pp. 291-312.

Pellegrino, E. (1991). 'Trust and distrust in professional ethics'. In: E. Pellegrino, R. Veatch and J. Langan (eds). *Ethics, Trust, and the Professions: Philosophical and Cultural Aspects*. Washington DC: Georgetown University Press.

Peplau, E. (1998). 'Psychodynamic nursing'. In: A. Marriner Tooney and M. Alligood (eds). *Nursing Theorists and Their Work*. St Louis: Mosby.

Pfeiffer, J. (2004). 'Condom social marketing, Pentacostalism, and structural adjustment in Mozambique: a clash of AIDS prevention messages'. *Medical Anthropology Quarterly Washington* **18**: 77-103.

Pillitteri, A. (ed.) (1999). *Maternal and Child Health Nursing*, 3rd edn. Philadelphia: Lippincott.

Portenoy, R. K. (1991). 'Issues in the management of neuropathic pain'. In: A. Basbaum and J.-M. Besson (eds). *Towards a New Pharmocotherapy of Pain*. Chichester: John Wiley, pp. 393-416.

Portenoy, R. K. and Kanner, R. M. (1996a). 'Definition and assessment of pain'. In: R. K. Portenoy and R. M. Kanner (eds). *Pain Management: Theory and Practice*, Chapter 6. Philadelphia, PA: F. A. Davis.

Portenoy, R. K. and Kanner, R. M. (1996b). 'Pain management'. In: R. K. Portenoy and R. M. Kanner (eds). *Pain Management: Theory and Practice*, Chapter 7. Philadelphia, PA: F. A. Davis.

Potts, A. (2005). 'Cyborg masculinity in the Viagra era'. *Sexualities, Evolution and Gender* 7: 3-16.

Purtillo, R. (1990). *Health Professional and Patient Interaction*. Philadelphia, PN: Saunders.

R

Ranney, D. (2001). *The Anatomy of Pain*. Paper presented at the Ontario Inter-Urban Pain Conference. University of Waterloo 29/11/1996. Updated 30/10/2001. Retrieved 24/02/2006 from http://www.ahs.uwaterloo.ca/~ranney/painanat.html

Rawls, J. A. (1971). *A Theory of Justice*. Cambridge, MA: Harvard University Press.

Rees, N. (1997). 'Moral aspects of pain and pain management'. In: G. Hawley (ed.). *Ethics Workbook for Nurses: Issues, Problems and Resolutions*. Sydney: Social Science Press.

Report of the Cervical Cancer Inquiry (1988). Prepared by the Committee of Inquiry into Allegations Concerning the Treatment of Cervical Cancer at National Women's Hospital and Other Related Matters. Auckland: Government Printing Office.

Report of The Royal Liverpool Children's Inquiry (2001). London: Ministry of the Crown Publishing. Retrieved 08/09/2006 from http://rlcinquiry.org./uk

Reynolds, M. A. and Schieve, L. A. (2003). 'Trends in multiple births conceived using assisted reproductive technology'. *Pediatrics* 111: 1159-1162.

Robinson, S. (Rev.) (2005). *Ethics and Employability. Learning and Employability Series 2*. York: The Higher Education Academy.

Robinson, D. S. and McKenna, H. P. (1998). 'Loss: an analysis of a concept of particular interest to nursing'. *Journal of Advanced Nursing* 27: 779-784.

Rogers, W. H., Wittick, H. M. and Ashburn, M. A. (2000). 'Using the "TOPS", an outcomes instrument for multidisciplinary outpatient pain treatment'. *Journal of Pain Medicine* 1: 55-67.

Royal College of Nursing (1996). *The RCN Code of Practice for Patient Handling*. London: RCN.

S

Sabo, D. (1999). *Understanding Men's Health: A Relational and Gender Sensitive Approach*. hppt://www.hsph.harvard.edu/grh/HUpapers/gender/sabo.html

Sanger, A. (2004). *Beyond Choice*. New York: Public Affairs.

Santhya, K. G. and Verma, S. (2004). 'Induced abortion: the current scenario in India'. *Regional Health Forum* 8: 1-14.

Schechtman, M. (1990). 'Personhood and personal identity'. *The Journal of Philosophy* 87: 71-92.

Scheper-Hughes, N. (2005). 'Police hunt for masterminds of cash-for-kidney scandal'. *The Standard*. Monday, 22 August 2005. Retrieved 01/12/2005 from www.eastandard.net/archives/cl/hm_news/news.php?articleid=27667&date=22/8/2005

Schwartz, D. A. (2004). 'Postmortem sperm retrieval: an ethical analysis'. *Clinical Excellence in Nursing Practice* 8: 183-188.

Schwartz, L. L. (2003). 'A nightmare for King Solomon: the new reproductive technologies'. *Journal of Family Psychology* 17: 229-237.

Scott, S. (2001). *Out of the Shadows*. Dorset: Russel Lane.

Sculenberg, J., Maggs, J. L. and Hurrelman, K. (eds) (1999). *Health Risks and Developmental Transitions During Adolescence*. New York: Cambridge University Press.

Sealy, R. (2004). 'Speaking out. One patient's search for antidotes to nihilism in psychiatry'. *Psychiatric Rehabilitation Journal* **27**: 291-294.

Settelmaier, E. (2002). 'Exploring the efficacy of dilemma stories as a way of addressing ethical issues in science education'. Western Australian Institute for Educational Research, Edith Cowan University, Mt. Lawley, WA.

Settelmaier, E. (2003). 'Transforming the culture of teaching and learning in science: the promise of moral dilemma stories'. *Science and Mathematics Education Centre*. Perth, Australia, Curtin University of Technology, p. 416.

Singleton, J. and McLaren, S. (1995). *Ethical Foundations of Health Care: Responsibilties in Decision Making*. London: Mosby.

Sleath, B., Svarstad, B. and Roter, D. (1998). 'Patient race and psychotropic prescribing during medical encounters'. *Patient Education and Counselling* **34**: 227-238.

Spross, J. A. (1985). 'Cancer pain and suffering: clinical lessons from life, literature and legend'. *Journal of Oncology Nurse Forum* **12**: 23-31.

Statman, D. (1997). *Virtue Ethics: A Critical Reader*. Edinburgh: Edinburgh University Press.

Staunton, P. and Chiarella, M. (2004). *Nursing and the Law*, 5th edn. Sydney: Churchill Livingstone.

Staunton, P. and Whyburn, B. (1997). *Nursing and the Law*, 4th edn. Sydney: W. B. Saunders-Bailliere Tindall.

Steinberg, A. (2003). 'Abortion of CNS malformations; religious aspects'. *Childs Nervous System* **19**: 592-595.

Stroebe, M. and Schut, H. (1999). 'The dual process model of coping with bereavement: rationale and description'. *Death Studies* **23**: 197-224.

T

TC Health Administration Pty Ltd (2001). *An Introduction. Diagnosis Related Groups (DRGs) Medical Record Coding and Casemix Management. 'Preparing your Hospital'*. TC Health Administration Pty Ltd: South Australia. Retrieved 29/09/2006 from http://www.casemix.com.au

Terry, L. (2007). 'Ethics and contemporary challenges in health and social care'. In: A. Leathard and S. McLaren, *Ethics: Contemporary Challenges in Health and Social Care*. Bristol: The Policy Press.

Terry, L. M. P. (2001). 'Saying no: Withholding and withdrawing life-prolonging treatment from non-PVS patients'. Unpublished PhD dissertation, Bristol: University of Bristol.

Tiefer, L. (1987). 'In pursuit of the perfect penis - the medicalisation of male sexuality'. In: M. S. Kimmel (ed.). *Changing Men: New Directions on Research on Men and Masculinity*. California: Sage Publications.

The Royal Commission Inquiry into Chelmsford Hospital. Report of the Royal Commission into Deep Sleep Therapy (1990). Sydney: Government Printing Office.

Thomas, K. and Kilmann, R. (2002). *Thomas Kilmann Conflict Mode Instrument*. Palo Alto, CA: Davies Black.

Thompson, I. E., Melia, K. M. and Boyd, K. M. (1992). *Nursing Ethics*, 2nd edn. Edinburgh: Churchill Livingstone.

Thornycroft, S. (2006). 'The long-ruling despot is to stage a lavish party as his nation collapes around him'. *The West Australian*, 23 February, West Australian Newspapers Pty Ltd.

Tollison, C. D., Satterthwaithe, J. R. and Tollison, J. W. (eds) (2002). *Practical Pain Management*, 3rd edn. Philadelphia, PA: Lippincott Williams & Wilkins, pp. 720-759.

U

University of Minnesota's Center for Bioethics (2004). 'Ethics for organ transplantation'. Retrieved 09/11/2005 from www.bioethics.umn.edu

V

Van Delvin, J. J. M., Wrakking, A. M., van der Heide, A. and van der Maas, P. J. (2004). 'Medical decision making in scarcity situations'. *Journal of Medical Ethics* 30: 207-211. Retrieved 21/10/2005 from www.jmejjournals.com

Van Gelder, S. (2005). 'Making sense of health care'. In context. A Quarterly of Humane Sustainable Culture. Retrieved 02/12/2005 from http://www.context.org/ICLIB/IC39/vanGldr.htm

Vearnelo, S. and Campbell, T. (2001). 'Male victims of male sexual assault: a review of psychological consequences and treatment'. *Sexual and Relationship Therapy* 16: 279-286.

Veatch, R. M. (1989). *Cross Cultural Perspectives in Medical Ethics: Readings*. Boston: Jones, Bartlett Publishers.

Victoria Climbie Inquiry. 'Report of the Victoria Climbie Inquiry' (2001). London: Crown Law. Archived transcript for 09/10/2001. Retrieved 22/12/05 from http://www.victoria-climbie-inquiry.org.uk/Evidence/Archive/Oct01/09100latestp1.htm

W

Waithe, M. E. (1989). 'Twenty-three hundred years of women philosophers: toward a gender differentiated moral theory'. In: M. M. Braback (ed.). *Who Cares? Theory, Research, and Educational Implications of the Ethic of Care*. New York: Praeger.

Wallace, M. (1995). *Health Care and the Law*, 2nd edn. Sydney: The Law Book Company.

Wallace, M. (2001). *Health Care and the Law*, 4th edn. Melbourne: Thomson Legal & Regulatory-Asia Pacific.

Warnock, M. (2002). *Making Babies. Is There a Right Way to have Children?* Oxford: Oxford University Press.

Watson, G. (1997). 'On the primacy of character'. In: D. Statman (ed.). *Virtue Ethics: A Critical Reader*. Edinburgh: Edinburgh University Press.

Wells, M., Dryden, H., Guild, P., Levack, P., Farrer, K. and Mowat, P. (2001). 'The knowledge and attitudes of surgical staff towards the use of opioids in cancer pain management: can the hospital palliative care team make a difference?' *European Journal of Cancer Care* 10: 201-211.

WHO (1978). 'United Nations International Children's Emergency Fund 1978 Primary Care'. Report of the International Conference on Primary Health Care. Alma Ata: WHO.

WHO (1999). 'Abortion in the developing world'. Press release 17 May. http://www.who.int/inf-pr-1999/en/pr99-28.html

WHO (2003). 'Health resources'. Retrieved 11/10/2005 from www.whosea.org

WHO (2005). 'Report on transmission and effects of HIV/AIDS'. Alma Ata: WHO.

WHO (2006). 'United Nations Report on Child Abuse'. Retrieved 10/10/2006 from http://www.violencestudy/IMG/pdf/English.pdf

Williams, A. (2005). 'Thinking about equity in health care'. *Journal of Nursing Management* **13**: 397–402.

Williams, B. (1985). *Ethics and the Limits of Philosophy*. London: Fontana/Collins.

Worden, W. (1991). *Grief Counselling and Grief Therapy: a Handbook for the Mental Health Practitioner*. London: Routledge.

World Bank (2001). 'World Development Report'. Retrieved 18/01/2007 from www.worldbank.org./ WEBSITE/EXTERNAL/DATASTATISTICS/0,,contentMDK:2042058~menupk:64133156~piPK: 64133175~thesitePK:239419,00.html

Wright, D. (1971). *The Psychology of Moral Behaviour*. Middlesex: Penguin Books.

Y

Yoder-Wise, P. S. and Kowalski, K. E. (2006). *Beyond Leading and Managing: Nursing Administration for the Future*. St Louis: Mosby Elsevier.

Z

Zanner, K. (1993). In: A. Bishop and J. Scudder (2001). *Nursing Ethics: Holistic Caring Practice*. National League of Nurses. 2nd edn. Massachusetts: Jones and Bartlett Publishers.

Complementary reading

The complementary reading that we have listed below come from chapters of books, journal articles or an internet site. These either:

- reflect the meaning; or
- enable you to read more about one of the topics in the chapter.

Please be aware that this complementary reading should not take the place of your own search for additional reading. What is listed (and chosen by the authors) for each of the chapters is just a small example of what is currently available in libraries and the internet.

Codes of practice

Chartered Society of Physiotherapists (2001). *Rules of Professional Conduct*. 2nd edn. London: CSP.

College of Occupational Therapists (2005). *Code of Ethics and Professional Conduct*. London: COT.

General Medical Council (2001). *Good Medical Practice*. London: GMC.

General Osteopathic Council (2005). *Code of Practice*. London: GOsC.

General Social Care Council (2002). *Code of Practice for Social Care Workers and Code of Practice for Employers of Social Care Workers*. London: GSCC.

Health Professions Council (2004). *Standards of Conduct, Performance and Ethics*. London: Health Professions Council.

Nursing and Midwifery Council (2004). *The NMC Code of Professional Conduct: Standards for Conduct Performance and Ethics*. London: NMC.

Chapter 1 Start at Go!

If you would like to learn more about reflection try Rolfe, G., Freshwater, D. and Jasper, M. (2001). *Critical Reflection for Nursing: A Users Guide*. Basingstoke: Palgrave Macmillan.

If you would like to get a feel for bioethics try reading some of the articles in *The Hastings Center Report*. This journal is published by one of the world's most important bioethics centres. The name of the journal is that of the centre, that is, The Hastings Center. Read any of the issues of the journal and you will find the articles fascinating.

If you would like to know more about interprofessional care, try the book written by Barret, G., Sellman, D. and Thomas, J. (2005). *Interprofessional Working in Health and Social Care*. Basingstoke: Palgrave Macmillan.

If you would like to know more about cultural sensitive care, try the book written by Papadopoulos, I., Tikki, M. and Taylor, G. (1998). *Transcultural Care: A Guide for Health Professionals*. Dinton: Quay Books.

If you would like to know more about the multicultural and multidisciplinary approach to health care there is an online magazine that you can access: www.themedicalnetwork.org

Chapter 2 Values, and culture

The BBC has an various sites for culture and religion. These can be accessed at www.bbc.co.uk/religions

Davidhizer, R., Dowd, S. and Giger, J. (1998). 'Educating the culturally diverse healthcare student'. *Nurse Educator* **23**(2) March/April.

Klessig, J. (1992). 'Cross-cultural medicine a decade later: the effect of values and culture on life-support decisions'. *Western Journal of Medicine* September **157**: 316-322.

Lawton, J. (2003). 'Lay experiences of health and illness: past research and future agendas'. *Sociology of Health and Illness* **25**(3): 23-40.

Leininger, M. and McFarland, M. (2002). *Transcultural Nursing*, 3rd edn. New York: McGraw Hill.

Papadopoulos, I., Tikki, M. and Taylor, G. (1998). *Transcultural Care: A Guide for Health Professionals*. Dinton: Quay Books.

Chapter 3 Ethical issues

Bishop, A. and Scuder, J. (2001). *Nursing Ethics Holistic Caring Practice*. 2nd edn. National League for Nurses. Massachusetts: Jones and Bartlett Publishers.

Bramley, S. and Cockshutt, G. (2005). 'Listening, not just talking'. *Occupational Therapy News* **13**(5): 24-25.

Dyson, S. and Smaje, C. (2001). 'The health status of minority ethnic groups'. In: L. Cully and S. Dyson (eds). *Ethnicity and Nursing Practice*. Buckingham: Palgrave Publishing.

Dyer, C. (2002a, Wednesday 20 March). Diane Pretty makes final 'death with dignity' plea. *Guardian*. Access from http://society.guardian.co.uk/print/0,3858,4377648-105965,00.html

Dyer, C. (2002b, Saturday 23 March). Paralysed woman wins right to die. *Guardian*. Access from http://www.guardian.co.uk/print/0,3858,4380281-103690,00.html

Hendrick, J. (2000). *Law and Ethics in Nursing and Health Care*. Cheltenham: Nelson Thornes Ltd.

Chapter 4 Client and patient rights

Kissane, D. W. and Kelly, B. J. (2000). 'Demoralisation, depression and desire for death: problems with the Dutch guidelines for euthanasia of the mentally ill'. *Australian and New Zealand Journal of Psychiatry* **34**: 325-333.

Larcher, V. (1999). 'Role of clinical ethics committees'. *Archives of Disease in Childhood* **81**: 104-106.

Maslach, C. (2003). 'Job burnout: new direction in research and intervention', *Current Directions in Psychological Science* **12**(5): 189-192.

Pang, M. S. (1999). 'Protective truthfulness: the Chinese way of safeguarding patients in informed treatment decisions'. *Journal of Medical Ethics* **25**: 247-253.

There is a massive collection of information on alternative medicine, complementary therapy and natural health care at www.internethealthlibrary.com

The journal of nursing ethics can be accessed at www.nursing-ethics.com

World Health Organisation (2003). Health resources. Access from www.whosea.org

Chapter 5 Western philosophy

Beachamp, T. L. and Childress, J. K. (2001). *Principles of Biomedical Ethics*. 5th edn. Oxford: Oxford University Press.

Gillon, R. (2003). 'Ethics needs principles – four can encompass the rest – and respect for auto-nomy "should be the first among equals"'. *Journal of Medical Ethics* **29**: 307-312.

Johnston, M.-J. (1996). *Bioethics: A Nursing Perspective*. Chapter 4. Sydney: W. B. Saunders.

Noddings, N. (1984). *Caring: A Feminist Approach to Ethics and Morality of Education*. Los Angeles: University of California Press.

Chapter 6 Eastern philosophy

Craig, E. (ed.) (1998). *Routledge Encyclopaedia of Philosophy*. London: Routledge Publishing. Access from www.rep.rputledge.com

Information about the safe and effective use of complementary medicines can be found at *Prince of Wales Foundation for Integrated Health* and accessed at www.fimed.org

Knott, K. (2000). *Hinduism: A Very Short Introduction*. Oxford: Oxford University Press.

Ruthven, M. (1997). *Islam: A Very Short Introduction*. Oxford: Oxford University Press.

Sheikh, A. and Gatrad, A. R. (2000). *Caring for Muslim Patients*. Oxford: Radcliffe Medical Press.

Chapter 7 Team work

Csikai, E. L. (2004). 'Social workers' participation in the resolution of ethical dilemmas in hospice care'. *Health and Social Work* **29**: 67-76.

Irvine, R., Kerridge, I., McPhee, J. and Freeman, S. (2002). 'Interprofessionalism and ethics: consensus or clash of cultures?' *Journal of Interprofessional Care* **16**: 199-210.

Goodman, B. (2004). 'Ms B and legal competence: interprofessional collaboration and nurse autonomy'. *Nursing in Critical Care 2004* **9**: 271-276.

Healy, T. C. (2003). 'Ethical decision-making: pressure and uncertainty as complicating factors'. *Health and Social Work* **28**: 293-301.

Shoefield, R. F. and Amodeo, M. (1999). 'Interdisciplinary teams in health care and human services settings'. *Health & Social Work* **24**: 210-219.

Victoria Climbe Inquiry (2001). Access from www.victoria-climbie-inquiry.org.uk

Chapter 8 Pain and resuscitation

Blackhall, L. J., Frank, G., Murphy, S. T., Michel, V., Palmer, J. M. and Azen, S. P. (1999). 'Ethnicity and attitudes towards life sustaining technology'. *Social Science and Medicine* **48**: 1779-1789.

Oberle K. and Hughes, D. (2001) 'Doctors' and nurses' perceptions of ethical problems in end-of-life decisions'. Journal of Advanced Nursing 33: 705-715.

Sheikh, A. and Gatrad, A. R. (2000). *Caring for Muslim Patients*. Chapter 8. Oxford: Radcliffe Medical Press.

The national discussion forum and community for UK health care professionals with an interest in acute, chronic, or palliative pain management. Access from www.pain-talk.co.uk

The Pain Society is the representative body for all professionals involved in the management and understanding of pain in the United Kingdom. Access from www.painsociety.org

Thompson, T. D. B., Barbour, R. S. and Schwartz, L. (2003). Health professionals' views on advance directives: a qualitative interdisciplinary study. *Palliative Medicine* **17**: 403-409.

Wells, M., Dryden, H., Guild, P., Levack, P., Farrer, K. and Mowat, P. (2001). 'The knowledge and attitudes of surgical staff towards the use of opioids in cancer pain management: can the hospital palliative care team make a difference?' *European Journal of Cancer Care* **10**: 201-211.

Chapter 9 Illness and loss

Davies, E. and Higginson, I. J. (eds) (2004). *The Solid Facts: Palliative Care*. Copenhagen: World Health Organization Europe.

Kylma, J. (2005). 'Dynamics of hope in adults living with HIV/AIDS: a substantive theory'. *Journal of Advanced Nursing* **52**(6): 620-630.

Moore, S. L. (2005). 'Hope makes a difference'. *Journal of Psychiatric and Mental Health Nursing* **12**: 100-105.

Murray, J. A. (2001). 'Loss as a universal concept: a review of the literature to identify common aspects of loss in diverse situations'. *Journal of Loss and Trauma* **6**: 219-241.

Stroebe, M. and Schut, H. (1999). 'The dual process model of coping with bereavement: rationale and description'. *Death Studies* **23**(3): 197-224.

The National Cancer Institute can be accessed at www.cancernet.nci.nih.gov

Chapter 10 Decision making

Cook, G., Gerrish, K. and Clarke, C. (2001). 'Decision making in teams: issues arising from two UK evaluations'. *Journal of Interprofessional Care* **15**: 141-151.

An internet site regarding ethical decision making can be accessed at www.ethics - network.org.uk

Healy, T. C. (2003). 'Ethical decision making: pressure and uncertainty as complicating factors'. *Health and Social Work* **28**: 293-301.

Van Delvin, J. J. M., Wrakking, A. M., van der Heide, A. and van der Maas, P. J. (2004). 'Medical decision making in scarcity situation'. *Journal of Medical Ethics* **30**: 207-211.

Jonsen, A. R., Siegler, M. and Winslade, W. J. (1998). *Clinical Ethics: A Practical Approach to Ethical Decisionmaking in Clinical Medicine*. 4th edn. New York: McGraw-Hill, Inc.

The website www.blackwellnursing.com promotes evidence based nursing practice by supporting worldwide research, clinical practice and professional development.

Chapter 11 Primary care

Blackie, C. (ed.) (2000). *Community Health Care Nursing*. London: Churchhill Livingston.

Community Health Services website http://www.cre.gov.uk/gdpract/health_care_cop_def.html

Edelman, C. L. and Mandle, C. L. (2002). *Health Promotion Through the Lifespan*. St Louis: Mosby.

Helman, C. G. (2001). *Culture Health and Illness*. 4th edn. London: Arnold Hodder Headline Group.

Henley, A. and Schott, J. (2000). *Culture, Religion and Patient Care in a Multi-ethnic Society: A Handbook for Professionals*. London: Age Concern.

Williams, A. (2005). 'Thinking about equity in health care'. *Journal of Nursing Management* **13**(5): 397-402.

Chapter 12 Mental health

Psychology and Mental Health Information. The psychology web directory for mental health professional, students, and those wanting assistance or seeking to know more about the areas of mental health can be accessed at www.psychnet-uk.com

The UK's senior psychiatry journal can be accessed at wwww.bjp.co.uk

Bancroft, J. (1999). 'Ethical aspects of sexuality and sex therapy'. In: S. Bloch and P. Chodoff (eds). *Psychiatric Ethics*. 4th edn. Oxford: Oxford University Press, pp. 215-242.

Kuhn, D. (2002). 'Intimacy, sexuality, and residents with dementia'. *Alzheimer's Care Quarterly* **3**(2): 165-176.

Brown, P. (1999). 'Ethical aspects of drug treatment'. In: S. Bloch and P. Chodoff (eds). *Psychiatric Ethics*. 4th edn. Oxford: Oxford University Press, pp. 167-184.

Carson, V. and Arnold, E. (2004). *Mental Health Nursing. The Health Professionals/Patient Journey*. Philadelphia: W. B. Saunders.

Gorman, J. and Davis, J. (2005). 'Antianxiety drugs'. In: H. Kaplan and B. Saddock. *Comprehensive Textbook of Psychiatry*. 5th edn. Baltimore: Williams & Wilkins, pp. 209-231.

Heyd, D. and Bloch, S. (1999). 'The ethics of suicide'. In: S. Bloch and P. Chodoff (eds). *Psychiatric Ethics*. 4th edn. Oxford: Oxford University Press, pp. 243-264.

Merskey, H. (1999). 'Ethical aspects of the physical manipulation of the brain'. In: S. Bloch and P. Chodoff (eds). *Psychiatric Ethics*. 4th edn. Oxford: Oxford University Press, pp. 185-214.

Peele, R. (1999). 'The ethics of deinstitutionalisation'. In: S. Bloch and P. Chodoff (eds). *Psychiatric Ethics*. 4th edn. Oxford: Oxford University Press, pp. 291-312.

Chapter 13 Complex care

British Medical Association (2001). *Withholding and Withdrawing Life-prolonging Medical Treatment: Guidance for Decision Making,* 2nd edn. London: BMA.

General Medical Council (2002). *Withholding and Withdrawing Life-prolonging Treatments: Good Practice in Decision-making*. London: General Medical Council.

Marsden, A. K., Ng, A., Dalziel, K. and Cobbe, S. M. (1995). 'When is it futile for ambulance personnel to initiate cardiopulmonary resuscitation?' *British Medical Journal* **311**(6996): pp. 49-51.

Maslach C. (2003). 'Job burnout: new directions in research and intervention'. *Current Directions in Psychological Science* **12**(5): 189-192.

Tassano, F. (1995). *The Power of Life or Death: a Critique of Medical Tyranny*. London: Duckworth.

Terry, L. (2007). 'Ethics and Contemporary Challenges in Health and Social Care'. In: A. Leathard and S. Mclaren (eds). *Ethics: Contemporary Challenges in Health and Social Care*. Bristol: Policy Press.

Chapter 14 Allocation of resources and organ transplantation

Arras, J. D. and Steinbock, B. (1995). 'Allocation, social justice and health policy'. In: J. D. Aras and B. Steinbock. *Ethical Issues in Modern Medicine*. 4th edn. Mountain View, Ca: Mayfield Publishing Company, pp. 585-592.

Asthana, S., Gibson, A., Moon, G., Dicker, J. and Brigham, P. (2004). 'The pursue in NHS resource allocation: Should morbidity replace utilization as the basis for setting health care capitations?' *Social Science & Medicine* **58**(3): 539-551.

Gillette, M. A. (2000). *Introduction to Micro-allocation*. Virginia: Bioethical Services of Virginia, Inc. Access from www.bsvinc.com/articles/allocation/micro-allocation.htm

Lott, J. P. (2005). 'Direct organ solicitation deserves reconsideration'. *Journal of Medical Ethics* **31**: 1136. Access from www.jme.bmijournals.com

University of Minnesota Center of Bioethics (2004). Ethics for Organ Transplantation. Access from ww.bioethics.umn.edu

Van Delvin, J. J. M., Wrakking, A. M., van der Heide, A. and van der Maas, P. J. (2004). 'Medical decision making in scarcity situation'. *Journal of Medical Ethics* **30**: 207-211.

Chapter 15 Sexuality

Alesi, R. (2005). 'Infertility and its treatment: an emotional roller coaster'. *Australian Family Physician* **34**(3): 135-138.

King, M., Coxell, A. and Mezey, G. (2000). 'The prevalence and characteristics of male sexual assessment'. In: G. Mezey and M. King (eds). *Male Victims of Sexual Assault*. Oxford: Oxford University Press.

Kirkman, M. (2005). 'Going home and forgetting about it: donor insemination and the secrecy debate'. In: H. G. Jones and M. Kirkman (eds). *Sperm Wars*. Australia: ABC Books, pp. 153-169.

Murphy, T. F. and White, G. B. (2005). 'Dead sperm and world hunger: are bioethicists studying the rights stuff?' *The Hastings Center Report* **35**: 2.

Pector, E. A. (2005). 'Ethical issues of high order multiple births'. *Newborn Infant Nurses Review* **5**(2): 69-76.

Schwartz, D. A. (2004). 'Postmortem sperm retrieval: an ethical analysis'. *Clinical Excellence in Nursing Practice* **8**(4): 183-188.

Vearnelo, S. and Campbell, T. (2001). 'Male victims of male sexual assault: A review of psychological consequences and treatment'. *Sexual and Relationship Therapy* **16**(3): 279-286.

Warnock, M. (2002). *Making Babies. Is There a Right Way to have Children*? UK: Oxford University Press.

Chapter 16 Research

Braunholz, D. A., Edwards, S. J. L. and Lilford, R. J. (2001). 'Are clinical trials good for us (in the short term?) Evidence for a "trial effect"'. *Journal of Clinical Epidemiology* **54**: 217-224.

Department of Health (2005). NHS Central Office for Research Ethics Committees. Access at www.corec.nhs.uk

Department of Health (2005). NHS Research and Development Forum. Access at www.rdforum. nhs.uk

Edwards, S., Lilford, R. J. and Hewison, J. (1998). 'The ethics of randomised controlled trials from the perspective of patients, the public and the health care professionals'. *British Medical Journal* **317**: 1209-1212.

Grodin, M. A. (1992). 'Historical origins of the Nuremberg Code'. In: G. Annas and M. A. Grodin. *The Nazi Doctors and the Nuremberg Code*. Oxford: Oxford University Press.

Hornblum, A. M. (1997). '"They were cheap and available": prisoners as research subjects in Twentiest Century America'. *British Medical Journal* **315**: 1437-1441.

O'Neill, O. (2003). 'Some limits of informed consent'. *Journal of Medical Ethics* **29**: 4-7.

Chapter 17 It isn't easy, but it is essential!

Freeman, J. M. and McDonnell, K. (2001). *Tough Decisions: Cases in Medical Ethics*: 2nd edn. New York: Oxford University Press.

Jonsen, A. R., Siegler, M. and Winslade, W. J. (1998). *Clinical Ethics: A Practical Approach to Ethical Decisionmaking in Clinical Medicine*. 4th edn. New York: McGraw-Hill, Inc.

Papadopoulos, I., Tikki, M. and Taylor, G. (1998). *Transcultural Care: A Guide for Health Professionals*. Dinton: Quay Books.

Richardson, R. (2006). 'Justice and sustainability in health care'. *Bulletin of Medical Ethics* March **213**: 15-28.

Van Delvin, J. J. M., Wrakking, A. M., van der Heide, A. and van der Maas, P. J. (2004). 'Medical decision making in scarcity situation'. *Journal of Medical Ethics* **30**: 207-211.

Wolf, S. M. (ed.). (1996). *Feminism and Bioethics: Beyond Reproduction*. Oxford: Oxford University Press.

Index

General Social Care Council (GSCC), code of professional conduct 28, 143, 144, 392
genetic counsellors 140-1
genetic testing 257, 324
Giger and Davidhizer's transcultural assessment model 29, 30-1
Giger and Davidhizer's transcultural care model 253-4
Gilligan's ethics of care 22, 93, 322
government control, health care research 361-3
government spending, factors influencing 301-2
gratitude
    as prima facie duty 90
        application in decision making 226, 232, 239
grief 196
gross national product (GNP)
    allocation to health care 303
    per capita 301
group behaviour 47
group work, confidentiality within 273
'groupie' moral standards, problems caused by 47, 230
gut response 39

Hare Krishna movement 107
harmony 92, 103, 125
    compared with Western concept of autonomy 103
health care, right to 57, 99, 154, 248-9, 307
Health Care Commission 305
health care research 348-65
    approval steps for 362-3
    benefits v. risks 351, 352, 353
    case study 358-9
    data collection and analysis 358
    difficulties experienced by researchers 363
    ethical principles applied 359-61
    governance of 361-3
    importance of ethics in 349-53
    informed consent for 351-2
    methodology 356-7
    non-participative 350
    non-therapeutic 351, 353
    participants 348
        clients/patients declining to be 353
        confidentiality for 352-3
        information given to 352, 354, 357
        informed consent by 351-2
        protection of 353-5, 353-6
        recruitment of 350-1, 358
        vulnerable people as 349, 355-6

participative 350-3
research process 356-9
Health Consumers Network (Australia) 234
health professionals
    apologising for mistakes 60
    behaviour 10
    cultural variation 254
    culturally sensitive practice 29-30
    differences of opinion among 48-9
    dual responsibility 64-5
    duties 70
    emotional and psychological burden of 297-8
    group behaviour 47
    ideal moral behaviours 60-1, 297
    oppositional views 49
    responsibilities 59-61
    rights 70-3, 210-11
        autonomy in providing care 71-2
        conflict with patients' rights 70-1
        identification using ethical grid 72-3
        refusal to provide care 71-2, 210
        safety at work 71
        support 72, 210-11
    standards of conduct/practice 7, 10-11, 28, 37, 392
    stress in intensive care environments 295
    values 28
Health Professions Council (HPC), code of professional conduct 28, 143, 144, 392
health resources
    demand for 301-3
    meaning of term 300
    see also allocation of resources
health and social care teams 138-42
Hegel, Georg Wilhelm Friedrich 132
high-dependency unit (HDU) 277
Hindu philosophy 105-12
    main principles 106
    modern philosophies 107
    spirituality and religion 107-8
Hindu society 106-7
Hinduism
    beliefs and practices 108
        relevance in health care 108-10
HIV/AIDS 341, 342
    modes of transmission 342
    social losses due to 193
Hobbes, Thomas 59, 86
holy water (Hinduism) 110
homeless people 64
homosexual clients 67, 340
    treatment of 272

sperm donation 333
spiritual beliefs
   in intensive care situation 291-2
   rights of dying person 114, 117, 127, 185, 201
stem cell transplantation 312
stereotyping
   gender roles 336-7
   pregnant teenagers 284
stillbirth, losses resulting from 195
structured reflection, model for 32, 52
students, ways to ask questions 44
subcultures 24
suffering, and euthanasia 207, 208
suicide 173
   and DNR request 181
   ethical aspects 268, 273-4
   and male peer pressure 345
   physician-assisted 206
   young men 345
Sunrise Model 45, 112
superior's orders 37-8
support, health professional's right 72, 210-11
surgery
   ethical decisions 280-1
   refusal by children 289-90
   refusal by elderly patient 287-9
   see also operating department/theatre
surrogacy 335-6
   laws in various countries 335-6
surrogate embryo transfer 334, 335
symbols used [in this book] 4

Taoism 122-3, 132
team working 7, 137-53
   see also interprofessional teams
teleological theories 85-8, 223
   applications, decision making 225, 231, 238
   compared with deontological theories 85
   see also utilitarianism
terminally ill client/patient, assisted dying for 171,
      172, 173
termination of pregnancy
   ethical/moral conflict 49, 56, 62-3, 148,
      325-30
   selective (in IVF) 83, 128, 335
   see also abortion
tertiary care 246
   interprofessional teams 141
therapeutic relationship 249-52, 270, 271
therapists 139-40
therapy
   ethical considerations 270-3

   see also aversion therapy; behavioural
      modification; group work; psychotherapy;
      sex therapy
Thomas and Kilmann's conflict
      (avoidance/resolution) model 151
totality, doctrine of 203, 210
traditional Chinese medicine 124
tranquillisers, withdrawal symptoms 264
transcultural assessment model 29, 30-1
transcultural care model 253-4
transference (in therapy) 270
transformative learning 22
traumatic events, unexpected losses due to 194
triage 279
truth telling 82, 197, 250-1
Tuskegee (USA), syphilis 'experiment' 5, 35, 37,
      55, 349

understanding
   ethical problems 41-2
      application in case studies 43-4, 111
   meaning of term 41
uniqueness 16-17
   of other people 20-1
United Nations Declaration of Human Rights
      55-6, 61, 266
United Network for Organ Sharing (UNOS) 312
utilitarianism 86-8, 306-7
   applications
      allocation of resources 307
      decision making 225, 231, 238
      psychiatric care 269

values and beliefs 8, 15-34
   case study 26-7
   changing 22-3, 251
   and culture 23-6
   of health professionals 28
   learning 21-2
   of other people 21
   perception based on 10
   sources 19-20
   and team working 142
veracity 82, 197-8, 250
   applications 84, 284
very ill people, as research participants 356
violent behaviour, ethical aspects 266-8
virtue ethics 95-6, 223
   application to case study 97
vulnerability 17, 54
vulnerable clients/patients 55, 61-9, 340-1
   unethical experiments/studies 5-6, 349

"You'll be up all night with **DIVERGENT**, a brainy thrill-ride of a novel."

"The imaginative action and g⟨...⟩es of a sprawling conspiracy are serious atte⟨...⟩bbers, and the portrait of a shattered, ⟨...⟩vergrown, and abandoned Chic⟨...⟩ ⟨...⟩ative as ever."

"Author Roth tells the riveting and complex story of a teenage girl forced to choose between her routinized, selfless family and the adventurous, unrestrained future she longs for. A memorable, unpredictable journey from which it is nearly impossible to turn away."

"With brisk pacing and lavish flights of imagination, **DIVERGENT** clearly has thrills, but it also movingly explores a more common adolescent anxiety—the painful realization that coming into one's own sometimes means leaving family behind, both ideologically and physically."

"Nonstop, adrenaline-heavy action. Packed with stunning twists and devastating betrayals."

—BCCB

"**DIVERGENT** is really an extended metaphor about the trials of modern adolescence: constantly having to take tests that sort and rank you among your peers, facing separation from your family, agonizing about where you fit in, and deciding when (or whether) to reveal the ways you may diverge from the group."

—WALL STREET JOURNAL

"This gritty, paranoid world is built with careful details and intriguing scope. The plot clips along at an addictive pace, with steady jolts of brutal violence and swoony romance. Fans snared by the ratcheting suspense will be unable to resist speculating on their own factional allegiance."

—KIRKUS REVIEWS

"Roth knows how to write. The novel's love story, intricate plot, and unforgettable setting work in concert to deliver a novel that will rivet fans of the first book."

—PUBLISHERS WEEKLY

Also by Veronica Roth

DIVERGENT

INSURGENT

ALLEGIANT

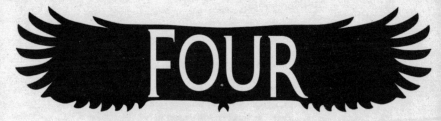

FOUR

A DIVERGENT COLLECTION

VERONICA ROTH

HarperCollins*Publishers*

First published in hardback in the US by HarperCollins Publishers Inc., in 2014
First published in Great Britain by HarperCollins *Children's Books* in 2014
This edition published in 2015
HarperCollins *Children's Books*, a division of HarperCollins *Publishers* Ltd,
HarperCollins*Publishers*
1 London Bridge Street,
London SE1 9GF

www.harpercollins.co.uk

14 15 16 17 18 10 9 8 7 6 5 4 3 2 1

ISBN: 978-0-00-755014-2

Printed and bound in Great Britain by Clays Ltd, St Ives plc
Typography by Joel Tippie

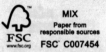

Find out more about HarperCollins and the environment at
www.harpercollins.co.uk/green

To my readers, who are wise and brave.

CONTENTS

INTRODUCTION

I FIRST STARTED writing *Divergent* from the perspective of Tobias Eaton, a boy from Abnegation with peculiar tension with his father who longed for freedom from his faction. I reached a standstill at thirty pages because the narrator wasn't quite right for the story I wanted to tell; four years later, when I picked up the story again, I found the right character to drive it, this time a girl from Abnegation who wanted to find out what she was made of. But Tobias never disappeared—he entered the story as Four, Tris's instructor, friend, boyfriend, and equal. He has always been a character I was interested in exploring further because of the way he came alive for me every time he was on the page. He is powerful for me largely because of the way he continues to overcome adversity, even managing, on several occasions, to flourish in it.

The first three stories, "The Transfer," "The Initiate,"

and "The Son," take place before he ever meets Tris, following his path from Abnegation to Dauntless as he earns his own strength. In the last, "The Traitor," which overlaps chronologically with the middle of *Divergent*, he meets Tris. I wanted very much to include the moment when they meet, but unfortunately, it didn't fit into the story's timeline—you can find it instead at the back of this book.

The series follows Tris from the moment she seized control of her own life and identity; and with these stories, we can follow Four as he does the same. And the rest, as they say, is history.

—*Veronica Roth*

THE TRANSFER

I EMERGE FROM the simulation with a yell. My lip stings, and when I take my hand away from it, there is blood on my fingertips. I must have bitten it during the test.

The Dauntless woman administering my aptitude test—Tori, she said her name was—gives me a strange look as she pulls her black hair back and ties it in a knot. Her arms are marked up and down with ink, flames and rays of light and hawk wings.

"When you were in the simulation . . . were you aware that it wasn't real?" Tori says to me as she turns off the machine. She sounds and looks casual, but it's a studied casualness, learned from years of practice. I know it when I see it. I always do.

Suddenly I'm aware of my own heartbeat. This is what

my father said would happen. He told me that they would ask me if I was aware during the simulation, and he told me what to say when they did.

"No," I say. "If I was, do you think I would have chewed through my lip?"

Tori studies me for a few seconds, then bites down on the ring in her lip before she says, "Congratulations. Your result was textbook Abnegation."

I nod, but the word "Abnegation" feels like a noose wrapped around my throat.

"Aren't you pleased?" she says.

"My faction members will be."

"I didn't ask about them, I asked about you." Tori's mouth and eyes turn down at the corners like they bear little weights. Like she's sad about something. "This is a safe room. You can say whatever you want here."

I knew what my choices in the aptitude test would add up to before I arrived at school this morning. I chose food over a weapon. I threw myself in the path of the dog to save the little girl. I knew that after I made those choices, the test would end and I would receive Abnegation as a result. And I don't know that I would have made different choices if my father hadn't coached me, hadn't controlled every part of my aptitude test from afar. So what was I expecting? What faction did I want?

Any of them. Any of them but Abnegation.

"I'm pleased," I say firmly. I don't care what she says—this isn't a safe room. There are no safe rooms, no safe truths, no safe secrets to tell.

I can still feel the dog's teeth closing around my arm, tearing my skin. I nod to Tori and start toward the door, but just before I leave, her hand closes around my elbow.

"You're the one who has to live with your choice," she says. "Everyone else will get over it, move on, no matter what you decide. But you never will."

I open the door and walk out.

+ + +

I return to the cafeteria and sit down at the Abnegation table, among the people who barely know me. My father doesn't permit me to come to most community events. He claims that I'll cause a disruption, that I'll do something to hurt his reputation. I don't care. I'm happier in my room, in the silent house, than surrounded by the deferential, apologetic Abnegation.

The consequence of my constant absence, though, is that the other Abnegation are wary of me, convinced there's something wrong with me, that I'm ill or immoral or strange. Even those willing to nod at me in greeting don't quite meet my eyes.

I sit with my hands clenching my knees, watching the other tables, while the other students finish their aptitude tests. The Erudite table is covered in reading material, but they aren't all studying—they're just making a show of it, trading conversation instead of ideas, their eyes snapping back to the words every time they think someone's watching them. The Candor are talking loudly, as always. The Amity are laughing, smiling, pulling food from their pockets and passing it around. The Dauntless are raucous and loud, slung over the tables and chairs, leaning on one another and poking one another and teasing.

I wanted any other faction. Any other faction but mine, where everyone has already decided that I am not worth their attention.

Finally an Erudite woman enters the cafeteria and holds up a hand for silence. The Abnegation and Erudite quiet down right away, but it takes her shouting "Quiet!" for the Dauntless, Amity, and Candor to notice her.

"The aptitude tests are now finished," she says. "Remember that you are not permitted to discuss your results with *anyone*, not even your friends or family. The Choosing Ceremony will be tomorrow at the Hub. Plan to arrive at least ten minutes before it begins. You are dismissed."

Everyone rushes toward the doors except our table,

where we wait for everyone else to leave before we even get to our feet. I know the path my fellow Abnegation will take out of here, down the hallway and out the front doors to the bus stop. They could be there for over an hour letting other people get on in front of them. I don't think I can bear any more of this silence.

Instead of following them, I slip out a side door and into an alley next to the school. I've taken this route before, but usually I creep along slowly, not wanting to be seen or heard. Today all I want to do is run.

I sprint to the end of the alley and into the empty street, leaping over a sinkhole in the pavement. My loose Abnegation jacket snaps in the wind, and I peel it from my shoulders, letting it trail behind me like a flag and then letting it go. I push the sleeves of my shirt up to my elbows as I run, slowing to a jog when my body can no longer stand the sprint. It feels like the entire city is rushing past me in a blur, the buildings blending together. I hear the slap of my shoes like the sound is separate from me.

Finally I have to stop, my muscles burning. I'm in the factionless wasteland that lies between the Abnegation sector and Erudite headquarters, Candor headquarters, and our common places. At every faction meeting, our leaders, usually speaking through my father, urge us not to be afraid of the factionless, to treat them like human beings instead of broken, lost creatures. But it never occurred to me to be afraid of them.

I move to the sidewalk so I can look through the windows of the buildings. Most of the time all I see is old furniture, every room bare, bits of trash on the floor. When most of the city's residents left—as they must have, since our current population doesn't fill every building—they must not have left in a hurry, because the spaces they occupied are so clean. Nothing of interest remains.

When I pass one of the buildings on the corner, though, I see something inside. The room just beyond the window is as bare as any of the others I've walked by, but past the doorway inside I can see a single ember, a lit coal.

I frown and pause in front of the window to see if it will open. At first it won't budge, and then I wiggle it back and forth, and it springs upward. I push my torso through first, and then my legs, toppling to the ground inside in a heap of limbs. My elbows sting as they scrape the floor.

The building smells like cooked food and smoke and sweat. I inch toward the ember, listening for voices that will warn me of a factionless presence here, but there's only silence.

In the next room, the windows are blacked out by paint and dirt, but a little daylight makes it through them, so I can see that there are curled pallets scattered on the floor all over the room, and old cans with bits of dried food stuck inside them. In the center of the room is a small charcoal grill. Most of the coals are white, their fuel spent, but one is still lit, suggesting that whoever was here was here recently. And judging by the smell and the abundance of old cans and blankets, there were quite a few of them.

I was always taught that the factionless lived without community, isolated from one another. Now, looking at this place, I wonder why I ever believed it. What would be stopping them from forming groups, just like we have? It's in our nature.

"What are you doing here?" a voice demands, and it travels through me like an electric shock. I wheel around and see a smudged, sallow-faced man in the next room, wiping his hands on a ragged towel.

"I was just . . ." I look at the grill. "I saw fire. That's all."

"Oh." The man tucks the corner of the towel into his back pocket. He wears black Candor pants, patched with blue Erudite fabric, and a gray Abnegation shirt, the same as the one I'm wearing. He's lean as a rail, but he looks strong. Strong enough to hurt me, but I don't think he will.

"Thanks, I guess," he says. "Nothing's on fire here, though."

"I can see that," I say. "What is this place?"

"It's my house," he says with a cold smile. He's missing one of his teeth. "I didn't know I would be having guests, so I didn't bother to tidy up."

I look from him to the scattered cans. "You must toss and turn a lot, to require so many blankets."

"Never met a Stiff who pried so much into other people's business," he says. He moves closer to me and frowns. "You look a little familiar."

I know I can't have met him before, not where I live, surrounded by identical houses in the most monotonous neighborhood in the city, surrounded by people in identical gray clothing with identical short hair. Then it occurs to me: hidden as my father tries to keep me, he's still the leader of the council, one of the most prominent people in our city, and I still resemble him.

"I'm sorry to have bothered you," I say in my best Abnegation voice. "I'll be going now."

"I do know you," the man says. "You're Evelyn Eaton's son, aren't you?"

I stiffen at her name. It's been years since I heard it, because my father won't speak it, won't even acknowledge it if he hears it. To be connected to her again, even just in facial resemblance, feels strange, like putting on an old piece of clothing that doesn't quite fit anymore.

"How did you know her?" He must have known her

well, to see her in my face, which is paler than hers, the eyes blue instead of dark brown. Most people didn't look closely enough to see all the things we had in common: our long fingers, our hooked noses, our straight, frowned eyebrows.

He hesitates a little. "She volunteered with the Abnegation sometimes. Handing out food and blankets and clothes. Had a memorable face. Plus, she was married to a council leader. Didn't everyone know her?"

Sometimes I know people are lying just because of the way the words feel when they press into me, uncomfortable and wrong, the way an Erudite feels when she reads a grammatically incorrect sentence. However he knew my mother, it's not because she handed him a can of soup once. But I'm so thirsty to hear more about her that I don't press the issue.

"She died, did you know?" I say. "Years ago."

"No, I didn't know." His mouth slants a little at one corner. "I'm sorry to hear that."

I feel strange, standing in this dank place that smells like live bodies and smoke, among these empty cans that suggest poverty and the failure to fit in. But there is something appealing about it here too, a freedom, a refusal to belong to these arbitrary categories we've made for ourselves.

"Your Choosing must be coming up tomorrow, for you to look so worried," the man says. "What faction did you get?"

"I'm not supposed to tell anyone," I say automatically.

"I'm not anyone," he says. "I'm nobody. That's what being factionless is."

I still don't say anything. The prohibition against sharing my aptitude test result, or any of my other secrets, is set firmly in the mold that makes me and remakes me daily. It's impossible to change now.

"Ah, a rule follower," he says, like he's disappointed. "Your mother said to me once that she felt like inertia had carried her to Abnegation. It was the path of least resistance." He shrugs. "Trust me when I tell you, Eaton boy, that resisting is worth doing."

I feel a rush of anger. He shouldn't be telling me about my mother like she belongs to him and not to me, shouldn't be making me question everything I remember about her just because she may or may not have served him food once. He shouldn't be telling me anything at all—he's nobody, factionless, separate, nothing.

"Yeah?" I say. "Look where resisting got you. Living out of cans in broken-down buildings. Doesn't sound so great to me." I start toward the doorway the man emerged from. I know I'll find an alley door somewhere back there;

I don't care where as long as I can get out of here quickly.

I pick a path across the floor, careful not to step on any of the blankets. When I reach the hallway, the man says, "I'd rather eat out of a can than be strangled by a faction."

I don't look back.

+++

When I get home, I sit on the front step and take deep breaths of the cool spring air for a few minutes.

My mother was the one who taught me to steal moments like these, moments of freedom, though she didn't know it. I watched her take them, slipping out the door after dark when my father was asleep, creeping back home when sunlight was just appearing behind the buildings. She took them even when she was with us, standing over the sink with her eyes closed, so distant from the present that she didn't even hear me when I spoke to her.

But I learned something else from watching her too, which is that the free moments always have to end.

I get up, brushing flecks of cement from my gray slacks, and push the door open. My father sits in the easy chair in the living room, surrounded by paperwork. I pull up straight, tall, so that he can't scold me for slouching. I move toward the stairs. Maybe he will let me go to my room unnoticed.

"Tell me about your aptitude test," he says, and he points at the sofa for me to sit.

I cross the room, stepping carefully over a stack of papers on the carpet, and sit where he points, right on the edge of the cushion so I can stand up quickly.

"Well?" He removes his glasses and looks at me expectantly. I hear tension in his voice, the kind that only develops after a difficult day at work. I should be careful. "What was your result?"

I don't even think about refusing to tell him. "Abnegation."

"And nothing else?"

I frown. "No, of course not."

"Don't give me that look," he says, and my frown disappears. "Nothing strange happened with your test?"

During my test, I knew where I was—I knew that while I felt like I was standing in the cafeteria of my secondary school, I was actually lying prostrate on a chair in the aptitude test room, my body connected to a machine by a series of wires. That was strange. But I don't want to talk to him about it now, not when I can see the stress brewing inside him like a storm.

"No," I say.

"Don't lie to me," he says, and he seizes my arm, his fingers tight like a vise. I don't look at him.

"I'm not," I say. "I got Abnegation, just as expected. The woman barely looked at me on my way out of the room. I promise."

He releases me. My skin pulses from where he gripped it.

"Good," he says. "I'm sure you have some thinking to do. You should go to your room."

"Yes, sir."

I get up and cross the room again, relieved.

"Oh," he says. "Some of my fellow council members are coming over tonight, so you should eat dinner early."

"Yes, sir."

+ + +

Before the sun goes down, I snatch food from the cupboards and the refrigerator: two dinner rolls and raw carrots with the greens still attached, a hunk of cheese and an apple, leftover chicken without any seasoning on it. The food all tastes the same, like dust and paste. I keep my eyes fixed on the door so I don't collide with my father's coworkers. He wouldn't like it if I was still down here when they came.

I am finishing off a glass of water when the first council member appears on the doorstep, and I hurry through the living room before my father reaches the door. He waits with his hand on the knob, his eyebrows raised at me as I slip around the banister. He points up the stairs and I climb them, fast, as he opens the door.

"Hello, Marcus." I recognize the voice as Andrew Prior's. He's one of my father's closest friends at work, which means nothing, because no one *really* knows my father. Not even me.

From the top of the stairs I look down at Andrew. He's wiping his shoes on the mat. I see him and his family sometimes, a perfect Abnegation unit, Natalie and Andrew, and the son and daughter—not twins, but both two years younger than I am in school—all walking sedately down the sidewalk and bobbing their heads at passersby. Natalie organizes all the factionless volunteer efforts among the Abnegation—my mother must have known her, though she rarely attended Abnegation social events, preferring to keep her secrets like I keep mine, hidden away in this house.

Andrew meets my eyes, and I rush down the hallway to my bedroom, closing the door behind me.

To all appearances, my room is as sparse and clean as every other Abnegation room. My gray sheets and blankets are tucked tightly around the thin mattress, and my schoolbooks are stacked in a perfect tower on my plywood desk. A small dresser that contains several identical sets of clothing stands next to the small window, which lets in only the barest sliver of sunlight in the evenings. Through it I can see the house next door, which is just the same as the one I'm in, except five feet to the east.

I know how inertia carried my mother to Abnegation, if indeed that man was speaking the truth about what she'd told him. I can see it happening to me, too, tomorrow when I stand among the bowls of faction elements with a knife in my hand. There are four factions I don't know or trust, with practices I don't understand, and only one that is familiar, predictable, comprehensible. If choosing Abnegation won't lead me to a life of ecstatic happiness, at least it will lead me to a comfortable place.

I sit on the edge of the bed. *No, it won't,* I think, and then I swallow the thought down, because I know where it comes from: the childish part of me that is afraid of the man holding court in the living room. The man whose knuckles I know better than his embrace.

I make sure the door is closed and wedge the desk chair under the knob just in case. Then I crouch next to the bed and reach under it to the trunk I keep there.

My mother gave it to me when I was young, and told my father it was for spare blankets, that she had found it in an alley somewhere. But when she put it in my room, she didn't fill it with spare blankets. She closed my door and touched her fingers to her lips and set it on my bed to open it.

Inside the unlocked trunk was a blue sculpture. It looked like falling water, but it was really glass, perfectly clear, polished, flawless.

"What does it do?" I asked her at the time.

"It doesn't do anything obvious," she said, and she smiled, but the smile was tight, like she was afraid of something. "But it might be able to do something in here." She tapped her chest, right over the sternum. "Beautiful things sometimes do."

Since then I have filled the trunk with objects that others would call useless: old spectacles without glass in them, fragments of discarded motherboards, spark plugs, stripped wires, the broken neck of a green bottle, a rusted knife blade. I don't know if my mother would have called them beautiful, or even if I would, but each of them struck me the same way that sculpture did, as secret things, and valuable ones, if only because they were so overlooked.

Instead of thinking about my aptitude test result, I pick up each object and turn it in my hands so I've memorized every part of every one.

+++

I wake with a start to Marcus's footsteps in the hallway just outside the bedroom. I'm lying on the bed with the objects strewn on the mattress around me. His footsteps are slowing down as he comes closer to the door, and I pick up the spark plugs and motherboard pieces and wires and throw them back into the trunk and lock it, stowing the key in my pocket. I realize at the last second, as the doorknob starts to move, that the sculpture is still out, so I shove it under the pillow and slide the trunk under the bed.

Then I dive toward the chair and pull it from under the knob so my father can enter.

When he does, he eyes the chair in my hands with suspicion.

"What was that doing over here?" he says. "Are you trying to keep me out?"

"No, sir."

"That's the second time you've lied to me today," Marcus says. "I didn't raise my son to be a liar."

"I—" I can't think of a single thing to say, so I just close my mouth and carry the chair back to my desk where it belongs, right behind the perfect stack of schoolbooks.

"What were you doing in here that you didn't want me to see?"

I clutch the back of the chair, hard, and stare at my books.

"Nothing," I say quietly.

"That's three lies," he says, and his voice is low but hard as flint. He starts toward me, and I back up instinctively. But instead of reaching for me, he bends down and pulls the trunk from beneath the bed, then tries the lid. It doesn't budge.

Fear slides into my gut like a blade. I pinch the hem of my shirt, but I can't feel my fingertips.

"Your mother claimed this was for blankets," he says. "Said you got cold at night. But what I've always wondered is, if it still has blankets in it, why do you keep it locked?"

He holds out his hand, palm up, and raises his eyebrows at me. I know what he wants—the key. And I have to give it to him, because he can see when I'm lying; he can see everything about me. I reach into my pocket, then drop the key in his hand. Now I can't feel my palms, and the breathing is starting, the shallow breathing that always comes when I know he's about to explode.

I close my eyes as he opens the trunk.

"What is this?" His hand moves through the treasured objects carelessly, scattering them to the left and right. He takes them out one by one and thrusts them toward me. "What do you need with *this*, or *this* . . . !"

I flinch, over and over again, and don't have an answer. I don't need them. I don't need any of them.

"This is *rank* with self-indulgence!" he shouts, and he shoves the trunk off the edge of the bed so its contents scatter all over the floor. "It poisons this house with selfishness!"

I can't feel my face, either.

His hands collide with my chest. I stumble back and hit the dresser. Then he draws his hand back by his face to hit me, and I say, my throat tight with fear, "The Choosing Ceremony, Dad!"

He pauses with his hand raised, and I *cower*, shrinking back against the dresser, my eyes too blurry to see out of. He usually tries not to bruise my face, especially for days like tomorrow, when so many people will be staring at me, watching me choose.

He lowers his hand, and for a second I think the violence is over, the anger stalled. But then he says, "Fine. Stay here."

I sag against the dresser. I know better than to think he'll leave and mull things over and come back apologizing. He never does that.

He will return with a belt, and the stripes he carves into my back will be easily hidden by a shirt and an obedient Abnegation expression.

I turn around, a shudder claiming my body. I clutch the edge of the dresser and wait.

+ + +

That night I sleep on my stomach, pain biting each thought, with my broken possessions on the floor around me. After he hit me until I had to stuff my fist into my mouth to muffle a scream, he stomped on each object until it was broken or dented beyond recognition, then threw the trunk into the wall so the lid broke from the hinges.

The thought surfaces: *If you choose Abnegation, you will never get away from him.*

I push my face into my pillow.

But I'm not strong enough to resist this Abnegation-inertia, this fear that drives me down the path my father has set for me.

+ + +

The next morning I take a cold shower, not to conserve resources as the Abnegation instruct, but because it numbs my back. I dress slowly in my loose, plain Abnegation clothes, and stand in front of the hallway mirror to cut my hair.

"Let me," my father says from the end of the hallway. "It's your Choosing Day, after all."

I set the clippers down on the ledge created by the sliding panel and try to straighten up. He stands behind me, and I avert my eyes as the clippers start to buzz. There's only one guard for the blade, only one length of hair acceptable for an Abnegation male. I wince as his fingers stabilize my head, and hope he doesn't see it, doesn't see how even his slightest touch terrifies me.

"You know what to expect," he says. He covers the top of my ear with one hand as he drags the clippers over the side of my head. Today he's trying to protect my ear from getting nicked by clippers, and yesterday he took a belt to me. The thought feels like poison working through me. It's almost funny. I almost want to laugh.

"You'll stand in your place; when your name is called, you'll go forward to get your knife. Then you'll cut yourself and drop the blood into the right bowl." Our eyes meet in the mirror, and he presses his mouth into a near-smile. He touches my shoulder, and I realize that we are about the same height now, about the same size, though I still feel so much smaller.

Then he adds gently, "The knife will only hurt for a moment. Then your choice will be made, and it will all be over."

I wonder if he even remembers what happened yesterday, or if he's already shoved it into a separate compartment in his mind, keeping his monster half separate from his father half. But I don't have those compartments, and I can see all his identities layered over one another, monster and father and man and council leader and widower.

And suddenly my heart is pounding so hard, my face is so hot, I can barely stand it.

"Don't worry about me handling the pain," I say. "I've had a lot of practice."

For a second his eyes are like daggers in the mirror, and my strong anger is gone, replaced by familiar fear. But all he does is switch off the clippers and set them on the ledge and walk down the stairs, leaving me to sweep up the trimmed hair, to brush it from my shoulders and neck, to put the clippers away in their drawer in the bathroom.

Then I go back into my room and stare at the broken objects on the floor. Carefully, I gather them into a pile and put them in the wastebasket next to my desk, piece by piece.

Wincing, I come to my feet. My legs are shaking.

In that moment, staring at the bare life I've made for myself here, at the destroyed remnants of what little I had, I think, *I have to get out.*

It's a strong thought. I feel its strength ringing inside me like the toll of a bell, so I think it again. *I have to get out.*

I walk toward the bed and slide my hand under the pillow, where my mother's sculpture is still safe, still blue and gleaming with morning light. I put it on my desk, next to the stack of books, and leave my bedroom, closing the door behind me.

Downstairs, I'm too nervous to eat, but I stuff a piece of toast into my mouth anyway so my father won't ask me any questions. I shouldn't worry. Now he's pretending I don't exist, pretending I'm not flinching every time I have to bend down to pick something up.

I have to get out. It's a chant now, a mantra, the only thing I have left to hold on to.

He finishes reading the news the Erudite release every morning, and I finish washing my own dishes, and we walk out of the house together without speaking. We walk down the sidewalk, and he greets our neighbors with a smile, and everything is always in perfect order for Marcus Eaton, except for his son. Except for me; I am not in order, I am in constant disarray.

But today, I'm glad for that.

We get on the bus and stand in the aisle to let others sit down around us, the perfect picture of Abnegation deference. I watch the others get on, Candor boys and girls with loud mouths, Erudite with studious stares. I watch the other Abnegation rise from their seats to give them away. Everyone is going to the same place today—the Hub, a black pillar in the distance, its two prongs stabbing the sky.

When we get there, my father puts a hand on my shoulder as we walk to the entrance, sending shocks of pain through my body.

I have to get out.

It's a desperate thought, and the pain only spurs it on with each footstep as I walk the stairs to the Choosing Ceremony floor. I struggle for air, but it's not because of my aching legs; it's because of my weak heart, growing stronger with each passing second. Beside me, Marcus wipes beads of sweat from his forehead, and all the other Abnegation close their lips to keep from breathing too loudly, lest they appear to be complaining.

I lift my eyes to the stairs ahead of me, and I am on fire with this thought, this need, this chance to escape.

We reach the right floor, and everyone pauses to catch their breath before entering. The room is dim, the windows blocked off, the seats arranged around the circle of bowls that hold glass and water and stones and coal and earth. I find my place in line, between an Abnegation girl and an Amity boy. Marcus stands in front of me.

"You know what to do," he says, and it's more like he's

telling himself than me. "You know what the right choice is. I know you do."

I just stare somewhere south of his eyes.

"I'll see you soon," he says.

He moves toward the Abnegation section and sits in the front row, with some of the other council leaders. Gradually people fill the room, those who are about to choose standing in a square at the edge, those watching sitting in the chairs in the middle. The doors close, and there's a moment of quiet as the council representative from Dauntless moves to the podium. Max is his name. He wraps his fingers around the edge of the podium, and I can see, even from here, that his knuckles are bruised.

Do they learn to fight in Dauntless? They must.

"Welcome to the Choosing Ceremony," Max says, his deep voice filling the room easily. He doesn't need the microphone; his voice is loud enough and strong enough to penetrate my skull and wrap around my brain. "Today you will choose your factions. Until this point you have followed your parents' paths, your parents' rules. Today you will find your own path, make your own rules."

I can almost see my father pressing his lips together with disdain at such a typical Dauntless speech. I know his habits so well, I almost do it myself, though I don't share the feeling. I have no particular opinions about Dauntless.

"A long time ago our ancestors realized that each of us, each individual, was responsible for the evil that exists in the world. But they didn't agree on exactly what that evil was," Max says. "Some said that it was dishonesty. . . ."

I think of the lies I have told, year after year, about this bruise or that cut, the lies of omission I told when I kept Marcus's secrets.

"Some said that it was ignorance, some aggression. . . ."

I think of the peace of the Amity orchards, the freedom I would find there from violence and cruelty.

"Some said selfishness was the cause."

This is for your own good is what Marcus said before the first blow fell. As if hitting me was an act of self-sacrifice. As if it hurt him to do it. Well, I didn't see *him* limping around the kitchen this morning.

"And the last group said that it was cowardice that was to blame."

A few hoots rise up from the Dauntless section, and the rest of the Dauntless laugh. I think of the fear swallowing me last night until I couldn't feel, until I couldn't breathe. I think of the years that have ground me into dust beneath my father's heel.

"That is how we came by our factions: Candor, Erudite,

Amity, Abnegation, and Dauntless." Max smiles. "In them we find administrators and teachers and counselors and leaders and protectors. In them we find our sense of belonging, our sense of community, our very lives." He clears his throat. "Enough of that. Let's get to it. Come forward and get your knife, then make your choice. First up, Zellner, Gregory."

It seems fitting that pain should follow me from my old life into my new one, with the knife digging into my palm. Still, even this morning I didn't know which faction I would choose as a haven. Gregory Zellner holds his bleeding hand over the bowl of dirt, to choose Amity.

Amity seems like the obvious choice for a haven, with its peaceful life, its sweet-smelling orchards, its smiling community. In Amity I would find the kind of acceptance I've craved my entire life, and maybe, over time, it would teach me to feel steady in myself, comfortable with who I am.

But as I look at the people sitting in that section, in their reds and yellows, I see only whole, healed people, capable of cheering one another, capable of supporting one another. They are too perfect, too kind, for someone like me to be driven into their arms by rage and fear.

The ceremony is moving too fast. "Rogers, Helena."

She chooses Candor.

I know what happens in Candor's initiation. I heard whispers about it in school one day. There, I would have to expose every secret, dig it out with my fingernails. I would have to flay myself alive to join Candor. No, I can't do that.

"Lovelace, Frederick."

Frederick Lovelace, dressed all in blue, cuts his palm and lets his blood drip into the Erudite water, turning it a deeper shade of pink. I learn easily enough for Erudite, but I know myself well enough to understand that I am too volatile, too emotional, for a place like that. It would strangle me, and what I want is to be free, not to be shuffled into yet another prison.

It takes no time at all for the name of the Abnegation girl beside me to be called. "Erasmus, Anne."

Anne—another one who never found more than a few words to speak to me—stumbles forward and walks the aisle to Max's podium. She accepts her knife with shaking hands and cuts her palm, and holds her hand over the Abnegation bowl. It's easy for her. She doesn't have anything to run from, just a welcoming, kind community to rejoin. And besides, no one from Abnegation has transferred in years. It's the most loyal faction, in terms of Choosing Ceremony statistics.

"Eaton, Tobias."

I don't feel nervous as I walk down the aisle to the bowls, though I still haven't chosen my place. Max passes me the knife, and I wrap my fingers around the handle. It's smooth and cool, the blade clean. A new knife for each person, and a new choice.

As I walk to the center of the room, to the center of the bowls, I pass Tori, the woman who administered my aptitude test. *You're the one who has to live with your choice,* she said. Her hair is pulled back, and I can see a tattoo creeping over her collarbone, toward her throat. Her eyes touch mine with peculiar force, and I stare back, unflinching, as I take my place among the bowls.

What choice can I live with? Not Erudite, or Candor. Not Abnegation, the place I am trying to get away from. Not even Amity, where I am too broken to belong.

The truth is, I want my choice to drive a knife right through my father's heart, to pierce him with as much pain and embarrassment and disappointment as possible.

There is only one choice that can do that.

I look at him, and he nods, and I cut deep into my own palm, so deep the pain brings tears to my eyes. I blink them away and curl my hand into a fist to let the blood collect there. His eyes are like my eyes, such a dark blue that in light like this they always look black, just pits in his skull. My back throbs and pinches, my collared shirt scratching at the raw skin there, the skin he wore into with that belt.

I open my palm over the coals. I feel like they're burning in my stomach, filling me to the brim with fire and smoke.

I am free.

+ + +

I don't hear the cheers of the Dauntless; all I hear is ringing.

My new faction is like a many-armed creature, stretching toward me. I move toward it, and I don't dare to look back to see my father's face. Hands slap my arms, commending me on my choice, and I move to the rear of the group, blood wrapping around my fingers.

I stand with the other initiates, next to a black-haired Erudite boy who appraises and dismisses me with one glance. I must not look like much, in my Abnegation grays, tall and scrawny after last year's growth spurt. The cut in my hand is gushing, the blood spilling onto the floor and running down my wrist. I dug too deep with the knife.

As the last of my peers choose, I pinch the hem of my loose Abnegation shirt between my fingers and rip. I tear a strip of fabric from the front and wrap it around my hand to stop the bleeding. I won't need these clothes anymore.

The Dauntless sitting in front of us come to their feet as soon as the last person chooses, and they rush toward the doors, carrying me with them. I turn back right before the doors, unable to stop myself, and I see my father sitting in the front row still, a few other Abnegation huddled around him. He looks stunned.

I smirk a little. I did it, *I* put that expression on his face. I am not the perfect Abnegation child, doomed to be swallowed whole by the system and dissolved into obscurity. Instead, I am the first Abnegation-Dauntless transfer in more than a decade.

I turn and run to catch up with the others, not wanting to be left behind. Before I exit the room, I unbutton my ripped long-sleeved shirt and let it fall on the ground. The gray T-shirt I am wearing beneath it is still oversized, but it's darker, blends in better with the black Dauntless clothes.

They storm down the stairs, flinging doors open, laughing, shouting. I feel burning in my back and shoulders and lungs and legs, and suddenly I am unsure of this choice I've made, of these people I've claimed. They are so loud and so wild. Can I possibly make a place for myself among them? I don't know.

I guess I don't have a choice.

I push my way through the group, searching for my

fellow initiates, but they seem to have disappeared. I move to the side of the group, hoping to get a glimpse of where we're headed, and I see the train tracks suspended over the street in front of us, in a cage of latticed wood and metal. The Dauntless climb the stairs and spill out onto the train platform. At the foot of the stairs, the crowd is so dense that I can't find a way to get in, but I know if I don't climb the stairs soon, I might miss the train, so I decide to push my way in. I have to clench my teeth to keep myself from apologizing as I elbow people aside, and the momentum of the crowd presses me up the steps.

"You're not a bad runner," Tori says as she sidles up to me on the platform. "At least for an Abnegation kid."

"Thanks," I say.

"You know what's going to happen next, right?" She turns and points at a light in the distance, fixed to the front of an oncoming train. "It's not going to stop. It's just going to slow down a little. And if you don't make it on, that's it for you. Factionless. It's that easy to get kicked out."

I nod. I'm not surprised that the trial of initiation has already begun, that it began the second we left the Choosing Ceremony. And I'm not surprised that the Dauntless expect me to prove myself either. I watch the train come closer—I can hear it now, whistling on the tracks.

She grins at me. "You're going to do just fine here, aren't you?"

"What makes you say that?"

She shrugs. "You strike me as someone who's ready to fight, that's all."

The train thunders toward us, and the Dauntless start piling on. Tori runs toward the edge, and I follow her, copying her stance and her movements as she prepares to jump. She grabs a handle at the edge of the door and swings herself inside, so I do the same thing, fumbling at first for my grip and then yanking myself in.

But I'm unprepared for the turning of the train, and I stumble, smacking my face against the metal wall. I grab my aching nose.

"Smooth," one of the Dauntless inside says. He's younger than Tori, with dark skin and an easy smile.

"Finesse is for Erudite show-offs," Tori says. "He made it on the train, Amar, that's what counts."

"He's supposed to be in the other car, though. With the other initiates," Amar says. He eyes me, but not the way the Erudite transfer did a few minutes ago. He seems more curious than anything else, like I'm an oddity he needs to examine carefully in order to understand it. "If he's friends with you, I guess it's okay. What's your name, Stiff?"

The name is in my mouth the second he asks me the question, and I am about to answer like I always do, that I am Tobias Eaton. It should be natural, but in that moment I can't bear to say my name out loud, not here, among the people I hoped would be my new friends, my new family. I can't—I *won't*—be Marcus Eaton's son anymore.

"You can call me 'Stiff' for all I care," I say, trying out the cutting Dauntless banter I've only listened to across hallways and classrooms until now. Wind rushes into the train car as it picks up speed, and it's *loud*, roaring in my ears.

Tori gives me a strange look, and for a moment I am afraid that she's going to tell Amar my name, which I'm sure she remembers from my aptitude test. But she just nods a little, and relieved, I turn toward the open doorway, my hand still on the handle.

It never occurred to me before that I could refuse to give my name, or that I could give a false one, construct a new identity for myself. I'm free here, free to snap at people and free to refuse them and free even to lie.

I see the street between the wooden beams that support the train tracks, just a story beneath us. But up ahead, the old tracks give way to new ones, and the platforms go higher, wrapping around the roofs of buildings. The climb happens gradually, so I wouldn't have noticed it was happening if I hadn't been staring at the ground as we traveled farther and farther away from it, farther and farther into the sky.

Fear makes my legs go weak, so I back away from the doorway and sink into a crouch by one wall as I wait to get to wherever we're going.

+++

I am still in that position—crouched by the wall, my head in my hands—when Amar nudges me with his foot.

"Get up, Stiff," he says, not unkindly. "It's almost time to jump."

"Jump?" I say.

"Yeah." He smirks. "This train stops for no one."

I press myself up. The fabric I wrapped around my hand is soaked through with red. Tori stands right behind me and pushes me toward the doorway.

"Let the initiate off first!" she shouts.

"What are you doing?" I demand, scowling at her.

"I'm doing you a favor!" she answers, and she shoves me toward the opening again. The other Dauntless step back for me, each one of them grinning like I'm a meal. I shuffle toward the edge, grabbing the handle so hard the tips of my fingers start to go numb. I see where I'm supposed to jump—up ahead, the tracks hug the roof of a building and then turn. The gap looks small from here, but as the train gets closer, it seems larger and larger, and my imminent death seems more and more likely.

My entire body shakes as the Dauntless in the cars ahead of us make the jump. None of them miss the roof, but that doesn't mean I won't be the first. I pry my fingers from the handle and stare at the rooftop and push off as hard as I can.

The impact shudders through me, and I fall forward onto my hands and knees, the gravel on the roof digging into my wounded palm. I stare at my fingers. I feel like time just lurched forward, the actual jump disappearing from sight and memory.

"Damn," someone behind me says. "I was hoping we would get to scrape some Stiff pancake off the pavement later."

I glare at the ground and sit back on my heels. The roof is tilting and bobbing beneath me—I didn't know a person could be dizzy with fear.

Still, I know I just passed two initiation tests: I got on a moving train, and I made it to the roof. Now the question is, how do the Dauntless get *off* the roof?

A moment later Amar steps up on the ledge, and I have my answer:

They're going to make us jump.

I close my eyes and pretend that I'm not here, kneeling on this gravel with these insane ink-marked people surrounding me. I came here to escape, but this is not an escape, it's just a different kind of torture and it's too late to get out of it. My only hope, then, is to survive it.

"Welcome to Dauntless!" Amar shouts. "Where you either face your fears and try not to die in the process, or you leave a coward. We've got a record low of faction transfers this year, unsurprisingly."

The Dauntless around Amar punch the air and whoop, bearing the fact that no one wants to join them as a banner of pride.

"The only way to get into the Dauntless compound from this rooftop is to jump off this ledge," Amar says, opening his arms wide to indicate the empty space around him. He tilts back on his heels and waves his arms around, like he's about to fall, then catches himself and grins. I pull a deep breath in through my nose and hold it.

"As usual, I offer the opportunity to go first to our initiates, Dauntless-born or not." He hops down from the ledge and gestures to it, eyebrows raised.

The cluster of young Dauntless near the roof exchange looks. Standing off to the side are the Erudite boy from before, an Amity girl, two Candor boys, and a Candor girl. There are only six of us.

One of the Dauntless steps up, a dark-skinned boy who beckons cheers from his friends with his hands.

"Go, Zeke!" one of the girls shouts.

Zeke hops onto the ledge but misjudges the jump and tips forward right away, losing his balance. He yells something unintelligible and disappears. The Candor girl nearby gasps, covering her mouth with one hand, but Zeke's Dauntless friends burst into laughter. I don't think that was the dramatic, heroic moment he had in mind.

Amar, grinning, gestures to the ledge again. The Dauntless-borns line up behind it, and so do the Erudite boy and the Amity girl. I know I have to join them, I have to jump, it doesn't matter how I feel about it. I move toward the line, stiff like my joints are rusted bolts. Amar looks at his watch and cues each jumper at thirty-second intervals.

The line is shrinking, dissolving.

Suddenly it's gone, and I am all that is left. I step onto the ledge and wait for Amar's cue. The sun is setting behind the buildings in the distance, their jagged line unfamiliar from this angle. The light glows gold near the horizon, and wind rushes up the side of the building, lifting my clothes away from my body.

"Go ahead," Amar says.

I close my eyes, and I'm frozen; I can't even push myself

off the roof. All I can do is tilt and fall. My stomach drops and my limbs fumble in the air for something, anything to hold on to, but there is nothing, only the drop, the air, the frantic search for the ground.

Then I hit a net.

It curls around me, wrapping me in strong threads. Hands beckon to me from the edge. I hook my fingers in the net and pull myself toward them. I land on my feet on a wooden platform, and a man with dark brown skin and bruised knuckles grins at me. Max.

"The Stiff!" He claps me on the back, making me flinch. "Nice to see you made it this far. Go join your fellow initiates. Amar will be down in a second, I'm sure."

Behind him is a dark tunnel with rock walls. The Dauntless compound is underground—I assumed it would be dangling from a high building from a series of flimsy ropes, a manifestation of my worst nightmares.

I try to walk down the steps and over to the other transfers. My legs seem to be working again. The Amity girl smiles at me. "That was surprisingly fun," she says. "I'm Mia. You okay?"

"It looks like he's trying not to throw up," one of the Candor boys says.

"Just let it happen, man," the other Candor boy adds. "We'd love to see a show."

My response comes out of nowhere. "Shut up," I snap.

To my surprise, they do. I guess they haven't been told to shut up by many of the Abnegation.

A few seconds later, I see Amar rolling over the edge of the net. He descends the steps, looking wild and rumpled and ready for the next insane stunt. He beckons all the initiates closer to him, and we gather at the opening of the yawning tunnel in a semicircle.

Amar brings his hands together in front of him.

"My name is Amar," he says. "I'm your initiation instructor. I grew up here, and three years ago, I passed initiation with flying colors, which means I get to be in charge of the newcomers for as long as I want. Lucky you.

"Dauntless-borns and transfers do most physical training separately, so that the Dauntless-borns don't break the transfers in half right away—" At this, the Dauntless-borns on the other side of the semicircle grin. "But we're trying something different this year. The Dauntless leaders and I want to see if knowing your fears before you begin training will better prepare you for the rest of initiation. So before we even let you into the dining hall to have dinner, we're going to do some self-discovery. Follow me."

"What if I don't want to discover myself?" Zeke asks.

All Amar has to do is look at him for him to sink back

into the group of Dauntless-borns again. Amar is like no one I've ever met—affable one minute and stern the next, and sometimes both at once.

He leads the way down the tunnel, then stops at a door built into the wall and shoves it open with his shoulder. We follow him into a dank room with a giant window in the back wall. Above us the fluorescent lights flicker and twitch, and Amar busies himself at a machine that looks a lot like the one used to administer my aptitude test. I hear a dripping sound—water from the ceiling is leaking into a puddle in the corner.

Another large, empty room stretches out beyond the window. There are cameras in each corner—are there cameras all over the Dauntless compound?

"This is the fear landscape room," Amar announces without looking up. "A fear landscape is a simulation in which you confront your worst fears."

Arranged on the table next to the machine is a line of syringes. They look sinister to me in the flickering light, like they might as well be instruments of torture, knives and blades and hot pokers.

"How is that possible?" the Erudite boy says. "You don't know our worst fears."

"Eric, right?" Amar says. "You're correct, I don't know your worst fears, but the serum I am going to inject you with will stimulate the parts of your brain that process fear, and you will come up with the simulation obstacles yourself, so to speak. In this simulation, unlike in the aptitude test simulation, you will be aware that what you are seeing is not real. Meanwhile, I will be in this room, controlling the simulation, and I get to tell the program embedded in the simulation serum to move on to the next obstacle once your heart rate reaches a particular level—once you calm down, in other words, or face your fear in a significant way. When you run out of fears, the program will terminate and you will 'wake up' in that room again with a greater awareness of your own fears."

He picks up one of the syringes and beckons to Eric.

"Allow me to satisfy your Erudite curiosity," he says. "You get to go first."

"But—"

"But," Amar says smoothly, "I am your initiation instructor, and it's in your best interest to do as I say."

Eric stands still for a moment, then removes his blue jacket, folds it in half, and drapes it over the back of a chair. His movements are slow and deliberate—designed, I suspect, to irritate Amar as much as possible. Eric approaches Amar, who sticks the needle almost savagely into the side of Eric's neck. Then he steers Eric toward the next room.

Once Eric is standing in the middle of the room behind the glass, Amar attaches himself to the simulation machine with electrodes and presses something on the computer screen behind it to start the program.

Eric is still, his hands by his sides. He stares at us through the window, and a moment later, though he hasn't moved, it looks like he's staring at something else, like the simulation has begun. But he doesn't scream or thrash or cry, like I would expect of someone who is staring down his worst fears. His heart rate, recorded on the monitor in front of Amar, rises and rises, like a bird taking flight.

He's afraid. He's afraid, but he's not even moving.

"What's going on?" Mia asks me. "Is the serum working?"

I nod.

I watch Eric take a deep breath into his gut and release it through his nose. His body shakes, shivers, like the ground is rumbling beneath him, but his breaths are slow and even, his muscles clenching and then relaxing every few seconds, like he keeps tensing up by accident and then correcting his mistake. I watch his heart rate on the monitor in front of Amar, watch it slow down more and more until Amar taps the screen, forcing the program to move on.

This happens over and over again with each new fear. I

count the fears as they pass in silence, ten, eleven, twelve. Then Amar taps the screen one last time, and Eric's body relaxes. He blinks, slowly, then smirks at the window.

I notice that the Dauntless-borns, usually so quick to comment on everything, are silent. That must mean that what I'm feeling is correct—that Eric is someone to watch out for. Maybe even someone to be afraid of.

+ + +

For more than an hour I watch the other initiates face their fears, running and jumping and aiming invisible guns and, in some cases, lying facedown on the floor, sobbing. Sometimes I get a sense of what they see, of the crawling, creeping fears that torment them, but most of the time the villains they're warding off are private ones, known only to them and Amar.

I stay near the back of the room, shrinking down every time he calls on the next person. But then I'm the last one in the room, and Mia is just finishing, pulled out of her fear landscape when she's crouching against the back wall, her head in her hands. She stands, looking worn, and shuffles out of the room without waiting for Amar to dismiss her. He glances at the last syringe on the table, then at me.

"Just you and me, Stiff," he says. "Come on, let's get this over with."

I stand in front of him. I barely feel the needle go in; I've never had a problem with shots, though some of the other initiates got teary-eyed before the injection. I walk into the next room and face the window, which looks like a mirror on this side. In the moment before the simulation takes effect, I can see myself the way the others must have seen me, slouched and buried in fabric, tall and bony and bleeding. I try to straighten up, and I'm surprised by the difference it makes, surprised by the shadow of strength I see in myself right before the room disappears.

Images fill the space in pieces, the skyline of our city, the hole in the pavement seven stories below me, the line of the ledge beneath my feet. Wind rushes up the side of the building, stronger than it was when I was here in real life, whipping my clothes so hard they snap, and pushing against me from all angles. Then the building grows with me on top of it, moving me far away from the ground. The hole seals up, and hard pavement covers it.

I cringe away from the edge, but the wind won't let me move backward. My heart pounds harder and faster as I confront the reality of what I have to do; I have to jump again, this time not trusting that there won't be pain when I slam into the ground.

A Stiff pancake.

I shake out my hands, squeeze my eyes shut, and

scream into my teeth. Then I follow the push of the wind and I drop, fast. I hit the ground.

Searing, white-hot pain rushes through me, just for a second.

I stand up, wiping dust from my cheek, and wait for the next obstacle. I have no idea what it will be. I haven't taken much time to consider my fears, or even what it would mean to be free from fear, to conquer it. It occurs to me that without fear, I might be strong, powerful, unstoppable. The idea seduces me for just a second before something hits my back, hard.

Then something hits my left side, and my right side, and I'm enclosed in a box large enough only for my body. Shock protects me from panic, at first, and then I breathe the close air and stare into the empty darkness, and my insides squeeze tighter and tighter. I can't breathe anymore. I can't breathe.

I bite down on my lip to keep from sobbing—I don't want Amar to see me cry, don't want him to tell the Dauntless that I'm a coward. I have to think, can't think, through the suffocation of this box. The wall against my back here is the same as the one in my memory, from when I was young, shut in the darkness in the upstairs hallway as punishment. I was never sure when it would end, how many hours I would be stuck there with imaginary monsters creeping up on me in the dark, with the sound of my mother's sobs leaking through the walls.

I slam my hands against the wall in front of me, again and again, then claw at it, though the splinters stab the skin under my fingernails. I put up my forearms and hit the box with the full weight of my body, again and again, closing my eyes so I can pretend I'm not in here, I'm not in here. *Let me out let me out let me out let me out.*

"Think it through, Stiff!" a voice shouts, and I go still. I remember that this is a simulation.

Think it through. What do I need to get out of this box? I need a tool, something stronger than I am. I nudge something with my toes and reach down to pick it up. But when I reach down, the top of the box moves with me, and I can't straighten again. I swallow a scream and find the pointy end of a crowbar with my fingers. I wedge it between the boards that form the left corner of the box and push as hard as I can.

All the boards spring apart at once and fall on the ground around me. I breathe the fresh air, relieved.

Then a woman appears in front of me. I don't recognize her face, and her clothes are white, not belonging to any faction. I move toward her, and a table springs up in front of me, with a gun and a bullet on it. I frown at it.

Is this a fear?

"Who are you?" I ask her, and she doesn't answer.

It's clear what I'm supposed to do—load the gun, fire the bullet. Dread builds inside of me, as powerful as any fear. My mouth goes dry, and I fumble for the bullet and the gun. I've never held a gun before, so it takes me a few seconds to figure out how to open the chamber of the pistol. In those seconds I think of the light leaving her eyes, this woman I don't know, don't know enough to care about her.

I am afraid—I am afraid of what I will be asked to do in Dauntless, of what I will want to do.

Afraid of some kind of hidden violence inside of me, wrought by my father and by the years of silence my faction forced on me.

I slide the bullet into the chamber, then hold the gun in both hands, the cut in my palm throbbing. I look at the woman's face. Her lower lip wobbles, and her eyes fill with tears.

"I'm sorry," I say, and I pull the trigger.

I see the dark hole the bullet creates in her body, and she falls to the floor, evaporating into a cloud of dust on contact.

But the dread doesn't go away. I know that something's coming; I can feel it building inside me. Marcus has not appeared yet, and he will, I know it as surely as I know my own name. Our name.

A circle of light envelops me, and at its edge, I see worn gray shoes pacing. Marcus Eaton steps into the edge of the light, but not the Marcus Eaton I know. This one has pits for eyes and a gaping black maw instead of a mouth.

Another Marcus Eaton stands beside him, and slowly, all around the circle, more and more monstrous versions of my father step forward to surround me, their yawning, toothless mouths open wide, their heads tilting at odd angles. I squeeze my hands into fists. It's not real. It's obviously not real.

The first Marcus undoes his belt and then slides it out from around his waist, loop by loop, and as he does, so do the other Marcuses. As they do, the belts turn into ropes made of metal, barbed at the ends. They drag their belts in lines across the floor, their oily black tongues sliding over the edges of their dark mouths. At once they draw back the metal ropes, and I scream at the top of my lungs, wrapping my arms around my head.

"This is for your own good," the Marcuses say in metallic, united voices, like a choir.

I feel pain, tearing, ripping, shredding. I fall to my knees and squeeze my arms against my ears like they can protect me, but nothing can protect me, nothing. I scream again and again but the pain continues, and so does his voice. "I will not have self-indulgent behavior in my house!" "I did not raise my son to be a liar!"

I can't hear, I won't hear.

An image of the sculpture my mother gave me rises into my mind, unbidden. I see it where I placed it on my desk, and the pain starts to recede. I focus all my thoughts on it and the other objects scattered around my room, broken, the top of the trunk loose from its hinges. I remember my mother's hands, with their slim fingers, closing the trunk and locking it and handing me the key.

One by one, the voices disappear, until there are none left.

I let my arms fall to the ground, waiting for the next obstacle. My knuckles brush the stone floor, which is cold and grainy with dirt. I hear footsteps and brace myself for what's coming, but then I hear Amar's voice:

"That's it?" he says. "That's all there is? God, Stiff."

He stops next to me and offers me his hand. I take it and let him pull me to my feet. I don't look at him. I don't want to see his expression. I don't want him to know what he knows, don't want to become the pathetic initiate with the messed-up childhood.

"We should come up with another name for you," he says casually. "Something tougher than 'Stiff.' Like 'Blade' or 'Killer' or something."

At that I do look at him. He's smiling a little. I do see

some pity in that smile, but not as much as I thought I would.

"I wouldn't want to tell people my name either," he says. "Come on, let's get some food."

+++

Amar walks me over to the initiates' table once we're in the dining hall. There are a few Dauntless already sitting at the surrounding tables, eyeing the other side of the room, where pierced and tattooed cooks are still setting out the food. The dining hall is a cavern lit from beneath by blue-white lamps, giving everything an eerie glow.

I sit down in one of the empty chairs.

"Jeez, Stiff. You look like you're about to faint," Eric says, and one of the Candor boys grins.

"You all made it out alive," Amar says. "Congratulations. You made it through the first day of initiation, with varying degrees of success." He looks at Eric. "None of you did as well as Four over here, though."

He points at me as he speaks. I frown—four? Is he talking about my fears?

"Hey, Tori," Amar calls over his shoulder. "You ever hear of anyone having only four fears in their fear landscape?"

"Last I heard, the record was seven or eight. Why?" Tori calls back.

"I've got a transfer over here with only four fears."

Tori points at me, and Amar nods.

"That's gotta be a new record," Tori says.

"Well done," Amar says to me. Then he turns and walks toward Tori's table.

All the other initiates stare at me, wide-eyed and quiet. Before the fear landscape, I was just someone they could step on, on their way to Dauntless membership. Now I'm like Eric—someone worth watching out for, maybe even someone worth being afraid of.

Amar gave me more than a new name. He gave me power.

"What's your real name, again? Starts with an *E* . . . ?" Eric asks me, narrowing his eyes. Like he knows something but isn't sure that now is the time to share it.

The others might remember my name too, vaguely, from the Choosing Ceremony, the way I remember theirs—just letters in an alphabet, buried under a nervous haze as I anticipated my own choice. If I strike at their memories now, as hard as I can, become as memorable as my Dauntless self as possible, I can maybe save myself.

I hesitate for a moment, then put my elbows on the table

and raise an eyebrow at him.

"My name is Four," I say. "Call me 'Stiff' again and you and I will have a problem."

He rolls his eyes, but I know I've made myself clear. I have a new name, which means I can be a new person. Someone who doesn't put up with cutting comments from Erudite know-it-alls. Someone who can cut back.

Someone who's finally ready to fight.

Four.

THE INITIATE

THE TRAINING ROOM smells like effort, like sweat and dust and shoes. Every time my fist hits the punching bag it stings my knuckles, which are split open from a week of Dauntless fights.

"So I guess you saw the boards," Amar says, leaning against the door frame. He crosses his arms. "And realized that you're up against Eric tomorrow. Or else you would be in the fear landscape room instead of in here."

"I come in here, too," I say, and I back away from the bag, shaking out my hands. Sometimes I clench my hands so hard I start to lose feeling in my fingertips.

I almost lost my first fight, against the Amity girl, Mia. I didn't know how to beat her without hitting her, and I couldn't hit her—at least, not until she had me in a choke hold and my vision was starting to go black at the edges. My instincts took over, and just one hard elbow to her jaw knocked her down. I still feel guilt curling up inside me when I think about it.

I almost lost the second fight, too, against the bigger Candor boy Sean. I wore him out, crawling to my feet every time he thought I was finished. He didn't know that pushing through pain is one of my oldest habits, learned young, like chewing on my thumbnail, or holding my fork in my left hand instead of my right. Now my face is patchworked with bruises and cuts, but I proved myself.

Tomorrow my opponent is Eric. Beating him will take more than a clever move, or persistence. It will take skill I don't have, strength I haven't earned.

"Yeah, I know." Amar laughs. "See, I spend a lot of time trying to figure out what your deal is, so I've been asking around. Turns out you're in here every morning and in the fear landscape room every night. You never spend any time with the other initiates. You're always exhausted and you sleep like a corpse."

A drop of sweat rolls down the back of my ear. I wipe it away with my taped-up fingers, then drag my arm across my forehead.

"Joining a faction is about more than getting through initiation, you know," Amar says, and he hooks his fingers in the chain that the punching bag dangles from, testing its strength. "For most of the Dauntless, they meet their best friends during initiation, their girlfriends, boyfriends, whatever. Enemies, too. But you seem determined not to have any of those things."

I've seen the other initiates together, getting pierced together and showing up to training with red, studded noses and ears and lips, or building towers out of food scraps at the breakfast table. It never even occurred to me that I could be one of them, or that I should try to be.

I shrug. "I'm used to being alone."

"Well, I feel like you're about to snap, and I don't really want to be there when it happens," he says. "Come on. A bunch of us are going to play a game tonight. A Dauntless game."

I pick at the tape covering one of my knuckles. I shouldn't go out and play games. I should stay here and work, and then sleep, so I'm ready to fight tomorrow.

But that voice, the one that says "should," now sounds to me like my father's voice, requiring me to behave, to isolate myself. And I came here because I was ready to *stop* listening to that voice.

"I'm offering you some Dauntless status for no particular reason other than that I feel bad for you," he says. "Don't be stupid and miss this opportunity."

"Fine," I say. "What's the game?"

Amar just smiles.

+ + +

"The game is Dare." A Dauntless girl, Lauren, is holding on to the handle on the side of the train car, but she keeps swaying so she almost falls out, then giggling and pulling herself back in, like the train isn't suspended two stories above the street, like she wouldn't break her neck if she fell out.

In her free hand is a silver flask. It explains a lot.

She tilts her head. "First person picks someone and dares them to do something. Then that person has a drink, does the dare, and gets a chance to dare someone else to do something. And when everyone has done their dare—or died trying—we get a little drunk and stumble home."

"How do you win?" one of the Dauntless calls out from the other side of the train car. A boy who sits slouched against Amar like they're old friends, or brothers.

I'm not the only initiate in the train car. Sitting across from me is Zeke, the first jumper, and a girl with brown hair and bangs cut straight across her forehead, and a pierced lip. The others are older, Dauntless members all. They have a kind of ease with one another, leaning into one another, punching one another's arms, tousling one another's hair. It's camaraderie and friendship and flirtation, and none of it is familiar to me. I try to relax, bending my arms around my knees.

I really am a Stiff.

"You win by not being a little pansycake," Lauren says. "And, hey, new rule, you also win by not asking dumb questions.

"I'm gonna go first, as the keeper of the alcohol," she adds. "Amar, I dare you to go into the Erudite library while all the Noses are studying and scream something obscene."

She screws the cap on the flask and tosses it to him. Everyone cheers as Amar takes the cap off and takes a swallow of whatever liquor is inside.

"Just tell me when we get to the right stop!" he shouts over the cheering.

Zeke waves a hand at me. "Hey, you're a transfer, right? Four?"

"Yeah," I say. "Nice first jump."

I realize, too late, that it might be a sore spot for him— his moment of triumph, stolen by a misstep and loss of balance. But he just laughs.

"Yeah, not my finest moment," he says.

"Not like anyone else stepped up," the girl at his side says. "I'm Shauna, by the way. Is it true you only had four fears?"

"Hence the name," I say.

"Wow." She nods. She looks impressed, which makes me sit up straighter. "Guess you were born Dauntless."

I shrug, like what she says might be true, even though I'm sure it's not. She doesn't know that I came here to escape the life I was meant for, that I'm fighting so hard to get through initiation so I don't have to admit that I'm an imposter. Abnegation-born, Abnegation result, in a Dauntless haven.

The corners of her mouth turn down, like she's sad about something, but I don't ask what it is.

"How are your fights going?" Zeke asks me.

"All right," I say. I wave a hand over my bruised face. "As you can clearly tell."

"Check it out." Zeke turns his head, showing me a large bruise on the underside of his jaw. "That's thanks to this girl over here."

He indicates Shauna with his thumb.

"He beat me," Shauna says. "But I got a good shot in, for once. I keep losing."

"It doesn't bother you that he hit you?" I say.

"Why would it?" she says.

"I don't know," I say. "Because . . . you're a girl?"

She raises her eyebrows. "What, you think I can't take it just like every other initiate, just because I have girl parts?" She gestures to her chest, and I catch myself staring, just for a second, before I remember to look away, my face flushing.

"Sorry," I say. "I didn't mean it that way. I'm just not used to this. Any of it."

"Sure, I get it," she says, and she doesn't sound angry. "But you should know that about Dauntless—girl, guy, whatever, it doesn't matter here. What matters is what you've got in your gut."

Then Amar gets up, putting his hands on his hips in a dramatic stance, and marches toward the open doorway. The train dips down and Amar doesn't even hold on to anything, he just shifts and sways with the car's movement. Everyone gets up, and Amar is the first one to jump, launching himself into the night. The others stream out behind him, and I let the people behind me carry me toward the opening. I'm not afraid of the speed of the train, just the heights, but here the train is close to the ground, so when I jump, I do it without fear. I land on two feet, stumbling for a few steps before I stop.

"Look at you, getting your train legs," Amar says, elbowing me. "Here, have a sip. You look like you need it."

He holds out the flask.

I've never tasted alcohol. The Abnegation don't drink it, so it wasn't even available. But I've seen how comfortable it seems to make people, and I desperately want to feel like I'm not wrapped up in skin that's too tight for me to wear, so I don't hesitate: I take the flask and drink.

The alcohol burns and tastes like medicine, but it goes down fast, leaving me warm.

"Good job," Amar says, and he moves on to Zeke, hooking his arm around Zeke's neck and dragging Zeke's head against his chest. "I see you've met my young friend Ezekiel."

"Just because my mom calls me that doesn't mean you have to," Zeke says, throwing Amar off. He looks at me. "Amar's grandparents were friends with my parents."

"Were?"

"Well, my dad's dead, and so are the grandparents," Zeke says.

"What about your parents?" I ask Amar.

He shrugs. "Died when I was young. Train accident. Very sad." He grins like it's not. "And my grandparents took the jump after I became an official member of Dauntless." He makes a careening gesture with his hand, suggesting a dive.

"The jump?"

"Oh, don't tell him while I'm here," Zeke says, shaking his head. "I don't want to see the look on his face."

Amar doesn't pay attention. "Elderly Dauntless sometimes take a flying leap into the unknown of the chasm when they hit a certain age. It's that or be factionless," Amar says. "And my grandpa was really sick. Cancer. Grandma didn't care to go on without him."

He tilts his head up to the sky, and his eyes reflect the moonlight. For a moment I feel like he is showing me a secret self, one carefully hidden beneath layers of charm and humor and Dauntless bravado, and it scares me, because that secret self is hard, and cold, and sad.

"I'm sorry," I say.

"At least this way, I got to say my good-byes," Amar says. "Most of the time death just comes whether you've said good-bye or not."

The secret self vanishes with the flash of a smile, and Amar jogs toward the rest of the group, flask in hand. I stay back with Zeke. He lopes along, somehow clumsy and graceful at once, like a wild dog.

"What about you?" Zeke says. "You have parents?"

"One," I say. "My mother died a long time ago."

I remember the funeral, with all the Abnegation filling our house with quiet chatter, staying with us in our grief. They carried us meals on metal trays, covered with tinfoil, and cleaned our kitchen, and boxed up all my mother's clothes for us, so there were no traces of her left. I remember them murmuring that she died from complications with another child. But I had a memory of her, a few months before her death, standing in front of her dresser, buttoning up her loose second shirt over the tight undershirt, her stomach flat. I shake my head a little, banishing the memory. She's dead. It's a child's memory, unreliable.

"And your dad, is he okay with your choice?" he says. "Visiting Day is coming up, you know."

"No," I say distantly. "He's not okay with it at all."

My father will not come on Visiting Day. I'm sure of it. He will never speak to me again.

The Erudite sector is cleaner than any other part of the city, every scrap of trash or rubble cleared from the pavement, every crack in the street shored up with tar. I feel like I need to step carefully rather than mar the sidewalk with my sneakers. The other Dauntless walk along carelessly, the soles of their shoes making slapping sounds like pattering rain.

Every faction headquarters is allowed to have the lights on in its lobby at midnight, but everything else is supposed to be dark. Here, in the Erudite sector, each building that makes up Erudite headquarters is like a pillar of light. The windows we walk past feature the Erudite sitting at long tables, their noses buried in books or screens, or talking quietly to one another. The young and the old mix together at every table, in their impeccable blue clothing, their smooth hair, more than half of them with gleaming spectacles. *Vanity,* my father would say. *They are so concerned with looking intelligent that they make themselves fools for it.*

I pause to watch them. They don't look vain to me. They look like people who make every effort to feel as smart as they are supposed to be. If that means wearing glasses with no prescription, it isn't my place to judge. They are a haven I might have chosen. Instead I chose the haven that mocks them through the windows, that sends Amar into their lobby to cause a stir.

Amar reaches the doors of the central Erudite building and pushes through them. We watch from just outside, snickering. I peer through the doors at the portrait of Jeanine Matthews hanging on the opposite wall. Her yellow hair is pulled back tight from her face, her blue jacket buttoned just beneath her throat. She's pretty, but that's not the first thing I notice about her. Her sharpness is.

And beyond that—it could just be my imagination, but does she look a little afraid?

Amar runs into the lobby, ignoring the protests of the Erudite at the front desk, and yells, "Hey, Noses! Check this out!"

All the Erudite in the lobby look up from their books or screens, and the Dauntless burst into laughter as Amar turns, mooning them. The Erudite behind the desk run around it to catch him, but Amar pulls up his pants and runs toward us. We all start running, too, sprinting away from the doors.

I can't help it—I'm laughing too, and it surprises me, how my stomach aches with it. Zeke runs at my shoulder, and we go toward the train tracks because there's nowhere else to run. The Erudite chasing us give up after a block, and we all stop in an alley, leaning against the brick to catch our breath.

Amar comes into the alley last, his hands raised, and we cheer for him. He holds up the flask like it's a trophy and points at Shauna.

"Young one," he says. "I dare you to scale the sculpture in front of the Upper Levels building."

She catches the flask when he throws it and takes a swig.

"You got it," she says, grinning.

+++

By the time they get to me, almost everyone is drunk, lurching with each footstep and laughing at every joke, no matter how stupid it is. I feel warm, despite the cool air, but my mind is still sharp, taking in everything about the night, the rich smell of marsh and the sound of bubbling laughter, the blue-black of the sky and the silhouette of each building against it. My legs are sore from running and walking and climbing, and still I haven't fulfilled a dare.

We're close to Dauntless headquarters now. The buildings are sagging where they stand.

"Who's left?" Lauren says, her bleary eyes skipping over each face until she reaches mine. "Ah, the numerically named initiate from Abnegation. Four, is it?"

"Yeah," I say.

"A Stiff?" The boy who sat so comfortably beside Amar looks at me, his words running together. He's the one holding the flask, the one determining the next dare. So far I've watched people scale tall structures, I've watched them jump into dark holes and wander into empty buildings to retrieve a faucet or a desk chair, I've watched them run naked down alleyways and stick needles through their earlobes without numbing them first. If I was asked to concoct a dare, I would not be able to think of one. It's a good thing I'm the last person to go.

I feel a tremor in my chest, nerves. What will he tell me to do?

"Stiffs are uptight," the boy says plainly, like it's a fact. "So, to prove you're really Dauntless now . . . I dare you to get a tattoo."

I see their ink, creeping over wrists and arms and shoulders and throats. The metal studs through ears and noses and lips and eyebrows. My skin is blank, healed, whole. But it doesn't match who I am—I should be scarred, marked, the way they are, but marked with memories of pain, scarred with the things I have survived.

I lift a shoulder. "Fine."

He tosses me the flask, and I drain it, though it stings my throat and lips and tastes bitter as poison.

We start toward the Pire.

+++

Tori is wearing a pair of men's underwear and a T-shirt when she answers the door, her hair hanging over the left half of her face. She raises an eyebrow at me. We clearly woke her from a sound sleep, but she doesn't seem angry— just a little grouchy.

"Please?" Amar says. "It's for a game of Dare."

"Are you sure you want a tired woman to tattoo your

skin, Four? This ink doesn't wash off," she says to me.

"I trust you," I say. I'm not going to back out of the dare, not after watching everyone else do theirs.

"Right." Tori yawns. "The things I do for Dauntless tradition. I'll be right back, I'm going to put on pants."

She closes the door between us. On the way here I racked my brain for what I might want tattooed, and where. I couldn't decide—my thoughts were too muddled. Still are.

A few seconds later Tori emerges wearing pants, her feet still bare. "If I get in trouble for turning on lights at this hour, I'm going to claim it was vandals and name names."

"Got it," I say.

"There's a back way. Come on," she says, beckoning to us. I follow her through her dark living room, which is tidy except for the sheets of paper spread over her coffee table, each one marked with a different drawing. Some of them are harsh and simple, like most of the tattoos I've seen, and others are more intricate, detailed. Tori must be the Dauntless approximation of an artist.

I pause by the table. One of the pages depicts all the faction symbols, without the circles that usually bind them. The Amity tree is at the bottom, forming a kind of root system for the eye of Erudite and the Candor scales. Above them, the Abnegation hands seem almost to cradle the Dauntless flames. It's like the symbols are growing into one another.

The others have moved past me. I jog to catch up, walking through Tori's kitchen—also immaculate, though the appliances are out of date, the faucet rusted, and the refrigerator door held closed by a large clamp. The back door is open and leads into a short, dank hallway that opens up to the tattoo parlor.

I've walked past it before but never cared to go inside, sure I wasn't going to find a reason to attack my own body with needles. I guess I have one now—those needles are a way for me to separate myself from my past, not just in the eyes of my fellow Dauntless, but in my own eyes, every time I look at my own reflection.

The room's walls are covered in pictures. The wall by the door is entirely dedicated to Dauntless symbols, some black and simple, some colorful and barely recognizable. Tori turns on the light over one of the chairs and arranges her tattoo needles on a tray next to it. The other Dauntless gather on benches and chairs around us, like they're getting ready to see a performance of some kind. My face gets hot.

"Basic principles of tattooing," Tori says. "The less cushion under the skin, or the bonier you are in a particular area, the more painful the tattoo. For your first one it's probably best to get it done on, I don't know, your arm, or—"

"Your butt cheek," Zeke suggests, with a snort of laughter.

Tori shrugs. "It wouldn't be the first time. Or the last."

I look at the boy who dared me. He raises his eyebrows at me. I know what he expects, what they all expect—that I'll get something small, on an arm or a leg, something that's easily hidden. I glance at the wall with all the symbols. One of the drawings in particular catches my eye, an artistic rendering of the flames themselves.

"That one," I say, pointing to it.

"Got it," Tori says. "Got a location in mind?"

I have a scar—a faint gouge in my knee from when I fell down on the sidewalk as a child. It's always seemed stupid to me that none of the pain I've experienced has left a visible mark; sometimes, without a way to prove it to myself, I began to doubt that I had lived through it at all, with the memories becoming hazy over time. I want to have some kind of reminder that while wounds heal, they don't disappear forever—I carry them everywhere, always, and that is the way of things, the way of scars.

That is what this tattoo will be, for me: a scar. And it seems fitting that it should document the worst memory of pain that I have.

I rest my hand on my rib cage, remembering the bruises that were, and the fear I felt for my own life. My father had a series of bad nights right after my mother died.

"You sure?" Tori says. "That's maybe the most painful place possible."

"Good," I say, and I sit down in the chair.

The crowd of Dauntless cheer and start passing around another flask, this one bigger than the last, and bronze instead of silver.

"So we have a masochist in the chair tonight. Lovely." Tori sits on the stool next to me and puts on a pair of rubber gloves. I sit forward, lifting up the hem of my shirt, and she soaks a cotton ball in rubbing alcohol, covering my ribs with it. She's about to move away when she frowns and pulls at my skin with her fingertip. Rubbing alcohol bites into the still-healing skin of my back, and I wince.

"How did this happen, Four?" she asks.

I look up and notice that Amar is staring at me, frowning.

"He's an initiate," Amar says. "They're *all* cut and bruised at this point. You should see them all limping around together. It's sad."

"I have a giant one on my knee," volunteers Zeke. "It's the sickest blue color—"

Zeke rolls up his pant leg to display his bruise to the others, and they all start sharing their own bruises, their own scars: "Got this when they *dropped* me after the zip line." "Well, I've got a stab wound from your grip slipping during knife-throwing, so I think we're even." Tori eyes me for a few seconds, and I'm sure she doesn't accept Amar's explanation for the marks on my back, but she doesn't ask again. Instead, she turns on the needle, filling the air with the sound of buzzing, and Amar tosses me the flask.

The alcohol is still burning my throat when the tattoo needle touches my ribs, and I wince, but somehow I don't mind the pain.

I relish it.

+++

The next day, when I wake up, everything hurts. Especially my head.

Oh God, my head.

Eric is perched on the edge of the mattress next to mine, tying his shoelaces. The skin around the rings in his lip looks red—he must have pierced it recently. I haven't been paying attention.

He looks at me. "You look like hell."

I sit up, and the sudden motion makes my head throb more.

"I hope that when you lose, you don't use it as an excuse," he says, sneering a little. "Because I would have beat you anyway."

He gets up, stretches, and leaves the dormitory. I cradle my head in my hands for a few seconds, then get up to take a shower. I have to stand with half my body under the water and half out, because of the ink on my side. The Dauntless stayed with me for hours, waiting for the tattoo to be finished, and by the time we left, all the flasks were empty. Tori gave me a thumbs-up as I stumbled out of the tattoo parlor, and Zeke slung an arm across my shoulders and said, "I think you're Dauntless now."

Last night I found myself relishing the words. Now I wish I could have my old head back, the one that was focused and determined and didn't feel like tiny men with hammers had taken up residence inside it. I let the cool water spill over me for a few more minutes, then check the clock on the bathroom wall.

Ten minutes to the fight. I'm going to be late. And Eric is right—I'm going to lose.

I push my hand into my forehead as I run toward the training room, my feet halfway out of my shoes. When I burst through the doors, the transfer initiates and some of the Dauntless-born initiates are standing around the edge of the room. Amar is in the center of the arena, checking his watch. He gives me a pointed look.

"Nice of you to join us," he says. I see in his raised eyebrows that the camaraderie of the night before does not extend to the training room. He points at my shoes. "Tie your shoes, and don't waste any more of my time."

Across the arena, Eric cracks each one of his knuckles, carefully, staring at me the whole time. I tie my shoes in a hurry and tuck the ends of the laces under so they don't get in my way.

As I face Eric I can feel only the pounding of my heart, the throbbing of my head, the burning in my side. Then Amar steps back, and Eric rushes forward, fast, his fist hitting me square in the jaw.

I stumble back, holding my face. All the pain runs together in my mind. I put up my hands to block the next punch. My head throbs and I see his leg move. I try to twist away from the kick, but his foot hits me hard in the ribs. I feel a sensation like an electric shock through the left side of my body.

"This is easier than I thought it would be," Eric says.

I feel hot with embarrassment, and in the arrogant opening he leaves me, I uppercut him in the stomach.

The flat of his hand smacks into my ear, making it ring, and I lose my balance, my fingers touching the ground to steady me.

"You know," Eric says quietly, "I think I've figured out your real name."

My eyes are blurry with half a dozen different kinds of pain. I didn't know it came in so many varieties, like flavors, acid and fire and ache and sting.

He hits me again, this time trying for my face but getting my collarbone instead. He shakes out his hand and says, "Should I tell them? Get everything out in the open?"

He has my name between his teeth, *Eaton*, a far more threatening weapon than his feet or his elbows or his fists. The Abnegation say, in hushed voices, that the problem with many Erudite is their selfishness, but I think it is their arrogance, the pride they take in knowing things that others do not. In that moment, overwhelmed with fear, I recognize it as Eric's weakness. He doesn't believe that I can hurt him as much as he can hurt me. He believes that I am everything he assumed me to be at the outset, humble and selfless and passive.

I feel my pain disappear into rage, and I grab his arm to hold him in place as I swing at him again, and again, and again. I don't even see where I'm hitting him; I don't see or feel or hear anything. I am empty, alone, nothing.

Then I finally hear his screams, see him clutching his face with both hands. Blood soaks his chin, runs into his teeth. He tries to wrench away but I am holding on as hard as I can, holding on for dear life.

I kick him hard in the side, so he topples. Over his clutched hands, I meet his eyes.

His eyes are glassy and unfocused. His blood is bright against his skin. It occurs to me that I did that, it was me, and fear creeps back in, a different kind of fear this time. A fear of what I am, what I might be becoming.

My knuckles throb, and I walk out of the arena without being dismissed.

+++

The Dauntless compound is a good place to recover, dark and full of secret, quiet places.

I find a hallway near the Pit and sit against the wall, letting the cold from the stone seep into me. My headache has returned, as well as various aches and pains from the fight, but I barely register any of them. My knuckles are tacky with blood, Eric's. I try to rub it off but it's been drying too long. I won the fight, and that means my place in Dauntless is secure for the time being—I should feel satisfied, not afraid. Maybe even happy, to finally belong somewhere, to be among people whose eyes don't skirt mine at the lunch table. But I know that for every good thing that comes along, there is always a cost. What is the cost of being Dauntless?

"Hey." I look up and see Shauna knocking on the stone

wall like it's a door. She grins. "This is not quite the victory dance I was expecting."

"I don't dance," I say.

"Yeah, I should have known better." She sits across from me, her back against the opposite wall. She draws her knees up to her chest and wraps her arms around them. Our feet are just a few inches apart. I don't know why I notice that. Well, yes I do—she's a girl.

I don't know how to talk to girls. Especially not a Dauntless girl. Something tells me you can never know what to expect from a Dauntless girl.

"Eric's in the hospital," she says, and there's a grin on her face. "They think you broke his nose. You definitely knocked out one of his teeth."

I look down. I knocked out someone's tooth?

"I was wondering if you could help me," she says, nudging my shoe with her toe.

As I suspected: Dauntless girls are unpredictable. "Help you with what?"

"Fighting. I'm no good at it. I keep getting humiliated in the arena." She shakes her head. "I have to face off with this girl in two days, her name's Ashley but she makes everyone call her Ash." Shauna rolls her eyes. "You know, Dauntless flames, ash, whatever. Anyway, she's one of the best people in our group, and I'm afraid she's going to kill me. Like actually kill me."

"Why do you want my help?" I say, suddenly suspicious. "Because you know I'm a Stiff and we're supposed to help people?"

"What? No, of course not," she says. Her eyebrows furrow in confusion. "I want your help because you're the best in *your* group, obviously."

I laugh. "No, I'm not."

"You and Eric were the only undefeated ones and you just beat him, so yeah, you are. Listen, if you don't want to help me, all you have to do is—"

"I'll help," I say. "I just don't really know how."

"We'll figure it out," she says. "Tomorrow afternoon? Meet you in the arena?"

I nod. She grins, gets up, and starts to leave. But a few steps away and she turns around, moving backward down the hallway.

"Quit sulking, Four," she says. "Everyone's impressed with you. Embrace it."

I watch her silhouette turn the corner at the end of the hallway. I was so disturbed by the fight that I never thought about what beating Eric meant—that I am now first in my initiate class. I may have chosen Dauntless as a haven, but I'm not just surviving here, I'm excelling.

I stare at Eric's blood on my knuckles and smile.

+ + +

The next morning I decide to take a risk. I sit with Zeke and Shauna at breakfast. Shauna mostly just slumps over her food and answers questions in grunts. Zeke yawns into his coffee, but he points out his family to me: his little brother, Uriah, sits at one of the other tables with Lynn, Shauna's little sister. His mother, Hana—the tamest Dauntless I've ever seen, her faction indicated only by the color of her clothing—is still in the breakfast line.

"Do you miss living at home?" I say.

The Dauntless have a proclivity for baked goods, I've noticed. There are always at least two different kinds of cake at dinner, and a mountain of muffins rests on a table near the end of the breakfast line. When I got there, all the good flavors were gone, so I was left with bran.

"Not really," he says. "I mean, they're right there. Dauntless-born initiates aren't really supposed to talk to family until Visiting Day, but I know if I really needed something, they'd be there."

I nod. Beside him, Shauna's eyes close, and she falls asleep with her chin resting on her hand.

"What about you?" he says. "Do you miss home?"

I am about to answer no, but right at that moment Shauna's chin slips off her hand and she smashes her chocolate muffin with her face. Zeke laughs so hard he cries, and I can't help but grin as I finish my juice.

+ + +

Later that morning I meet Shauna in the training room. She has her short hair pulled back from her face, and her Dauntless boots, normally untied and flapping when she walks, laced up tight. She's punching at nothing, pausing between each hit to adjust her position, and for a moment I watch her, not sure how to start. I only just learned to throw a punch myself; I'm hardly qualified to teach her anything.

But as I watch her, I start to notice things. How she stands with her knees locked, how she doesn't hold up a hand to protect her jaw, how she punches from her elbow instead of throwing her body weight behind each hit. She stops, wiping her forehead with the back of her hand. When she notices me, she jumps like she just touched a live wire.

"Rule number one for not being creepy," she says. "Announce your presence in a room if another person doesn't see you come in."

"Sorry," I say. "I was coming up with some pointers for you."

"Oh." She chews on the inside of her cheek. "What are they?"

I tell her what I noticed, and then we face off in the

fighting arena. We begin slowly, pulling back on each hit so we don't hurt each other. I have to keep tapping her elbow with my fist to remind her to keep her hand up by her face, but a half hour later, she's at least moving better than she was before.

"This girl you have to fight tomorrow," I say. "I'd get her right here, in the jaw." I touch the underside of my jaw. "A good uppercut should do it. Let's practice those."

She squares off, and I notice with satisfaction that her knees are bent, and there's a bounce in her stance that wasn't there before. We shuffle around each other for a few seconds, and then she punches up. As she does, her left hand drops from her face. I block the first punch, then start to attack the hole she left in her guard. At the last second, I stop my fist in the air and raise my eyebrows at her.

"You know, maybe I would learn my lesson if you actually hit me," she says, straightening. Her skin is flushed from exertion, and sweat shines along her hairline. Her eyes are bright and critical. It occurs to me, for the first time, that she's pretty. Not in the way I usually think of—she's not soft, delicate—but in a way that's strong, capable.

I say, "I would really rather not."

"What you think is some kind of lingering Abnegation chivalry is really kind of insulting," she says. "I can take care of myself. I can take a little pain."

"It's not that," I say. "It's not because you're a girl. I just . . . I'm not really into violence for no reason."

"Some kind of Stiff thing, huh?" she says.

"Not really. Stiffs aren't into violence, period. Put a Stiff in Dauntless and they just let themselves get punched a lot," I say, letting myself smile a little. I'm not used to using Dauntless slang, but it feels good to claim it as my own, to let myself relax into their rhythms of speech. "It just doesn't feel like a game to me, that's all."

It's the first time I've expressed that to anyone. I know why it doesn't feel like a game—because for so long, it was my reality, it was my waking and my sleeping. Here, I've learned to defend myself, I've learned to be stronger, but one thing I haven't learned, won't let myself learn, is how to enjoy causing someone else pain. If I'm going to become Dauntless, I'm going to do it on my terms, even if that means that a part of me will always be a Stiff.

"All right," she says. "Let's go again."

We spar until she's mastered the uppercut and we've almost missed dinner. When we leave, she thanks me, and casually, she wraps an arm around me. It's just a quick embrace, but she laughs at how tense it makes me.

"How to Be Dauntless: An Introductory Course," she says. "Lesson one: It's okay to hug your friends here."

"We're friends?" I say, only halfway joking.

"Oh, shut up," she says, and she jogs down the hallway toward the dormitory.

+++

The next morning, all the transfer initiates follow Amar past the training room to a grim hallway with a heavy door at the end of it. He tells us to sit against the wall, and then disappears behind the door without saying anything. I check my watch. Shauna will be fighting any minute now— it's taking the Dauntless-borns longer to get through the first phase of initiation than us, since there are more of them.

Eric sits as far away from me as he can, and I am glad for the distance. The night after I fought him, it occurred to me that he might tell everyone that I'm Marcus Eaton's son just to spite me for beating him, but he hasn't done it. I wonder if he's just waiting for the right opportunity to strike, or if he's holding back for another reason. No matter what, it's probably better for me to stay away from him as much as possible.

"What do you think is in there?" Mia, the Amity transfer, sounds nervous.

No one answers. For some reason I don't feel nervous. There's nothing behind that door that can hurt me. So when Amar steps into the hallway again and calls my name first, I don't cast desperate looks at my fellow initiates. I just follow him in.

The room is dim and grungy, with just a chair and a computer in it. The chair is reclined, like the one I sat in for my aptitude test. The computer screen is bright and running a program that amounts to lines of dark text on a white background. When I was younger, I used to volunteer at the school in the computer labs, maintaining the facilities, and sometimes even fixing the computers themselves when they failed. I worked under the supervision of an Erudite woman named Katherine, and she taught me far more than she had to, happy to share her knowledge with someone who was willing to listen. So I know, looking at that code, what kind of program I'm looking at, though I would never be able to do much with it.

"A simulation?" I say.

"The less you know, the better," he says. "Sit down."

I sit, leaning back in the chair and setting my arms on the armrests. Amar prepares a syringe, holding it up to the light to make sure the vial is locked in place. He sticks the needle into my neck without warning and presses down on the plunger. I flinch.

"Let's see which of your four fears comes up first," he

says. "You know, I'm getting kind of bored of them, you might try to show me something new."

"I'll work on it," I say.

The simulation swallows me.

+ + +

I am sitting on the hard wooden bench at an Abnegation kitchen table, an empty plate in front of me. All the shades are drawn over the windows, so the only light comes from the bulb dangling over the table, its filament glowing orange. I stare at the dark fabric covering my knee. *Why am I wearing black instead of gray?*

When I lift my head, he—Marcus—is across from me. For a split second, he's just like the man I saw across the Choosing Ceremony hall not long ago, his eyes dark blue to match mine, his mouth pressed into a frown.

I'm wearing black because I'm Dauntless now, I remind myself. *So why am I in an Abnegation house, sitting across from my father?*

I see the outline of the lightbulb reflected in my empty plate. *This must be a simulation,* I think.

Then the light above us flickers, and he turns into the man I always see in my fear landscape, a twisted monster with pits for eyes and a wide, empty mouth. He lunges across the table with both hands outstretched, and instead of fingernails he has razor blades embedded in his fingertips.

He swipes at me, and I lurch back, falling off the bench. I scramble on the floor for my balance, then run into the living room. There is another Marcus there, reaching for me from the wall. I search for the front door, but someone has sealed it with cinder blocks, trapping me.

Gasping, I sprint up the stairs. At the top I trip, and sprawl on the wooden floor in the hallway. A Marcus opens the closet door from the inside; another one walks out of my parents' bedroom; yet another one claws across the floor from the bathroom. I shrink back against the wall. The house is dark. There are no windows.

This place is full of him.

Suddenly one of the Marcuses is right in front of me, pressing me to the wall with both hands around my throat. Another one drags his fingernails down my arms, provoking a stinging pain that brings tears to my eyes.

I am paralyzed, panicking.

I swallow air. I can't scream. I feel pain and my pounding heart and I kick as hard as I can, hitting only air. The Marcus with his hands around my throat shoves me up the wall, so my toes drag along the floor. My limbs are limp, like a rag doll's. I can't move.

This place, this place is full of him. *It's not real*, I realize.

It's a simulation. It's just like the fear landscape.

There are more Marcuses now, waiting below me with their hands outstretched, so I'm staring down at a sea of blades. Their fingers clutch at my legs, cutting me, and I feel a hot trail down the side of my neck as the Marcus who is choking me digs in harder.

Simulation, I remind myself. I try to send life into every one of my limbs. I imagine my blood on fire, racing through me. I slap my hand against the wall, searching for a weapon. One of the Marcuses reaches up, his fingers poised over my eyes. I scream and thrash as the blades dig into my eyelids.

My hands find not a weapon but a doorknob. I twist it, hard, and fall back into another closet. The Marcuses lose their hold on me. In the closet is a window, just big enough for my body. As they chase me into the darkness, I throw my shoulder against the glass, and it shatters. Fresh air fills my lungs.

I sit upright in the chair, gasping.

I put my hands against my throat, on my arms, on my legs, checking for wounds that aren't there. I can still feel the cuts and the unfurling of blood from my veins, but my skin is intact.

My breaths slow down, and with them, my thoughts.

Amar is sitting at the computer, hooked up to the simulation, and he's staring at me.

"What?" I say, breathless.

"You were in there for five minutes," Amar says.

"Is that long?"

"No." He frowns at me. "No, it's not long at all. It's very good, actually."

I put my feet on the floor and hold my head in my hands. I may not have panicked for that long during the simulation, but the image of my warped father trying to claw my eyes out keeps flashing in my mind, causing my heart rate to spike again and again.

"Is the serum still in effect?" I say, clenching my teeth. "Making me panic?"

"No, it should have gone dormant when you exited the simulation," he says. "Why?"

I shake my hands, which are tingling, like they're going numb. I shake my head. *It wasn't real,* I tell myself. *Let it go.*

"Sometimes the simulation causes lingering panic, depending on what you see in it," Amar says. "Let me walk you back to the dormitory."

"No." I shake my head. "I'll be fine."

He gives me a hard look.

"It wasn't a request," he says. He gets up and opens a

door behind the chair. I follow him down a short, dark hallway and into the stone corridors that lead back to the transfer dormitory. The air is cool there, and moist, from being underground. I hear our footsteps echo, and my own breaths, but nothing else.

I think I see something—movement—on my left, and I flinch away from it, pulling back against the wall. Amar stops me, putting his hands on my shoulders so I have to look at his face.

"Hey," he says. "Get it together, Four."

I nod, heat rushing into my face. I feel a deep twinge of shame in my stomach. I am supposed to be Dauntless. I am not supposed to be afraid of monster Marcuses creeping up on me in the dark. I lean against the stone wall and take a deep breath.

"Can I ask you something?" Amar says. I cringe, thinking he's going to ask me about my father, but he doesn't. "How did you get out of that hallway?"

"I opened a door," I say.

"Was there a door behind you the whole time? Is there one in your old house?"

I shake my head.

Amar's usually amiable face is serious. "So you created one out of nowhere?"

"Yeah," I say. "Simulations are all in your head. So my

head made a door so I could get out. All I had to do was concentrate."

"Strange," he says.

"What? Why?"

"Most initiates can't make something impossible happen in these simulations, because unlike in the fear landscape, they don't recognize that they are *in* a simulation," he says. "And they don't get out of simulations that fast, as a result."

I feel my pulse in my throat. I didn't realize these simulations were supposed to be different from the fear landscape—I thought everyone was aware of this simulation while they were in it. But judging by what Amar is saying, this was supposed to be like the aptitude test, and before the aptitude test, my father warned me against my simulation awareness, coached me to hide it. I still remember how insistent he was, how tense his voice was and how he grabbed my arm a little too hard.

At the time, I thought that he would never speak that way unless he was worried about me. Worried for my safety.

Was he just being paranoid, or is there still something dangerous about being aware during simulations?

"I was like you," Amar says quietly. "I could change the simulations. I just thought I was the only one."

I want to tell him to keep it to himself, to protect his secrets. But the Dauntless don't care about secrets the way the Abnegation do, with their tight-lipped smiles and identical, orderly houses.

Amar is giving me a strange look—eager, like he expects something from me. I shift, uncomfortable.

"It's probably not something you should brag about," Amar says. "The Dauntless are all about conformity, just like every other faction. It's just not as obvious here."

I nod.

"It's probably just a fluke," I say. "I couldn't do that during my aptitude test. Next time I'll probably be more normal."

"Right." He doesn't sound convinced. "Well, next time, try not to do anything impossible, all right? Just face your fear in a logical way, a way that would always make sense to you whether you were aware or not."

"Okay," I say.

"You're okay now, right? You can get back to the dorms on your own?"

I want to say that I could always get back to the dormitory on my own; I never needed him to take me there. But I just nod again. He claps me on the shoulder, good-naturedly, and walks back to the simulation room.

I can't help but think that my father wouldn't have

warned me against displaying my simulation awareness just because of faction norms. He scolded me for embarrassing him in front of the Abnegation all the time, but he had never hissed warnings in my ears or taught me how to avoid a misstep before. He never stared at me, wide-eyed, until I promised to do as he said.

It feels strange, to know that he must have been trying to protect me. Like he's not quite the monster I imagine, the one I see in my worst nightmares.

As I start toward the dorms, I hear something at the end of the hallway we just walked down—something like quiet, shuffling footsteps, moving in the opposite direction.

+++

Shauna runs up to me in the cafeteria at dinner and punches me hard in the arm. She's wearing a smile so wide it looks like it's cutting into her cheeks. There's some swelling just beneath her right eye—she'll have a black eye later.

"I won!" she says. "I did what you said—got her right in the jaw within the first sixty seconds, and it totally threw her off her game. She still hit me in the eye because I let my guard down, but after that I pummeled her. She has a bloody nose. It was awesome."

I grin. I'm surprised by how satisfying it is, to teach

someone how to do something and then to hear that it actually worked.

"Well done," I say.

"I couldn't have done it without your help," she says. Her smile changes, softens, less giddy and more sincere. She stands on her tiptoes and kisses my cheek.

I stare at her as she pulls away. She laughs and drags me toward the table where Zeke and some of the other Dauntless-born initiates sit. My problem, I realize, isn't that I'm a Stiff, it's that I don't know what these gestures of affection mean to the Dauntless. Shauna is pretty, and funny, and in Abnegation I would go over to her house for dinner with her family if I was interested in her, I would find out what volunteering project she was working on and insinuate myself into it. In Dauntless I have no idea how to go about that, or how to know if I even like her that way.

I decide not to let it distract me, at least not now. I get a plate of food and sit down to eat it, listening to the others talk and laugh together. Everyone congratulates Shauna on her win, and they point out the girl she beat up, sitting at one of the other tables, her face still swollen. At the end of the meal, when I'm poking at a piece of chocolate cake with my fork, a pair of Erudite women walk into the room.

It takes a lot to make the Dauntless go quiet. Even the sudden appearance of the Erudite doesn't quite do it—there are still mutters everywhere, like the distant sound of running footsteps. But gradually, as the Erudite sit down with Max and nothing else happens, conversations pick up again. I don't participate in them. I keep stabbing the cake with the fork tines, watching.

Max stands and approaches Amar. They have a tense conversation between the tables, and then they start walking in my direction. Toward *me*.

Amar beckons to me. I leave my almost-empty tray behind.

"You and I have been called in for an evaluation," Amar says. His perpetually smiling mouth is now a flat line, his animated voice a monotone.

"Evaluation?" I say.

Max smiles at me, a little. "Your fear simulation results were a little abnormal. Our Erudite friends behind us—" I look over his shoulder at the Erudite women. With a start, I realize that one of them is Jeanine Matthews, representative of Erudite. She's dressed in a crisp blue suit, with a pair of spectacles dangling from a chain around her neck, a symbol of Erudite vanity pushed so far as to be illogical. Max continues, "Will observe another simulation to make sure that the abnormal result wasn't an error in the simulation program. Amar will take you all to the fear simulation room now."

I feel my father's fingers clamped around my arm, hear his hissing voice, warning me not to do anything strange in my aptitude test simulation. I feel tingling in my palms, the sign that I'm about to panic. I can't speak, so I just look at Max, and then at Amar, and nod. I don't know what it means, to be aware during a simulation, but I know it can't be good. I know that Jeanine Matthews would never come here just to observe my simulation if something wasn't seriously wrong with me.

We walk to the fear simulation room without speaking, Jeanine and her assistant—I'm assuming—talking quietly behind us. Amar opens the door and lets us file in.

"I'll go get the extra equipment so you can observe," Amar says. "Be right back."

Jeanine paces around the room with a thoughtful expression. I'm wary of her, as all Abnegation are, taught to distrust Erudite vanity, Erudite greed. It occurs to me, though, as I watch her, that what I was taught might not be right. The Erudite woman who taught me how to take apart a computer when I was volunteering in the computer labs at school wasn't greedy or vain; maybe Jeanine Matthews isn't, either.

"You were logged into the system as 'Four,'" Jeanine says after a few seconds. She stops pacing, folding her hands in front of her. "Which I found perplexing. Why do you not go by 'Tobias' here?"

She already knows who I am. Well, of course she does. She knows everything, doesn't she? I feel like my insides are shriveling up, collapsing into each other. She knows my name, she knows my father, and if she's seen one of my fear simulations, she knows some of the darkest parts of me, too. Her clear, almost watery eyes touch mine, and I look away.

"I wanted a clean slate," I say.

She nods. "I can appreciate that. Especially given what you've gone through."

She sounds almost . . . *gentle*. I bristle at her tone, staring her straight in the face. "I'm fine," I say coldly.

"Of course you are." She smiles a little.

Amar wheels a cart into the room. It carries more wires, electrodes, computer parts. I know what I'm supposed to do; I sit down in the reclining chair and put my arms on the armrests as the others hook themselves up to the simulation. Amar approaches me with a needle, and I stay still as it pinches my throat.

I close my eyes, and the world falls away again.

+ + +

When I open my eyes, I am standing on the roof of an impossibly high building, right near the ledge. Beneath me is the hard pavement, the streets all empty, no one around to help me down. Wind buffets me from all angles, and I tilt back, falling on my back on the gravel roof.

I don't even like being up here, seeing the wide, empty sky around me, reminding me that I am at the tallest point in the city. I remember that Jeanine Matthews is watching; I throw myself against the door to the roof, trying to pull it open as I form a strategy. My usual way to face this fear would be to leap off the ledge of the building, knowing that it's just a simulation and I won't actually die. But someone else in this simulation would never do that; they would find a safe way to get down.

I evaluate my options. I can try to get this door open, but there are no tools that will help me do that around here, just the gravel roof and the door and the sky. I can't create a tool to get through the door, because that's exactly the kind of simulation manipulation that Jeanine is probably looking for. I back up, kicking the door hard with my heel, and it doesn't budge.

My heart pounding in my throat, I walk to the ledge again. Instead of looking all the way down at the minuscule sidewalks beneath me, I look at the building itself. There are windows with ledges beneath me, hundreds of them. The fastest way down, the most Dauntless way, is to scale the side of the building.

I put my face in my hands. I know this isn't real, but it feels real, the wind whistling in my ears, crisp and cool, the concrete rough beneath my hands, the sound of the gravel scattered by my shoes. I put one leg over the ledge, shuddering, and turn to face the building as I lower myself down, one leg at a time, until I'm hanging by my fingertips from the ledge.

Panic bubbles up inside me, and I scream into my teeth. *Oh God.* I hate heights—I *hate* them. I blink tears from my eyes, internally blaming them on the wind, and feel with my toes for the window ledge beneath me. Finding it, I feel for the top of the window with one hand, and press up to keep my balance as I lower myself onto the balls of my feet on the windowsill below me.

My body tilts back, over the empty space, and I scream again, clenching my teeth so hard they squeak.

I have to do that again. And again. And again.

I bend, holding the top of the window with one hand and the bottom with the other. When I have a good grip, I slide my toes down the side of the building, listening to them scrape on the stone, and let myself dangle again.

This time, when I let myself drop onto the other ledge, I don't hold on hard enough with my hands. I lose my footing on the windowsill and tip back. I scramble, scratching at the concrete building with my fingertips, but it's too late; I plummet, and another scream rises up inside me, tearing from my throat. I could create a net beneath me; I could create a rope in the air to save me—no, I shouldn't create anything or they will know what I can do.

I let myself fall. I let myself die.

I wake with pain—created by my mind—singing in every part of my body, screaming, my eyes blurry with tears and terror. I jerk forward, gasping. My body is shaking; I'm ashamed to be acting this way with this audience, but I know that it's a good thing. It will show them that I'm not special—I'm just another reckless Dauntless who thought he could scale a building and failed.

"Interesting," Jeanine says, and I can barely hear her over my own breathing. "I never tire of seeing inside a person's mind—every detail suggests so much."

I put my legs—still shaking—over the edge of the chair and plant my feet on the ground.

"You did well," Amar says. "Your climbing skills are maybe a little wanting, but you still got out of the simulation quickly, like last time."

He smiles at me. I must have succeeded at pretending to be normal, because he doesn't look worried anymore.

I nod.

"Well, it appears that your abnormal test result was a program error. We will have to investigate the simulation program to find the flaw," Jeanine says. "Now, Amar. I'd like to see one of *your* fear simulations, if you wouldn't mind obliging."

"Mine? Why mine?"

Jeanine's mild smile doesn't change. "Our information suggests that you were not alarmed by Tobias's abnormal result—that you were quite familiar with it, in fact. So I would like to see if that familiarity comes from experience."

"Your information," Amar says. "Information from where?"

"An initiate came forward to express his concerns for your and Tobias's well-being," Jeanine says. "I would like to respect his privacy. Tobias, you may leave now. Thank you for your assistance."

I look at Amar. He nods a little. I push myself to my feet, still a little unsteady, and walk out, leaving the door cracked open so I can stay and eavesdrop. But as soon as I'm in the hallway, Jeanine's assistant pushes the door shut, and I can't hear anything behind it, even when I press my ear to it.

An initiate came forward to express his concerns—and I'm sure I know who that initiate is. Our only former Erudite: Eric.

+ + +

For a week, it seems that nothing will come of Jeanine Matthews's visit. All the initiates, Dauntless-born and transfer alike, go through fear simulations every day, and every day, I allow myself to be consumed by my own fears: heights, confinement, violence, Marcus. Sometimes they blur together, Marcus at the top of tall buildings, violence in confined spaces. I always wake half-delirious, shaking, embarrassed that even though I am the initiate with only four fears, I am also the one who can't dispel them when the simulations are done. They creep up on me when I least expect them, filling my sleep with nightmares and my waking with shudders and paranoia. I grind my teeth, I jump at small noises, my hands go numb without warning. I worry that I will go insane before initiation is done.

"You okay?" Zeke asks me at breakfast one morning. "You look . . . exhausted."

"I'm fine," I say, harsher than I mean to be.

"Oh, clearly," Zeke says, grinning. "It's okay to not be okay, you know."

"Yeah, right," I say, and I force myself to finish my food, even though it all tastes like dust to me, these days. If I have to feel like I'm losing my mind, I'm at least putting on weight—muscle, mostly. It's strange to take up so much space just by existing when I used to disappear so easily.

It makes me feel just a little stronger, a little more stable.

Zeke and I put our trays away. When we're on our way out to the Pit, Zeke's little brother—Uriah is his name, I remember—runs up to us. He's taller than Zeke already, with a bandage behind his ear that covers up a fresh tattoo. Usually he looks like he's constantly on the verge of making a joke, but not right now. Right now he just looks stunned.

"Amar," he says, a little breathless. "Amar is . . ." He shakes his head. "Amar is dead."

I laugh a little. Distantly I'm aware that that's not an appropriate reaction, but I can't help it. "What? What do you mean, he's *dead*?"

"A Dauntless woman found a body on the ground near the Pire early this morning," Uriah says. "They just identified it. It was Amar. He . . . he must have . . ."

"Jumped?" Zeke says.

"Or fell, no one knows," Uriah says.

I move toward the paths climbing the walls of the Pit. Usually I almost press my body to the wall when I do this, afraid of the height, but this time I don't even think about what's below me. I brush past running, shrieking children and the people going into shops, coming out of them. I climb the staircase that dangles from the glass ceiling.

A crowd is gathered in the lobby of the Pire. I elbow my way through it. Some people curse at me, or elbow me back, but I don't really notice. I make my way to the edge of the room, to the glass walls above the streets that surround the Dauntless compound. Out there, there's an area sectioned off with tape, and a streak of dark red on the pavement.

I stare at the streak for a long time, until I feel myself comprehending that that streak comes from Amar's blood, from his body colliding with the ground.

Then I walk away.

+ + +

I didn't know Amar well enough to feel grief, in the way I've taught myself to think of it. Grief was what I felt after my mother's death, a weight that made it impossible to move through each day. I remember stopping in the middle of simple tasks to rest, and forgetting to start them again, or waking up in the middle of the night with tears on my face.

I don't carry Amar's loss like that. I find myself feeling it every now and then, when I remember how he gave me my name, how he protected me when he didn't even know me. But most of the time I just feel angry. His death had something to do with Jeanine Matthews and the evaluation of his fear simulation, I know it. And that means that whatever happened is also Eric's responsibility, because he overheard our conversation and told his former faction leader about it.

They killed Amar, the Erudite. But everyone thinks that he jumped, or fell. It's something a Dauntless would do.

The Dauntless have a memorial service for him that evening. Everyone is drunk by late afternoon. We gather by the chasm, and Zeke passes me a cup of dark liquid, and I swallow it all without thinking. As the liquid calm moves through me, I sway a little on my feet and pass the empty cup back to him.

"Yeah, that seems about right," Zeke says, staring into the empty cup. "I'm going to get some more."

I nod and listen to the roar of the chasm. Jeanine Matthews seemed to accept that my own abnormal results were just a problem with the program, but what if that was just an act? What if she comes after me the way she came after Amar? I try to push the thought down where I won't find it again.

A dark, scarred hand falls on my shoulder, and Max stands beside me.

"You all right, Four?" he says.

"Yeah," I say, and it's true, I am all right. I am all right because I'm still on my feet and I'm not yet slurring my words.

"I know Amar took a particular interest in you. I think

he saw strong potential." Max smiles a little.

"I didn't really know him," I say.

"He was always a little troubled, a little unbalanced. Not like the rest of the initiates in his class," Max says. "I think losing his grandparents really took a toll on him. Or maybe the problem was deeper. . . . I don't know. It could be that he's better off this way."

"Better off *dead*?" I say, scowling at him.

"That's not exactly what I meant," Max says. "But here in Dauntless, we encourage our members to choose their own paths through life. If this is what he chose . . . so much the better." He puts his hand on my shoulder again. "Depending on how you do in your final examination tomorrow, you and I should talk about the future you'd like to have here in Dauntless. You're by far our most promising initiate, despite your background."

I just keep staring at him. I don't even understand what he's saying, or why he's saying it here, at Amar's memorial service. Is he trying to *recruit* me? For what?

Zeke returns with two cups, and Max melts into the crowd like nothing ever happened. One of Amar's friends stands on a chair and shouts something meaningless about Amar being brave enough to explore the unknown.

Everyone lifts their glasses and chants his name. *Amar, Amar, Amar.* They say it so many times that it loses all meaning, the noise relentless and repetitive and all-consuming.

Then we all drink. This is how the Dauntless mourn: by chasing grief into the oblivion of alcohol and leaving it there.

All right. Fine. I can chase it too.

+++

My final examination, my fear landscape, is administered by Tori and observed by the Dauntless leaders, including Max. I go somewhere in the middle of the pack of the initiates, and for the first time, I'm not even a little bit nervous. In the fear landscape, everyone is aware during the simulation, so I have nothing to hide. I jab myself in the neck with the needle and let reality disappear.

I've done it dozens of times. I find myself at the top of a high building and run off the edge. I get shut into a box and allow myself a brief moment of panic before slamming my shoulder into the right wall, shattering the wood with the impact, impossibly. I pick up a gun and shoot an innocent person—this time a faceless man dressed in Dauntless black—in the head without even thinking about it.

This time, when the Marcuses surround me, they look more like him than they did before. His mouth is a mouth, though his eyes are still empty pits. And when he draws back his arm to hit me, he's holding a belt, not a barbed chain or some other weapon that can tear me apart piece by piece. I take a few hits, then dive at the nearest Marcus, wrapping my hands around his throat. I punch wildly at his face, and the violence gives me just a brief moment of satisfaction before I wake up, crouched on the floor of the fear landscape room.

The lights go on in the room beyond this one, so I can see the people inside it. There are two rows of waiting initiates, including Eric, who now has so many piercings in his lip that I find myself daydreaming about yanking them out one by one. Sitting in front of them are the three Dauntless leaders, including Max, all of whom are nodding and smiling. Tori gives me a thumbs-up.

I went into the examination thinking I didn't care anymore, not about passing, not about doing well, not about being Dauntless. But Tori's thumbs-up makes me swell with pride, and I let myself smile a little when I walk out. Amar may be dead, but he always wanted me to do well. I can't say I did it for him—I didn't really do it for anyone, not even myself. But at least I didn't embarrass him.

All the initiates who are finished with their final examination wait for the results in the transfer dormitory, Dauntless-borns and transfers alike. Zeke and

Shauna whoop when I come in, and I sit down on the edge of my bed.

"How'd it go?" Zeke asks me.

"Fine," I say. "No surprises. Yours?"

"Awful, but I made it out alive," he says, shrugging. "Shauna got some new ones, though."

"I handled them," Shauna says with exaggerated nonchalance. She has a pillow across her knees, one of Eric's. He won't like that.

Her act breaks, and she grins. "I was pretty awesome."

"Yeah, yeah," Zeke says.

Shauna smacks him with the pillow, right in the face. He snatches it from her.

"What do you want me to say? Yes, you were awesome. Yes, you're the best Dauntless ever. Happy?" He hits her in the shoulder with the pillow. "She's been bragging nonstop since we started the fear sims because she's better at them than I am. It's annoying."

"It's just revenge for how much you bragged during combat training," she says. "'Did you see that great hit I got right in the beginning?' Blah, blah, blah."

She pushes him, and he grabs her wrists. She breaks free and flicks his ear, and they're laughing, fighting.

I may not understand Dauntless affection, but

apparently I know flirtation when I see it. I smirk. I guess that resolves the Shauna question, not that it was really plaguing me. That was probably an answer in and of itself.

We sit around for another hour as the others finish their final exams, trickling in one after another. The last one to come in is Eric, and he just stands in the doorway, looking smug.

"Time to get our results," he says.

The others all get up and walk past him on their way out. Some of them seem nervous; others look cocky, sure of themselves. I wait until they're all gone before I walk to the doorway, but I don't go through it. I stop, crossing my arms and staring at Eric for a few seconds.

"Got something to say?" he says.

"I know it was you," I say. "Who told the Erudite about Amar. I know."

"I don't know what you're talking about," he says, but it's obvious that he does.

"You're the reason he's dead," I say. I'm surprised by how quickly the anger comes on. My body quakes with it, my face hot.

"Did you get hit in the head during your exam, Stiff?" Eric says, smirking. "You're not making any sense."

I shove him back, hard, against the door. Then I hold

him there with one arm—I'm surprised, for a moment, how much stronger I am—and lean in close to his face. "I know it was you," I say, searching his black eyes for something, anything. I see nothing, just dead-fish eyes, impenetrable. "You're the reason he's dead, and you won't get away with it."

I let him go and walk down the hallway toward the cafeteria.

+++

The dining hall is *packed* with people dressed in their Dauntless best—all piercings exaggerated by flashier rings, all tattoos on display, even if it means going without clothing. I try to keep my eyes on people's faces as I navigate through the crush of bodies. The scents of cake and cooked meat and bread and spices are on the air, making my mouth water—I forgot to eat lunch.

When I reach my usual table, I steal a roll from Zeke's plate when he's not looking and stand with the others to wait for our results. I hope they won't make us wait too long. I feel like I'm holding a live wire, my hands twitching and my thoughts frantic, scattered. Zeke and Shauna try to talk to me, but none of us can shout loud enough over the noise for them to hear me, so we resign ourselves to waiting without speaking.

Max gets on one of the tables and holds up his hands for quiet. He mostly gets it, though even he can't completely silence the Dauntless, some of whom go on talking and joking like nothing ever happened. Still, I can hear him as he gives his speech.

"A few weeks ago, a group of scrawny, scared initiates gave their blood to the coals and made the big jump into Dauntless," Max says. "To be honest, I didn't think any of them would make it through the first day"—he pauses to allow for laughter, and it comes, even though it wasn't a very good joke—"but I'm pleased to announce that this year, all of our initiates attained the required scores necessary to become Dauntless!"

Everyone cheers. Despite the assurance that they won't be cut, Zeke and Shauna exchange nervous looks—the order in which we are ranked still determines what kind of job we can choose in Dauntless. Zeke puts his arm across Shauna's shoulders and squeezes.

I feel suddenly alone again.

"No more delays," Max says. "I know our initiates are jumping out of their skin. So, here are our twelve new Dauntless members!"

The initiates' names appear on a large screen behind him, large enough even for people at the back of the room to see. I search the list automatically for their names:

Instantly, some of my tension disappears. I follow the list up, and panic stabs me for just a second when I can't find my own name. But then, there it is, right at the top.

Shauna lets out a yell, and she and Zeke crush me into a sloppy hug, their weight almost knocking me to the ground. I laugh and bring my arms up to return the gesture.

Somewhere in the chaos, I dropped my dinner roll—I crush it under my heel and smile as people surround me, people I don't even know, slapping my shoulders and grinning and saying my name. My name, which is only "Four" now, all suspicions about my origin and my identity forgotten now that I am one of them, now that I am Dauntless.

I am not Tobias Eaton, not anymore, never again. I am Dauntless.

+ + +

That night, dizzy with excitement and so full of food I can hardly walk, I slip away from the celebration and climb the paths to the top of the Pit, to the lobby of the Pire. I walk out of the doors and suck in a deep breath of the night air, which is cool and refreshing, unlike the hot, close air in the cafeteria.

I walk toward the train tracks, too full of manic energy to stay still. There is a train coming, the light fixed to its front car blinking as it comes toward me. It charges past with power and energy, loud as thunder in my ears. I lean closer to it, for the first time savoring the thrill of fear in my stomach, to be so close to such a dangerous thing.

Then I see something dark and human-like standing in one of the last cars. A tall, lean female figure, leaning out of the car, holding on to one of the handles. For just a second as the blur of the train passes me, I see dark, curly hair and a hooked nose.

She looks almost like my mother.

And then she's gone, gone with the train.

THE SON

THE SMALL APARTMENT is bare, the floor still streaked with broom strokes at the corners. I don't own anything to fill the space except my Abnegation clothes, which are stuffed into the bottom of the bag at my side. I throw it on the bare mattress and check the drawers beneath the bed for sheets.

The Dauntless lottery was kind to me, because I was ranked first, and because unlike my outgoing fellow initiates, I wanted to live alone. The others, like Zeke and Shauna, grew up surrounded by Dauntless community, and to them the silence and the stillness of living alone would be unbearable.

I make the bed quickly, pulling the top sheet taut, so it almost has corners. The sheets are worn in places, from moths or from prior use, I'm not sure. The blanket, a blue quilt, smells like cedar and dust. When I open the bag that contains my meager possessions, I hold the Abnegation shirt—torn, from where I had to tear away fabric to bind the wound in my hand—in front of me. It looks small—I doubt I could even fit into it if I tried to put it on now, but I don't try, I just fold it and drop it in the drawer.

I hear a knock, and I say, "Come in!" thinking it's Zeke or Shauna. But Max, a tall man with dark skin and bruised knuckles, walks into my apartment, his hands folded in front of him. He surveys the room once and curls his lip with disgust at the gray slacks folded on my bed. The reaction surprises me a little—there aren't many in this city who would choose Abnegation as their faction, but there aren't many who hate it, either. Apparently I've found one of them.

I stand, unsure what to say. There's a faction leader in my apartment.

"Hello," I say.

"Sorry to interrupt," he says. "I'm surprised you didn't choose to room with your fellow former initiates. You did make some friends, didn't you?"

"Yeah," I say. "This just feels more normal."

"I guess it'll take you some time to let go of your old faction." Max skims the counter in my small kitchen with a fingertip, looks at the dust he collected, then wipes his hand on his pants. He gives me a critical look—one that tells me to let go of my old faction faster. If I was still an initiate, I might worry about that look, but I'm a Dauntless member now, and he can't take that away from me, no matter how "Stiff" I seem.

Can he?

"This afternoon you'll pick your job," Max says. "Did you have anything in mind?"

"I guess it depends on what's available," I say. "I'd like to do something with teaching. Like what Amar did, maybe."

"I think the first-ranked initiate can do a little better than 'initiation instructor,' don't you?" Max's eyebrows lift, and I notice that one doesn't move as much as the other—it's crossed with a scar. "I came because an opportunity has opened up."

He pulls a chair out from under the small table near the kitchen counter, turns it, and sits on it backward. His black boots are caked with light-brown mud and the laces are knotted and fraying at the ends. He might be the oldest Dauntless I've ever seen, but he may as well be made of steel.

"To be honest, one of my fellow leaders of Dauntless is getting a little old for the job," Max says. I sit on the edge of the bed. "The remaining four of us think it would be a good idea to get some new blood in leadership. New ideas for new Dauntless members and initiation, specifically. That task is usually given to the youngest leader anyway, so it's a good fit. We were thinking of drawing from the more recent initiate classes for a training program to see if anyone is a good candidate. You're a natural choice."

I feel like my skin is too tight for me, suddenly. Is he really suggesting that at the age of sixteen I could qualify as a Dauntless leader?

"The training program will last at least a year," Max says. "It will be rigorous and it will test your skills in a lot of areas. We both know you'll do just fine in the fear landscape portion."

I nod without thinking. He must not mind my self-assuredness, because he smiles a little.

"You won't need to go to the job selection meeting later today," Max says. "Training will start very soon—tomorrow morning, in fact."

"Wait," I say, a thought breaking through the muddle in my mind. "I don't have a choice?"

"Of course you have a choice." He looks puzzled. "I just assumed someone like you would rather train to be a leader than spend all day standing around a fence with a gun on his shoulder, or lecturing initiates about good fighting technique. But if I was wrong . . ."

I don't know why I'm hesitating. I don't want to spend my days guarding the fence, or patrolling the city, or even pacing the training room floor. I may have an aptitude for fighting, but that doesn't mean I want to do it all day, every day. The chance to make a difference in Dauntless appeals to the Abnegation parts of me, the parts that are lingering around, occasionally demanding attention.

I think I just don't like when I'm not given a choice.

I shake my head. "No, you weren't wrong." I clear my throat and try to sound stronger, more determined. "I want to do it. Thank you."

"Excellent." Max gets up and cracks one of his knuckles idly, like it's an old habit. He holds out his hand for me to shake, and I take it, though the gesture is still unfamiliar to me—the Abnegation would never touch each other so casually. "Come to the conference room near my office tomorrow morning at eight. It's in the Pire. Tenth floor."

He leaves, scattering bits of dried earth from the bottom of his shoes as he walks out. I sweep them up with the broom that leans against the wall near the door. It's not until I'm scooting the chair back under the table that I realize—if I become a Dauntless leader, a representative of my faction, I'll have to come face-to-face with my father again. And not just once but constantly, until he finally retires into Abnegation obscurity.

My fingers start to go numb. I've faced my fears so many times in simulations, but that doesn't mean I'm ready to face them in reality.

+++

"Dude, you missed it!" Zeke is wide-eyed, concerned. "The only jobs left by the end were the gross jobs, like scrubbing toilets! Where *were* you?"

"It's fine," I say as I carry my tray back to our table near the doors. Shauna is there with her little sister, Lynn, and Lynn's friend Marlene. When I first saw them there, I wanted to turn around and leave immediately—Marlene is too cheerful for me even on a good day—but Zeke had already seen me, so it was too late. Behind us, Uriah jogs to catch up, his plate loaded with more food than he can possibly pack into his stomach. "I didn't miss anything— Max came to see me earlier."

As we take our seats at the table, under one of the bright-blue lamps that hang from the wall, I tell him about Max's offer, careful not to make it sound too impressive. I only just found friends; I don't want to create jealous tension between us for no reason. When I finish, Shauna leans her face into one of her hands and says to Zeke, "I guess we should have tried harder during initiation, huh?"

"Or killed him before he could take his final test."

"Or both." Shauna grins at me. "Congrats, Four. You deserve it."

I feel everyone's eyes on me like distinct, powerful beams of heat, and hurry to change the subject. "Where did you guys end up?"

"Control room," Zeke says. "My mom used to work there, and she taught me most of what I'll need to know already."

"I'm in the patrol leadership track . . . thing," Shauna says. "Not the most exciting job ever, but at least I'll get to be outside."

"Yeah, let's hear you say that in the dead of winter when you're trudging through a foot of snow and ice," Lynn says sourly. She stabs at a pile of mashed potatoes with her fork. "I better do well in initiation. I don't want to get stuck at the fence."

"Didn't we talk about this?" Uriah says. "Don't say the 'I' word until at most two weeks before it happens. It makes me want to throw up."

I look at the pile of food on his tray. "Stuffing yourself up to your eyeballs with food, though, that's fine?"

He rolls his eyes at me and bends over his tray to keep eating. I poke at my own food—I haven't had any appetite since this morning, too worried about tomorrow to stand a full stomach.

Zeke spots someone across the cafeteria. "I'll be right back."

Shauna watches him cross the room to greet a few young Dauntless members. They don't look much older than he is, but I don't recognize them from initiation, so they must be a year or two older. Zeke says something to the group—mostly made up of girls—that sends them into fits of laughter, and he jabs one of the girls in the ribs, making her squeal. Beside me, Shauna glowers and misses her mouth with her fork, smearing sauce from the chicken all over her cheek. Lynn snorts into her food, and Marlene kicks her—audibly—under the table.

"So," Marlene says loudly. "Do you know of anyone else who's doing that leadership program, Four?"

"Come to think of it, I didn't see Eric there today, either," Shauna says. "I was hoping he tripped and fell into the chasm, but . . ."

I shove a bite of food in my mouth and try not to think about it. The blue light makes my hands look blue, too, like the hands of a corpse. I haven't spoken to Eric since I accused him of being indirectly responsible for Amar's death—someone reported Amar's simulation aware-ness to Jeanine Matthews, leader of Erudite, and as a former Erudite, Eric is the most likely suspect. I haven't decided what I'll do the next time I have to talk to him, either. Beating him up again isn't going to prove that he's a faction traitor. I'll have to find some way to connect his recent activities to the Erudite and take the information to one of the Dauntless leaders—Max, probably, since I know him best.

Zeke walks back to the table and slides into his seat. "Four. What are you doing tomorrow night?"

"I don't know," I say. "Nothing?"

"Not anymore," he says. "You're coming with me on a date."

I choke on my next bite of potatoes. "What?"

"Um, hate to tell you this, big brother," Uriah says, "but you're supposed to go on dates alone, not bring a friend."

"It's a double date, obviously," Zeke says. "I asked Maria out, and she said something about finding a date for her friend Nicole, and I indicated that you would be interested."

"Which one's Nicole?" Lynn says, craning her neck to look at the group of girls.

"The redhead," Zeke says. "So, eight o'clock. You're in, I'm not even asking."

"I don't—" I say. I look at the redheaded girl across the room. She's fair-skinned, with wide eyes smeared with black, and wearing a tight shirt, which shows off the bend in her waist and . . . other things my inner Abnegation voice tells me not to notice. I do anyway.

I've never been on a date, thanks to my former faction's strict courtship rituals, involving engaging in acts of service together and maybe—*maybe*—having dinner with someone else's family and helping them clean up afterward. I've never even thought about whether I wanted to date anyone; it was such an impossibility. "Zeke, I've never—"

Uriah frowns and pokes my arm, hard, with one finger. I slap his hand away. *"What?"*

"Oh, nothing," Uriah says cheerfully. "You were just sounding *Stiffer* than usual, so I thought I would check—"

Marlene laughs. "Yeah, right."

Zeke and I exchange a look. We've never explicitly talked about not sharing my faction of origin, but as far as I know, he's never mentioned it to anyone. Uriah knows, but despite his loud mouth, he seems to understand when to withhold information. Still, I'm not sure why Marlene hasn't figured it out—maybe she's not very observant.

"It's not a big deal, Four," Zeke says. He eats his last bite of food. "You'll go, you'll talk to her like she's a normal human being—which she *is*—maybe she'll let you—*gasp*—hold her hand—"

Shauna gets up suddenly, her chair screeching on the stone floor. She tucks her hair behind one ear and walks toward the tray return, head down. Lynn glares at Zeke—which hardly looks different from her normal facial expression—and follows her sister across the cafeteria.

"Okay, you don't have to hold hands with anyone," Zeke says, like nothing happened. "Just go, all right? I'll owe you one."

I look at Nicole. She's sitting at a table near the tray return and laughing at someone else's joke again. Maybe Zeke's right—maybe it's not that big a deal, and maybe this is another way that I can unlearn my Abnegation past and learn to embrace my Dauntless future. And besides—she's pretty.

"Okay," I say. "I'll go. But if you make some kind of joke about hand holding, I'm going to break your nose."

+ + +

When I get back to my apartment that night, it still smells like dust and a hint of mold. I turn on one of the lamps, and a glimmer of light reflects off the countertop. I run my hand over it, and a small piece of glass pricks my finger, making it bleed. I pinch it between my fingertips and carry it to the trash can, which I put a bag in this morning. But resting at the bottom of the bag now is a pile of shards in the shape of a drinking glass.

I haven't used one of those yet.

A shiver goes down my spine, and I scan the rest of the apartment for signs of disruption. The sheets aren't rumpled, none of the drawers are open, none of the chairs seem to have moved. But I would know if I had broken a glass that morning.

So who was in my apartment?

+++

I don't know why, but the first thing my hands find in the morning when I stumble into the bathroom is the set of hair clippers I got with my Dauntless credits yesterday. And then while I'm still blinking the clouds from my eyes, I turn them on and touch them to my head the way I've done since I was young. I bend my ear forward to protect it from the blades; I know just how to twist and shift so that I can see as much of the back of my head as possible. The ritual calms my nerves, makes me feel focused and steady. I brush the trimmed hairs from my shoulders and neck and sweep them into the wastebasket.

It's an Abnegation morning. A quick shower, a plain breakfast, a clean house. Except I'm wearing Dauntless black, boots and pants and shirt and jacket. I avoid looking in the mirror on my way out, and it makes me grit my teeth, knowing how deep these Stiff roots go, and how hard it will be to excise them from my mind, as tangled up in everything as they are. I left that place out of fear and defiance, and that will make it harder to assimilate than anyone knows, harder than if I had actually chosen Dauntless for the right reasons.

I walk quickly toward the Pit, emerging through an arch halfway up the wall. I stay away from the edge of the path, though Dauntless children, shrieking with laughter, sometimes run right along it, and I should be braver than they are. I'm not sure bravery is something you acquire more of with age, like wisdom—but maybe here, in Dauntless, bravery is the highest form of wisdom, the acknowledgment that life can and should be lived without fear.

It's the first time I've found myself being thoughtful about Dauntless life, so I hold on to the thought as I ascend the paths around the Pit. I reach the staircase that hangs from the glass ceiling and keep my eyes up, away from the space opening up beneath me, so I don't start to panic. But my heart is pounding by the time I reach the top anyway; I can feel it even in my throat. Max said his office was on the tenth floor, so I ride the elevator up with a group of Dauntless going to work. They don't all seem to know one another, unlike the Abnegation—it's not as important to them to memorize names and faces and needs and wants, so maybe they just keep to their friends and families, forming rich but separate communities within their faction. Like the one I'm forming myself.

When I reach the tenth floor, I'm not sure where to go, but then I spot a dark head turning a corner in front of me. Eric. I follow him, partly because he probably knows where he's going, but partly because I want to know what he's doing even if he's not going to the same place I am. But when I turn the corner, I see Max standing in a conference room that has glass walls, surrounded by young Dauntless. The oldest one is maybe twenty, and the youngest is probably not much older than I am. Max sees me through the glass and motions for me to come in. Eric sits close to him—*Suck-up*, I think—but I sit at the other end of the table, between a girl with a ring through her nostrils and a boy whose hair is such a bright shade of green I can't look straight at him. I feel plain by comparison—I may have gotten Dauntless flames tattooed on my side during initiation, but it's not like they're on display.

"I think everyone is here, so let's get started." Max closes the door to the conference room and stands before us. He looks strange in such an ordinary environment, like he's here to break all the glass and cause chaos rather than lead this meeting. "You're all here because you've shown potential, first, but also because you've displayed enthusiasm for our faction and its future." I don't know how I've done that. "Our city is changing, faster now than ever before, and in order to keep up with it, we'll have to change, too. We'll have to become stronger, braver, better than we are now. And among you are the people who can get us there, but we'll have to figure out who they are. We'll be doing a combination of instruction and skills tests for the next several months, to teach you what you'll need to know if you make it through this program, but also to see how quickly you learn." That sounds a little like something the Erudite would value, not the Dauntless—strange.

"The first thing you'll do is fill out this info sheet," he says, and I almost laugh. There's something ridiculous about a tough, hardened Dauntless warrior with a stack of papers he calls "info sheets," but of course some things have to be ordinary, because it's more efficient that way. He sends the stack around the table, along with a bundle of pens. "All this will do is tell us more about you and give us a starting point by which to measure your progress. So it's in your best interest to be honest, and not to make yourself sound better than you are."

I feel unsettled, staring at the sheet of paper. I fill out my name—which is the first question—and my age—the second. The third asks for my faction of origin, and the fourth asks for my number of fears. The fifth asks what those fears are.

I'm not sure how to describe them. The first two are easy—heights, confinement—but the next one? And what am I supposed to write about my father, that I'm afraid of Marcus Eaton? Eventually I scribble *losing control* for my third fear and *physical threats in confined spaces* for my fourth, knowing that that's far from true.

But the next few questions are strange, confusing. They're statements, trickily worded, that I'm supposed to agree or disagree with. *It's okay to steal if it's to help someone else.* Well, that's easy enough—agree. *Some people are more deserving of rewards than others.* Maybe. It depends on the rewards. *Power should be given only to those who earn it. Difficult circumstances form stronger people. You don't know how strong a person really is until they're tested.* I glance around the table at the others. Some people seem puzzled, but no one looks the way I feel—disturbed, almost afraid to circle an answer beneath each statement.

I don't know what to do, so I circle "agree" for each one and pass my sheet back with everyone else's.

+++

Zeke and his date, Maria, are pressed up against a wall in a hallway next to the Pit. I can see their silhouettes from here. It looks like they're still just as pressed-up-against-each-other as they were five minutes ago when they first went back there, giggling like idiots the whole time. I cross my arms and look back at Nicole.

"So," I say.

"So," she says, tipping forward onto the balls of her feet and back onto her heels again. "This is a little awkward, right?"

"Yeah," I say, relieved. "It is."

"How long have you been friends with Zeke?" she says. "I haven't seen you around much."

"A few weeks," I say. "We met during initiation."

"Oh," she says. "Were you a transfer?"

"Um . . ." I don't want to admit that I transferred from Abnegation, partly because whenever I admit that, people start thinking I'm uptight, and partly because I don't like to toss out hints about my parentage when I can avoid it. I decide to lie. "No, just . . . kept to myself before then, I guess."

"Oh." She narrows her eyes a little. "You must have been really good at it."

"One of my specialties," I say. "How long have you been friends with Maria?"

"Since we were kids. She could trip and fall and land on a date with someone," Nicole says. "Others of us aren't as talented."

"Yeah." I shake my head. "Zeke had to push me into this a little."

"Really." Nicole raises an eyebrow. "Did he at least show you what you were in for?"

She points at herself.

"Um, yeah," I say. "I wasn't sure if you were my type, but I thought maybe—"

"Not your type." She sounds cold, suddenly. I try to backtrack.

"I mean, I don't think that's that important," I say. "Personality is much more important than—"

"Than my unsatisfactory looks?" She raises both eyebrows.

"That's not what I said," I say. "I'm . . . really terrible at this."

"Yeah," she says. "You are."

She grabs the small black bag that was resting against her feet and tucks it under her arm. "Tell Maria I had to go home early."

She stalks away from the railing and disappears into one of the paths next to the Pit. I sigh and look at Zeke and Maria again. I can tell by the faint movements I'm able to detect that they haven't slowed down at all. I tap my fingers against the railing. Now that our double date has become an awkward, triangle-shaped date, it must be all right for me to leave.

I spot Shauna coming out of the cafeteria and wave to her.

"Isn't tonight your big date night with Ezekiel?" she says.

"*Ezekiel*," I say, cringing. "I forgot that was his whole name. Yeah, my date just stormed off."

"Good one," she says, laughing. "What'd you last, ten minutes?"

"Five," I say, and I find myself laughing, too. "Apparently I'm insensitive."

"No," she says with mock surprise. "You? But you're so sentimental and sweet!"

"Funny," I say. "Where's Lynn?"

"She started arguing with Hector. Our little brother," she says. "And I've been listening to them do that for, oh, my whole life. So I left. I thought I'd go to the training room, get some exercise in. Want to go?"

"Yeah," I say. "Let's go."

We head toward the training room, but then I realize that we have to walk down the same hallway that Zeke and Maria currently occupy to get there. I try to stop Shauna with a hand, but I'm too late—she sees their two bodies pressed together, her eyes wide. She pauses for a moment, and I hear smacking noises I wish I hadn't heard. Then she moves down the hallway again, walking so fast I have to jog to catch up to her.

"Shauna—"

"Training room," she says.

When we get there, she starts immediately on the punching bag, and I've never seen her hit so hard before.

+ + +

"Though it might seem strange, it's important for high-level Dauntless to understand how a few programs work," Max says. "The surveillance program in the control room is an obvious one—a Dauntless leader will sometimes have to monitor the things happening in the faction. Then there's the simulation programs, which you have to understand in order to evaluate Dauntless initiates. Also the currency tracking program, which keeps commerce in our faction running smoothly, among others. Some of these programs are pretty sophisticated, which means you'll have to be able to learn computer skills easily, if you don't already have them. That's what we'll be doing today."

He gestures to the woman standing at his left shoulder. I recognize her from the game of Dare. She's young, with purple streaks in her short hair and more piercings than I can easily count.

"Lauren here will be teaching you some of the basics, and

then we'll test you," Max says. "Lauren is one of our initiation instructors, but in her downtime she works as a computer technician in Dauntless headquarters. It's a little Erudite of her, but we'll let it slide for the sake of convenience."

Max winks at her, and she grins.

"Go ahead," he says. "I'll be back in an hour."

Max leaves, and Lauren claps her hands together.

"Right," she says. "Today we're going to talk about how programming works. Those of you who already have some experience with this, please feel free to tune out. The rest of you better keep focused because I'm not going to repeat myself. Learning this stuff is like learning a language—it's not enough to memorize the words; you also have to understand the rules and why they work the way they do."

When I was younger, I volunteered in the computer labs in the Upper Levels building to meet my faction-mandated volunteer hours—and to get out of the house—and I learned how to take a computer apart and put it back together. But I never learned about this. The next hour passes in a blur of technical terms I can barely keep up with. I try to jot some notes on a piece of scrap paper I found on the floor, but she's moving so fast it's hard for my hand to keep up with my ears, so I abandon the effort after a few minutes and just try to pay attention. She shows examples of what she's talking about on a screen at the front of the room, and it's hard not to be distracted by the view from the windows behind her—from this angle, the Pire displays the city's skyline, the prongs of the Hub piercing the sky, the marsh peeking from between the glimmering buildings.

I'm not the only one who seems overwhelmed—the other candidates lean over to one another to whisper frantically, asking for definitions they missed. Eric, however, sits comfortably in his chair, drawing on the back of his hand. Smirking. I recognize that smirk. Of course he already knows all this stuff. He must have learned it in Erudite, probably when he was a child, or else he wouldn't look quite so smug.

Before I can really register the passage of time, Lauren is pressing a button for the display screen to withdraw into the ceiling.

"On the desktop of your computer, you'll find a file marked 'Programming Test,'" she says. "Open it. It will take you to a timed exam. You'll go through a series of small programs and mark the errors you find that are causing them to malfunction. They might be really big things, like the order of the code, or really small things, like a misplaced word or marking. You don't have to fix them right now, but you do have to be able to spot them. There will be one error per program. Go."

Everyone starts frantically tapping at their screens.

Eric leans over to me and says, "Did your Stiff house even *have* a computer, Four?"

"No," I say.

"Well, you see, this is how you open a file," he says with an exaggerated tap on the file on his screen. "See, it looks like paper, but it's really just a picture on a screen—you know what a screen is, right?"

"Shut up," I say as I open the test.

I stare at the first program. *It's like learning a language,* I say to myself. *Everything has to start in the right order and finish in the reverse order. Just make sure that everything is in the right place.*

I don't start at the beginning of the code and make my way down—instead, I look for the innermost kernel of code inside all the wrappers. There, I notice that the line of code finishes in the wrong place. I mark the spot and press the arrow button that will allow me to continue the exam if I'm right. The screen changes, presenting me with a new program.

I raise my eyebrows. I must have absorbed more than I thought.

I start the next one in the same way, moving from the center of the code to the outside, checking the top of the program with the bottom, paying attention to quotation marks and periods and backslashes. Looking for code errors is strangely soothing, just a way of making sure that the world is still in the same order it's supposed to be, and as long as it is, everything will run smoothly.

I forget about all the people around me, even about the skyline beyond us, about what finishing this exam will mean. I just focus on what's in front of me, on the tangle of words on my screen. I notice that Eric finishes first, long before anyone else looks ready to complete their exam, but I try not to let it worry me. Even when he decides to stay next to me and look over my shoulder as I work.

Finally I touch the arrow button and a new image pops up. *EXAM COMPLETE*, it says.

"Good job," Lauren says, when she comes by to check my screen. "You're the third one to finish."

I turn toward Eric.

"Wait," I say. "Weren't you about to explain what a screen was? Obviously I have *no* computer skills at all, so I really need your help."

He glowers at me, and I grin.

+++

My apartment door is open when I return. Just an inch, but I know I closed it before I left. I nudge it open with the toe of my shoe and enter with a pounding heart, expecting to find an intruder rifling through my things, though

I'm not sure who—one of Jeanine's lackeys, searching for evidence that I'm different in the same way Amar was, maybe, or Eric, looking for a way to ambush me. But the apartment is empty and unchanged.

Unchanged—except for the piece of paper on the table. I approach it slowly, like it might burst into flames, or dissolve into the air. There's a message written on it in small, slanted handwriting.

> *On the day you hated most*
> *At the time when she died*
> *In the place where you first jumped on.*

At first the words are nonsense to me, and I think they're a joke, something left here to rattle me, and it worked, because I feel unsteady on my feet. I sit in one of the rickety chairs, hard, without moving my eyes from the paper. I read it over and over again, and the message starts to take shape in my mind.

In the place where you first jumped on. That must mean the train platform I ascended after I had just joined Dauntless.

At the time when she died. There's only one "she" this could be: my mother. My mother died in the dead of night, so that by the time I awoke, her body was already gone, whisked away by my father and his Abnegation friends. Her time of death was estimated to be around two in the morning, he said.

On the day you hated most. That's the hardest one—is it referring to a day of the year, a birthday or a holiday? None of those are coming up, and I don't see why someone would leave a note that far in advance. It must be referring to a day of the week, but what day of the week did I hate most? That's easy—council meeting days, because my father was out late and would return home in a foul mood. Wednesday.

Wednesday, two a.m., at the train platform near the Hub. That's tonight. And there's only one person in the world who would know all that information: Marcus.

+++

I'm clutching the folded piece of paper in my fist, but I can't feel it. My hands have been tingling and mostly numb since I first thought his name.

I left my apartment door wide open, and my shoes are untied. I move along the walls of the Pit without noticing how high up I am and run up the stairs to the Pire without even feeling tempted to look down. Zeke mentioned the control room's location in passing a few days ago. I can only hope he's still there now, because I'll need his help if I want to access the footage of the hallway outside my apartment. I know where the camera is, hidden in the corner where they think no one will notice it. Well, I noticed it.

My mother used to notice things like that, too. When we walked through the Abnegation sector, just the two of us, she would point out the cameras, hidden in bubbles of dark glass or fixed to the edges of buildings. She never said anything about them, or seemed worried about them, but she always knew where they were, and when she passed them, she made a point to look directly at them, as if to say, *I see you, too.* So I grew up searching, scanning, watching for details in my surroundings.

I ride the elevator to the fourth floor, then follow signs for the control room. It's down a short corridor and around the bend, the door wide open. A wall of screens greets me—a few people sit behind it, at desks, and then there are other desks along the walls where more people sit, each one with a screen of their own. The footage rotates every five seconds, showing different parts of the city—the Amity fields, the streets around the Hub, the Dauntless compound, even the Merciless Mart, with its grand lobby. I glimpse the Abnegation sector on one of the screens, then pull myself out of the daze, looking for Zeke. He's sitting at a desk on the right wall, typing something into a dialog box on the left half of his screen while footage of the Pit plays on the right half. Everyone in the room is wearing headphones—listening, I assume, to whatever they're supposed to be watching.

"Zeke," I say quietly. Some of the others look at me, as if scolding me for intruding, but no one says anything.

"Hey!" he says. "I'm glad you came, I'm bored out of my—what's wrong?"

He looks from my face to my fist, still clenched around the piece of paper. I don't know how to explain, so I don't try.

"I need to see footage from the hallway outside my apartment," I say. "From the last four or so hours. Can you help?"

"Why?" Zeke says. "What happened?"

"Someone was in my place," I say. "I want to know who it was."

He looks around, checking to make sure no one is watching. Or listening. "Listen, I can't do that—even we aren't allowed to pull up specific things unless we see something weird, it's all on a rotation—"

"You owe me a favor, remember?" I say. "I would never ask unless it was important."

"Yeah, I know." Zeke looks around again, then closes the dialog box he had open and opens another one. I watch the code he types in to call up the right footage, and I'm surprised to find that I understand some of it, after the day's lesson. An image appears on the screen, of one of the Dauntless corridors near the cafeteria. He taps it, and another image replaces it, this one of the inside of the cafeteria; the next one is of the tattoo parlor, then the hospital.

He keeps scrolling through the Dauntless compound, and I watch the images as they go past, showing momentary glimpses of ordinary Dauntless life, people playing with their piercings as they wait in line for new clothing, people practicing punches in the training room. I see a flash of Max in what appears to be his office, sitting in one of the chairs, a woman sitting across from him. A woman with blond hair tied back in a tight knot. I put my hand on Zeke's shoulder.

"Wait." The piece of paper in my fist seems a little less urgent. "Go back."

He does, and I confirm what I suspected: Jeanine Matthews is in Max's office, a folder in her lap. Her clothes are perfectly pressed, her posture straight. I take the headphones from Zeke's head, and he scowls at me but doesn't stop me.

Max's and Jeanine's voices are quiet, but I can still hear them.

"I've narrowed it down to six," Max is saying. "I'd say that's pretty good for, what? The second day?"

"This is inefficient," Jeanine says. "We already have the candidate. I ensured it. This was always the plan."

"You never asked me what I thought of the plan, and this is my faction," Max says tersely. "I don't like him, and I don't want to spend all my days working with someone I don't like. So you'll have to let me at least try to find someone else who meets all the criteria—"

"Fine." Jeanine stands, pressing her folder to her stomach. "But when you fail to do so, I expect you to admit it. I have no patience for Dauntless pride."

"Yeah, because the Erudite are the picture of humility," Max says sourly.

"Hey," Zeke hisses. "My supervisor is looking. Give me back the headphones."

He snatches them from my head, and they snap around my ears in the process, making them sting.

"You have to get out of here or I'll lose my job," Zeke says.

He looks serious, and worried. I don't object, even though I didn't find out what I needed to know—it was my own fault for getting distracted anyway. I slip out of the control room, my mind racing, half of me still terrified at the thought that my father was in my apartment, that he wants me to meet him alone on an abandoned street in the middle of the night, the other half confused by what I just heard. *We already have the candidate. I ensured it.* They must have been talking about the candidate for Dauntless leadership.

But why is Jeanine Matthews concerned with who is appointed as the next leader of Dauntless?

I make it all the way back to my apartment without noticing, then sit on the edge of the bed and stare at the opposite wall. I keep thinking separate but equally frantic thoughts. *Why does Marcus want to meet with me? Why are the Erudite so involved in Dauntless politics? Does Marcus want to kill me without witnesses, or does he want to warn me about something, or threaten me . . . ? Who was the candidate they were talking about?*

I press the heels of my hands to my forehead and try to calm down, though I feel each nervous thought like a prickle at the back of my head. I can't do anything about Max and Jeanine now. What I have to decide now is whether I'm going to this meeting tonight.

On the day you hated most. I never knew that Marcus even noticed me, noticed the things I liked or hated. He just seemed to view me as an inconvenience, an irritant. But didn't I learn a few weeks ago that he knew the simulations wouldn't work on me, and he tried to help me stay out of danger? Maybe, despite all the horrible things he's done and said to me, there's a part of him that is actually my father. Maybe that's the part of him that's inviting me to this meeting, and he's trying to show me by telling me he knows me, he knows what I hate, what I love, what I fear.

I'm not sure why that thought fills me with such hope when I've hated him for so long. But maybe, just as there's a part of him that's actually my father, there's also a part of me that's actually his son.

+++

The sun's heat is still coming off the pavement at one thirty in the morning when I leave the Dauntless compound. I can feel it on my fingertips. The moon is covered in clouds, so the streets are darker than usual, but I'm not afraid of the dark, or the streets, not anymore. That's one thing beating up a bunch of Dauntless initiates can teach you.

I breathe in the smell of warm asphalt and set off at a slow run, my sneakers slapping the ground. The streets that surround the Dauntless sector of the city are empty; my faction lives huddled together, like a pack of sleeping dogs. That's why, I realize, Max seemed so concerned about my living alone. If I'm really Dauntless, shouldn't

I want my life to overlap with theirs as much as possible, shouldn't I be looking for ways to fold myself into my faction until we are inextricable?

I consider it as I run. Maybe he's right. Maybe I'm not doing a very good job of integrating myself; maybe I'm not pushing myself hard enough. I find a steady rhythm, squinting at the street signs as I pass them, to keep track of where I'm going. I know when I reach the ring of buildings the factionless occupy because I can see their shadows moving around behind blacked-out and boarded windows. I move to run under the train tracks, the latticed wood stretching out far ahead of me and curving away from the street.

The Hub grows larger and larger in my sight as I get closer. My heart is pounding, but I don't think it's from the running. I stop abruptly when I reach the train platform, and as I stand at the foot of the stairs, catching my breath, I remember when I first climbed these steps, the sea of hooting Dauntless moving around me, pressing me forward. It was easy to be carried by their momentum then. I have to carry myself forward now. I start to climb, my footsteps echoing on the metal, and when I reach the top, I check my watch.

Two o'clock.

But the platform is empty.

I walk back and forth over it, to make sure no dark figures are hiding in dark corners. A train rumbles in the distance, and I pause to look for the light fixed to its nose. I didn't know the trains ran this late—all power in the city is supposed to shut off after midnight, to conserve energy. I wonder if Marcus asked the factionless for a special favor. But why would he travel on the train? The Marcus Eaton I know would never dare to associate himself so closely with Dauntless. He would sooner walk the streets barefoot.

The train light flashes, just once, before it careens past the platform. It pounds and churns, slowing but not stopping, and I see a person leap from the second-to-last car, lean and lithe. Not Marcus. A woman.

I squeeze the paper tighter into my fist, and tighter, until my knuckles ache.

The woman strides toward me, and when she's a few feet away, I can see her. Long curly hair. Prominent hooked nose. Black Dauntless pants, gray Abnegation shirt, brown Amity boots. Her face is lined, worn, thin. But I know her, I could never forget her face, my mother, Evelyn Eaton.

"Tobias," she breathes, wide-eyed, like she's as stunned by me as I am by her, but that's impossible. She knew I was alive, but I remember how the urn containing her ashes looked as it stood on my father's mantel, marked with his fingerprints.

I remember the day I woke to a group of grave-faced Abnegation in my father's kitchen, and how they all looked up when I entered, and how Marcus explained to me, with sympathy I knew he didn't feel, that my mother had passed in the middle of the night, complications from early labor and a miscarriage.

She was pregnant? I remember asking.

Of course she was, son. He turned to the other people in our kitchen. *Just shock, of course. Bound to happen, with something like this.*

I remember sitting with a plate full of food, in the living room, with a group of murmuring Abnegation around me, the whole neighborhood packing my house to the brim and no one saying anything that mattered to me.

"I know this must be . . . alarming for you," she says. I hardly recognize her voice; it's lower and stronger and harder than in my memories of her, and that's how I know the years have changed her. I feel too many things to manage, too powerfully to handle, and then suddenly I feel nothing at all.

"You're supposed to be dead," I say, flat. It's a stupid thing to say. Such a stupid thing to say to your mother when she comes back from the dead, but it's a stupid situation.

"I know," she says, and I think there are tears in her eyes, but it's too dark to tell. "I'm not."

"Obviously." The voice coming from my mouth is snide, casual. "Were you ever even pregnant?"

"Pregnant? Is that what they told you, something about dying in childbirth?" She shakes her head. "No, I wasn't. I had been planning my exit for months—I needed to disappear. I thought he might tell you when you were old enough."

I let out a short laugh, like a bark. "You thought that *Marcus Eaton* would admit that his wife left him. To me."

"You're his son," Evelyn says, frowning. "He loves you."

Then all the tension of the past hour, the past few weeks, the past few *years* builds inside me, too much to contain, and I really laugh, but it comes out sounding strange, mechanical. It scares me even though I'm the one doing it.

"You have a right to be angry that you were lied to," she says. "I would be angry, too. But Tobias, I had to leave, I know you understand why. . . ."

She reaches for me, and I grab her wrist, push her away. "Don't touch me."

"All right, all right." She puts her palms up and backs away. "But you do understand, you must."

"What I *understand* is that you left me alone in a house with a sadistic maniac," I say.

It looks like something inside her is collapsing. Her hands fall to her sides like two weights. Her shoulders slump. Even her face goes slack, as it dawns on her what I mean, what I must mean. I cross my arms and put my shoulders back, trying to look as big and strong and tough as possible. It's easier now, in Dauntless black, than it ever was in Abnegation gray, and maybe *that's* why I chose Dauntless as a haven. Not out of spite, not to hurt Marcus, but because I knew this life would teach me a stronger way to be.

"I—" she starts.

"Stop wasting my time. What are we doing here?" I toss the crumpled note on the ground between us and raise my eyebrows at her. "It's been seven years since you died, and you never tried to do this dramatic reveal before, so what's different now?"

At first she doesn't answer. Then she pulls herself together, visibly, and says, "We—the factionless—like to keep an eye on things. Things like the Choosing Ceremony. This time, our eye told me that you chose Dauntless. I would have gone myself, but I didn't want to risk running into *him*. I've become . . . kind of a leader to the factionless, and it's important that I don't expose myself."

I taste something sour.

"Well, well," I say. "What important parents I have. I'm so very lucky."

"This isn't like you," she says. "Is even a part of you happy to see me again?"

"Happy to see you again?" I say. "I barely remember you, Evelyn. I've almost lived as long without you as I did with you."

Her face contorts. I wounded her. I'm glad.

"When you chose Dauntless," she continues slowly, "I knew it was time to reach out to you. I've always been planning to find you, after you chose and you were on your own, so that I could invite you to join us."

"Join you," I say. "Become factionless? Why would I want to do that?"

"Our city is changing, Tobias." It's the same thing Max said yesterday. "The factionless are coming together, and so are Dauntless and Erudite. Sometime soon, everyone will have to choose a side, and I know which one you would rather be on. I think you can really make a difference with us."

"*You* know which one I'd rather be on. Really," I say. "I'm not a faction traitor. I chose Dauntless; that's where I belong."

"You aren't one of those mindless, danger-seeking fools," she snaps. "Just like you weren't a suffocated

Stiff drone. You can be more than either, more than any faction."

"You have no idea what I am or who I can be," I say. "I was the first-ranked initiate. They want me to be a Dauntless leader."

"Don't be naive," she says, narrowing her eyes at me. "They don't want a new leader; they want a pawn they can manipulate. That's why Jeanine Matthews frequents Dauntless headquarters, that's why she keeps planting minions in your faction to report on their behavior. You haven't noticed that she seems to be aware of things she has no right to be aware of, that they keep shifting Dauntless training around, experimenting with it? As if the Dauntless would ever change something like that on their own."

Amar told us the fear landscapes didn't usually come first in Dauntless initiation, that it was something new they were trying. An experiment. But she's right; the Dauntless don't do experiments. If they were really concerned with practicality and efficiency, they wouldn't bother teaching us to throw knives.

And then there's Amar, turning up dead. Wasn't I the one who accused Eric of being an informant? Haven't I suspected for weeks that he was still in touch with the Erudite?

"Even if you're right," I say, and all the malicious energy has gone out of me. I move closer to her. "Even if you're right about Dauntless, I would never join you." I try to keep my voice from wavering as I add, "I never want to see you again."

"I don't believe you," she says quietly.

"I don't care what you believe."

I move past her, toward the stairs I climbed to get up to the platform.

She calls after me, "If you change your mind, any message given to one of the factionless will go to me."

I don't look back. I run down the stairs and sprint down the street, away from the platform. I don't even know if I'm moving in the right direction, just that I want to be as far away from her as possible.

+++

I don't sleep.

I pace my apartment, frantic. I pull the remnants of my Abnegation life out of my drawers and dump them in the trash, the ripped shirt, the pants, the shoes, the socks, even my watch. At some point, around sunrise, I hurl the electric shaver against the shower wall, and it breaks into several pieces.

An hour after daybreak, I walk to the tattoo parlor. Tori

is already there—well, "there" might be too strong a word, because her eyes are swollen from sleep and unfocused, and she's just started on her coffee.

"Something wrong?" she said. "I'm not really here. I'm supposed to go for a run with Bud, that maniac."

"I'm hoping you'll make an exception," I say.

"Not many people come in here with urgent tattoo requests," she says.

"There's a first time for everything."

"Okay." She sits up, more alert now. "You have something in mind?"

"You had a drawing in your apartment when we walked through it a few weeks ago. It was of all the faction symbols together. Still have it?"

She stiffens. "You weren't supposed to see that."

I know why I wasn't supposed to see it, why that drawing isn't something she wants made public. It suggests leanings toward other factions instead of asserting Dauntless supremacy, like her tattoos are supposed to. Even established Dauntless members are worried about seeming Dauntless enough, and I don't know why that is, what kind of threats are leveled at people who could be called "faction traitors," but that's exactly why I'm here.

"That's sort of the point," I say. "I want that tattoo."

I thought of it on the way home, while I was cycling

through what my mother said, over and over again. *You can be more than either, more than any faction.* She thought that in order to be more than any faction, I would have to abandon this place and the people who have embraced me as their own; I would have to forgive her and let myself be swallowed by her beliefs and her lifestyle. But I don't have to leave, and I don't have to do anything I don't want to do. I can be more than any faction right here in Dauntless; maybe I already am more, and it's time to show it.

Tori looks around, her eyes jumping up to the camera in the corner, one I noticed when I walked in. She is the type who notices cameras, too.

"It was just a stupid drawing," she says loudly. "Come on, you're clearly upset—we can talk about it, find something better for you to get."

She beckons me to the back of the parlor, through the storage room behind it, and into her apartment again. We walk through the dilapidated kitchen to the living room, where her drawings are still stacked on the coffee table.

She sorts through the pages until she finds a drawing like the one I was talking about, the Dauntless flames being cupped by Abnegation hands, the Amity tree roots growing beneath an Erudite eye, which is balanced under the Candor scales. All the faction symbols stacked on top of each other. She holds it up, and I nod.

"I can't do this in a place that people will see all the time," she says. "That'll make you a walking target. A suspected faction traitor."

"I want it on my back," I say. "Covering my spine."

The hurts from my last day with my father are healed now, but I want to remember where they were; I want to remember what I escaped for as long as I live.

"You really don't do things halfway, do you." She sighs. "It'll take a long time. Several sessions. We'll have to do them in here, after hours, because I'm not going to let those cameras catch it, even if they don't bother to look in here most of the time."

"Fine," I say.

"You know, the kind of person who gets this tattoo is probably the kind that should keep it very quiet," she says, looking at me from the corner of her eye. "Or else someone will start thinking they're Divergent."

"Divergent?"

"That's a word we have for people who are aware during simulations, who refuse categorization," she says. "A word you don't speak without care, because those people often die in mysterious circumstances."

She has her elbows resting on her knees, casual, as she sketches the tattoo I want on transfer paper. Our eyes meet, and I realize: Amar. Amar was aware during simulations, and now he's dead.

Amar was Divergent.

And so am I.

"Thanks for the vocabulary lesson," I say.

"No problem." She returns to her drawing. "I'm getting the feeling you enjoy putting yourself through the wringer."

"So?" I say.

"Nothing, it's just a pretty Dauntless quality for someone who got an Abnegation result." Her mouth twitches. "Let's get started. I'll leave a note for Bud; he can jog alone just this once."

+++

Maybe Tori is right. Maybe I do enjoy putting myself "through the wringer"; maybe there is a masochistic streak inside me that uses pain to cope with pain. The faint burning that follows me to my next day of leadership training certainly makes it easier to focus on what I'm about to do, instead of on my mother's cold, low voice and the way I pushed her away when she tried to comfort me.

In the years after her death, I used to dream that she would come back to life in the middle of the night and run a hand over my hair and say something comforting but nonsensical, like "It will be all right" or "It will get better someday." But then I stopped allowing myself to dream, because it was more painful to long for things and never get them than to deal with whatever was in front of me. Even now I don't want to imagine what reconciling with her would be like, what having a mother would be like. I'm too old to hear comforting nonsense anymore. Too old to believe that everything will be all right.

I check the top of the bandage that protrudes over my collar to make sure it's secure. Tori outlined the first two symbols this morning, Dauntless and Abnegation, which will be larger than the others, because they are the faction I chose and the faction I actually have aptitude for, respectively—at least, I think I have aptitude for Abnegation, but it's hard to be sure. She told me to keep them covered. The Dauntless flame is the only symbol that shows with my shirt on, and I'm not in the position to remove my shirt in public very often, so I doubt that will be a problem.

Everyone else is already in the conference room, and Max is speaking to them. I feel a kind of reckless weariness as I walk through the door and take my seat. Evelyn was wrong about quite a few things, but she wasn't wrong about the Dauntless—Jeanine and Max don't want a leader of Dauntless, they want a pawn, and that's why they're selecting from the youngest of us, because young people are easier shaped and molded. I will not be molded and shaped by Jeanine Matthews. I will not be a pawn, not for them and not for my mother and not for my father; I will not belong to anyone but myself.

"Nice of you to join us," Max says. "Did this meeting interrupt your sleep?"

The others titter with laughter, and Max continues.

"As I was saying, today I would like to hear your thoughts about how to improve Dauntless—the vision you have for our faction in the coming years," he says. "I'll be meeting with you in groups by age, the oldest first. The rest of you, think of something good to say."

He leaves with the three oldest candidates. Eric is right across from me, and I notice that he has even more metal in his face than the last time I saw him—now there are rings through his eyebrows. Soon he's going to look more like a pincushion than a human being. Maybe that's the point—strategy. No one looking at him now could ever mistake him for being Erudite.

"Do my eyes deceive me, or are you really late because you were getting a tattoo?" he says, pointing to the corner of the bandage that's visible just over my shoulder.

"Lost track of time," I say. "A lot of metal appears to have attached itself to your face recently. You may want to get that checked out."

"Funny," Eric says. "Wasn't sure someone with your background could ever develop a sense of humor. Your father doesn't seem like the type to allow it."

I feel a stab of fear. He's dancing awfully close to saying my name in front of this room full of people, and he wants me to know it—he wants me to remember that he knows who I am, and that he can use it against me whenever he pleases.

I can't pretend that it doesn't matter to me. The power dynamic has shifted, and I can't make it shift back.

"I think I know who told you that," I say. Jeanine Matthews knows both my name and my alias. She must have given him both.

"I was already fairly sure," he says in a low voice. "But my suspicions were confirmed by a credible source, yes. You aren't as good at keeping secrets as you think, Four."

I would threaten him, tell him that if he reveals my name to the Dauntless, I'll reveal his lasting connections to Erudite. But I don't have any evidence, and the Dauntless dislike Abnegation more than Erudite anyway. I sit back in my chair to wait.

The others file out as they're called, and soon we're the only ones left. Max makes his way down the hallway, then beckons to us from the door, without a word. We follow him back to his office, which I recognize from yesterday's footage of his meeting with Jeanine Matthews. I use my memory of that conversation to steel myself against what's coming next.

"So." Max folds his hands on his desk, and again I'm struck by how strange it is to see him in such a clean, formal environment. He belongs in a training room, hitting a bag, or next to the Pit, leaning over the railing. Not sitting at a low wooden table surrounded by paper.

I look out the windows of the Pire at the Dauntless sector of the city. A few yards away I can see the edge of the hole I jumped into when I first chose Dauntless, and the rooftop that I stood on just before that. *I chose Dauntless,* I told my mother yesterday. *That's where I belong.*

Is that really true?

"Eric, let's begin with you," Max says. "Do you have ideas for what might be good for Dauntless, moving forward?"

"I do." Eric sits up. "I think we need to make some changes, and I think they should start during initiation."

"What kind of changes do you have in mind?"

"Dauntless has always embraced a spirit of competition," Eric says. "Competition makes us better; it brings out the best, strongest parts of us. I think initiation should foster that sense of competition more than it currently does, so that it produces the best initiates possible. Right now initiates are competing only against the system, striving for a particular score in order to move forward. I think they should be compet-ing against each other for spots in Dauntless."

I can't help it; I turn and stare at him. A limited num-ber of spots? In a faction? After just *two weeks* of initiation training?

"And if they don't get a spot?"

"They become factionless," Eric says. I swallow a deri-sive laugh. Eric continues, "If we believe that Dauntless truly is the superior faction to join, that its aims are more important than the aims of other factions, then becoming one of us should be an honor and a privilege, not a right."

"Are you kidding?" I say, unable to contain myself any longer. "People choose a faction because they value the same things that faction values, not because they're already proficient in what a faction teaches. You'd be kicking people out of Dauntless just for not being strong enough to jump on a train or win a fight. You would favor the big, strong, and reckless more than the small, smart, and brave—you wouldn't be improving Dauntless at all."

"I'm sure the small, smart ones would be better off in Erudite, or as little gray-clad Stiffs," Eric says with a wry smile. "And I don't think you're giving our potential new Dauntless members enough credit, Four. This system would favor only the most determined."

I glance at Max. I expect him to look unimpressed by Eric's plan, but he doesn't. He's leaning forward, focused on Eric's pierced face like something about it has inspired him.

"This is an interesting debate," Max says. "Four, how would you improve Dauntless, if not by making initiation more competitive?"

I shake my head, looking out the window again. *You aren't one of those mindless, danger-seeking fools,* my mother said to me. But those are the people Eric wants in Dauntless: mindless, danger-seeking fools. If Eric is one of Jeanine Matthew's lackeys, then why would Jeanine encourage him to propose this kind of plan?

Oh. Because mindless, danger-seeking fools are easier to control, easier to manipulate. Obviously.

"I would improve Dauntless by fostering true bravery instead of stupidity and brutality," I say. "Take out the knife throwing. Prepare people physically and mentally to defend the weak against the strong. That's what our manifesto encourages—ordinary acts of bravery. I think we should return to that."

"And then we can all hold hands and sing a song together, right?" Eric rolls his eyes. "You want to turn Dauntless into Amity."

"No," I say. "I want to make sure we still know how to think for ourselves, think about more than the next surge of adrenaline. Or just think, period. That way we can't be taken over or . . . controlled from the outside."

"Sounds a little Erudite to me," Eric says.

"The ability to think isn't exclusive to Erudite," I snap. "The ability to think in stressful situations is what the fear simulations are supposed to develop."

"All right, all right," Max says, holding up his hands. He looks troubled. "Four, I'm sorry to say this, but you sound a little paranoid. Who would take us over, or try to control us? The factions have coexisted peacefully for longer than you've been alive, there's no reason that's going to change now."

I open my mouth to tell him he's wrong, that the second he let Jeanine Matthews get involved in the affairs of our faction, the second he let her plant Erudite-loyal transfers into our initiation program, the second he started consulting with her on who to appoint as the next Dauntless leader, he compromised the system of checks and balances that has allowed us to coexist peacefully for so long. But then I realize that to tell him those things would be to accuse him of treason, and to reveal just how much I know.

Max looks at me, and I read disappointment in his face.

I know that he likes me—likes me more than Eric, at least. But my mother was right yesterday—Max doesn't want someone like me, someone who can think for himself, develop his own agenda. He wants someone like Eric, who will help him establish the new Dauntless agenda, who will be easy to manipulate simply because he's still under the thumb of Jeanine Matthews, someone with whom Max is closely aligned.

My mother presented me with two options yesterday: be a pawn of Dauntless, or become factionless. But there's a third option: to be neither. To align myself with no one in particular. To live under the radar, and free. That's what I really want—to shed all the people who want to form and shape me, one by one, and learn instead to form and shape myself.

"To be honest, sir, I don't think this is the right place for me," I say calmly. "I told you when you first asked me that I'd like to be an instructor, and I think I'm realizing more and more that that's where I belong."

"Eric, will you excuse us, please?" Max says. Eric, barely able to suppress his glee, nods and leaves. I don't watch him go, but I would bet all my Dauntless credits that there's a little skip in his step as he walks down the hallway.

Max gets up and sits next to me, in the chair Eric just vacated.

"I hope you're not saying this because I accused you of being paranoid," Max says. "I was just concerned about you. I feared that the pressure was getting to you, making you stop thinking straight. I still think you're a strong candidate for leadership. You fit the right profile, you've demonstrated proficiency with everything we've taught you—and beyond that, quite frankly, you're more likable than some of our other promising candidates, which is important in a close working environment."

"Thank you," I say. "But you're right, the pressure is getting to me. And the pressure if I was actually a leader would be much worse."

Max nods sadly. "Well." He nods again. "If you'd like to be an initiation instructor, I will arrange that for you. But that's seasonal work—where would you like to be placed for the rest of the year?"

"I was thinking maybe the control room," I say. "I've discovered that I enjoy working with computers. I don't think I would enjoy patrolling nearly as much."

"Okay," Max says. "Consider it done. Thank you for being honest with me."

I get up, and all I feel is relief. He seems concerned,

sympathetic. Not suspicious of me or my motives or my paranoia.

"If you ever change your mind," Max says, "please don't hesitate to tell me. We could always use someone like you."

"Thank you," I say, and even though he's the worst faction traitor of anyone I've met, and probably responsible at least in part for Amar's death, I can't help but feel a little grateful to him for letting me go so easily.

+++

Eric is waiting for me around the corner. As I try to walk past him, he grabs my arm.

"Careful, Eaton," he murmurs. "If anything about my involvement with Erudite escapes you, you won't like what happens to you."

"You won't like what happens to you, either, if you ever call me by that name again."

"Soon I'm going to be one of your leaders," Eric says, smirking. "And believe me, I am going to keep a very, very close eye on you and how well you implement my new training methods."

"He doesn't like you, you know that?" I say. "Max, I mean. He'd rather have anyone else but you. He's not going to give you more than an inch in any direction. So good luck with your short leash."

I wrench my arm from his grasp and walk toward the elevators.

+++

"Man," Shauna says. "That *is* a bad day."

"Yeah."

She and I are sitting next to the chasm with our feet over the edge. I rest my head against the bars of the metal barrier that's keeping us from falling to our deaths, and feel the spray of water against my ankles as one of the larger waves hits a wall.

I told her about my departure from leadership training, and Eric's threat, but I didn't tell her about my mother. How do you tell someone that your mother came back from the dead?

All my life, someone has been trying to control me. Marcus was the tyrant of our house, and nothing happened without his permission. And then Max wanted to recruit me as his Dauntless yes-man. And even my mother had a plan for me, for me to join up with her when I reached a certain age to work against the faction system that *she* has a vendetta against, for whatever reason. And just when I thought that I had escaped control altogether, Eric swooped in to remind me that if he became a

Dauntless leader, he would be watching me.

All I have, I realize, are the small moments of rebellion I'm able to manage, just like when I was in Abnegation, collecting objects I found on the street. The tattoo that Tori is drawing on my back, the one that might declare me to be Divergent, is one of those moments. I'll have to keep looking for more of them, more brief moments of freedom in a world that refuses to allow it.

"Where's Zeke?" I say.

"I don't know," she says. "I haven't wanted to hang out with him much recently."

I look sideways at her. "You could just tell him that you like him, you know. I honestly don't think he has a clue."

"That's obvious," she says, snorting. "But what if this is what he wants—to just bounce around from girl to girl for a while? I don't want to be one of those girls he bounces to."

"I seriously doubt you would be," I say, "but fair enough."

We sit quietly for a few seconds, both of us staring down at the raging water below.

"You'll be a good instructor," she says. "You were really good at teaching me."

"Thanks."

"*There* you are," Zeke says from behind us. He's carrying a large bottle full of some kind of brown liquid, holding it by the neck. "Come on. I found something."

Shauna and I look at each other and shrug, then follow him to the doors on the other side of the Pit, the ones we first went through after jumping into the net. But instead of leading us toward the net, he takes us through another door—the lock is taped down with duct tape—and down a pitch-black corridor and a flight of stairs.

"Should be coming up—ouch!"

"Sorry, I didn't know you were stopping," Shauna says.

"Hold on, almost got it—"

He opens a door, letting faint light in so we can see where we are. We're on the other side of the chasm, several feet above the water. Above us, the Pit seems to go on forever, and the people milling around near the railing are small and dark, impossible to distinguish from this distance.

I laugh. Zeke just led us into another small moment of rebellion, probably without meaning to.

"How did you *find* this place?" Shauna says with obvious wonder as she jumps down onto one of the lower rocks. Now that I'm here, I see a path that would carry us up and across the wall, if we wanted to walk to the other side of the chasm.

"That girl Maria," Zeke says. "Her mom works in chasm maintenance. I didn't know there was such a thing, but apparently there is."

"You still seeing her?" Shauna asks, trying to be casual.

"Nah," Zeke says. "Every time I was with her I just kept getting the itch to be with friends instead. That's not a good sign, right?"

"No," Shauna agrees, and she seems more cheerful than before.

I lower myself more carefully onto the rock Shauna is standing on. Zeke sits next to her, opening his bottle and passing it around.

"I heard you're out of the running," Zeke says when he passes it to me. "Thought you might need a drink."

"Yeah," I say, and then I take a swig.

"Consider this act of public drunkenness a big—" He makes an obscene gesture toward the glass ceiling above the Pit. "You know, to Max and Eric."

And Evelyn, I think, as I take another swallow.

"I'll be working in the control room when I'm not training initiates," I say.

"Awesome," Zeke says. "It'll be good to have a friend in

there. Right now no one talks to me."

"Sounds like me in my old faction," I say with a laugh. "Imagine an entire lunch period in which no one even looks at you."

"Ouch," Zeke says. "Well, I bet you're glad to be here now, then."

I take the bottle from him again, drink another mouthful of stinging, burning alcohol, and wipe my mouth with the back of my hand. "Yeah," I say. "I am."

If the factions are deteriorating, as my mother would have me believe, this is not a bad place to watch them fall apart. At least here I have friends to keep me company while it happens.

+++

It's just after dark, and I have my hood up to hide my face as I run through the factionless area of the city, right by the border it shares with the Abnegation sector. I had to go to the school to get my bearings, but now I remember where I am, and where I ran, that day that I barged into a factionless warehouse in search of a dying ember.

I reach the door I walked through when I exited, and tap on it with my first knuckle. I can hear voices just beyond it and smell food coming from one of the open windows, where smoke from the fire within is leaking into the alley. Footsteps, as someone comes to see what the knocking is about.

This time the man is wearing a red Amity shirt and black Dauntless pants. He still has a towel tucked into his back pocket, the same as the last time I spoke to him. He opens the door just enough to look at me, and no farther.

"Well, look who made a change," he said, eyeing my Dauntless clothes. "To what do I owe this visit? Did you miss my charming company?"

"You knew my mother was alive when you met me," I say. "That's how you recognized me, because you've spent time with her. That's how you knew what she said about inertia carrying her to Abnegation."

"Yeah," the man said. "Didn't think it was my business to be the one to tell you she was still alive. You here to demand an apology, or something?"

"No," I say. "I'm here to hand off a message. You'll give it to her?"

"Yeah, sure. I'll be seeing her in the next couple days."

I reach into my pocket and take out a folded piece of paper. I offer it to him.

"Go ahead and read it, I don't care," I say. "And thanks."

"No problem," he says. "Want to come in? You're starting to seem more like one of us than one of them, Eaton."

I shake my head.

I make my way back down the alley, and before I turn the corner, I see him opening up the note to read what it says.

> *Evelyn,*
> *Someday. Not yet.*
> *—4*
> *P.S. I'm glad you're not dead.*

THE TRAITOR

ANOTHER YEAR, ANOTHER Visiting Day.

Two years ago, when I was an initiate, I pretended my own Visiting Day didn't exist, holed up in the training room with a punching bag. I was there for so long that I smelled the dust-sweat for days afterward. Last year, the first year I taught initiates, I did the same thing, though Zeke and Shauna both invited me to spend the day with their families instead.

This year I have more important things to do than punch a bag and mope about my family dysfunction. I'm going to the control room.

I walk through the Pit, dodging tearful reunions and shrieks of laughter. Families can always come together on Visiting Day, even if they're from different factions, but over time, they usually stop coming. "Faction before blood," after all. Most of the mixed clothing I see belongs to transfer families: Will's Erudite sister is dressed in light blue, Peter's Candor parents are in black and white. For a moment I watch his parents, and wonder if they made him into the person he is. But most of the time, people aren't that easy to explain, I guess.

I'm supposed to be on a mission, but I pause next to the chasm, pressing into the railing. Bits of paper float in the water. Now that I know where the steps cut into the stone in the opposite wall are, I can see them right away, and the hidden doorway that leads to them. I smile a little, thinking of the nights I've spent on those rocks with Zeke or Shauna, sometimes talking and sometimes just sitting and listening to the water move.

I hear footsteps approaching, and look over my shoulder. Tris is walking toward me, tucked under the gray-clad arm of an Abnegation woman. Natalie Prior. I stiffen, suddenly desperate to escape—what if Natalie knows who I am, where I came from? What if she lets it slip, here, surrounded by all these people?

She can't possibly recognize me. I don't look anything like the boy she knew, lanky and slouched and buried in fabric.

When she's close enough, she extends her hand. "Hello,

my name is Natalie. I'm Beatrice's mother."

Beatrice. That name is so wrong for her.

I clasp Natalie's hand and shake it. I've never been fond of Dauntless hand-shaking. It's too unpredictable—you never know how tightly to squeeze, how many times to shake.

"Four," I say. "It's nice to meet you."

"Four," Natalie says, and she smiles. "Is that a nickname?"

"Yes," I say. I change the subject. "Your daughter is doing well here. I've been overseeing her training."

"That's good to hear," she says. "I know a few things about Dauntless initiation, and I was worried about her."

I glance at Tris. There's color in her cheeks—she looks happy, like seeing her mother is doing her some good. For the first time I fully appreciate how much she's changed since I first saw her, tumbling onto the wooden platform, fragile-looking, like the impact with the net should have shattered her. She doesn't look fragile anymore, with the shadows of bruises on her face and a new stability in the way she stands, like she's ready for anything.

"You shouldn't worry," I say to Natalie.

Tris looks away. I think she's still angry with me for the way I nicked her ear with that knife. I guess I don't really blame her.

"You look familiar for some reason, Four," Natalie says. I would think her comment was lighthearted if not for the way she's looking at me, like she's pinning me down.

"I can't imagine why," I say, as coldly as I can manage. "I don't make a habit of associating with the Abnegation."

She doesn't react the way I expect her to, with surprise or fear or anger. She just laughs. "Few people do, these days. I don't take it personally."

If she does recognize me, she doesn't seem eager to say so. I try to relax.

"Well, I'll leave you to your reunion," I say.

+++

On my screen, the security footage switches from the lobby of the Pire to the hole hemmed in by four buildings, the initiate entrance to Dauntless. A crowd is gathered around the hole, climbing in and out of it, I assume to test the net.

"Not into Visiting Day?" My supervisor, Gus, stands at my shoulder, sipping from a mug of coffee. He's not that old, but there's a bald spot at the crown of his head. He keeps the rest of his hair short, even shorter than mine. His earlobes are stretched around wide discs. "I didn't think I'd see you again until initiation was over."

"Figured I might as well do something productive."

On my screen, everyone crawls out of the hole and

stands aside, their backs against one of the buildings. A dark figure inches toward the edge of the roof high above the hole, runs a few steps, and jumps off. My stomach drops like I'm the one falling, and the figure disappears beneath the pavement. I'll never get used to seeing that.

"They seem to be having a good time," Gus says, sipping his coffee again. "Well, you're always welcome to work when you're not scheduled to, but it's not a crime to go have some mindless fun, Four."

He walks away, and I mumble, "So I'm told."

I look over the control room. It's almost empty—on Visiting Day, only a few people are required to work, and it's usually the oldest ones. Gus is hunched over his screen. Two others flank him, scanning through footage with their headphones half on, half off. And then there's me.

I type in a command, calling up the footage I saved last week. It shows Max in his office, sitting at his computer. He pokes at the keys with an index finger, hunting for the right ones for several seconds between jabs. Not many of the Dauntless know how to type properly, especially Max, who I'm told spent most of his Dauntless time patrolling the factionless sector with a gun at his side—he must not have anticipated that he would ever need to use a computer. I lean close to the screen to make sure that the numbers I took down earlier are accurate. If they are, I have Max's account password written on a piece of paper in my pocket.

Ever since I realized that Max was working closely with Jeanine Matthews, and began to suspect that they had something to do with Amar's death, I've been looking for a way to investigate further. When I saw him type in his password the other day, I found one.

084628. Yes, the numbers look right. I call up the live security footage again, and cycle through the camera feeds until I find the ones that show Max's office and the hallway beyond it. Then I type the command to take the footage of Max's office out of the rotation, so Gus and the others won't see it; it will only play on my screen. The footage from the whole city is always divided by however many people are in the control room, so we aren't all looking at the same feeds. We're only supposed to pull footage from the general rotation like that for a few seconds at a time, if we need a closer look at something, but hopefully this won't take me long. I slip out of the room and walk toward the elevators.

This level of the Pire is almost empty—everyone is gone. That will make it easier for me to do what I have to do. I ride the elevator up to the tenth floor, and walk purposefully toward Max's office. I've found that when you're sneaking around, it's best not to look like you're sneaking around. I tap the flash drive in my pocket as I walk, and turn the corner toward Max's office.

I nudge the door open with my shoe—earlier today, after I was sure he had gone to the Pit to start Visiting Day preparations, I'd crept up here and taped the lock. I close the door quietly behind me, not turning on the lights, and crouch next to his desk. I don't want to move the chair to sit in it; I don't want him to see that anything about this room has changed when he gets back.

The screen prompts me for a password. My mouth feels dry. I take the paper from my pocket and press it flat to the desk top while I type it in. 084628.

The screen shifts. I can't believe it worked.

Hurry. If Gus discovers that I'm gone, that I'm in here, I don't know what I'll say, what excuse I could possibly give that would sound reasonable. I insert the flash drive and transfer the program I put there earlier. I asked Lauren, one of the Dauntless technical staff and my fellow initiation instructor, for a program that would make one computer mirror another, under the pretense that I wanted to prank Zeke when we're at work. She was happy to help—another thing I've discovered is that the Dauntless are always up for a prank, and rarely looking for a lie.

With a few simple keystrokes, the program is installed

and buried somewhere in Max's computer that I'm sure he would never bother to access. I put the flash drive back in my pocket, along with the piece of paper with his password on it, and leave the office without getting my fingerprints on the glass part of the door.

That was easy, I think, as I walk toward the elevators again. According to my watch, it only took me five minutes. I can claim that I was on a bathroom break if anyone asks.

But when I get back to the control room, Gus is standing at my computer, staring at my screen.

I freeze. How long has he been there? Did he see me break into Max's office?

"Four," Gus says, sounding grave. "Why did you isolate this footage? You're not supposed to take feeds out of rotation, you know that."

"I . . ." *Lie! Lie now!* "I thought I saw something," I finish lamely. "We're allowed to isolate footage if we see something out of the ordinary."

Gus moves toward me.

"So," he says, "then why did I just see you on this screen coming out of that same hallway?"

He points to the hallway on my screen. My throat tightens.

"I thought I saw something, and I went upstairs to

investigate it," I say. "I'm sorry, I just wanted to move around."

He stares at me, chewing the inside of his cheek. I don't move. I don't look away.

"If you ever see something out of the ordinary again, you follow the protocol. You report it to your supervisor, who is . . . who, again?"

"You," I say, sighing a little. I don't like to be patronized.

"Correct. I see you *can* keep up," he says. "Honestly, Four, after over a year of working here there shouldn't be so many irregularities in your job performance. We have very clear rules, and all you have to do is follow them. This is your last warning. Okay?"

"Okay," I say. I've been chastised a few times for pulling feeds out of rotation to watch meetings with Jeanine Matthews and Max, or with Max and Eric. It never gave me any useful information, and I almost always got caught.

"Good." His voice lightens up a little. "Good luck with the initiates. You got transfers again this year?"

"Yeah," I say. "Lauren gets the Dauntless-borns."

"Ah, too bad. I was hoping you would get to know my little sister," Gus says. "If I were you, I'd go do something to wind down. We're fine in here. Just let that footage loose before you go."

He walks back to his computer, and I unclench my jaw. I wasn't even aware that I was doing it. My face throbbing, I shut down my computer and leave the control room. I can't believe I got away with it.

Now, with this program installed on Max's computer, I can go through every single one of his files from the relative privacy of the control room. I can find out exactly what he and Jeanine Matthews are up to.

+++

That night I dream that I'm walking through the hallways of the Pire, and I'm alone, but the corridors don't end, and the view from the windows doesn't change, lofted train tracks curving into tall buildings, the sun buried in clouds. I feel like I'm walking for hours, and when I wake with a start, it's like I never slept at all.

Then I hear a knock, and a voice shouting, "Open up!"

This feels more like a nightmare than the tedium I just escaped—I'm sure it's Dauntless soldiers coming to my door because they found out I'm Divergent, or that I'm spying on Max, or that I've been in touch with my faction-less mother in the past year. All things that say "faction traitor."

Dauntless soldiers coming to kill me—but as I walk to the door, I realize that if they were going to do that, they wouldn't make so much noise in the hallway. And besides, that's Zeke's voice.

"Zeke," I say when I open the door. "What's your problem? It's the middle of the night."

There's a line of sweat on his forehead, and he's out of breath. He must have run here.

"I was working the night shift in the control room," Zeke says. "Something happened in the transfer dorm."

For some reason, my first thought is *her*, her wide eyes staring at me from the recesses of my memory.

"What?" I say. "To who?"

"Walk and talk," Zeke says.

I put on my shoes and pull on my jacket and follow him down the hall.

"The Erudite guy. Blond," Zeke says.

I have to suppress a sigh of relief. It's not her. Nothing happened to her. "Will?"

"No, the other one."

"Edward."

"Yeah, Edward. He was attacked. Stabbed."

"Dead?"

"Alive. Got hit in the eye."

I stop. "In the *eye*?"

Zeke nods.

"Who did you tell?"

"Night supervisor. He went to tell Eric, Eric said he would handle it."

"Sure he will." I veer to the right, away from the transfer dormitory.

"Where are you going?" Zeke says.

"Edward's already in the infirmary?" I walk backward as I talk.

Zeke nods.

I say, "Then I'm going to see Max."

+++

The Dauntless compound isn't so large that I don't know where people live. Max's apartment is buried deep in the underground corridors of the compound, near a back door that opens up right next to the train tracks outside. I march toward it, following the blue emergency lamps run by our solar generator.

I pound on the metal door with my fist, waking Max the same way Zeke woke me. He yanks the door open a few seconds later, his feet bare and his eyes wild.

"What happened?" he says.

"One of my initiates was stabbed in the eye," I say.

"And you came here? Didn't someone inform Eric?"

"Yeah. That's what I want to talk to you about. Mind if I come in?"

I don't wait for an answer—I brush past him and walk into his living room. He flips on the lights, displaying the messiest living space I've ever seen, used cups and plates strewn across the coffee table, all the couch cushions in disarray, the floor gray with dust.

"I want initiation to go back to what it was before Eric made it more competitive," I say, "and I want him out of my training room."

"You don't really think it's Eric's fault that an initiate got hurt," Max says, crossing his arms. "Or that you're in any position to make demands."

"Yes, it's his fault, of course it's his fault!" I say, louder than I mean to be. "If they weren't all fighting for one of ten slots, they wouldn't be so desperate they're ready to attack each other! He has them wound up so tight, of course they're bound to explode eventually!"

Max is quiet. He looks annoyed, but he isn't calling me ridiculous, which is a start.

"You don't think the initiate who did the attacking should be held responsible?" Max says. "You don't think he or she is the one to blame, instead of Eric?"

"Of course he—she—whoever—should be held responsible," I say. "But this never would have happened if Eric—"

"You can't say that with any certainty," Max says.

"I can say it with the certainty of a reasonable person."

"I'm not reasonable?" His voice is low, dangerous, and suddenly I remember that Max is not just the Dauntless leader who likes me for some inexplicable reason—he's the Dauntless leader who's working closely with Jeanine Matthews, the one who appointed Eric, the one who probably had something to do with Amar's death.

"That's not what I meant," I say, trying to stay calm.

"You should be careful to communicate exactly what you mean," Max says, moving closer to me. "Or someone will start to think you're insulting your superiors."

I don't respond. He moves still closer.

"Or questioning the values of your faction," he says, and his bloodshot eyes drift to my shoulder, where the Dauntless flames of my tattoo stick out over the collar of my shirt. I have hidden the five faction symbols that cover my spine since I got them, but for some reason, at this moment, I am terrified that Max knows about them. Knows what they mean, which is that I am not a perfect Dauntless member; I am someone who believes that more than one virtue should be prized; I am Divergent.

"You had your shot to become a Dauntless leader," Max says. "Maybe you could have avoided this incident had you not backed out like a coward. But you did. So now you have to deal with the consequences."

His face is showing his age. It has lines it didn't have

last year, or the year before, and his skin is grayish brown, like it was dusted with ash.

"Eric is as involved in initiation as he is because you refused to follow orders last year—" Last year, in the training room, I stopped all the fights before the injuries became too severe, against Eric's command that the fighting only stop when one person was unable to continue. I nearly lost my position as initiation instructor as a result; I would have, if Max hadn't gotten involved.

"—and I wanted to give you another chance to make it right, with closer monitoring," Max says. "You're failing to do so. You've gone too far."

The sweat I worked up on my way here has turned cold. He steps back and opens his door again.

"Get out of my apartment and deal with your initiates," Max says. "Don't let me see you step out of line again."

"Yes, sir," I say quietly, and I leave.

+++

I go to see Edward in the infirmary early in the morning, when the sun is rising, shining through the glass ceiling of the Pit. His head is wrapped in white bandages, and he's not moving, not speaking. I don't say anything to him, just sit by his head and watch the minutes tick by on the wall clock.

I've been an idiot. I thought I was invincible, that Max's desire to have me as a fellow leader would never waver, that on some level he trusted me. I should have known better. All Max ever wanted was a pawn—that's what my mother said.

I can't be a pawn. But I'm not sure what I should be instead.

+++

The setting Tris Prior invents is eerie and almost beautiful, the sky yellow-green, yellow grass stretching for miles in every direction.

Watching someone else's fear simulation is strange. Intimate. I don't feel right about forcing other people to be vulnerable, even if I don't like them. Every human being is entitled to her secrets. Watching my initiates' fears, one after another, makes me feel like my skin has been scraped raw with sandpaper.

In Tris's simulation, the yellow grass is perfectly still. If the air wasn't stagnant, I would say this was a dream, not a nightmare—but still air means only one thing to me, and that is a coming storm.

A shadow moves across the grass, and a large black bird lands on her shoulder, curling its talons into her shirt. My fingertips prickle, remembering how I touched her shoulder when she walked into the simulation room, how I brushed her hair away from her neck to inject her. Stupid. Careless.

She hits the black bird, hard, and then everything happens at once. Thunder rumbles; the sky darkens, not with storm clouds, but with *birds*, an impossibly huge swarm of them, moving in unison like many parts of the same mind.

The sound of her scream is the worst sound in the world, desperate—she's desperate for help and I am desperate to help her, though I know what I'm seeing isn't real, I know it. The crows keep coming, relentless, surrounding her, burying her alive in dark feathers. She screams for help and I can't help her and I don't want to watch this, I don't want to watch another second.

But then, she starts to move, shifting so she's lying in the grass, relenting, relaxing. If she's in pain now she doesn't show it; she just closes her eyes and surrenders, and that is worse than her screaming for help, somehow.

Then it's over.

She lurches forward in the metal chair, smacking at her body to get the birds off, though they're gone. Then she curls into a ball and hides her face.

I reach out to touch her shoulder, to reassure her, and she hits my arm, hard. "Don't touch me!"

"It's over," I say, wincing—she punches harder than she realizes. I ignore the pain and run a hand over her hair, because I'm stupid, and inappropriate, and stupid . . .

"Tris."

She just shifts back and forth, soothing herself.

"Tris, I'm going to take you back to the dorms, okay?"

"No! They can't see me . . . not like this. . . ."

This is what Eric's new system creates: A brave human being has just defeated one of her worst fears in less than five minutes, an ordeal that takes most people at least twice that time, but she's terrified to go back into the hallway, to be seen as weak or vulnerable in any way. Tris is Dauntless, plain and simple, but this faction isn't really Dauntless anymore.

"Oh, calm down," I say, more irritable than I mean to be. "I'll take you out the back door."

"I don't need you to . . ." I can see her hands trembling even as she shrugs off my offer.

"Nonsense," I say. I take her arm and help her to her feet. She wipes her eyes as I move toward the back door. Amar once took me through this door, tried to walk me back to the dormitory even when I didn't want him to, the way she probably doesn't want me to now. How is it possible to live the same story twice, from different vantage points?

She yanks her arm from mine, and turns on me. "Why

did you do that to me? What was the point of that, huh? I wasn't aware that when I chose Dauntless, I was signing up for weeks of torture!"

If she was anyone else, any of the other initiates, I would have yelled at her for insubordination a dozen times by now. I would have felt threatened by her constant assaults against my character, and tried to squelch her uprisings with cruelty, the way I did to Christina on the first day of initiation. But Tris earned my respect when she jumped first, into the net; when she challenged me at her first meal; when she wasn't deterred by my unpleasant responses to questions; when she spoke up for Al and stared me right in the eye as I threw knives at her. She's not my subordinate, couldn't possibly be.

"Did you think overcoming cowardice would be easy?" I say.

"That isn't overcoming cowardice! Cowardice is how you decide to be in real life, and in real life, I am not getting pecked to death by crows, Four!"

She starts to cry, but I'm too struck by what she just said to feel uncomfortable with her tears. She's not learning the lessons Eric wants her to learn. She's learning different things, wiser ones.

"I want to go home," she says.

I know where the cameras are in this hallway. I hope

none of them have picked up on what she just said.

"Learning how to think in the midst of fear is a lesson that everyone, even your Stiff family, needs to learn," I say. I doubt a lot of things about Dauntless initiation, but the fear simulations aren't one of them; they are the most straightforward way for a person to engage their own fears and conquer them, far more straightforward than the knife throwing or the fighting. "That's what we're trying to teach you. If you can't learn it, you'll need to get the hell out of here, because we won't want you."

I'm hard on her because I know she can handle it. And also because I don't know any other way to be.

"I'm trying. But I failed. I'm failing."

I almost feel like laughing. "How long do you think you spent in that hallucination, Tris?"

"I don't know. A half hour?"

"Three minutes," I say. "You got out three times faster than any of the other initiates. Whatever you are, you're not a failure."

You might be Divergent, I think. But she didn't do anything to change the simulation, so maybe she's not. Maybe she's just that brave.

I smile at her. "Tomorrow you'll be better at this. You'll see."

"Tomorrow?"

She's calmer now. I touch her back, right beneath her shoulders.

"What was your first hallucination?" she asks me.

"It wasn't a 'what' so much as a 'who.'" As I'm saying it, I think I should have just told her the first obstacle in my fear landscape, fear of heights, though it's not exactly what she's asking about. When I'm around her I can't control what I say the way I do around other people. I say vague things because that's as close as I can get to stopping myself from saying anything, my mind addled by the feeling of her body through her shirt. "It's not important."

"And are you over that fear now?"

"Not yet." We're at the dormitory door. The walk has never gone by so quickly. I put my hands in my pockets so I don't do anything stupid with them again. "I may never be."

"So they don't go away?"

"Sometimes they do. And sometimes new fears replace them. But becoming fearless isn't the point. That's impossible. It's learning how to control your fear, and how to be free from it, *that's* the point."

She nods. I don't know what she came here for, but if I had to guess, it would be that she chose Dauntless for its freedom. Abnegation would have stifled the spark in her until it died out. Dauntless, for all its faults, has kindled the spark into a flame.

"Anyway," I say. "Your fears are rarely what they appear to be in the simulation."

"What do you mean?"

"Well, are you really afraid of crows?" I grin. "When you see one, do you run away screaming?"

"No, I guess not."

She moves closer to me. I felt safer when there was more space between us. Even closer, and I think about touching her, and my mouth goes dry. I almost never think about people that way, about girls that way.

"So what am I really afraid of?" she says.

"I don't know," I say. "Only you can know."

"I didn't know Dauntless would be this difficult."

I'm glad to have something else to think about, other than how easy it would be to fit my hand to the arch of her back.

"It wasn't always like this, I'm told. Being Dauntless, I mean."

"What changed?"

"The leadership. The person who controls training sets the standard of Dauntless behavior. Six years ago Max and the other leaders changed the training methods to make them more competitive and more brutal." Six years ago, the combat portion of training was brief and didn't include bare-knuckled sparring. Initiates wore padding. The emphasis was on being strong and capable, and on developing camaraderie with the other initiates. And even when I was an initiate, it was better than this—an unlimited potential for initiates to become members, fights that stopped when one person conceded. "Said it was to test people's strength. And that changed the priorities of Dauntless as a whole. Bet you can't guess who the leaders' new protégé is."

Of course, she does immediately. "So if you were ranked first in your initiate class, what was Eric's rank?"

"Second."

"So he was their second choice for leadership. And you were their first."

Perceptive. I don't know that I was the first choice, but I was certainly a better option than Eric. "What makes you say that?"

"The way Eric was acting at dinner the first night. Jealous, even though he has what he wants."

I've never thought of Eric that way. Jealous? Of what? I've never taken anything from him, never posed a real threat to him. He's the one who came after Amar, who came after me. But maybe she's right—maybe I never saw how frustrated he was to be second to a transfer from Abnegation, after all his hard work, or that I was favored by Max for leadership even when he was positioned here specifically to take the leadership role.

She wipes her face.

"Do I look like I've been crying?"

The question seems almost funny to me. Her tears vanished almost as quickly as they came, and now her face is fair again, her eyes dry, her hair smooth. Like nothing ever happened—like she didn't just spend three minutes overwhelmed by terror. She's stronger than I was.

"Hmm." I lean in closer, making a joke of examining her, but then it's not a joke, and I'm just close, and we're sharing a breath.

"No, Tris," I say. "You look . . ." I try a Dauntless expression. "Tough as nails."

She smiles a little. So do I.

+++

"Hey," Zeke says sleepily, leaning his head into his fist. "Want to take over for me? I practically need to tape my eyes open."

"Sorry," I say. "I just need to use a computer. You do know it's only nine o'clock, right?"

He yawns. "I get tired when I'm bored out of my mind. Shift's almost over, though."

I love the control room at night. There are only three people monitoring the footage, so the room is silent except for the hum of computers. Through the windows I see only a sliver of the moon; everything else is dark. It's hard to find peace in the Dauntless compound, and this is the place where I find it most often.

Zeke turns back to his screen. I sit at a computer a few seats over from him, and angle the screen away from the room. Then I log in, using the fake account name I set up several months ago, so no one would be able to track this back to me.

Once I'm logged in, I open the mirroring program that lets me use Max's computer remotely. It takes a second to kick in, but when it does, it's like I'm sitting in Max's office, using the same machine he uses.

I work quickly, systematically. He labels his folders with numbers, so I don't know what each one will contain. Most are benign, lists of Dauntless members or schedules of events. I open them and close them in seconds.

I go deeper into the files, folder after folder, and then I find something strange. A list of supplies, but the supplies don't involve food or fabric or anything else I would expect for mundane Dauntless life—the list is for weapons. Syringes. And something marked *Serum D2*.

I can imagine only one thing that would require the Dauntless to have so many weapons: an attack. But on who?

I check the control room again, my heartbeat pounding in my head. Zeke is playing a computer game that he wrote himself. The second control-room operator is slumped to one side, her eyes half-closed. The third is stirring his glass of water idly with his straw, staring out the windows. No one is paying attention to me.

I open more files. After a few wasted efforts, I find a map. It's marked mostly with letters and numbers, so at first I don't know what it's showing.

Then I open a map of the city on the Dauntless database to compare them, and sit back in my chair as I realize what streets Max's map is focusing on.

The Abnegation sector.

The attack will be against Abnegation.

+++

It should have been obvious, of course. Who else would Max and Jeanine bother to attack? Max and Jeanine's vendetta is against Abnegation, and it always has been. I should have realized that when the Erudite released that story about my father, the monstrous husband and father. The only true thing they've written, as far as I can tell.

Zeke nudges my leg with his foot. "Shift's over. Bedtime?"

"No," I say. "I need a drink."

He perks up noticeably. It's not every night I decide I want to abandon my sterile, withdrawn existence for an evening of Dauntless indulgence.

"I'm your man," he says.

I close down the program, my account, everything. I try to leave the information about the Abnegation attack behind, too, until I can figure out what to do about it, but it chases me all the way into the elevator, through the lobby, and down the paths to the bottom of the Pit.

+++

I surface from the simulation with a heavy feeling in the pit of my stomach. I detach from the wires and get up. She's still recovering from the sensation of almost drowning, shaking her hands and taking deep breaths. I watch her for a moment, not sure how to say what I need to say.

"What?" she says.

"How did you do that?"

"Do what?"

"Crack the glass."

"I don't know."

I nod, and offer her my hand. She gets up without any trouble, but she avoids my eyes. I check the corners of the room for cameras. There is one, just where I thought it would be, right across from us. I take her elbow and lead her out of the room, to a place where I know we won't be observed, in the blind spot between two surveillance points.

"What?" she says irritably.

"You're Divergent," I say. I haven't been very nice to her today. Last night I saw her and her friends by the chasm, and a lapse in judgment—or sobriety—led me to lean in too close, to tell her she looked good. I'm worried that I went too far. Now I'm even more worried, but for different reasons.

She cracked the glass. She's Divergent. She's in danger.

She stares.

Then she sinks against the wall, adopting an almost-convincing aura of casualness. "What's Divergent?"

"Don't play stupid," I say. "I suspected it last time, but this time it's obvious. You manipulated the simulation; you're Divergent. I'll delete the footage, but unless you want to wind up dead at the bottom of the chasm, you'll figure out how to hide it during the simulations! Now, if you'll excuse me."

I walk back to the simulation room, pulling the door closed behind me. It's easy to delete the footage—just a few keystrokes and it's done, the record clean. I double-check her file, making sure the only thing that's in there is the data from the first simulation. I'll have to come up with a way to explain where the data from this session went. A good lie, one that Eric and Max will actually believe.

In a hurry, I take out my pocketknife and wedge it between the panels covering the motherboard of the computer, prying them apart. Then I go into the hallway, to the drinking fountain, and fill my mouth with water.

When I return to the simulation room, I spit some of the water into the gap between the panels. I put my knife away and wait.

A minute or so later, the screen goes dark. Dauntless headquarters is basically a leaky cave—water damage happens all the time.

+++

I was desperate.

I sent a message through the same factionless man I used as a messenger last time I wanted to get in touch with my mother. I arranged to meet her inside the last car of the ten-fifteen train from Dauntless headquarters. I assume she'll know how to find me.

I sit with my back against the wall, an arm curled around one of my knees, and watch the city pass. Night trains don't move as fast as day trains between stops. It's easier to observe how the buildings change as the train draws closer to the center of the city, how they grow taller but narrower, how pillars of glass stand next to smaller, older stone structures. Like one city layered on top of another on top of another.

Someone runs alongside the train when it reaches the north side of the city. I stand up, holding one of the railings along the wall, and Evelyn stumbles into the car wearing Amity boots, an Erudite dress, and a Dauntless jacket. Her hair is pulled back, making her already-severe face even harsher.

"Hello," she says.

"Hi," I say.

"Every time I see you, you're bigger," she says. "I guess there's no point in worrying that you're eating well."

"Could say the same to you," I say, "but for different reasons."

I know she's not eating well. She's factionless, and the Abnegation haven't been providing as much aid as they usually do, with the Erudite bearing down on them the way they are.

I reach behind me and grab the backpack I brought with cans from the Dauntless storeroom.

"It's just bland soup and vegetables, but it's better than nothing," I say when I offer it to her.

"Who says I need your help?" Evelyn says carefully. "I'm doing just fine, you know."

"Yeah, that's not for you," I say. "It's for all your skinny friends. If I were you, I wouldn't turn down food."

"I'm not," she says, taking the backpack. "I'm just not used to you caring. It's a little disarming."

"I'm familiar with the feeling," I say coldly. "How long was it before you checked in on my life? Seven years?"

Evelyn sighs. "If you asked me to come here just to start this argument again, I'm afraid I can't stay long."

"No," I say. "No, that's not why I asked you to come here."

I didn't want to contact her at all, but I knew I couldn't tell any of the Dauntless what I had learned about the Abnegation attack—I don't know how loyal to the faction and its policies they are—and I had to tell someone. The last time I spoke to Evelyn, she seemed to know things about the city that I didn't. I assumed she might know how to help me with this, before it's too late.

It's a risk, but I'm not sure where else to turn.

"I've been keeping an eye on Max," I say. "You said the Erudite were involved with the Dauntless, and you were right. They're planning something together, Max and Jeanine and who knows who else."

I tell her what I saw on Max's computer, the supply lists and the maps. I tell her what I've observed about the Erudite's attitude toward Abnegation, the reports, how they're poisoning even Dauntless minds against our former faction.

When I finish, Evelyn doesn't look surprised, or even grave. In fact, I have no idea how to read her expression. She's quiet for a few seconds, and then she says, "Did you see any indication of when this might happen?"

"No," I say.

"How about numbers? How large a force do Dauntless and Erudite intend to use? Where do they intend to summon it from?"

"I don't know," I say, frustrated. "I don't really care, either. No matter how many recruits they get, they'll mow down the Abnegation in seconds. It's not like they're trained to defend themselves—not like they would even if they knew how, either."

"I knew something was going on," Evelyn says, furrowing her brow. "The lights are on at Erudite headquarters all the time now. Which means that they're not afraid of getting in trouble with the council leaders anymore, which . . . suggests something about their growing dissent."

"Okay," I say. "How do we warn them?"

"Warn who?"

"The Abnegation!" I say hotly. "How do we warn the Abnegation that they're going to be killed, how do we warn the Dauntless that their leaders are conspiring against the council, how—"

I pause. Evelyn is standing with her hands loose at her sides, her face relaxed and passive. *Our city is changing, Tobias.* That's what she said to me when we first saw each other again. *Sometime soon, everyone will have to choose a side, and I know which one you would rather be on.*

"You already knew," I say slowly, struggling to process the truth. "You knew they were planning something like this, and have been for a while. You're waiting for it. Counting on it."

"I have no lingering affection for my former faction. I don't want them, or any faction, to continue to control this city and the people in it," Evelyn says. "If someone wants to take out my enemies for me, I'm going to let them."

"I can't believe you," I say. "They're not all Marcus, Evelyn. They're *defenseless*."

"You think they're so innocent," she says. "You don't know them. I know them, I've *seen* them for who they really are."

Her voice is low, throaty.

"How do you think your father managed to lie to you about me all those years? You think the other Abnegation leaders didn't help him, didn't perpetuate the lie? *They* knew I wasn't pregnant, that no one had called a doctor, that there *was no body*. But they still told you I was dead, didn't they?"

It hadn't occurred to me before. There was no body. No body, but still all the men and women sitting in my father's house on that awful morning and at the funeral the following evening played the game of pretend for me, and for the rest of the Abnegation community, saying even in their silence, *No one would ever leave us. Who would want to?*

I shouldn't be so surprised to find that a faction is full of liars, but I guess there are parts of me that are still naive, still like a child.

Not anymore.

"Think about it," Evelyn said. "Are those people—the kind of people who would tell a child that his mother was dead just to save face—are they the ones you want to help? Or do you want to help remove them from power?"

I thought I knew. Those innocent Abnegation, with their constant acts of service and their deferent head-bobbing, they needed to be saved.

But those *liars*, who forced me into grief, who left me alone with the man who caused me pain—should they be saved?

I can't look at her, can't answer her. I wait for the train to pass a platform, and then jump off without looking back.

+++

"Don't take this the wrong way, but you look awful."

Shauna sinks into the chair next to mine, setting her tray down. I feel like yesterday's conversation with my mother was a sudden, earsplitting noise, and now every other sound is muffled. I've always known that my father was cruel. But I always thought the other Abnegation were innocent; deep down, I've always thought of myself as weak for leaving them, as a kind of traitor to my own values.

Now it seems like no matter what I decide, I'll be betraying someone. If I warn the Abnegation about the attack plans I found on Max's computer, I'll be betraying Dauntless. If I don't warn them, I betray my former faction again, in a much greater way than I did before. I have no choice but to decide, and the thought of deciding makes me feel sick.

I went through today the only way I knew how: I got up and went to work. I posted the rankings—which were a source of some contention, with me advocating for giving heavier weight to improvement, and Eric advocating for consistency. I went to eat. I put myself through the motions as if by muscle memory alone.

"You going to eat any of that?" Shauna says, nodding to my plate full of food.

I shrug. "Maybe."

I can tell she's about to ask what's wrong, so I introduce a new topic. "How's Lynn doing?"

"You would know better than I do," she says. "Getting to see her fears and all that."

I cut a piece from my hunk of meat and chew it.

"What's that like?" she asks cautiously, raising an eyebrow at me. "Seeing all their fears, I mean."

"Can't talk to you about her fears," I say. "You know that."

"Is that your rule, or Dauntless's rule?"

"Does it matter?"

Shauna sighs. "Sometimes I feel like I don't even know her, that's all."

We eat the rest of our meals without speaking. That's what I like most about Shauna: she doesn't feel the need to fill the empty spaces. When we're done, we leave the dining hall together, and Zeke calls out to us from across the Pit.

"Hey!" he says. He's spinning a roll of tape around his finger. "Want to go punch something?"

"Yes," Shauna and I say in unison.

We walk toward the training room, Shauna updating Zeke on her week at the fence—"Two days ago the idiot I was on patrol with started freaking out, swearing he saw something out there.... Turns out it was a *plastic bag*"—and

Zeke sliding his arm across her shoulders. I run my fingers over my knuckles and try not to get in their way.

When we get closer to the training room, I think I hear voices inside. Frowning, I push the door open with my foot. Standing inside are Lynn, Uriah, Marlene, and . . . Tris. The collision of worlds startles me a little.

"I thought I heard something in here," I say.

Uriah is firing at a target with one of the plastic pellet guns the Dauntless keep around for fun—I know for a fact that he doesn't own it, so this one must be Zeke's—and Marlene is chewing on something. She grins at me and waves when I walk in.

"Turns out it's my idiot brother," says Zeke. "You're not supposed to be here after hours. Careful, or Four will tell Eric, and then you'll be as good as scalped."

Uriah tucks the gun under his waistband, against the small of his back, without turning on the safety. He'll probably end up with a welt on his butt later from the gun firing into his pants. I don't mention it to him.

I hold the door open to usher them through it. As she passes me, Lynn says, "You wouldn't tell Eric."

"No, I wouldn't," I say. When Tris passes me I put out a hand, and it fits automatically in the space between her shoulder blades. I don't even know if that was intentional or not. And I don't really care.

The others start down the hallway, our original plan of spending time in the training room forgotten once Uriah and Zeke start bickering and Shauna and Marlene share the rest of a muffin.

"Wait a second," I say to Tris. She turns to me, looking worried, so I try to smile, but it's hard to feel like smiling right now.

I noticed tension in the training room when I posted the rankings earlier this evening—I never thought, when I was tallying up the points for the rankings, that maybe I should mark her down for her protection. It would have been an insult to her skill in the simulations to put her any lower on the list, but maybe she would have preferred the insult to the growing rift between her and her fellow transfers.

Even though she's pale and exhausted, and there are little cuts around each of her nail beds, and a wavering look in her eyes, I know that's not the case. This girl would never want to be tucked safely in the middle of the pack, never.

"You belong here, you know that?" I say. "You belong with us. It'll be over soon, so . . . just hold on, okay?"

The back of my neck suddenly feels hot, and I scratch at it with one hand, unable to meet her eyes, though I can *feel* them on me as the silence stretches.

Then she slips her fingers between mine, and I stare at her, startled. I squeeze her hand, lightly, and it registers through my turmoil and my exhaustion that though I've touched her half a dozen times—each one a lapse in judgment—this is the first time she's ever done it back.

Then she turns and runs to catch up with her friends.

And I stand in the hallway, alone, grinning like an idiot.

+++

I try to sleep for the better part of an hour, twisting under the covers to find a comfortable position. But it seems like someone has replaced my mattress with a bag of rocks. Or maybe it's just that my mind is too busy for sleep.

Eventually I give up, putting on my shoes and jacket and walking to the Pire, the way I do every time I can't sleep. I think about running the fear landscape program again, but I didn't think to replenish my supply of simulation serum this afternoon, and it would be a hassle to get some now. Instead I walk to the control room, where Gus greets me with a grunt and the other two on staff don't even notice me come in.

I don't try to go through Max's files again—I feel like I know everything I need to know, which is that something bad is coming and I have no idea whether I'll try to stop it.

I need to tell *someone*, I need *someone* to share in this with me, to tell me what to do. But there's no one that I would trust with something like this. Even my friends here were born and raised in Dauntless; how can I know that they wouldn't trust their leaders implicitly? I can't know.

For some reason, Tris's face comes to mind, open but stern as she clasps my hand in the hallway.

I scroll through the footage, looking over the city streets and then returning to the Dauntless compound. Most of the hallways are so dark, I couldn't see anything even if it was there. In my headphones, I hear only the rush of water in the chasm or the whistle of wind through the alleys. I sigh, leaning my head into my hand, and watch the changing images, one after another, and let them lull me into something like sleep.

"Go to bed, Four," Gus says from across the room.

I jerk awake, and nod. If I'm not actually looking at the footage it's not a good idea for me to be in the control room. I log out of my account and walk down the hallway to the elevator, blinking myself awake.

As I walk across the lobby, I hear a scream coming from below, coming from the Pit. It's not a good-natured Dauntless shout, or the shriek of someone who is scared but delighted, or anything but the particular tone, the particular pitch of terror.

Small rocks scatter behind me as I run down to the bottom of the Pit, my breathing fast and heavy, but even.

Three tall, dark-clothed people stand near the railing below. They are crowded around a fourth, smaller target, and even though I can't see much about them, I know a fight when I see one. Or, I would call it a fight, if it wasn't three against one.

One of the attackers wheels around, sees me, and sprints in the other direction. When I get closer I see one of the remaining attackers holding the target up, over the chasm, and I shout, "Hey!"

I see her hair, blond, and I can hardly see anything else. I collide with one of the attackers—Drew, I can tell by the color of his hair, orange-red—and slam him into the chasm barrier. I hit him once, twice, three times in the face, and he collapses to the ground, and then I'm kicking him and I can't think, can't think at all.

"Four." Her voice is quiet, ragged, and it's the only thing that could possibly reach me in this place. She's hanging from the railing, dangling over the chasm like a piece of bait from a fishing hook. The other one, the last attacker, is gone.

I run toward her, grabbing her under her shoulders, and pull her over the edge of the railing. I hold her against me. She presses her face to my shoulder, twisting her fingers into my shirt.

Drew is on the ground, collapsed. I hear him groan as I carry her away—not to the infirmary, where the others who went after her would think to look for her, but to my apartment, in its lonely, removed corridor. I shove my way through the apartment door and lay her down on my bed. I run my fingers over her nose and cheekbones to check for breaks, then I feel for her pulse, and lean in close to listen to her breathing. Everything seems normal, steady. Even the bump on the back of her head, though swollen and scraped, doesn't seem serious. She isn't badly injured, but she could have been.

My hands shake when I pull away from her. *She* isn't badly injured, but Drew might be. I don't even know how many times I hit him before she finally said my name and woke me up. The rest of my body starts to shake, too, and I make sure there's a pillow supporting her head, then leave the apartment to go back to the railing next to the Pit. On the way, I try to replay the last few minutes in my mind, try to recall what I punched and when and how hard, but the whole thing is lost to a dizzy fit of anger.

I wonder if this is what it was like for him, I think, remembering the wild, frantic look in Marcus's eyes every time he got angry.

When I reach the railing, Drew is still there, lying in a strange, crumpled position on the ground. I pull his arm across my shoulders and half lift, half drag him to the infirmary.

+ + +

When I make it back to my apartment, I immediately walk to the bathroom to wash the blood from my hands—a few of my knuckles are split, cut from the impact with Drew's face. If Drew was there, the other attacker had to be Peter, but who was the third? Not Molly—the shape was too tall, too big. In fact, there's only one initiate that size.

Al.

I check my reflection, like I'm going to see little pieces of Marcus staring back at me there. There's a cut at the corner of my mouth—did Drew hit me back at some point? It doesn't matter. My lapse in memory doesn't matter. What matters is that Tris is breathing.

I keep my hands under the cool water until it runs clear, then dry them on the towel and go to the freezer for an ice pack. As I carry it toward her, I realize she's awake.

"Your hands," she says, and it's a ridiculous thing to say, so stupid, to be worried about my *hands* when she was just dangled over the chasm by her throat.

"My hands," I say irritably, "are none of your concern."

I lean over her, slipping the ice pack under her head, where I felt a bump earlier. She lifts her hand and touches her fingertips lightly to my mouth.

I never thought you could feel a touch this way, like a jolt of energy. Her fingers are soft, curious.

"Tris," I say. "I'm all right."

"Why were you there?"

"I was coming back from the control room. I heard a scream."

"What did you do to them?"

"I deposited Drew at the infirmary a half hour ago. Peter and Al ran. Drew claimed they were just trying to scare you. At least, I think that's what he was trying to say."

"He's in bad shape?"

"He'll live. In what condition, I can't say," I spit.

I shouldn't let her see this side of me, the side that derives savage pleasure from Drew's pain. I shouldn't *have* this side.

She reaches for my arm, squeezes it. "Good," she says.

I look down at her. She has that side, too, she must have it. I saw the way she looked when she beat Molly, like she was going to keep going whether her opponent was unconscious or not. Maybe she and I are the same.

Her face contorts, twists, and she starts to cry. Most of the time, when someone has cried in front of me, I've felt squeezed, like I needed to escape their company in order to breathe. I don't feel that way with her. I don't worry, with her, that she expects too much from me, or that she needs anything from me at all. I sink down to the floor so we're on the same plane, and watch her carefully for a moment. Then I touch my hand to her cheek, careful not to press against any of her still-forming bruises. I run my thumb over her cheekbone. Her skin is warm.

I don't have the right word for how she looks, but even now, with parts of her face swollen and discolored, there's something striking about her, something I haven't seen before.

In that moment I'm able to accept the inevitability of how I feel, though not with joy. I need to talk to someone. I need to trust someone. And for whatever reason, I know, I *know* it's her.

I'll have to start by telling her my name.

+ + +

I approach Eric in the breakfast line, standing behind him with my tray as he uses a long-handled spoon to scoop scrambled eggs onto his plate.

"If I told you that one of the initiates was attacked last night by a few of the other initiates," I say, "would you even care?"

He pushes the eggs to one side of his plate, and lifts a shoulder. "I might care that their instructor doesn't seem to be able to control his initiates," Eric says as I pick up a bowl of cereal for myself. He eyes my split knuckles. "I might care that this hypothetical attack would be the *second* under that instructor's watch . . . whereas the Dauntless-borns don't seem to have this problem."

"Tensions between the transfers are naturally higher—they don't know each other, or this faction, and their backgrounds are wildly different," I say. "And you're their leader, shouldn't you be responsible for keeping them 'under control'?"

He sets a piece of toast next to his eggs with some tongs. Then he leans in close to my ear and says, "You're on thin ice, *Tobias*," he hisses. "Arguing with me in front of the others. 'Lost' simulation results. Your obvious bias toward the weaker initiates in the rankings. Even Max agrees now. If there *was* an attack, I don't think he would be too happy with you, and he might not object when I suggest that you be removed from your post."

"Then you'd be out an initiation instructor a week before the end of initiation."

"I can finish it out myself."

"I can only *imagine* what it would be like under your watch," I say, narrowing my eyes. "We wouldn't even need to make any cuts. They would all die or defect on their own."

"If you're not careful you won't have to imagine anything." He reaches the end of the food line and turns to me. "Competitive environments create tension, Four. It's natural for that tension to be released somehow." He smiles a little, stretching the skin between his piercings. "An attack would certainly show us, in a real-world situation, who the strong ones and the weak ones are, don't you think? We wouldn't have to rely on the test results at all, that way. We could make a more informed decision about who doesn't belong here. That is . . . if an attack were to happen."

The implication is clear: As the survivor of the attack, Tris would be viewed as weaker than the other initiates, and fodder for elimination. Eric wouldn't rush to the aid of the victim, but would rather advocate for her expulsion from Dauntless, as he did before Edward left of his own accord. I don't want Tris to be forced into factionlessness.

"Right," I say lightly. "Well, it's a good thing no attacks have happened recently, then."

I dump some milk on top of my cereal and walk to my table. Eric won't do anything to Peter, Drew, or Al, and I can't do anything without stepping out of line and suffering the repercussions. But maybe—maybe I don't have to do this alone. I put my tray down between Zeke and Shauna and say, "I need your help with something."

+ + +

After the fear landscape explanation is over and the initiates are dismissed for lunch, I pull Peter aside into the observation room next to the bare simulation room. It contains rows of chairs, ready for the initiates to sit in as they wait to take their final test. It also contains Zeke and Shauna.

"We need to have a chat," I say.

Zeke lurches toward Peter, slamming him against the concrete wall with alarming force. Peter cracks the back of his head, and winces.

"Hey there," Zeke says, and Shauna moves toward them, spinning a knife on her palm.

"What is this?" Peter says. He doesn't even look a little afraid, even when Shauna catches the blade by the handle and touches the point to his cheek, creating a dimple. "Trying to *scare* me?" he sneers.

"No," I say. "Trying to make a point. You're not the only one with friends who are willing to do some harm."

"I don't think initiation instructors are supposed to threaten initiates, do you?" Peter gives me a wide-eyed look, one I might mistake for innocence if I didn't know what he was really like. "I'll have to ask Eric, though, just to be sure."

"I didn't threaten you," I say. "I'm not even touching you. And according to the footage of this room that's stored on the control room computers, we're not even in here right now."

Zeke grins like he can't help it. That was his idea.

"I'm the one who's threatening you," Shauna says, almost in a growl. "One more violent outburst and I'm going to teach you a lesson about justice." She holds the knife point over his eye, and brings it down slowly, pressing the point to his eyelid. Peter freezes, barely moving even to breathe. "An eye for an eye. A bruise for a bruise."

"Eric may not care if you go after your peers," Zeke says, "but we do, and there are a lot of Dauntless like us. People who don't think you should lay a hand on your fellow faction members. People who listen to gossip, and spread it like wildfire. It won't take long for us to tell them what kind of worm you are, or for them to make your life very, very difficult. You see, in Dauntless, reputations tend to stick."

"We'll start with all your potential employers," Shauna says. "The supervisors in the control room—Zeke can take them; the leaders out by the fence—I'll get those. Tori knows everyone in the Pit—Four, you're friends with Tori, right?"

"Yes I am," I say. I move closer to Peter, and tilt my head. "You may be able to cause pain, initiate . . . but we can cause you lifelong misery."

Shauna takes the knife away from Peter's eye. "Think about it."

Zeke lets go of Peter's shirt and smooths it down, still smiling. Somehow the combination of Shauna's ferocity and Zeke's cheerfulness is just strange enough to be threatening. Zeke waves at Peter, and we all leave together.

"You want us to talk to people anyway, right?" Zeke asks me.

"Oh yeah," I say. "Definitely. Not just about Peter. Drew and Al, too."

"Maybe if he survives initiation, I'll accidentally trip him and he'll fall right into the chasm," Zeke says hopefully, making a plummeting gesture with his hand.

+ + +

The next morning, there's a crowd gathered by the chasm, all quiet and still, though the smell of breakfast beckons us all toward the cafeteria. I don't have to ask what they're gathered for.

This happens almost every year, I'm told. A death.

Like Amar's, sudden and awful and wasteful. A body pulled out of the chasm like a fish on a hook. Usually someone young—an accident, because of a daredevil stunt gone wrong, or maybe not an accident, a wounded mind further injured by the darkness, pressure, pain of Dauntless.

I don't know how to feel about those deaths. Guilty, maybe, for not seeing the pain myself. Sad, that some people can't find another way to escape.

I hear the name of the deceased spoken up ahead, and both emotions strike me hard.

Al. Al. Al.

My initiate—my *responsibility*, and I failed, because I've been so obsessed with catching Max and Jeanine, or with blaming everything on Eric, or with my indecision about warning the Abnegation. No—none of those things so much as this: that I distanced myself from them for my own protection, when I should have been drawing them out of the dark places here and into the lighter ones. Laughing with friends on the chasm rocks. Late-night tattoos after a game of Dare. A sea of embraces after the rankings are announced. Those are the things I could have shown him—even if it wouldn't have helped him, I should have tried.

I know one thing: after this year's initiation is done,

Eric won't need to try so hard to oust me from this position. I'm already gone.

+ + +

Al. Al. Al.

Why do all dead people become heroes in Dauntless? Why do we need them to? Maybe they're the only ones we can find in a faction of corrupt leaders, competitive peers, and cynical instructors. Dead people can be our heroes because they can't disappoint us later; they only improve over time, as we forget more and more about them.

Al was unsure and sensitive, and then jealous and violent, and then gone. Softer men than Al have lived and harder men than Al have died and there's no explanation for any of it.

But Tris wants one, craves one, I can see it in her face, a kind of hunger. Or anger. Or both. I can't imagine it's easy to like someone, hate them, and then lose them before any of those feelings are resolved. I follow her away from the chanting Dauntless because I'm arrogant enough to believe I can make her feel better.

Right. Sure. Or maybe I follow her because I'm tired of being so removed from everyone, and I'm no longer sure it's the best way to be.

"Tris," I say.

"What are you doing here?" she says bitterly. "Shouldn't you be paying your respects?"

"Shouldn't you?" I move toward her.

"Can't pay respect when you don't have any." I'm surprised, for a moment, that she can manage to be so cold—Tris isn't always nice, but she's rarely cavalier about anything. It only takes her a second to shake her head. "I didn't mean that."

"Ah."

"This is ridiculous," she says, flushing. "He throws himself off a ledge and Eric's calling it brave? Eric, who tried to have you throw knives at Al's head?" Her face contorts. "He wasn't brave! He was depressed and a coward and he almost killed me! Is that the kind of thing we respect here?"

"What do you want them to do?" I say as gently as I can— which isn't saying much. "Condemn him? Al's already dead. He can't hear it, and it's too late."

"It's not *about* Al," she says. "It's about everyone watching! Everyone who now sees hurling themselves into the chasm as a viable option. I mean, why *not* do it if everyone calls you a hero afterward? Why not do it if everyone will remember your name?" But of course, it is about Al, and she knows that. "It's . . ." She's struggling, fighting with herself. "I can't . . . This would *never* have happened in Abnegation! None of it! Never. This place warped him and ruined him, and I don't care if saying that makes me a Stiff, I don't care, I don't *care*!"

My paranoia is so deeply ingrained, I look automatically at the camera buried in the wall above the drinking fountain, disguised by the blue lamp fixed there. The people in the control room can see us, and if we're unlucky, they could choose this moment to hear us, too. I can see it now, Eric calling Tris a faction traitor, Tris's body on the pavement near the railroad tracks . . .

"Careful, Tris," I say.

"Is that all you can say?" She frowns at me. "That I should be *careful*? That's *it*?"

I understand that my response wasn't exactly what she was expecting, but for someone who just railed against Dauntless recklessness, she's definitely acting like one of them.

"You're as bad as the Candor, you know that?" I say. The Candor are always running their mouths, never thinking about the consequences. I pull her away from the drinking fountain, and then I'm close to her face and I can see her dead eyes floating in the water of the underground river and I can't stand it, not when she was just attacked and who knows what would have happened if I hadn't heard her scream.

"I'm not going to say this again, so listen carefully." I put my hands on her shoulders. "They are watching you. *You*, in particular."

I remember Eric's eyes on her after the knife throwing. His questions about her deleted simulation data. I claimed water damage. He thought it was interesting that the water damage occurred not five minutes after Tris's simulation ended. *Interesting.*

"Let go of me," she says.

I do, immediately. I don't like hearing her voice that way.

"Are they watching you, too?"

Always have been, always will be. "I keep trying to help you, but you refuse to be helped."

"Oh, right. Your help," she says. "Stabbing my ear with a knife and taunting me and yelling at me more than you yell at anyone else, it sure is helpful."

"Taunting you? You mean when I threw the knives? I wasn't taunting you!" I shake my head. "I was reminding you that if you failed, someone else would have to take your place."

To me, at the time, it almost seemed obvious. I thought, since she seemed to understand me better than most people, she might understand that, too. But of course she didn't. She's not a mind reader.

"Why?" she says.

"Because . . . you're from Abnegation," I say. "And . . . it's when you're acting selflessly that you are at your bravest. And if I were you, I would do a better job of pretending that selfless impulse is going away, because if the wrong people discover it . . . well, it won't be good for you."

"Why? Why do they care about my intentions?"

"Intentions are the only thing they care about. They try to make you think they care about what you do, but they don't. They don't want you to act a certain way, they want you to *think* a certain way. So you're easy to understand. So you won't pose a threat to them."

I put my hand on the wall near her face and lean into it, thinking of the tattoos forming a line on my back. It wasn't getting the tattoos that made me a faction traitor. It was what they meant to me—an escape from the narrow thinking of any one faction, the thinking that slices away at all the different parts of me, paring me down to just one version of myself.

"I don't understand why they care what I think, as long as I'm acting how they want me to," she says.

"You're acting how they want you to now, but what happens when your Abnegation-wired brain tells you to do something else, something they don't want?"

Much as I like him, Zeke is the perfect example.

Dauntless-born, Dauntless-raised, Dauntless-chosen. I can count on him to approach everything the same way. He was trained to from birth. To him, there are no other options.

"I might not need you to help me. Ever think about that?" she says. I want to laugh at the question. Of course she doesn't need me. When was it ever about that? "I'm not weak, you know. I can do this on my own."

"You think my first instinct is to protect you." I shift so I'm a little closer to her. "Because you're small, or a girl, or a Stiff. But you're wrong."

Even closer. I touch her chin, and for a moment I think about closing this gap completely.

"My first instinct is to push you until you break, just to see how hard I have to press," I say, and it's a strange admission, and a dangerous one. I don't mean her any harm, and never have, and I hope she knows that's not what I mean. "But I resist it."

"Why is that your first instinct?" she says.

"Fear doesn't shut you down," I say. "It wakes you up. I've seen it. It's fascinating." Her eyes in every fear simulation, ice and steel and blue flame. The short, slight girl with the wire-taut arms. A walking contradiction. My hand slips over her jaw, touches her neck. "Sometimes I just want to see it again. Want to see you awake."

Her hands touch my waist, and she pulls herself against me, or pulls me against her, I can't tell which. Her hands move over my back, and I *want* her, in a way I haven't felt before, not just some kind of mindless physical drive but a real, specific desire. Not for "someone," just for *her*.

I touch her back, her hair. It's enough, for now.

"Should I be crying?" she asks, and it takes me a second to realize she's talking about Al again. Good, because if this embrace made her want to cry, I would have to admit to knowing absolutely nothing about romance. Which might be true anyway. "Is there something wrong with me?"

"You think I know anything about tears?" Mine come without prompting and disappear a few seconds later.

"If I had forgiven him . . . do you think he would be alive now?"

"I don't know." I set my hand on her cheek, my fingers stretching back to her ear. She really is small. I don't mind it.

"I feel like it's my fault," she says.

So do I.

"It isn't your fault." I bring my forehead to hers. Her breaths are warm against my face. I was right, this is better than keeping my distance, this is much better.

"But I should have. I should have forgiven him."

"Maybe. Maybe there's more we all could have done," I say, and then I spit out an Abnegation platitude without thinking. "But we just have to let the guilt remind us to do better next time."

She pulls away immediately, and I feel that familiar impulse, to be mean to her so she forgets what I said, so she doesn't ask me any questions.

"What faction did you come from, Four?"

I think you know. "It doesn't matter. This is where I am now. Something you would do well to remember for yourself."

I don't want to be close to her anymore; it's all I want to do.

I want to kiss her; now is not the time.

I touch my lips to her forehead, and neither of us moves. No turning back now, not for me.

+ + +

Something she said sticks with me all day. *This would never have happened in Abnegation.*

At first I find myself thinking, *She just doesn't know what they're really like.*

But I'm wrong, and she's right. Al would not have died in Abnegation, and he would not have attacked her there, either. They may not be as purely good as I once believed—or wanted to believe—but they certainly aren't evil, either.

I see the map of the Abnegation sector, the one I found on Max's computer, printed on my eyelids when I close my eyes. If I warn them, if I don't, I'm a traitor either way, to one thing or another. So if loyalty is impossible, what do I strive for instead?

+++

It takes me a while to figure out a plan, how to go about this. If she was a normal Dauntless girl and I was a normal Dauntless boy, I would ask her on a date and we would make out by the chasm and I might show off my knowledge of Dauntless headquarters. But that feels too ordinary, after the things we've said to each other, after I've seen into the darkest parts of her mind.

Maybe that's the problem—it's all one-sided right now, because I know her, I know what she's afraid of and what she loves and what she hates, but all she knows about me is what I've told her. And what I've told her is so vague as to be negligible, because I have a problem with specificity.

After that I know what to do, it's just the doing it that's the problem.

I turn on the computer in the fear landscape room and set it to follow my program. I get two syringes of simulation serum from the storeroom, and put them in the little black box I have for this purpose. Then I set out for the transfer dormitory, not sure how I'll get her alone long enough to ask her to come with me.

But then I see her with Will and Christina, standing by the railing, and I should call her name and ask her, but I can't do it. Am I crazy, thinking of letting her into my head? Letting her see Marcus, learn my name, know everything I've tried so hard to keep hidden?

I start up the paths of the Pit again, my stomach churning. I reach the lobby, and the city lights are starting to go out all around us. I hear her footsteps on the stairs. She came after me.

I turn the black box in my hand.

"Since you're here," I say, like it's casual, which is ridiculous, "you might as well go in with me."

"Into your fear landscape?"

"Yes."

"I can do that?"

"The serum connects you to the program, but the program determines whose landscape you go through. And right now, it's set to put us through mine."

"You would let me see that?"

I can't quite look at her. "Why else do you think I'm going in?" My stomach hurts even worse. "There are some things I want to show you."

I open the box and take out the first syringe. She tilts her head, and I inject the serum, just like we always do during fear simulations. But instead of injecting myself with the other syringe, I offer her the box. This is supposed to be my way of evening things out, after all.

"I've never done this before," she says.

"Right here." I touch the place. She shakes a little as she inserts the needle, and the deep ache is familiar, but it no longer bothers me. I've done this too many times. I watch her face. No turning back, no turning back. Time to see what we're both made of.

I take her hand, or maybe she takes mine, and we walk into the fear landscape room together.

"See if you can figure out why they call me Four."

The door closes behind us, and the room is black. She moves closer to me and says, "What's your real name?"

"See if you can figure that out, too."

The simulation begins.

The room opens up to a wide blue sky, and we are on the roof of the building, surrounded by the city, sparkling in the sun. It's beautiful for just a moment before the wind starts, fierce and powerful, and I put my arm around her because I know she's steadier than I am, in this place.

I'm having trouble breathing, which is normal for me,

here. I find the rush of air suffocating, and the height makes me want to curl into a ball and hide.

"We have to jump off, right?" she says, and I remember that I can't curl into a ball and hide; I have to face this now.

?"

l I have to do is follow her, that's all I

aree and drags me behind her as she
ailboat and I'm an anchor, pulling us
and I struggle against the sensation
me, terror shrieking in every nerve,
ground, clutching my chest.
my feet. I feel stupid, remembering
Ferris wheel with no hesitation.

's not a game; my fears aren't thrill-
o on. But she probably doesn't mean

The wall comes from nowhere, slamming into her back, my back, both our sides. Forcing us together, closer than we've ever been before.

"Confinement," I say, and it's worse than usual with her in here, taking up half the air. I groan a little, hunching over her. I hate it in here. I *hate* it in here.

"Hey," she says. "It's okay. Here—"

She pulls my arm around her. I've always thought of her as spare, not an ounce of extra anything on her. But her waist is soft.

"This is the first time I'm happy I'm so small," she says. "Mmhmm."

She's talking about how to get out. Fear-landscape strategy. I am trying to focus on breathing. Then she pulls us both down, to make the box smaller, and turns so her back is against my chest, so I'm completely wrapped around her.

"This is worse," I say, because with my nervousness about the box and my nervousness about touching her combined, I can't even think straight. "This is definitely . . ."

"Shh. Arms around me."

I wrap my arms around her waist, and bury my face in her shoulder. She smells like Dauntless soap, and sweet, like apple.

I'm forgetting where I am.

She's talking about the fear landscape again, and I'm listening, but I'm also focused on how she *feels*.

"So try to forget we're here," she finishes.

"Yeah?" I put my mouth right up against her ear, on purpose this time, to keep the distraction going, but also because I get the feeling I'm not the only one who's distracted. "That easy, huh?"

"You know, most boys would enjoy being trapped in close quarters with a girl."

"Not claustrophobic people, Tris!"

"Okay, okay." She guides my hand to her chest, right under where her collarbone dips. All I can think about is what I want, which has nothing to do with getting out of this box, suddenly. "Feel my heartbeat. Can you feel it?"

"Yes."

"Feel how steady it is?"

I smile into her shoulder. "It's fast."

"Yes, well, that has nothing to do with the box." Of course it doesn't. "Every time you feel me breathe, you breathe. Focus on that."

We breathe together, once, twice.

"Why don't you tell me where this fear comes from. Maybe talking about it will help us somehow."

I feel like this fear should have vanished already, but what she's doing is keeping me at a steady level of heightened uneasiness, not taking my fear away completely. I try to focus on where this box comes from.

"Um . . . okay." *Okay, just do it, just say something real.* "This one is from my . . . fantastic childhood. Childhood punishments. The tiny closet upstairs."

Shut in the dark to think about what I did. It was better than other punishments, but sometimes I was in there for too long, desperate for fresh air.

"My mother kept our winter coats in our closet," she says, and it's a silly thing to say after what I just told her, but I can tell she doesn't know what else to do.

"I don't really want to talk about it anymore," I say with a gasp. She doesn't know what to say because no one could possibly know what to say, because my childhood pain is too pathetic for anyone else to handle—my heart rate spikes again.

"Okay. Then . . . I can talk. Ask me something."

I lift my head. It was working before, focusing on her. Her racing heart, her body against mine. Two strong skeletons wrapped in muscle, tangled together; two Abnegation transfers working on leaving tentative flirtation behind. "Why is your heart racing, Tris?"

"Well, I . . . I barely know you." I can picture her scowling. "I barely know you and I'm crammed up against you in a box, Four, what do you think?"

"If we were in your fear landscape . . ." I say. "Would I be in it?"

"I'm not afraid of you."

"Of course you're not. That's not what I meant." I meant not *Are you afraid of me?* but *Am I important enough to you to feature in the landscape anyway?*

Probably not. She's right, she hardly knows me. But still: Her heart is racing.

I laugh, and the walls break as if my laugh shook them and broke them, and the air opens up around us. I swallow a deep breath of it, and we peel away from each other. She looks at me, suspicious.

"Maybe you were cut out for Candor, because you're a terrible liar," I say.

"I think my aptitude test ruled that one out pretty well."

"The aptitude test tells you nothing."

"What are you trying to tell me? Your test isn't the reason you ended up Dauntless?"

I shrug. "Not exactly, no. I . . ."

I see something out of the corner of my eye, and turn to face it. A plain-faced, forgettable woman stands alone at the other end of the room. Between her and us is a table with a gun on it.

"You have to kill her," Tris says.

"Every time."

"She isn't real."

"She looks real. It feels real."

"If she was real, she would have killed *you* already."

"It's okay. I'll just . . . do it." I start toward the table. "This one's not so bad. Not as much panic involved."

Panic and terror aren't the only kinds of fear. There are deeper kinds, more terrible kinds. Apprehension and heavy, heavy dread.

I load the gun without thinking about it, hold it out in front of me, and look at her face. She's blank, like she knows what I'm going to do and accepts it.

She's not dressed in the clothes of any faction, but she might as well be Abnegation, standing there waiting for me to hurt her, the way they would. The way they will, if Max and Jeanine and Evelyn all get their way.

I close one eye, to focus on my target, and fire.

She falls, and I think of punching Drew until he was almost unconscious.

Tris's hand closes around my arm. "Come on. Keep moving."

We walk past the table, and I shudder with fear. Waiting for this last obstacle might be a fear in itself.

"Here we go," I say.

Creeping into the circle of light we now occupy is a dark figure, pacing so just the edge of his shoe is visible. Then he steps toward us, Marcus with his black-pit eyes and his gray clothes and his close-cut hair, showing off the contours of his skull.

"Marcus," she whispers.

I watch him. Waiting for the first blow to fall. "Here's

the part where you figure out my name."

"Is he . . ." She knows, now. She'll know forever; I can't make her forget it if I wanted to. "Tobias."

It's been so long since someone said my name that way, like it was a revelation and not a threat.

Marcus unwinds a belt from his fist.

"This is for your own good," he says, and I want to scream.

He multiplies immediately, surrounding us, the belts dragging on white tile. I curl into myself, hunching my back, waiting, waiting. The belt pulls back and I flinch before it hits, but then it doesn't.

Tris stands in front of me, her arm up, tense from head to toe. She grits her teeth as the belt wraps around her arm, and then she pulls it free, and lashes out. The movement is so powerful I'm amazed by how strong it looks, by how *hard* the belt slaps Marcus's skin.

He lunges at Tris, and I step in front of her. I'm ready this time, ready to fight back.

But the moment never comes. The lights lift and the fear landscape is over.

"That's it?" she says as I watch the place where Marcus stood. "Those were your worst fears? Why do you only have four . . . oh."

She looks at me.

"That's why they call you . . ."

I was afraid that if she knew about Marcus, she would look at me with pity, and she would make me feel weak, and small, and empty.

But she saw Marcus and she looked at *him*, with anger and without fear. She made me feel, not weak, but powerful. Strong enough to fight back.

I tug her toward me by her elbow, and kiss her cheek, slowly, letting her skin burn into mine. I hold her tightly, slouching into her.

"Hey." She sighs. "We got through it."

I put my fingers through her hair.

"*You* got me through it," I say.

+++

I take her to the rocks that Zeke, Shauna, and I go to sometimes, late at night. Tris and I sit on a flat stone suspended over the water, and the spray soaks my shoes, but it's not so cold that I mind. Like all initiates, she's too focused on the aptitude test, and I'm struggling with talking to her about it. I thought that when I spilled one secret, the rest would come tumbling after, but openness is a habit you form over time, and not a switch you flip whenever you want to, I'm finding.

"These are things I don't tell people, you know. Not

even my friends." I watch the dark, murky water and the things it carries—pieces of trash, discarded clothing, floating bottles like small boats setting out on a journey. "My result was as expected. Abnegation."

"Oh." She frowns. "But you chose Dauntless anyway?"

"Out of necessity."

"Why did you have to leave?"

I look away, not sure I can give voice to my reasons, because admitting them makes me a faction traitor, makes me feel like a coward.

"You had to get away from your dad," she says. "Is that why you don't want to be a Dauntless leader? Because if you were, you might have to see him again?"

I shrug. "That, and I've always felt that I don't quite belong among the Dauntless. Not the way they are now, anyway." It's not quite the truth. I'm not sure this is the moment to tell her what I know about Max and Jeanine and the attack—selfishly, I want to keep this moment to myself, just for a little while.

"But . . . you're incredible," she says. I raise my eyebrows at her. She seems embarrassed. "I mean, by Dauntless standards. Four fears is unheard of. How could you not belong here?"

I shrug again. The more time goes by, the stranger I find it that my fear landscape isn't riddled with fears like everyone else's. A lot of things make me nervous, anxious, uncomfortable . . . but when confronted with those things, I can *act*, I'm never paralyzed. My four fears, if I'm not careful, will paralyze me. That's the only difference.

"I have a theory that selflessness and bravery aren't all that different." I look up at the Pit, rising high above us. From here I can see just a small slice of night sky. "All your life you've been training to forget yourself, so when you're in danger, it becomes your first instinct. I could belong in Abnegation just as easily."

"Yeah, well. I left Abnegation because I wasn't selfless enough, no matter how hard I tried to be."

"That's not entirely true," I say with a smile. "That girl who let someone throw knives at her to spare a friend, who hit my dad with a belt to protect me—that selfless girl, that's not you?"

In this light, she looks like she comes from another world, her eyes rendered so pale they almost seem to glow in the dark.

"You've been paying close attention, haven't you?" she asks, like she just read my mind. But she's not talking about me looking at her face.

"I like to observe people," I say slyly.

"Maybe you were cut out for Candor, Four, because you're a terrible liar."

I set my hand down next to hers and lean closer. "Fine."
Her long, narrow nose is no longer swollen from the
attack, and neither is her mouth. She has a nice mouth.
"I watched you because I like you. And . . . don't call me
'Four,' okay? It's . . . nice. To hear my name again."

She looks momentarily bewildered.

"But you're older than I am . . . Tobias."

It sounds so good when she says it. Like it's nothing to
be ashamed of.

"Yes, that whopping two-year gap really is *insurmount-
able*, isn't it?"

"I'm not trying to be self-deprecating," she says stub-
bornly. "I just don't get it. I'm younger. I'm not pretty. I—"

I laugh, and kiss her temple.

"Don't pretend," she says, sounding a little breathless.
"You know I'm not. I'm not ugly, but I am certainly not
pretty."

The word "pretty," and all that it represents, seems so
completely useless right now that I have no patience for it.

"Fine. You're not pretty. So?" I move my lips to her cheek,
trying to work up some courage. "I like how you look." I
pull back. "You're deadly smart. You're brave. And even
though you found out about Marcus . . . you aren't giving
me that look. Like I'm . . . a kicked puppy, or something."

"Well," she says factually. "You're not."

My instincts were right: She is worth trusting. With my secrets, with my shame, with the name that I abandoned. With the beautiful truths and the awful ones. I know it.

I touch my lips to hers. Our eyes meet, and I grin, and kiss her again, this time more sure of it.

It's not enough. I pull her closer, kiss her harder. She comes alive, putting her arms around me and leaning into me and it's still not enough, how can it be?

+++

I walk her back to the transfer dormitory, my shoes still damp from the river spray, and she smiles at me as she slips through the doorway. I start toward my apartment, and it doesn't take long for the giddy relief to give way to uneasiness again. Somewhere between watching that belt curl around her arm in my fear landscape and telling her that selflessness and bravery were often the same thing, I made a decision.

I turn at the next corner, not toward my apartment but toward a stairway that leads outside, right next to Max's place. I slow down when I pass his door, afraid that my footsteps will be loud enough to rouse him. Irrational.

My heart pounds when I reach the top of the stairs. A train is just passing, its silver side catching moonlight. I walk beneath the tracks and set out toward the Abnegation sector.

+ + +

Tris came from Abnegation—part of her innate power comes from them, whenever she's called upon to defend people who are weaker than she is. And I can't stand to think of the men and women who are like her falling to Dauntless-Erudite weapons. They may have lied to me, and maybe I failed them when I chose Dauntless, and maybe I'm failing Dauntless now, but I don't have to fail myself. And *I*, no matter what faction I'm in, know the right thing to do.

The Abnegation sector is so clean, not a scrap of trash on the streets, sidewalks, or lawns. The identical gray buildings are worn in places from where selfless people have refused to mend them when the factionless sector so badly needs the materials, but neat and unremarkable. The streets here could easily be a maze, but I haven't been gone long enough to forget the way to Marcus's house.

Strange, how quickly it became *his* house instead of mine, in my mind.

Maybe I don't have to tell him; I could tell another Abnegation leader, but he's the most influential one, and there's still a part of him that's my father, that tried to protect me because I'm Divergent. I try to remember the swell of power I felt in my fear landscape, when Tris showed me he was just a man, not a monster, and that I could face him. But she's not here with me now, and I feel flimsy, like I'm made of paper.

I walk up the path to the house, and my legs are rigid, like they don't have joints. I don't knock; I don't want to wake anyone else. I reach under the doormat for the spare key and unlock the front door.

It's late, but the light is still on in the kitchen. By the time I walk through the door, he's already standing where I can see him. Behind him, the kitchen table is covered with papers. He's not wearing his shoes—they're on the living room carpet, their laces undone—and his eyes are just as shadowed as they are in my nightmares about him.

"What are you doing here?" He looks me up and down. I wonder what he's looking at until I remember that I'm wearing Dauntless black, heavy boots and a jacket, tattoo ink on my neck. He comes a little closer, and I notice that I'm as tall as he is, and stronger than I ever have been.

He could never overpower me now.

"You're no longer welcome in this house," he says.

"I . . ." I stand up straighter, and not because he hates

bad posture. "I don't care," I say, and his eyebrows pop up like I just surprised him.

Maybe I did.

"I came to warn you," I say. "I found something. Attack plans. Max and Jeanine are going to attack Abnegation. I don't know when, or how."

He watches me for a second, in a way that makes me feel like I'm being measured, and then his expression shifts into a sneer.

"Max and Jeanine are going to attack," he says. "Just the two of them, armed with some simulation syringes?" His eyes narrow. "Did Max send you here? Have you become his Dauntless lackey? What, does he want to scare me?"

When I thought about warning the Abnegation, I was sure the hardest part would be getting myself through this door. It never occurred to me that he wouldn't *believe* me.

"Don't be stupid," I say. I would never have said that to him when I lived in this house, but two years of intentionally adopting Dauntless speech patterns make it come out of my mouth naturally. "If you're suspicious of Max, it's for a reason, and I'm telling you it's a good one. You're right to be suspicious. You're in danger—you all are."

"You dare to come to my house after you betrayed your

faction," he says, his voice low, "after you betrayed your *family* . . . and insult me?" He shakes his head. "I refuse to be intimidated into doing what Max and Jeanine want, and certainly not by my son."

"You know what?" I say. "Forget it. I should have gone to someone else."

I turn toward the door, and he says, "Don't walk away from me."

His hand closes around my arm, tightly. I stare at it, for a second feeling dizzy, like I'm outside of my own body, already separating myself from the moment so I can survive it.

You can fight him, I think, as I remember Tris drawing back the belt in my fear landscape to strike him.

I pull my arm free, and I'm too strong for him to hold on to. But I can only muster the strength to walk away, and he doesn't dare shout after me, not when the neighbors could hear. My hands shake a little bit, so I put them in my pockets. I don't hear the front door shut behind me, so I know he's watching me go.

It wasn't the triumphant return I pictured.

+ + +

I feel guilty when I pass through the doorway to the Pire, like there are Dauntless eyes all over me, judging me for what I just did. I went against the Dauntless leaders, and for what? For a man I hate, who didn't even believe me? It doesn't feel like it was worth it, worth being called a faction traitor.

I look through the glass floor to the chasm far beneath me, the water calm and dark, too far away to reflect any moonlight. A few hours ago I was standing right here, about to show a girl I hardly knew all the secrets I've fought so hard to protect.

She was equal to my trust, even if Marcus wasn't. *She*, and her mother, and the rest of the faction she believes in, are still worth protecting. So that's what I'm going to do.

READ ON FOR MORE EXCLUSIVE
SCENES FROM

DIVERGENT,

TOLD FROM TOBIAS'S
PERSPECTIVE!

"FIRST JUMPER—TRIS!"

"CAREFUL, TRIS."

"YOU LOOK GOOD, TRIS."

"FIRST JUMPER—TRIS!"

I CHECK MY watch. The first initiate should be jumping any minute now.

The net waits beside me, wide and sturdy and lit from above by the sun. The last time I was here was last year's Choosing Day, and before then, the day I jumped. I didn't want to remember the feeling of inching toward the edge of the building, my mind and my body going haywire with terror, the awful drop, the helpless flailing of limbs, the slap of the net fibers against my arms and neck.

"How'd the prank go?" Lauren says.

It takes me a second to figure out what she means: the program, and my supposed desire to prank Zeke. "Haven't done it yet. Our work time didn't overlap much today."

."You know, if you were up for some serious studying, we could use you in tech services," she says.

"If you're recruiting, you should talk to Zeke. He's much better than I am."

"Yeah, but Zeke doesn't know when to shut it," she says. "We don't recruit for skill so much as compatibility. We spend a lot of time together."

I grin. Zeke does like to surround himself with chatter, but that's never bothered me. Sometimes it's nice not to worry about providing any conversation.

Lauren plays with one of the rings in her eyebrow, and we wait. I try to crane my neck to see the top of the building from the ground, but all I can see is sky.

"Bet you it's one of my Dauntless-borns," she says.

"It's always a Dauntless-born. No bet."

They have an unfair advantage, the Dauntless-born. They usually know what's at the bottom of the jump, though we try to keep it from them as much as possible—the only time we use this entrance to headquarters is on Choosing Day, but the Dauntless are curious, they explore the compound when they think no one is watching. They also grow up cultivating in themselves the desire to make bold moves, to take drastic action, to commit themselves fully to whatever they decide to do. It would take a strange kind of transfer to know how to do that without having been taught.

Then I see her.

Not a black streak like I was expecting, but gray, tumbling through the air. I hear a *snap* of the net pulling taught around the metal supports, and it shifts to cradle her. For a second I stare, amazed, at the familiar clothing that she wears. Then I put my hand out, into the net, so she can reach it.

She wraps her fingers around mine, and I pull her across. As she tumbles over the side, I grab her arms to steady her. She's small, and thin—fragile-looking, like the impact with the net should have shattered her. Her eyes are wide and bright blue.

"Thank you," she says. She may look fragile, but her voice is steady.

"Can't believe it," Lauren says, with more Dauntless swagger than usual. "A Stiff, the first to jump? Unheard of."

She's right. It is unheard of. It's unheard of for a Stiff to join Dauntless, even. There were no Abnegation transfers last year. And before that, for a long time, there was only me.

"There's a reason why she left them, Lauren," I say,

feeling distant from the moment, from my own body. I pull myself back and say to the initiate, "What's your name?"

"Um . . ." She hesitates, and I feel, for a strange, brief moment, like I know her. Not from my time in Abnegation, not from school, but on a deeper level, somehow, her eyes and her mouth searching for a name, dissatisfied with the one she finds, just like I was. My initiation instructor gave me an escape from my old identity. I can give her one, too.

"Think about it," I say, smiling a little. "You don't get to pick again."

"Tris," she says, like she's already sure of it.

"Tris," Lauren says. "Make the announcement, Four."

She's my initiate, after all, this transfer from Abnegation.

I look over my shoulder, at the crowd of Dauntless members who have gathered to watch the initiates jump, and I announce, "First jumper—Tris!"

This way, they'll remember her, not for the gray she wears but for her first act of bravery. Or insanity. Sometimes they're the same thing.

Everyone cheers, and as the sound fills the cavern, another initiate plummets into the net with a blood-curdling scream. A girl dressed in Candor black and white. This time, Lauren is the one to reach across the net to help her. I touch a hand to Tris's back to guide her toward the stairs, in case she's not as steady as she seems. Before she takes the first step, I say, "Welcome to Dauntless."

"CAREFUL, TRIS."

ONE ABNEGATION, FIVE Candor, two Erudite. Those are my initiates.

I'm told that Candor and Dauntless have a fairly high mutual transfer rate—we usually lose as many to them as we gain. I consider it my job to get these eight initiates through at least the first round of cuts. Last year, when Eric and Max insisted on the cuts, I fought them as hard as I dared. But it seems the cuts are here to stay, all for the sake of the Dauntless Max and Eric want to create—a faction of mindless brutality.

But I intend to leave Dauntless as soon as I find out what Max and Jeanine are up to, and if that's in the middle of initiation, so much the better.

Once all the Dauntless-borns—including Uriah, Lynn,

and Marlene—are with us, I start down the tunnel, beckoning them to follow with one hand. We walk down the dark hallway toward the Pit doors.

"This is where we divide," Lauren says, when she reaches the doors. "The Dauntless-born initiates are with me. I assume *you* don't need a tour of the place."

She smiles, and the Dauntless-borns follow her down the hallway that bypasses the Pit, leading them right into the cafeteria. I watch them leave, and once they've disappeared, I straighten up. I learned last year that in order for them to take me seriously from the beginning, I have to be hard on them from the beginning. I don't have Amar's natural charm, which won people's loyalty with just a smile or a joke, so I have to compensate in other ways.

"Most of the time I work in the control room, but for the next few weeks, I'm your instructor," I say. "My name is Four."

One of the Candor girls—tall, with dark skin and an energetic voice—speaks up. "Four? Like the number?"

I sense the beginnings of an uprising. People who don't know what my name means often like to laugh at it, and I don't like to be laughed at, especially not by a group of initiates fresh from Choosing, who have no idea what they're in for.

"Yes," I say testily. "Is there a problem?"

"No," the girl says.

"Good. We're about to go into the Pit, which you will someday learn to love. It—"

The Candor girl interrupts again. "The Pit? Clever name."

I feel a swell of irritation, and I move toward her without really deciding to. I can't have someone cracking jokes about everything I say, especially not at the beginning of initiation, when everyone's attitudes are so malleable. I have to show them all that I'm not someone to be messed with, and I have to do it now.

I lean in close to her face and stare at her for a few seconds, until I see her smile falter.

"What's your name?" I say, keeping my voice quiet.

"Christina," she says.

"Well, Christina, if I wanted to put up with Candor smart-mouths, I would have joined their faction," I say. "The first lesson you will learn from me is to keep your mouth shut. Got that?"

She nods. I turn away, my heart throbbing in my ears. I think that did it, but I can't be sure, not until initiation really begins. I push through the double doors that open up to the Pit, and for a moment, I see it like it's for the first time, the impossibly huge space, bustling with life and energy, the pulse of water in the chasm, crashing against the rocks, the echoes of conversation everywhere. Most of the time I avoid it because it's so busy, but today I love it. I can't help it.

"If you follow me," I say. "I'll show you the chasm."

+++

The Abnegation transfer sits at my table. For a moment I wonder if she knows who I am, or if she's somehow magnetized to me by an invisible force of Stiff that I can't help but give off. But she doesn't look at me like she knows me. And she doesn't know what a hamburger is.

"You've never had a hamburger before?" Christina says. Incredulous. The Candor are like that, amazed that not everyone lives the way that they do. It's one of the reasons I don't like them. It's like the rest of the world doesn't exist to them, but for the Abnegation, the rest of the world is all that exists, and it is full of need.

"No," Tris says. For someone so small, she has a low voice. It always sounds serious, no matter what she says. "Is that what it's called?"

"Stiffs eat plain food," I say, trying out the slang. It feels unnatural, applied to Tris; I feel like I owe her the courtesies I would owe any woman in my former faction, deferential, averted eyes and polite conversation. I have to push myself to remember that I'm not in Abnegation anymore. And neither is she.

"Why?" Christina says.

"Extravagance is considered self-indulgent and un-necessary." She says it like she's reciting it from memory. Maybe she is.

"No wonder you left."

"Yeah." Tris rolls her eyes, which surprises me. "It was just because of the food."

I try not to smile. I'm not sure it works.

Then Eric walks in, and everything goes quiet.

Eric's appointment to Dauntless leader was met with confusion and, in some cases, anger. There had never been a leader so young before, and plenty of people spoke out against the decision, voiced concerns about his youth and his Erudite background. Max made sure to silence those concerns. And so did Eric. Someone would be out-spoken one day and silent, frightened the next, almost like he had threatened them. Knowing Eric, he probably did, with soft-spoken words that twisted together into malice, clever and calculated as always.

"Who's that?" Christina says.

"His name is Eric," I say. "He's a Dauntless leader."

"Seriously? But he's so young."

I set my jaw. "Age doesn't matter here." *Connections to Jeanine Matthews do.*

He comes toward us and drops into the seat next to me. I stare at my food.

"Well, aren't you going to introduce me?" he says lightly. Like we're friends.

"This is Tris and Christina," I say.

"Ooh, a Stiff," says Eric, smirking. I worry, for a moment, that he's about to tell her where *I* came from, and I curl a hand around my knee, clenching so I don't lash out and smack him. But all he says is, "We'll see how long you last."

I still want to smack him. Or remind him that the last transfer we had from Abnegation, who is sitting right next to him, managed to knock out one of his teeth, so who knows what this next one will do. But with these new practices in place—fighting until an opponent can't stand, cuts after just a week of combat training—he's right, it's unlikely that she'll last very long, small as she is. I don't like it, but there it is.

"What have you been doing lately, Four?" Eric says.

I feel a prickle of fear, worried, for a moment, that he

knows that I'm spying on him and Max. I shrug. "Nothing, really."

"Max tells me he keeps trying to meet with you, and you don't show up," Eric says. "He requested that I find out what's going on with you."

I find it easy to discard Max's messages, like they're bits of garbage blown toward me by the wind. The backlash from Eric's appointment as Dauntless leader may not bother Eric anymore, but it still bothers Max, who has never liked his protégé as much as he was supposed to. He liked me, though I'm not sure why, since I hole up alone while the other Dauntless pull together.

"Tell him I'm satisfied with the position I currently hold," I say.

"So he wants to give you a job."

There's that suspicious probing again, oozing from his mouth like pus from a new piercing.

"So it would seem."

"And you aren't interested."

"I haven't been interested for two years."

"Well. Let's hope he gets the point, then."

He hits my shoulder, like he means it to be casual, but the force of it almost pushes me into the table. I glare at him as he walks away—I don't like to be pushed around, especially not by scrawny Erudite-lovers.

"Are you two . . . friends?" Tris asks.

"We were in the same initiate class." I decide to make a preemptive strike, to poison them against Eric before he poisons them against me. "He transferred from Erudite."

Christina raises her eyebrows, but Tris disregards the word "erudite," disregards the suspicion that ought to be written into her very skin after a lifetime in Abnegation, and says, "Were you a transfer too?"

"I thought I would only have trouble with the Candor asking too many questions," I say. "Now I've got Stiffs, too?"

As it was with Christina before, my sharpness is intended to slam doors before they open too much. But Tris's mouth twists like she tastes something sour, and she says, "It must be because you're so approachable. You know. Like a bed of nails."

Her face flushes as I stare at her, but she doesn't look away. Something about her seems familiar to me, though I swear I would remember if I had ever met such a sharp Abnegation girl, even for just a second.

"Careful, Tris," I say. Careful what you say to me, is what I mean, careful what you say to anyone, in this faction that values all the wrong things, that doesn't understand that when you come from Abnegation, standing up for yourself, even in small moments, is the height of bravery.

As I say her name, I realize how I know her. She's Andrew Prior's daughter. Beatrice. Tris.

"YOU LOOK GOOD, TRIS."

I'M NOT SURE I remember what made me laugh, but Zeke said it, and it was hilarious. Around me, the Pit sways like I'm standing on a swing. I hold the railing to steady myself and tip the rest of whatever it is I'm drinking down my throat.

Abnegation attack? What Abnegation attack? I hardly remember.

Well, that's actually a lie, but it's never too late to get comfortable with lying to yourself.

I see a blond head bobbing in the crowd and follow it down to Tris's face. For once, she's not wearing multiple layers of clothing, and her shirt collar isn't pressed right up against the bottom of her throat. I can see her shape—*Stop it*, a voice in my head scolds me, before the thought can go any further.

"Tris!" The word is out of my mouth, no stopping it, don't even care to try. I walk toward her, ignoring the stares of Will, Al, and Christina. It's easy to do—her eyes seem brighter, more piercing than before.

"You look . . . different," I say. I mean to say "older," but I don't want to suggest that she looked young before. She may not bend in all the places that older women do, but no one could look at her face and see a child. No child has that ferocity.

"So do you," she says. "What are you doing?"

Drinking, I think, but she's probably noticed that.

"Flirting with death," I say, laughing. "Drinking near the chasm. Probably not a good idea."

"No, it isn't." She's not laughing. She looks wary. Wary of what, of me?

"Didn't know you had a tattoo," I say, scanning her collarbone. There are three black birds there—simple, but they almost look like they're flying across her skin. "Right. The *crows*."

I want to ask her why she would get one of her worst fears tattooed on her body, why she would want to wear the mark of her fear forever instead of burying it, ashamed. Maybe she's not ashamed of her fears the way I'm ashamed of mine.

I look back at Zeke and Shauna, who are standing with

shoulders touching at the railing.

"I'd ask you to hang out with us," I say, "but you're not supposed to see me this way."

"What way?" she says. "Drunk?"

"Yeah . . . well, no." Suddenly it doesn't seem that funny to me. "Real, I guess."

"I'll pretend I didn't."

"Nice of you." I lean in, closer than I mean to, and I can smell her hair, feel the cool, smooth, delicate skin of her cheek against mine. I would be embarrassed that I'm acting so foolish, so forward, if she had, even for a second, pulled away. But she doesn't—if anything, she moves a little closer. "You look good, Tris," I say, because I'm not sure she knows it, and she should.

This time she laughs.

"Do me a favor and stay away from the chasm, okay?"

"Of course."

She smiles. And I wonder, for the first time, if she likes me. If she can still grin at me when I'm like this . . . well, she might.

One thing I know: For helping me forget how awful the world is, I prefer her to alcohol.

ACKNOWLEDGMENTS

Thank you, thank you, thank you to:

My husband, family (Roth-Rydz-Rosses, Fitches, Krausses, Paquettes, Johnsons, and everyone in between), and friends (writers and non-writers alike, far and wide), for your constant support, generosity, and forgiveness, without which I would surely perish. No, seriously.

Joanna Volpe, friendgent, for unfailing kindness and wisdom and All the (Good) Things. Katherine Tegen, frienditor, for all kinds of editorial wisdom and hard, hard work. The whole team at HarperCollins, for continued awesomeness for all varieties: Joel Tippie, Amy Ryan, Barb Fitzsimmons, Brenna Franzitta, Josh Weiss, Mark Rifkin, Valerie Shea, Christine Cox, Joan Giurdanella, Lauren Flower, Alison Lisnow, Sandee Roston, Diane Naughton, Colleen O'Connell, Aubry Parks-Fried, Margot Wood, Patty Rosati, Molly Thomas, Onalee Smith, Andrea Pappenheimer, Kerry Moynagh, Kathy Faber, Liz Frew, Heather Doss, Jenny Sheridan, Fran Olson, Deb Murphy, Jessica Abel, Samantha Hagerbaumer, Andrea Rosen, David Wolfson, Jean McGinley, Alpha Wong, Sheala Howley, Ruiko Tokunaga, Caitlin Garing, Beth Ives, Katie Bignell, Karen Dziekonski, Sean McManus, Randy Rosema, Pam Moore, Rosanne Romanello, Melinda

Weigel, Gwen Morton, Lillian Sun, Rosanne Lauer, Erica Ferguson, and of course, Kate Jackson, Susan Katz, and Brian Murray. I could not have a better publishing home.

Danielle Barthel, for your patient mind and special encouragement with regard to these stories in particular. Pouya Shahbazian, for showing me how to be steady even in a storm (I'm working on it). Everyone at New Leaf Literary for working so damn hard and making that work so good. Steve Younger, for humor and legal prowess in equal measure.

And last but definitely, definitely not least: all the Divergent readers (Initiates!) across the globe. Your enthusiasm for these characters made me excited to sit down with these stories and propelled me through the hard parts.

I feel like it's only fitting to end with a

‹4

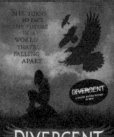
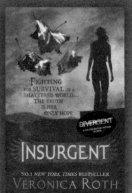
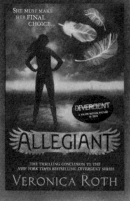
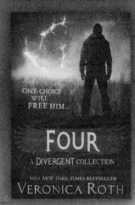

simulation serum from the storeroom, and put them in the little black box I have for this purpose. Then I set out for the transfer dormitory, not sure how I'll get her alone long enough to ask her to come with me.

But then I see her with Will and Christina, standing by the railing, and I should call her name and ask her, but I can't do it. Am I crazy, thinking of letting her into my head? Letting her see Marcus, learn my name, know everything I've tried so hard to keep hidden?

I start up the paths of the Pit again, my stomach churning. I reach the lobby, and the city lights are starting to go out all around us. I hear her footsteps on the stairs. She came after me.

I turn the black box in my hand.

"Since you're here," I say, like it's casual, which is ridiculous, "you might as well go in with me."

"Into your fear landscape?"

"Yes."

"I can do that?"

"The serum connects you to the program, but the program determines whose landscape you go through. And right now, it's set to put us through mine."

"You would let me see that?"

I can't quite look at her. "Why else do you think I'm going in?" My stomach hurts even worse. "There are some things I want to show you."

I open the box and take out the first syringe. She tilts her head, and I inject the serum, just like we always do during fear simulations. But instead of injecting myself with the other syringe, I offer her the box. This is supposed to be my way of evening things out, after all.

"I've never done this before," she says.

"Right here." I touch the place. She shakes a little as she inserts the needle, and the deep ache is familiar, but it no longer bothers me. I've done this too many times. I watch her face. No turning back, no turning back. Time to see what we're both made of.

I take her hand, or maybe she takes mine, and we walk into the fear landscape room together.

"See if you can figure out why they call me Four."

The door closes behind us, and the room is black. She moves closer to me and says, "What's your real name?"

"See if you can figure that out, too."

The simulation begins.

The room opens up to a wide blue sky, and we are on the roof of the building, surrounded by the city, sparkling in the sun. It's beautiful for just a moment before the wind starts, fierce and powerful, and I put my arm around her because I know she's steadier than I am, in this place.

I'm having trouble breathing, which is normal for me,

here. I find the rush of air suffocating, and the height makes me want to curl into a ball and hide.

"We have to jump off, right?" she says, and I remember that I can't curl into a ball and hide; I have to face this now.

I nod.

"On three, okay?"

I nod again. All I have to do is follow her, that's all I have to do.

She counts to three and drags me behind her as she runs, like she's a sailboat and I'm an anchor, pulling us both down. We fall and I struggle against the sensation with every inch of me, terror shrieking in every nerve, and then I'm on the ground, clutching my chest.

She helps me to my feet. I feel stupid, remembering how she scaled that Ferris wheel with no hesitation.

"What's next?"

I want to tell her it's not a game; my fears aren't thrilling rides she gets to go on. But she probably doesn't mean it that way.

"It's—"

The wall comes from nowhere, slamming into her back, my back, both our sides. Forcing us together, closer than we've ever been before.

"Confinement," I say, and it's worse than usual with her in here, taking up half the air. I groan a little, hunching over her. I hate it in here. I *hate* it in here.

"Hey," she says. "It's okay. Here—"

She pulls my arm around her. I've always thought of her as spare, not an ounce of extra anything on her. But her waist is soft.

"This is the first time I'm happy I'm so small," she says.

"Mmhmm."

She's talking about how to get out. Fear-landscape strategy. I am trying to focus on breathing. Then she pulls us both down, to make the box smaller, and turns so her back is against my chest, so I'm completely wrapped around her.

"This is worse," I say, because with my nervousness about the box and my nervousness about touching her combined, I can't even think straight. "This is definitely . . ."

"Shh. Arms around me."

I wrap my arms around her waist, and bury my face in her shoulder. She smells like Dauntless soap, and sweet, like apple.

I'm forgetting where I am.

She's talking about the fear landscape again, and I'm listening, but I'm also focused on how she *feels*.

"So try to forget we're here," she finishes.

"Yeah?" I put my mouth right up against her ear, on purpose this time, to keep the distraction going, but also